HISTORICAL ASPECTS OF THE NEUROSCIENCES

A Festschrift for Macdonald Critchley

RC
338
H57
1982

Historical Aspects of the Neurosciences

A Festschrift for Macdonald Critchley

Editors

F. Clifford Rose, F.R.C.P.
Department of Neurology
Charing Cross Hospital
London, England

W. F. Bynum, M.D., Ph.D.
Wellcome Institute for the History of Medicine
London, England

Raven Press ■ New York

Raven Press, 1140 Avenue of the Americas, New York, New York 10036

Library of Congress Cataloging in Publication Data
Main entry under title:

Historical aspects of the neurosciences.

Papers presented at the 1st meeting of the History of Neurosciences Group, held at the Medical Society of London in 1980.
Includes bibliographical references and index.
1. Neurology—History—Congresses. 2. Critchley, Macdonald. I. Critchley, Macdonald. II. Rose, F. Clifford (Frank Clifford) III. Bynum, William F. IV. History of Neurosciences Group. [DNLM: 1. Neurology —History—Congresses. WL 11.1 H673 1982]
RC338.H57 612′.8′09 81-40023
ISBN 0-89004-661-1 AACR2

Preface

In September 1979, there was a meeting of the Research Committee of the World Federation of Neurology in Newcastle-upon-Tyne, England under the chairmanship of Sir John Walton to prepare for the International Congress of Neurology to be held in Kyoto, Japan in September 1981. This Committee consists of representatives of the various research groups supported by the World Federation and, on the train back to London, three of them found that they had a common interest in medical history. They thought it was a pity that the History of Neurosciences Group had never met; they discussed where and when the first meeting could be held. It was felt that there could be no more suitable occasion than to honour the 80th year of Dr. Macdonald Critchley, Emeritus President of the World Federation of Neurology and one of the founders of the History of Neurosciences Group.

The symposium, on which this volume is based, was held at the Medical Society of London, and all those attending agreed that it was one of the most enjoyable meetings they had experienced. Dr. Macdonald Critchley's colleagues, students, and friends attended from all over the world, and the meeting received editorial praise from the *British Medical Journal*.

No book can recapture the happy sentiments of that occasion, but this volume, in honour of Macdonald Critchley, will not only serve as a permanent reminder, but will also make more widely available many historical aspects of the neurosciences.

F. Clifford Rose
W. F. Bynum

London 1981

Acknowledgments

We are grateful to the Wellcome Trustees for support, to Miss Frieda Houser of the Wellcome Institute for the History of Medicine for help in organising the symposium, and to Miss Patricia Pollock for secretarial assistance.

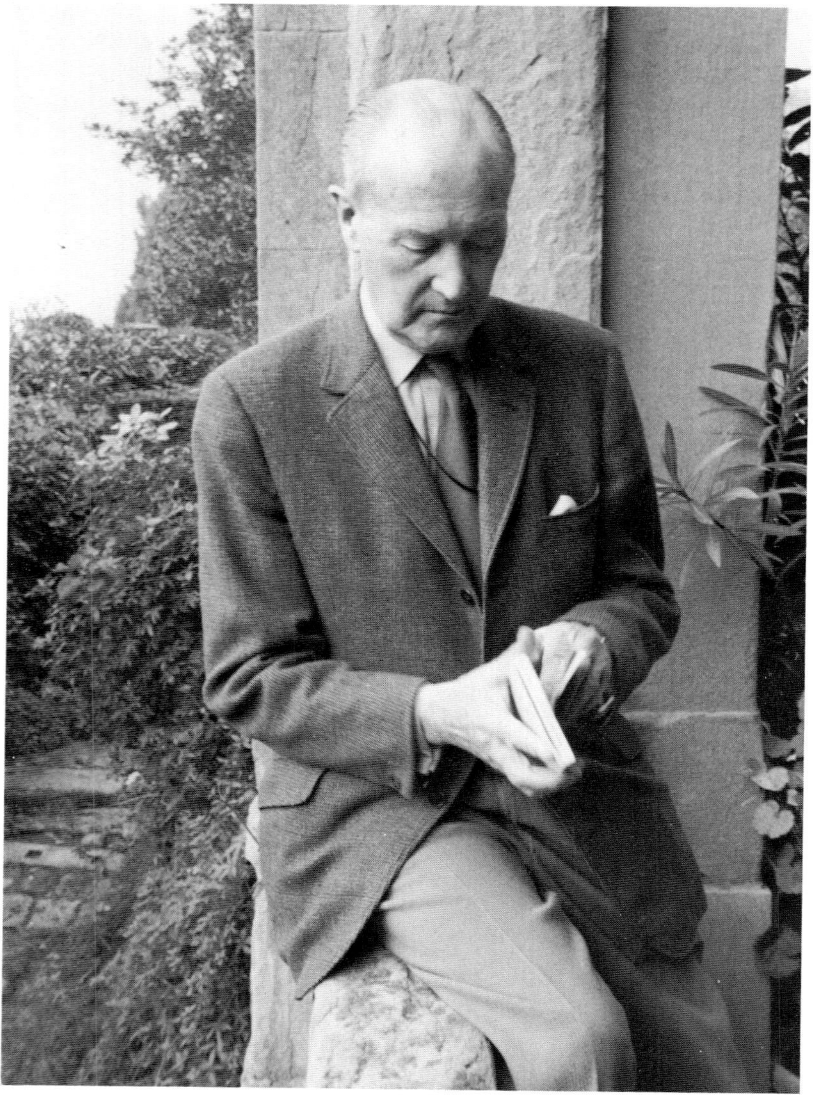

Dr. Macdonald Critchley

Macdonald Critchley

Macdonald Critchley was born in Bristol in 1900. He was educated at the Christian Brothers College, where he founded and edited the school magazine. He won a university place at the age of 15, but being too young to go to the university, he stayed at school for another year and filled in the time by learning Greek. Even before this, at the age of 11, he had won his first literary prize in a "Daily Mail" competition. It was in 1911, and with the prize of two guineas he bought a bookcase, which he still has in his study at home.

The year after he started Bristol University, at the age of 17, he volunteered to join the Army. Romantically, he wanted to be attached to the Russian Army, so he began to learn Russian. However, he was thwarted by the October Revolution, and he joined the Royal Flying Corps as a cadet. Within a month or two, the R.F.C. became the Royal Air Force, and his uniform changed. Next, the university wanted him to return to do his second M.B., after which he would be expected to join the Royal Navy as the Surgeon-Probationer. In order for Macdonald Critchley to become the Surgeon-Probationer, complicated regulations necessitated his being transferred to the Wiltshire Regiment as a private, and he served in Dublin during the "troubles." In his short career in the Army, he was in trouble twice. He was late on parade and was put on a charge. Asked what he did in civilian life, he replied that he was a medical student. He was then told to decapitate and fillet 500 bloaters. It may be that this experience put him off surgery for life. For another minor offence, that of being out of the guard room without permission, he was put in jail for a week and made to pick oakum. The task was not to his liking, so he volunteered to become the Governor's gardener. It is probable that this experience put him off gardening forever, for he has not done any more to this day.

Demobilised in 1918, Macdonald Critchley returned to Bristol University and gained a First Class Honours degree at the age of 21. He became a house physician at the Bristol General Hospital. His next appointment, as House Physician to the Hospital for Sick Children, Great Ormond Street, took him to London, where he has remained. The next year, in June 1923, he was appointed Resident Medical Officer at Maida Vale Hospital, after which he served for 3 years as House Physician at the National Hospital, Queen Square. Dr. Critchley has maintained his links with that hospital ever since, being appointed to the consultant staff at the early age of 27. Three weeks later, he was appointed Consultant Neurologist to another London teaching hospital, King's College Hospital.

Dr. Critchley is possibly the only British neurologist to have travelled extensively throughout Europe before the Second World War. He reads French and German fluently, having taught himself the latter language. With these languages, he was able to keep abreast with the neurological literature, and he made many friends in Europe, especially in France and Germany.

Before the outbreak of the Second World War, Dr. Critchley volunteered in the spring of 1939 for the Royal Navy and was called up for wartime service on September 1, 1939, 2 days before war was declared between England and Germany. He was Consultant in Neurology to the Royal Navy, with the rank of Surgeon Captain, and was consequently one of the few men to have been in all three armed services. During nearly 7 years of active service, he carried out the original research into hardships endured by shipwreck survivors. He also investigated living conditions in adverse climatic circumstances, which entailed extensive worldwide travel, including a winter's journey in an Arctic convoy of British ships carrying tanks, food, and medical supplies to the Russians, as well as tropical summers in the Persian Gulf and the Far East.

Dr. Critchley was demobilised in May 1946 and returned to the National Hospital, where he remained until retirement from the active staff in 1965. However, he stayed on in Queen Square in his consulting rooms next door to the hospital, and he continues to see patients and, from time to time, to teach. He was honoured for "services to neurology" by being made a Commander of the Order of the British Empire in 1958.

One of the high spots of Macdonald Critchley's career was being elected by his neurological colleagues throughout the world to become President of the World Federation of Neurology in 1965. He served for two 4-year terms.

Dr. Critchley's career spans more than 50 years of advances in neurology. He has written 15 books and more than 200 papers. Sixty of the latter are on aphasia, 16 on neuro-ophthalmology, 15 on developmental dyslexia, 12 on migraine, 10 on geriatric neurology, 7 on epilepsy, 6 on sleep, 6 on body image, 5 on boxing, 5 on the neurological effects of electric shock and lightning, 4 on epidemic encephalitis, as well as 66 papers on miscellaneous neurological subjects.

F. Clifford Rose

Making Rounds with Macdonald Critchley

What else can I write in honor of such a superb clinician and scholar of linguistics, literature, and aphasia as Macdonald Critchley but a memorial essay about the one and only time when he invited me to make rounds with him while he was a visitor at the University of California Medical Center in San Francisco.

All this happened in the early weeks of 1964, a few months after I had joined the faculty of that institution. At that time, my clinical experiences in the field of neurology were somewhat meager and left over from what I had learned in medical school, and I was not quite certain why a luminary of Dr. Critchley's stature would wish to have my help in a neurological diagnosis, as he had said. After a little while, I was to see the reasons for his choosing me as a consultant. We began, as was to be expected, with the usual series of neurological patients: some suffering from migraines, vertigo, or various such disturbances, sudden weakness in the extremities, and occasional fainting spells, which the patients insisted on describing as "blackouts." Then, after about half an hour, we arrived at the bedside of "my" patient, a young Oriental woman.

Dr. Critchley went through the usual typical neurological examination, using the reflex hammer and the inevitable pin with the same elegant dexterity that characterizes all his movements. When he lifted the patient's right leg and let go of it, it fell back on the bed without hesitancy or resistance; the same happened when he raised her right arm; it too plunged back down on the bed. The patient followed these procedures with a somewhat vague and unfocused look without saying a word or making a sound. Then Dr. Critchley said to me: "Now she is your patient, please speak to her."

This was a bit of a challenge in view of the fact that I did not have the vaguest clue whether the girl was Japanese, Korean, Chinese, or of any other Asian background. If she was Chinese, the complication of the respective dialect would pose a further problem, since I could speak only Mandarin. I asked to see her chart with the case history so as to deduce her national and regional background from the spelling of the name. This ruse did not work, as there was no name on the chart. So I began as well I could and asked her in Japanese: *"anata-no namae-wa nan desu-ka?"* which means "What is your name?" In reply I received a long drawn-out giggle; the giggle was repeated when I restated my question. So far as Dr. Critchley's question was concerned, I could not tell him whether the girl was aphasic, whether her laughter was due to her astonishment that I was addressing her in Japanese, or whether she was even able to recognize the language I was using. Well, I thought, let's try Chinese. I addressed her in my best Mandarin and asked her whether or not she could understand me. Again there was no response but extended laughter. Did she understand me? Did she even know that I was speaking Chinese? I noticed that Dr. Critchley and his neurological entourage, who had remained silent during my linguistic efforts, were beginning to show some signs of restlessness indicating impatience. From her total lack of effort to speak in whatever Oriental language was hers, they concluded that her aphasia was complete. Dr. Critchley suggested that she be given some speech and physical therapy and that we move on to the next patient. He thanked me for the pains I had taken, and I gathered that from now on my services were no longer needed, and I drifted away from the group making neurological rounds.

I was sorry for the poor speechless girl and returned to her bedside. When she saw me, there was none of the hysterical laughter that she had used to respond to my Japanese and Chinese addresses, but a happy smile and an evident attempt to speak. What she said was unclear, as she obviously was suffering from a severe dysarthria, but she repeated her sentence again and again until I finally understood her to say in English that she was Chinese, but unfortunately could not speak it. Here I had the answer to Dr. Critchley's question. The girl was not aphasic. I caught up with his rounds and reported my findings, whereupon he immediately returned to the patient's bed and, with his inimitable skill and elegance, elicited some response from the girl. The response, oddly enough, was in Chinese; it was a simple phrase that she must have been taught to use by her Chinese parents when she was a small child: *"Wo bu ming-bai. Wo bu ming-bai."* There we had our answer. She did not know Chinese, as she had been brought up in the United States; but she could not understand Macdonald Critchley's British accent and defended herself with the first sentence that came to her mind for such purposes, her first method of saying "I don't understand." I translated this for Dr. Critchley and explained to him the reasons for her sudden use of Chinese. So, finally I had proved my usefulness to our distinguished English visitor and his neurological following.

Whether or not the young Chinese-born American girl ever regained her ability to speak or to use her paralyzed extremities, I don't know. I do know, however, that on his next visit to San Francisco, about a month later, Dr. Critchley paid a private visit to another patient, a left hemiplegic who did not suffer from aphasia, and that it was I who was the recipient of his superb diagnostic skill and his charming bedside manner. I had read his writings about hemiplegia and could give him my first-hand reactions as to their accuracy. Suddenly, I knew at least as much about hemiplegia as he did, but I also knew that all his observations on partial paralysis had been all too correct. I had come to hate my paralyzed arm and the helplessness it imposed upon me, but I had not invented a pejorative name for it, nor have I done so in the intervening 16 years.

Ilza Veith

Contents

Neurophysiology

Higher Functions

Paroxysmal Disorders

Vascular Disorders

Spinal Disorders

Muscle

Neurosurgical Aspects

Other Neurosciences

The Development of Neurology in Various Countries

Miscellaneous

Contributors

Johan A. Aarli, Dr. med.
Head
Department of Neurology
University of Bergen
Bergen, Norway

Motoo Aki, M.D.
Counselor
Department of Neurology
Toranomon Hospital
Minato-ku
Tokyo, Japan

E. Bay, M.D.
Moorenstrasse 70
D–4000 Düsseldorf, West Germany

Peter O. Behan, M.D., F.A.C.P., F.R.C.P. (Glasgow), F.R.C.P. (London)
Reader in Neurology
Glasgow University
Glasgow G12, Scotland

Wilhelmina M. H. Behan, M.B., Ch.B., M.R.C.Path.
Senior Lecturer in Pathology
Glasgow University
Glasgow G12, Scotland

Simon Behrman, F.R.C.P.
Consultant Emeritus in Neurology
Guy's Hospital
London, England

Morris B. Bender, M.D.
Henry P. and Georgette Goldschmidt Professor and Chairman Emeritus
The Mount Sinai Medical Center
New York, New York 10029

E. P. Bharucha, M.D. (London), F.R.M.S. (India)
Emeritus Professor of Neurology
K.E.M. Hospital
G.S. Medical College
Bombay, India

Mary A. B. Brazier, Ph.D., D.Sc., M.D. (Hon.)
Professor of Anatomy and Physiology
Department of Anatomy
UCLA School of Medicine
Los Angeles, California 90024

George W. Bruyn, M.D., D.Sc.
Professor and Chairman
Department of Neurology
Academic Hospital
State University
Leyden, The Netherlands

J. W. D. Bull, M.D., F.R.C.P., F.R.C.S., F.R.C.R.
Honorary Consultant Neuroradiologist
National Hospital for Nervous Diseases
Queen Square
London WC1, England

W. F. Bynum, M.D., Ph.D.
Wellcome Institute for the History of Medicine
London NW1, England

Rudy Capildeo, M.B., M.R.C.P.
Senior Registrar
Department of Neurology
Charing Cross Hospital
London W6, England

Irving S. Cooper, M.D., Ph.D.
Professor of Physiologic Neurosurgery
New York Medical College
New York, New York 10029

Kenneth Dewhurst, T.D., M.D., M.Litt., D. Phil., F.R.C. Psych., D.P.M.
Professor of Psychiatry
University of the West Indies
Kingston, Jamaica

Victor Dubowitz, B.Sc., Ph.D., M.D., F.R.C.P., D.C.H.
Professor of Paediatrics
Department of Paediatrics and Neonatal Medicine
Co-director, Jerry Lewis Muscle Research Centre
Hammersmith Hospital
London W12, England

Eugene S. Flamm, M.D.
Associate Professor of Neurosurgery
New York University School of Medicine
New York, New York

J. B. Foster, M.D., F.R.C.P.
Hon. Reader in Neurology
Newcastle University
Consultant Neurologist
Newcastle General Hospital
Newcastle, England

Arnold P. Friedman, M.D.
Neurological Associates of Tucson
Tucson, Arizona 85712

Marek Gawel, M.A., M.B., M.R.C.P.
Lecturer
Department of Neurology
Charing Cross Hospital
London W6, England

William C. Gibson, M.D., D.Phil. (Oxon), F.R.C.P.
Professor of the History of Medicine and Science
University of British Columbia
Vancouver, British Columbia
Canada

William Gooddy, M.D., F.R.C.P.
Consultant Physician
National Hospital for Nervous Diseases
Queen Square
London WC1, England

Paul Guilly
Médecin Assistant des Hôpitaux
Ancien Interne des Hôpitaux de Paris
Ancien Chef de Clinique Neuro-Psychiatrique ā la Faculté
Paris 75004, France

Vladimir Hachinski, M.D., F.R.C.P. (C)
Chairman
Department of Clinical Neurological Sciences
University of Western Ontario
London, Ontario
Canada

J. Trevor Hughes, M.A., M.D., D.Phil.
Department of Neuropathology
Radcliffe Infirmary
Oxford OX2 6HE, England

Robin Illingworth, F.R.C.S.
Consultant Neurosurgeon
Charing Cross Hospital
The Regional Department of Neurosurgery, Central Middlesex Hospital
London, England

Robert J. Joynt, M.D., Ph.D.
Professor and Chairman
Department of Neurology
University of Rochester
Rochester, New York 14642

Harold L. Klawans, M.D., F.R.N.S.
Professor of Neurology
Rush-Presbyterian St. Luke's Medical Center
Chicago, Illinois

J. B. Lyons, M.D., F.R.C.P.I.
Professor of the History of Medicine
Royal College of Surgeons in Ireland
President of the Irish Epilepsy Association
Consultant Physician
Mercer's and St. Michael's Hospitals
Dublin, Ireland

Lawrence C. McHenry, Jr., M.D.
Professor of Neurology
Bowman Gray School of Medicine of Wake Forest University
Winston-Salem, North Carolina 27103

V. C. Medvei, C.B.E., M.D., F.R.C.P.
38 Westmoreland Terrace
London SW1V 3HL, England

Ian D. Melville, M.B., Ch.B., F.R.C.P. (London), F.R.C.P. (Glasgow)
Consultant Neurologist
The Institute of Neurological Sciences
Glasgow, Scotland

J. David Parkes, M.D., F.R.C.P.
University Department of Neurology
King's College Hospital and Institute of Psychiatry
London, England

B. Gerald Parsons-Smith, O.B.E., M.D., F.R.C.P.
Consultant Neurologist
Charing Cross Hospital
West End Hospital for Nervous Diseases
Western Ophthalmic Hospital (St. Mary's)
London, England

Andrew Peacock, B.Sc., M.Phil., M.R.C.P.
Nuffield Department of Clinical Medicine
John Radcliffe Hospital
Oxford OX3 9DU, England

J. M. S. Pearce, M.D., F.R.C.P.
Department of Neurology
Hull Royal Infirmary
Hull, England

G. D. Perkin, B.A., M.B., M.R.C.P.
Consultant Neurologist
Charing Cross Hospital
London W6, England

Ole J. Rafaelson, M.D.
Psykokemisk Institut
Rigshospitalet
Copenhagen, Denmark

Sigvald Refsum, M.D., Dr. med., Med. dr. (Honoris causa), Hondr. Med. Sc.
President, World Federation of Neurology
Emeritus Professor
Department of Neurology
University of Oslo
Oslo, Norway

F. Clifford Rose, F.R.C.P.
Physician in Charge
Department of Neurology
Charing Cross Hospital
London W6, England

Francis Schiller, M.D.
Clinical Professor Emeritus in Neurology
Senior Lecturer
Department of Neurology
University of California
San Francisco, California 94143

Franz Seitelberger
Professor and Director
The Neurological Institute
University of Vienna
Vienna, Austria

Stefan Shanzer, M.D.
Professor of Clinical Neurology
Mount Sinai Medical Center
Beth Israel Medical Center
New York, New York 10003

J. D. Spillane, M.D., F.R.C.P.
Prescelly
Newport
Pembrokeshire, Wales

T. J. Steiner, M.B., Ph.D.
Lecturer in Experimental Neurology
Department of Neurology
Charing Cross Hospital
London W6, England

William Elgin Swinton, Ph.D., D.Sc., LL.D., F.R.S.C., F.R.S.E., Hon. F.R.C.P.S. (C)
Senior Fellow
Massey College
University of Toronto
Honorary Curator
Academy of Medicine Museum
Toronto, Canada

John Todd, M.B., M.R.C.Psych., D.P.M.
Consultant Psychiatrist
High Royds Hospital
Menston, Ilkley
Yorkshire, England

Ilza Veith, M.A., Ph.D., M.D.
Professor Emeritus
Department of the History of Health Sciences and Department of Psychiatry
University of California
San Francisco, California 94143

Lucius Waites, M.D.
Texas Scottish Rite Hospital for Crippled Children
Dallas, Texas 75219

Marcia Wilkinson, D.M., F.R.C.P.
Regional Neurological Unit
Eastern Hospital
The City and East London Area Health Authority
London E9 6BY, England

Historical Aspects of the Neurosciences,
edited by F. Clifford Rose and W. F. Bynum.
Raven Press, New York ©

Neurology: The Electrical Root

Francis Schiller

Department of Neurology, University of California, San Francisco, California 94143

> . . . more nervous Disorders would be cured by this single Remedy, than the whole English Materia Medica will cure . . .[1]

The untidiness of roots is obvious to anyone who has lifted a plant out of the ground. And no matter how wide the circumference of his spade work, some rootlets at least will remain broken and still buried underground. The historian and his material share this unfortunate lot with the gardener and his plants.

The roots of what we today call neurology are, of course, multiple. The list—neuroanatomy, physiology, pathology, epidemiology, clinical diagnosis, gadgetry, therapy—could easily be lengthened, especially by subdividing the items. Changing the metaphor, yet still remaining in the realm of botany, you may want to call them branches, but the various techniques of, say, histology will again send the historian to look for their "roots." Our botanical metaphor will altogether break down with the necessary shift to other disciplines such as physics and chemistry, whether we wish to deal with neurophysiology or therapy, not to speak of our discomfort as we turn to psychiatry, psychology, or even sociology and economics: this may be taken as an apology to the reader who may scold the author for either his pedantry or his superficiality.

As to the fundamental role electricity came to play in the specialty of neurology, a threefold division into rootlets seems to be in order. First, in neurophysiology we have the recognition that the nature of those classical animal spirits was electrical, as well as the subsequent exploitation of this fact for clinical diagnosis. Second, we have the application of the electrical current in experiments carried out on the nervous system, and third, the treatment of its disorders in the clinic or at the bedside. The roots of the first two are well known, especially from Mary Brazier's writings (1,2), and too diffuse to deserve in the following more than a sketchy reminder. Less well-anchored in our historical awareness is the decisive role electrotherapy and diagnosis have played in emancipating neurology as a specialty.

But first, how did we begin to speak of specialties? Émile Littré (1801–1881) who, after an internship in medicine, proceeded to render into French the Hippocratic writings (10 volumes), to become a member of the French Academy and Senate, and to leave an unsurpassed lexicographic monument to his own language, defines in his Dictionary (3) *spécialité* "as a term in physiology, a special action performed by a special organ or tissue."

[1]Wesley, John (1760): *The Desideratum: Or, Electricity Made Plain and Useful. By a Lover of Mankind and of Common Sense*, London.

As an example, he quotes the neurophysiologist M. J. P. Flourens (1794–1867): "The great fact of speciality of action by various parts of the nervous system [is] a fact to the demonstration of which physiologists have devoted their noblest efforts for such a long time and with such ardor." Note that here, approximately in the 1840s, speciality or specialization appears, a little ponderously and self-servingly, as something nature herself does, in none of her creations more than in the nervous system—their epitome, as it were. And what is a *spécialiste*? According to Littré, the word was a *néologisme* in the 1860s. In support, he quotes from an article that appeared in the *Revue des Deux Mondes* of July 1856: "In science as in industry only specialists have perfection; while I regret this neologism, it does express a true idea so well that it will not perish." One senses the mid-Victorian fascination with the novel concept. Nineteenth-century industry, we hear, no less than science, had grasped the need for a division of labor, but to which enterprise we should give priority is hard to say. At all events, it was an idea whose time had not only come, but also one that would always remain with us. Still more pertinently, Littré made this statement to enlighten us regarding the type of person who best fits the new concept of a specialist: "in particular a physician who devotes himself principally or even exclusively to the treatment of certain diseases such as the eyes, the ears, the teeth, or the skin, the affections of the urinary tract, of mental alienation, etc." Neurology is not among them yet, unless we put it there ourselves, anachronistically, under "mental alienation," or "etc."

Sir James Murray and his collaborators of the Oxford English Dictionary (O.E.D.) (4) also refer us to the middle of the 19th century. Again the emphasis is on medicine in general, and the nervous system in particular. Thus, we find "specialist" related to "indications of scurvey" (1856); "specialty" to Czermak, one of the inventors of the laryngoscope (1861): "to make a specialty of laryngoscopy." Also quoted as an early user of the word is an editorialist of *Lancet* (8.8.1868, p. 17) who even, surprisingly, states that "Medicine is a specialism, but of a narrow kind." As neighbors to medicine, anthropology and zoology hold the field. Lewes wrote about a "specialized nervous system" (1853); Owen of the "modified or specialized character of the elements of the cranial vertebrae" (1854); Lubbock about our "specialized . . . modern instruments . . . such as a knife" (1865); Dana stressed the fact that "the general . . . (coming) before the special—is the law of all development" (1862). Specialization was a hallmark of 19th-century progress mirrored in, or driven by, the corollary preoccupation with evolution. For in the *Origin of Species* Charles Darwin (5), referring to Owen, associates "lowness" of organization with parts that "have been but little specialized for particular functions," whereas, operating to the advantage of each being, natural selection develops organs that serve a special purpose; to serve this purpose, they must have a particular shape.

Again we see how an epoch's insight into natural processes parallels its own practices and the principles underlying them. Now according to teleological thinking, it is a need, a desired function, that gives rise to the necessary tool. But the view that the reverse may be true—the tool preceding and determining its use—has often equal merit. Teleologically speaking, primitive man undeniably had a desire to move himself and his loads faster with less effort. But seen pragmatically, the invention of the wheel led as much to the establishment of the coachman as the discovery of x-rays led to the institution of radiologists and x-ray technicians. Without a passion for the dissecting knife, among other motivations, Morgagni would not have created morbid anatomy, nor would Bichat, a surgeon, have laid down the principle that organs are specialized tissues. The result is well known: the human body ceased to be regarded as a mere vessel for the interplay of arbitrary humors and became an assembly of organs or tissues, each of which deserved special study in health and disease.

Yet only to a limited extent was the organization and specialization of medical teaching, of hospitals and of office practice patterned after the organs illustrated in the anatomy books.

Not until recently were there any "gastroenterologists," "hepatologists," or "stethologists" (the author's suggestion for "chest specialist," or worse, "pulmonologist"). While the separation of practitioners inspecting the urine, feeling the pulse, and prescribing diets or drugs, from those working with the knife, cautery, and cannula is very old, only from the 17th century did some physicians and surgeons encroach on the midwife's territory and become obstetrician-gynecologists. Others, clever with the cataract knife, became ophthalmologists, yet only fully so when Helmholtz sent them off with ophthalmoscopes. We have already heard how the laryngoscope set up another specialty. Pediatricians seceded from the obstetricians. Somewhat earlier, the isolated men administering lunatic asylums became psychiatrists (6,7). (Let us remember here, in passing, that since antiquity practitioners who claimed special cures for this or that special human organ were, more rightly than wrongly, regarded as quacks by the learned profession. This attitude was reversed in the 19th century).

True, the brain and the spinal cord with its roots and appended nerves form a nicely defined system. But it is more hindsight than history, and we commit an anachronism when, with respect to nervous disease, we refer to Thomas Willis and the 17th century: Willis coined the word "neurology" merely to designate an anatomical category (8). Regarding the 18th century, when William Cullen considered most diseases being "nervous" in nature and was therefore called a "neurologist, i.e., a solidist" by his biographer in 1832 (9), it is obvious that the term there stood for the Edinburgh professor's repudiation of humoralism in general, remote from any specialized connotation. Otherwise, the word was hardly in use for two centuries. Cullen's and, in his wake, Pinel's nosology have saddled us with the endlessly confusing term "neurosis," standing for all those symptoms that to Cullen were not localizable nor associated with fever or cachexia. Almost as mysterious as the soul, to which it was indissolubly joined until about the mid-19th century, the nervous system remained dispersed in the various domains of anatomy, physiology, pathology, internal medicine, and psychiatry.

Then, how and when did *neurology*, word and concept, gain cohesion and a sovereign status? The story again unfolds over the latter decades of the 19th century. Romberg, in the 1840s and after, was still a Professor of Medicine. His successor in Berlin, Wilhelm Griesinger, best known as one of the founders of an "organic" psychiatry, became the first anywhere to occupy a chair for Psychiatry and Nervous Diseases. This pair of Siamese twins was born in 1867, i.e., the decade when Jean Martin Charcot began his work at the Salpêtrière, for which he attracted Duchenne de Boulogne to his service. In the year 1860, a charitable institution opened in London, the National Hospital, to serve, not as a haven yet of "neurology," for that was an almost unintelligible word and not to be found in contemporary dictionaries, but "for the Paralysed and Epileptic." (According to Cullen's nosology, they still could even then be said to suffer from a "neurosis.")

In contemporary Vienna, at that time the home of Europe's most prestigious medical school and one that pioneered specialization (10), Ludwig Türck, as early as 1846, was the first to be assigned to a "department" at the General Hospital, actually a small ward, reserved for *Nervenkranke*. This happened in recognition for his work leading him from "spinal irritation" to the naming of the "pyramidal" tract, thanks to his discovery of "secondary degeneration" affecting long tracts in the spinal cord. Türck's work reached the public one week after the Englishman A. V. Waller had submitted his better-known studies of cranial nerve degeneration to the French Académie des Sciences. (Nor was Türck luckier with his invention of the laryngoscope, where priority fell to a Viennese colleague, Johann Nepomuk Czermak, already quoted from the O.E.D.) For several decades after Türck's death in 1868, diseases of the nervous system essentially remained, at most German-speaking schools, in the hands of the psychiatrist. This was something of a paradox as most of these men were primarily neuroanatomists.

At the same time, during the 1860s and 1870s, the Viennese General Hospital, which served as the clinical teaching institution of the medical faculty, was blessed with no less than five young electrotherapists of academic standing. Three of them, Moriz Benedikt (1835–1920), Moriz Rosenthal (1833–1889), who was an assistant of Türck's, and Friedrich Fieber (1835–1882), published their own monographs on electrodiagnosis and therapy (11–13). These "young Turks" (as we cannot repress calling those clinical professors) also practiced and taught electrotherapy and "neuropathology" (as neurology then was actually called) at the *Poliklinik*, an outpatient department for the city's indigent, since 1872. The *Poliklinik* was established when the overcrowded General Hospital, run by the senior full-time academic staff, caused the younger men to secede. Here Benedikt became head of a Department of "Electrotherapy and Neuropathology" in 1875. Similar appointments involving electrodiagnosis and treatment were held at the Joseph's Academy and later at the Military Hospital by Franz Chvostek, Sr. (1835–1884), of tetany fame, and by his student Rudolf Lewandowski (1847–1902). The latter alone published four different texts on electrotherapy between 1875 and 1892.

Of course, these were not the only, nor the first, books on the subject. A bibliography collected in 1967 by the physiatrist S. Licht (14) gives no less than 923 titles on electrotherapy. Of these, 110 were published in the 18th century, and five times as many in the 19th century, the majority in its second half. This does not include the works by physicists. But let us briefly recall that early in the 18th century came the machines using friction and delivering the sparks of the "electric fire." Next, conduction, even by the human body, was discovered (Gray in London, 1720) and then insulation (Du Fay in Paris, 1733). In the 1740s, Benjamin Franklin, F. R. S., named Du Fay's "vitreous" and "resinous" kinds of electricity "positive" and "negative"; while experimenting with atmospheric electricity, he found that pointed metallic objects could catch lightning.

Ever since its invention by Pieter van Musschenbroek in 1746 in Leyden, after which place it took its name, the entertaining water jar charged with static electricity and connected to a condenser was also being used by both qualified and unqualified healers. They treated with this jar all and sundry ailments, most of which, in the broadest sense, were nervous.

From the multitude of 18th-century electrotherapists, let us pick only the most prominent figures who had published their medical observations and advice. These figures include a German-born Professor of Physics in Copenhagen by the name of Kratzenstein; the outstanding nosologist Boissier de Sauvages in Montpellier; John Wesley, the Methodist reformer and writer of popular medical tracts who devoted a separate pamphlet to the subject (several editions) (15) and expressed elsewhere that he was "firmly persuaded there is no remedy in nature for nervous disorders of every kind, comparable to the proper and constant use of the electrical machine," that "the palsy be electrified, daily, for three months, from the places wherein the nerves spring, which are brought to the paralytic part" (16); Jean Paul Marat, the assassinated physician and political "friend of the people," during a revolution that advocated "science for the people" and liquidated Lavoisier together with the French universities. Finally, there was in Bologna Dr. Luigi Galvani himself, a qualified physician, who not only experimented with frog muscles but also practiced electrotherapy and wrote about it (1792) (17). His "animal electricity" took its place alongside "animal magnetism" to share a low degree of respectability during the first half of the 19th century, thanks to Volta who, with metallic pile, thought he had disproved the validity of animal electricity. After Volta, in the 1820s and 1830s, the following physicists, who reported startling discoveries, held the stage: Oerstedt, Arago, Ampère, and Faraday (18). They proved the basic identity of magnetism and electricity; they also gave the world the galvanometer, the induction coil, and the dynamo.

In Berlin, meanwhile, Alexander von Humboldt, the influential naturalist, world traveler, and protector of seemingly lost causes in science, had kept Galvani's idea alive, and even coined the term "galvanism" (19). Physiology based on physics, the unity of the organic and the inorganic parts of nature, dear to the German mind, found new support in Du Bois-Reymond. For he, in the 1840s, showed the identity existing between electricity and the spontaneous conduction of the nervous impulse along the nerve fiber. "Animal electricity," part of the title of DuBois-Reymond's work (1,20), was vindicated, and with it those who, like Christian Reil, the neuroanatomist and romantic psychiatrist (the latter term is his), had opposed the belief in a special "life force" (21). Next, in 1858 galvanotherapy too was again made respectable in Berlin through a book with this title by Robert Remak (22). He significantly dedicated it to the 89th birthday of his protector, Alexander von Humboldt. Remak, the early protagonist of the neuron theory, believed in electrochemical influences on the body fluids and was inspired to experiment with electricity by a visit to Paris where he had watched Duchenne de Boulogne.

Before we return to Duchenne's towering figure, we must remember that in the 18th century, static apparatus was introduced in most London hospitals [Middlesex, 1767; Bartholomew's, 1777; St. Thomas's about 1799 (23)]. Later galvanotherapy, although under a cloud in many quarters during the early years of the 19th century, was also practiced, especially at Guy's Hospital, and by such men as Thomas Addison and Marshall Hall, of reflex fame, who was eminent if not generally accepted by his influential colleagues. (Hall, however, published nothing on the subject.) There even existed a doctor in London, La Beaume, who dared to call himself "Medical Galvanist to Her Majesty the Queen," if to raised professional eyebrows (14).

Now Duchenne's work (24) appeared in 1855, three years before Remak's *Galvanotherapy*. It was not based on galvanism. For over 10 years, Duchenne had used Faraday's induction coil, which had already appealed to some physicians in England, Italy, and France. What distinguished this intrepid free-lance doctor from Boulogne, haunting the Paris hospitals, from the rest? For one thing, he replaced electroacupuncture—Magendie too had stuck electrically charged needles into some of his patients (25)—by less painful moistened surface electrodes. More important, Duchenne also stimulated the precise points where nerves were known to enter muscle, much as John Wesley had advocated, and he was able to draw important conclusions as to the anatomy and pathology underlying the neuromuscular diseases that presented themselves. The title of Duchenne's book, *On localized electrification, and on its application to pathology and therapy*, indicates the author's methodical approach, almost a reversal of the therapeutic dilettantism then still current. Such expertise impressed Charcot to the extent that he referred to Duchenne as his "master," after appointing him to his permanent staff in 1862 (26).

This is how, in theory and practice, galvanism and faradism, now highly respected, gained a firm scientific footing in Western medicine. Revealing some of its mysteries, electrotherapy had lost none of its magic. We have seen it having its impact in Vienna, Berlin, and Paris, to name only those capitals. In London too, Gordon Holmes tells us (27) that the electrical apparatus was "urgently requested" at the National Hospital. An "electrical room," established in 1867, eventually contained, it was said, "every variety and perfection of scientific apparatus without parallel in Europe." The boast almost sounds defensive as we sense that, among the more famous of the Queen Square staff, electrotherapy never quite generated the serious dedication that prevailed on the Continent. Only Charles Bland Radcliffe, in his lectures printed in 1866, expressed an uncommon enthusiasm for electricity as the "nerve force" (28). Russell Reynold's book on diagnosis of 1855 (29), published before the great vogue set in, devotes barely and skeptically one of his 200 odd pages to "electrical irritability" for therapeutic use; yet he published *Lectures on clinical uses of electricity* in 1871 (30). Despite his "fondness for 'gadgets'," as pointed out by Critchley (31), Gowers, in his famous *Manual* of 1888, had little if any good to say about the value of electrotherapy. Reviewing in his text the conditions for which it was widely used elsewhere, such as tabes dorsalis (p. 322), chronic and other muscular atrophy (p. 373), ocular paralysis (p. 392), softening of the brain (p. 832), chorea (p. 987), paralysis agitans (p. 1013), writer's cramp (p. 1075), and migraine (p. 1189), we see that he found electrotherapy rather unacceptable. Gowers thought its cautious application justified only in the rehabilitation of poliomyelitis (p. 270), of "considerable value when properly employed" in neuralgia (pp. 1164–5), and "unsurpassed" in hysterical paralysis—the causes of which are "partly moral, partly physical" (pp. 1322, 1327) (32). The index to Hughlings Jackson's *Selected works* has no room for the subject. [Duchenne and galvanism are mentioned, as one would expect, only in reference to muscle physiology (33).] According to Gordon Holmes, the electrical department at Queen Square was soon left in the hands of the house staff. [By 1925, as Macdonald Critchley helpfully once recalled, the head nurse in charge of physiotherapy and radiology, a Miss Wintle—incidentally also the designer of the "Queen Square reflex hammer"—went by the nickname of "Sister Electrical" (34).]

Does this cool critical British climate of opinion make my claim seem exaggerated that applied electricity played a considerable role in promoting neurology to a clinical specialty, emancipated from both internal medicine and psychiatry? To answer the question and defend the claim, our inquiry must cross the Channel again eastward, the Atlantic westward.

It may be observed that on the European as well as on the American continents, labeling and legalism have played a larger role than in the British Isles. Academic titles particularly, so weighty and so characteristic for the birth and distinction of specialties, used to carry far less weight in England. After all, restless Brown-Séquard left Queen Square as a physician in 1863 to be appointed "Professor of Physiology and Pathology of the Nervous System" in the following year at Harvard (35). Gowers, knighted in 1897, only held the title of Professor of Clinical Medicine at University College Hospital (1883). There were no other professors at the National Hospital. And neurologists altogether did not officially exist in London before 1920; "professors" in this specialty, not before 1962 (36). By contrast, American professorships in this field, which did not go under the term "Neurology" but under "Nervous" (plus or minus "Mental") diseases, were established, aside from Harvard. In New York, William Alexander Hammond was already so appointed at the Bellevue Hospital in 1867; prior to his appointment, he had ordered into existence a United States Army Hospital for Diseases of the Nervous System in 1863, during the Civil War when he was Surgeon General.

Hammond's *Diseases of the Nervous System* (37), published in 1871, is usually considered to be the first English text exclusively and entirely devoted to the subject of neurology. How does he introduce it? With

> The Instruments and Apparatus Employed in the Diagnosis and Treatment of Diseases of the Nervous System.
>
> Diseases of the nervous system, like those of the heart, lungs, and larynx, require special means of investigation and treatment. In no department of medical science has progress been

> more decided during the last decade than in that class of affections considered in this treatise, and undoubtedly a great deal of the advancement is due to the instruments and apparatus by which scientific research in this direction has become practicable.

These are the first words of the book, and the "instruments and apparatus," besides the ophthalmoscope, are electrical.

Also in New York, Edward Constant Seguin became Professor of Nervous Disease at the College of Physicians and Surgeons in 1870. At Harvard, J. J. Putnam significantly started his academic career as "Lecturer on the Application of Electricity in Nervous Diseases" in 1872, similar to the development taking place in the 1860s, as mentioned before, in Vienna. Putnam was named "Lecturer of Diseases of the Nervous System" in 1872, Professor in 1893 (38).

The modern terms "neurology," "neurological," and "neurologist" did not yet figure in any academic positions nor in book titles. One of Moriz Benedikt's textbooks was from 1874 to 1876 typically called *Nervenpathologie und Electrotherapie*. In 1882 Charcot's first neurological chair in France was not given any name other than a professorship for *Maladies du Système Nerveux*. His quarterly journal, however, founded in 1880, did bear the title *Archives Neurologiques*. In Vienna again, Heinrich Obersteiner's *Institut* of 1882, i.e., at the time of its beginning, was one for "Anatomy and Physiology of the Central Nervous System" until it was renamed *Neurologisches Institut* in 1900 (39). In dictionaries, general or medical, English, French, or German, the word does not appear before the mid-1880s. Earlier than this, it was only in New York that a broadly assembled avant-garde of medical practitioners, led in 1872 by Hammond, formed the New York Neurological Society, and so officially initiated this term. Two years later, a rival society, also in New York, under the leadership of Austin Flint and George Beard, called itself the New York Society of Neurology and Electrology. In 1875 the American Neurological Association (Hammond, Seguin, Putnam, Hamilton, et al.) was founded (40). Yet the O.E.D. can find no earlier use than 1878 of "neurology" and "neurologist" in the clinical sense, and that was in a textbook on *Nervous Diseases* (41). Its author, Allan MacLane Hamilton, again an American, used the word as one being quite current. The grandson of the statesman Alexander Hamilton, he was a New York physician dealing, as much as the rest of the "neurologists" there, with functional as well as organic "nervous" complaints. At one New York neurological meeting in 1883, Hammond expressed regret that "a specialty so broad and comprehensive should not excite a still greater interest than it had done." *Medical Record* goes on to report that "the explanation suggested was that nearly every practising physician felt himself to be more or less of a neurologist" (42).

The name of George Beard is possibly better known than any of the foregoing, thanks to the publicity he sought and amply received, both nationally and internationally. For that very reason, he was somewhat less esteemed by his colleagues. Among them figured general practitioners who altogether resented specialization and the fashionable fuss made in particular over "nervousness" and "neurasthenia" (43), declared by Beard as the "American" disease. (This was not a far cry from the "English malady," as in the 18th century they used to call melancholy, with its offshoot hypochondria, or simply "the hyp.") Academic specialists saw in Beard "a kind of Barnum of American medicine" (44). Yet his *Practical Treatise on the Medical and Surgical Uses of Electricity*, first published in 1867, sold seven editions in the ensuing 17 years. Beard's coauthor, A. D. Rockwell, defended the application of electricity to the central nervous system—à la Remak. There had been British and Russian attacks by Anstie, Brown-Séquard, Cyon, and others. To them Rockwell replied that "electrotherapeutics, based on clinical experience is independent of, and in advance of, electrophysiology . . . this being an uncertain science, unreliable as far as it bears upon the practical employment . . . in . . . disease" (45).

"We-don't-know-how-but-it-works-so-let's-use-it" is, of course, a tradition in medical practice. The defensive attitude showed up in many texts on electrotherapy, including Wilhelm Erb's most prestigious work of 1882 and 1886 (46). Nevertheless, the day was not too distant when neurologists would find out that the various electrical methods were not worth their effort, could be left to physiotherapists (another developing if ancillary specialty), and eventually altogether almost abandoned.

And yet the therapeutic application of electrical currents to the human head (not of a voltage then, of course, to cause generalized convulsions) did in fact prompt what may well have been the most striking single historic moment in neurophysiology. In their report from Berlin, "On the electrical excitability of the cerebrum," Fritsch and Hitzig (47) challenged previous assertions that the cerebral cortex was unexcitable. Hitzig—he is probably the first person giving this account—proceeded to stimulate the dog's cortex, he tells us, because he had observed eye movements in somebody's head while he was "galvanizing" it. (He does not say that the subject so observed was a patient, or possibly Fritsch, which seems unlikely.) "Such facts show," Hitzig summed up, "that the origin of at least some function of the soul is bound up with circumscribed parts of the brain . . . [because] that part of the convexity of the cerebral hemisphere of the dog is motor." Five years later in Liverpool, Richard Caton was able to record electrical signs from the brain (48). In that very same year, but stirring the profession far more, appeared Westphal's, and independently Erb's, first description of the fundamental, and the emblematic, knee jerk (49,50).

Wilhelm Erb's work and fame, which was such as to make him Germany's first and foremost neurologist, consisted mainly in an extension of Duchenne's. Although Erb was officially still a Professor of Internal Medicine in Heidelberg, his writings on electrodiagnosis and therapy, together with his fervor as a propagandist, made him the greatest single force east of the Rhine in establishing neurology as the speciality of that name. His separatist drive caused neurology to become an obligatory subject, complete with examinations for medical students in Heidelberg, and to be the sole subject of *Deutsche Zeitschrift für Nervenheilkunde*, a journal he founded in 1891. Was the scientific productivity of the neurologists not vastly superior to that of the psychiatrists? [Or so he pointed out at a joint meeting in 1900 (51,52).] As to electrotherapy, he hails it almost as a panacea, and he sounds like a John Wesley when he asserts in his standard *Handbook* (53):

> We may state, unhesitatingly, that electricity is an extremely powerful and many sided remedy, and that more evident and undoubted curative effects may be attributed to it in diseases of the nervous system than to almost any other remedy. The experience of the last thirty years leaves not the least doubt that electricity is valuable in the treatment of neuralgia, anesthesia, spasms, and paralysis, in diseases of the peripheral nerves as in those of the central nervous system, and that its introduction into therapeutics has caused a more favorable prognosis in many forms of disease. I am not guilty of exaggeration when I say that the curative effects not infrequently astonish even the experienced physician by their magical rapidity and completeness. Despite these facts, however, we know extremely little of a positive nature with regard to the finer processes in electrical curative efforts, or their connection with the, to a certain extent, well-known physiological effects of electrical currents.

And he argues:

> The greatest authority was enjoyed by the electrotonic theory, according to which the majority

> of the curative effects of electricity are due to its modifying action (increase or diminution of irritability). What appeared more natural than that neuralgia and spasms could be relieved by the sedative action of the anode, with production of anelectrotonus, anaesthesia, and paralysis cured by the exciting action of the cathode, with production of catelectrotonus.

Alas, or rather, fortunately, any established creed has its dissenters. We all may agree with the fact, if not with the venal motivation, honestly expressed in this statement (54): "Anyone who wants to make a living from the treatment of nervous patients must clearly be able to do something to help them." The autobiographical writer who made this declaration in 1924, but which referred to the 1880s, is Sigmund Freud, and he goes on to say:

> My therapeutic arsenal contained only two weapons, electrotherapy and hypnotism, for prescribing a visit to a hydropathic establishment after a single consultation was an inadequate source of income. My knowledge of electrotherapy was derived from W. Erb's text-book (1882), which provided detailed instructions for the treatment of all the symptoms of nervous diseases. Unluckily I was soon driven to see that following these instructions was of no help whatever and that what I had taken for an epitome of exact observations was merely the construction of phantasy. The realization that the work of the greatest name in German neuropathology had no more relation to reality than some 'Egyptian' dream-book, such as is sold in cheap book-shops, was painful, but it helped to rid me of another shred of the innocent faith in authority from which I was not yet free. So I put my electrical apparatus aside, even before Moebius had saved the situation by explaining that the successes of electric treatment in nervous disorders (in so far as there were any) were the effect of suggestion on the part of the physician. With hypnotism the case was better.

Now Paul Julius Moebius (55), whom Freud mentioned in the above passage, had in 1879, like many other pre-neurologists, opened his practice for *Nervenheilkunde und Elektrotherapie*. This was in Leipzig where, as the coeditor of *Schmidt's Jahrbücher für die gesamte Medizin*, he also became the regular reviewer of the world literature in those two fields. One can imagine the shock and outcry of indignation when he flatly stated at a meeting in 1891: "Electrotherapy is four fifths psychotherapy" (56,57). Unlike Freud, Moebius did not abandon the treatment of organic nervous diseases, such as it was. An ardent philosophical monist and a skilled hypnotist, he did not endorse the split between psychiatry and neurology that inevitably ensued from the diametrically opposed endeavors of a Freud or an Erb.

As to organic nervous diseases, Freud continued (54):

> on the one hand the prospects in the treatment of such disorders were in any case never promising, while, on the other hand, in the private practice of a physician working in a large town, the quantity of such patients was nothing compared to the crowds of neurotics, whose number seemed further multiplied by the way in which they hurried, with their troubles unsolved, from one physician to another. And, apart from this, there was something positively seductive in working with hypnotism. . . . It was not until later that I was to discover the drawbacks of the procedure . . .

The result is well known: divorced from neurology, Freud was to give birth to psychoanalysis, a therapeutic method, not unlike electrotherapy or hypnotism, that many will classify with the placebos.

Yet electrodiagnosis and therapy were not quite passé. In the 1930s and 1940s, it seemed for a while that the electric current applied to the brain as a convulsant was going to cure patients afflicted with a psychosis. Still later, transcutaneous and spinal cord stimulation came in for analgesic or muscle-relaxing purposes, and the EEG is being used in biofeedback therapy. One hardly has to mention how much, since the 1930s, electroencephalography, electromyography, and nerve conduction velocity testing have lent a respectable background of precision to clinical neurology. But these applications of electricity are not the historical roots of the specialty.

Let us return then once more to 19th-century civilization. The last three decades were pervaded not only by the spread of electrical technology to affect every day life, but also by the vague yet vigorous notion, and not without due scientific backing, that electrical and nervous forms of energy are ubiquitous, inseparable, and in fact identical and indispensable. Hence, nervous disease of any kind—and this included the functional with the organic—could simply be explained as an electrical breakdown. Men with the expertise in understanding and handling these currents, installations, and systems, might be able to repair the damage. In medicine, only such experts could call themselves practicing neurologists. Like the proverbial phoenix, one might say, 19th-century neurology had risen from the ashes of the 18th-century "electric fire."

REFERENCES

1. Brazier, M. A. B. (1959): *Handbook of Neurophysiology*, Vol. 1, p. 1. Am. Physiol. Soc., Washington, D.C.
2. Brazier, M. A. B. (1963): The history of the electrical activity of the brain as a method for localizing sensory function. *Med. Hist.*, 7:199.
3. Littré, E. (1964): *Dictionnaire de la langue française*. Gallimard/Hachette, Paris.
4. Murray, J. A. H., Bradley, H., Craigie, W. A., Onions, C. T. (eds.) (1933): *A new English Dictionary on Historical Principles* (*O.E.D.*) Clarendon Press, Oxford, U.K.
5. Darwin, C. (1958): *The Origin of Species by Natural Selection or the Preservation of Favored Races in the Struggle for Life* (1859). New American Library (Mentor Books), New York.
6. Rosen, G. (1944): *The Specialization of Medicine with Particular Reference to Ophthalmology*. Froben, New York.
7. Eulner, H.-H. (1970): Die Entwicklung der medizinischen Spezialfächer an den Universitäten des deutschen Sprachgebietes. (*Studien zur Medizingeschichte des neunzehnten Jahrhunderts*), Vol. 4, Emke, Stuttgart.
8. Feindel, W. (1970): In: *The Founders of Neurology*, edited by W. Haymaker and F. Schiller, p. 91. Charles C. Thomas, Springfield, Illinois.
9. Thomson, J. (1832): *An Account of the Life, Lectures and Writings of William Cullen*, Vol. 1, p. 443. Blackwood, Edinburgh.
10. Lesky, E. (1976): *The Vienna Medical School of the 19th century* (1965), L. W. Williams and I. S. Levid (transl.), pp. 159,348. Johns Hopkins Press, Baltimore.
11. Benedikt, M. (1868): *Elektrotherapie*. Tendler, Vienna.
12. Rosenthal, M. (1865): *Die Elektrotherapie, ihre Begründer und Anwendung in der Medizin*. Braumüller, Vienna.
13. Fieber, F. (1869): *Compendium der Elektrotherapie*. Braumüller, Vienna.
14. Licht, S. (1967): *Therapeutic Electricity and Ultraviolet Radiation*, 2nd ed., p. 1. Waverly Press, Baltimore.
15. Wesley, J. (1871): *The Desideratum: Or, Electricity Made Plain and Useful. By a Lover of Mankind and of Common Sense* (1760). London.
16. Wesley, J. (1776): *Primitive Physick* (reprinted, 1973, as *Primitive Remedies*), p. 92. Woodbridge, Santa Barbara, Calif.
17. Benassi, E. (1961): In: *Essays on the History of Italian Neurology*, edited by L. Belloni, p. 131. Istituto di Storia della medicina, Milan.
18. Singer, C. (1941): *A Short History of Science to the 19th Century*, p. 302. Clarendon Press, Oxford, U.K.
19. Licht, S. (1967): *Therapeutic Electricity and Ultraviolet Radiation*, 2nd ed., p. 24. Waverly Press, Baltimore.
20. Gasser, H. S. (1970): In: *The Founders of Neurology*, edited by W. Haymaker and F. Schiller, p. 178. Charles C. Thomas, Springfield, Illinois.
21. Schiller, F. (1970): In: *The Founders of Neurology*, edited by W. Haymaker and F. Schiller, p.. 62. Charles C. Thomas, Springfield, Illinois.
22. Remak, R. (1858): *Galvanotherapie der Nerven- und Muskelkrankheiten*. Hirschwald, Berlin.
23. McHenry, L. (1969): *Garrison's History of Neurology*, p. 138. Charles C. Thomas, Springfield, Illinois.
24. Duchenne, G. B. A. (1855): *De l'électrisation localisée, et de son application à la pathologie et à la thérapeutique*. Baillière, Paris.
25. Licht, S. (1967): *Therapeutic Electricity and Ultraviolet Radiation*, 2nd ed., p. 27. Waverly Press, Baltimore.
26. Guillain, G. (1959): *Jean-Martin Charcot, 1825–1893. His Life—his work*, P. Bailey (transl.), p.101. Hoeber, New York.
27. Holmes, G. (1954): *The National Hospital Queen Square*, p. 21. Livingstone, London.

28. Radcliffe, C. B. (1866): *Lectures on Epilepsy, Pain, Paralysis, and Certain Other Disorders of the Nervous System*. Lindsay & Blakiston, Philadelphia.
29. Reynolds, R. (1855): *The Diagnosis of Diseases of the Brain, Spinal Cord, Nerves, and Their Appendages*. Churchill, London.
30. Reynolds, R. (1871): *Lectures on Clinical Uses of Electricity*. Churchill, London.
31. Critchley, M. (1949): *Sir William Gowers, 1845–1915*, p.88. Heinemann, London.
32. Gowers, W. R. (1888): *A Manual of Diseases of the Nervous System*. Blakiston, Philadelphia.
33. Jackson, J. H. (1931): *Selected Writings*, edited by J. Taylor. Hodder & Stoughton, London.
34. Schiller, F. (1967): The reflex hammer. *Med. Hist.*, 9:75.
35. Olmsted, J. M. D. (1946): *Charles-Edouard Brown-Séquard*, pp. 106,120,123,130. Johns Hopkins Press, Baltimore.
36. Haymaker, W., and Schiller, F. (1970): Introduction. In: *The Founders of Neurology*, edited by W. Haymaker and F. Schiller, p. XV. Charles C. Thomas, Springfield, Illinois.
37. Hammond, W. A. (1871): *A Treatise on the Diseases of the Nervous System*, p. 1. Appleton, New York.
38. Beecher, H. K., and Altschule, M. D. (1977): *Medicine at Harvard. The First 300 Years*, pp. 145,379. University Press New England, Hanover, N. H.
39. Seitelberger, F. (1963): In: *Grosse Nervenärtze*, Vol. 3, edited by K. Kolle, p. 21. Thieme, Stuttgart.
40. (1874): *J. Nerv. Ment. Dis.*, 1:74,228,370,535. (1875): *J. Nerv. Ment. Dis.*, 2:367.
41. Hamilton, A. M. (1878): *Nervous Diseases, Their Description and Treatment. A Manual for Students and Practitioners of Medicine*. Lea, Philadelphia.
42. (1883): *(Editorial)*. *Med. Record*, 23:710.
43. Blustein, B. E. (1979): New York neurologists and the specialization of American medicine. *Bull. Hist. Med.*, 53:170.
44. Rosenberg, C. E. (1962): The place of George Beard in 19th century psychiatry. *Bull. Hist. Med.*, 36:247.
45. Rockwell, A. D. (1873): On the application of electricity to the central nervous system. A reply to the objections of Anstie, Brown-Séquard, Cyon, and others. *N.Y. Med. J.*, 18:271.
46. Erb, W. H. (1883): *Handbook of Electrotherapeutics*, L. Pützel, (transl.). Wood, New York.
47. Fritsch, G., and Hitzig, E. (1960): In: *Some Papers on the Cerebral Cortex*, edited by G. Bonin, p. 78. Charles C. Thomas, Springfield, Ill.
48. Caton, R. (1875): The electric currents of the brain. *Brit. Med. J.*, 2:278.
49. Erb, W. H. (1875): Ueber Sehnenreflexe bei Gesunden und Rückenmarkskranken. *Arch. f. Psychiat. und Nervenkrankheiten*, 5:792.
50. Westphal, C. E. (1875): Ueber einige durch mechanische Einwirkung auf Sehnen und Muskeln hervorgebrachte Bewegungserscheinungen. *Arch. f. Psychiat. und Nervenkrankheiten*, 5:803.
51. Viets, H. R. (1970): In: *The Founders of Neurology*, edited by W. Haymaker and F. Schiller, p. 435. Charles C. Thomas, Springfield, Illinois.
52. Erb, W. H. (1900): Meeting of southwest German neurologists and alienists. *Arch. f. Psychiat. und Nervenkrankheiten*, 33:646.
53. Erb, W. H. (1883): *Handbook of Electrotherapeutics*, L. Pützel (transl.), p. 103. Wood, New York.
54. Freud, S. (1959): *An Autobiographical Study. The Standard Edition of the Complete Psychological Works*, Vol. 20, p. 16. Hogarth Press, London.
55. Bodenheimer, A. R. (1963): In: *Grosse Nervenärzte*, Vol. 3, edited by K. Kolle, p. 109. Thieme, Stuttgart.
56. Strümpell, A. (1925): *Aus dem Leben eines deutschen Klinikers, Erinnerungen und Beobachtungen*. Vogel, Leipzig. Pages 135, 138.
57. Möbius, P. J. (1891): *Schmidt's Jahrb. d. ges. Med.*, 229:81. Möbius, P. J. (1893): *Schmidt's Jahrb. d. ges. Med.*, 237:65.

Historical Aspects of the Neurosciences,
edited by F. Clifford Rose and W. F. Bynum.
Raven Press, New York ©

The Problem of Neuromuscular Action: Two 17th Century Dutchmen

Mary A. B. Brazier

Department of Anatomy, UCLA School of Medicine, Los Angeles, California 90024

The Renaissance was a long time coming to northern Europe and did not reach its students of the nervous system until the 17th century, but it is then that we find an explosion of interest. This chapter will concentrate on those aspects of the history of research on the brain in this period that deal with nervous transmission and muscular transaction.

Selected for description here are the contributions of two outstanding Dutchmen, Jan Swammerdam and Antoni van Leeuwenhoek, born within five years of each other in the third decade of that century. Both were to become concerned, in their separate ways, with the 1500-year-old Galenic dictum that animal spirits flowed down hollow nerves to inflate the muscle; both came to this subject from another field of study, namely entomology.

Let us first take Jan Swammerdam, for it was he who produced, as a scientist should, the experimental evidence for his hypothesis. Swammerdam was born in 1637, the son of an apothecary who had taken the family name from a village on a tributary of the Rhine near Leiden, the city whose university was and is an outstanding leader in science.

Swammerdam attended the Faculty of Medicine at Leiden from 1661 to 1663. Among his teachers was Franciscus de la Boë Sylvius, the distinguished anatomist, and incidentally, the originator of the famous Dutch gin, which he concocted as a disinfectant and all-around "medicine for the poor." Swammerdam, having earned the degree of Doctor of Physics from the University of Leiden, began extensive research into entomology, from which grew his interest in comparative anatomy. These studies led him to the experimentation that proved so important for the physiology of the nerve and muscle.

Swammerdam was a skilled dissector, even to the minutiae of small insects, using for his work magnifying glasses that he ground himself. In a letter (1) to his patron, Thévenot in Paris, he wrote:

> Nowadays I believe the magnifying glasses are in perfection, and so are the instruments that one has to use. And I found a very easy way to make all that myself, and I could teach it to another person in a quarter of an hour.

Swammerdam was one of the earliest biologists to work at all extensively with the frog, which later became the almost universally chosen animal for class work. It was in this animal that he identified the red corpuscles of the blood. A note (2) dated 1658 and found among his papers after his death shows that his observations antedated those of Malpighi, who is usually credited with their detection. Swammerdam, examining the frog, noted the following: "In the blood I perceived the serum in which floated an immense number of rounded particles, possessing the shape of as it were a flat oval but nevertheless wholly regular."

It was the frog that Swammerdam used for his search into neuromuscular action. He demonstrated many times that mechanical irritation of the nerve caused the muscle to contract, as others before had noted. Moreover, he had shown that stimulation of the spinal marrow had caused the contraction of the limbs.

These experiments brought Swammerdam to one that is a landmark in the development of biological sciences in the 17th century, for it introduced experiment as the test of hypothesis. Swammerdam would not accept the theory that the swelling of the muscle on contraction was due to an inflow of animal spirits. This age-old theory was being challenged by contemporaries, but not by a definitive experiment. Borelli (3), the distinguished professor of mathematics at Pisa, in an attempt to disprove spirits, slit the muscle of a struggling animal under water and demonstrated that no gaseous bubbles appeared. Unfortunately, he then concluded that the agent was a liquid, which on reaching the muscle caused a contraction by explosive fermentation. We find the same suggestion made by Thomas Willis (4), who described the meeting of spirits with the blood in the muscle as "like the explosion of gun powder."

Other distinguished contemporaries of Swammerdam still held to what later was to be irreverently called "the balloonist theory." René Descartes thought that the animal spirits were "like a wind or a very subtle flame"[1] and that "when they flow into a muscle they cause it to become stiff and swollen, just as air in a balloon makes it hard and stretches the substance in which it is contained."

A similar hypothesis was embraced by William Croone (5) in England, whose original idea differed little from that of Willis. He thought that a "spiritous liquid" flowed in and mixed with "the nourishing juice of the muscle" that then "swell'd like a bladder blown up." Later he was to modify this comparison to a number of small bladders for each muscle fiber.

Against this multitude of unproven hypotheses, Swammerdam demonstrated in critical experiments that the proposed ballooning effect did not take place. It is interesting to note that all of the dicta just quoted appeared during Swammerdam's most active scientific years, but as his critical experiments were not published until 58 years after his death, they were unknown to those who only speculated.

Among Swammerdam's several experiments on the frog that are germane to the elucidation of muscular contraction is one depicted on the right side of Fig. 1. The frog's muscle (b) was suspended in a vessel with a thin glass tube projecting from it, closed to the air by a very small drop of water (e). The nerve was threaded through a loop that could be pulled by a wire (c), thus mechanically stimulating the nerve, which then caused the muscle to contract.

The observation that the drop of water in the glass tube did not rise, although the muscle visibly swelled on contraction, convinced Swammerdam that the muscle did not inflate to an increased size, but changed its shape, contracting longitudinally and expanding transversely. This led Swammerdam to the recognition of the next step that would have to be taken, namely, proof of the relationship of the nerve to the muscle. Writing like an anatomist, he said:

---

[1]"Un vent très subtil, ou plutôt une flamme très vive et très pure, qu'on nomme les Esprits Animaux." Descartes, René (1664): Traité de l'Homme. Paris, (posthumous).

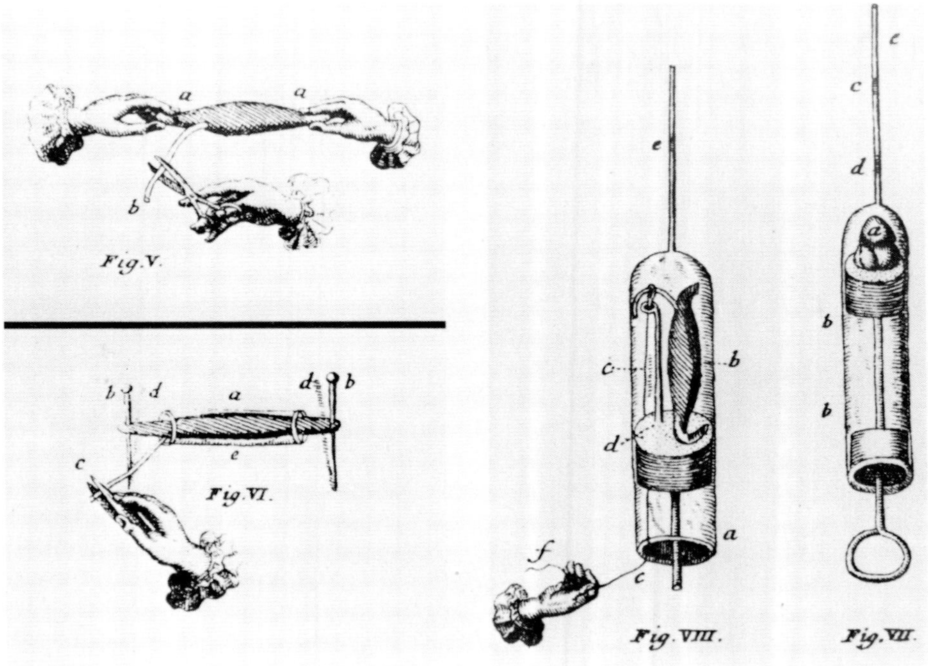

FIG. 1. Swammerdam's experiments, including the one by which he proved that muscles were not swollen by an influx of nervous fluid when they contracted. His Fig. V is of an experiment to show the change in shape of a muscle when stimulated by pinching its nerve. His Fig. VI illustrates the pulling together of the pins holding the tendons when the muscle contracts. The crucial one is Fig. VIII, in which a drop of water is imprisoned in the narrow tube projecting from the vessel enclosing the muscle. Swammerdam found that when he stimulated the nerve by pulling it down by a wire, the muscle contracted, but the drop of water did not rise. He concluded that the volume of the muscle did not expand on contraction. Some originals of Swammerdam's plates can be seen at the Boerhaave Museum for the History of Science in Leiden. [From *Biblia Naturae* (1738), Amsterdam.]

> In the construction and motion of the muscle it is of particular import to note in what manner the nerve is actually joined to the muscle; how it is constructed in the muscle; what its course, entrance, middle, distribution and end is; also how it communicates with the moving fiber, and what effect it produces in it; also what that very subtle matter properly is which is undoubtedly conveyed to the muscle through the nerve.

This is an outstanding example of a reasoned concept anticipating its proof for lack of the necessary technology. Swammerdam's primitive magnifying glasses could not enable him to see the neuromuscular ending, which is so familiar to us today. But he knew it must be there. It was unfortunate for the progress of neuromuscular understanding that these critical experiments were not published for nearly 70 years, long after his death.

Unaware of Swammerdam's experiments, one cruder test of the inflation theory was described by Glisson, the Regius Professor of Medicine at Cambridge. He reported in 1677 (7) that an experiment had been made demonstrating, by the immersion of a man's arm in water, that the level did not rise on contraction. The experiment he described may have been one reported earlier on two occasions to the Royal Society by Jonathan Goddard in 1669, for Glisson, who was a member of the Royal Society, does not claim to have done it himself. Goddard's (8) description and illustration are in the Register of the Royal Society.

Swammerdam, towards the end of his short life, had withdrawn from science into religious mysticism. The voluminous papers found after his death revealed his original intention to publish the experiments on muscle and nerve, for they included 52 prepared copper plates made from his own drawings. He was an excellent artist. After many vicissitudes, these papers came into the possession of Boerhaave, the famous professor at Leiden, who undertook to publish them.

Swammerdam died in 1680 at the early age of 43, and it was over half a century later that Boerhaave published his works in parallel columns in the original Dutch and a Latin translation. Another 20 years passed before this famous "Bible of Nature," as Boerhaave called it, was translated into English. Figure 2 reproduces the title page of this translation.

Some of the original copper plates, together with Boerhaave's Biblia Naturae, can be seen in the Boerhaave Museum for the History of Science in Leiden. The house in which he lived was preserved, and on the bicentenary of his death, to mark the house, a tablet was mounted that said (in Dutch) "His research of nature remains an example for ever." Today we are in the tricentenary of his death.

We have no portrait of Swammerdam. Perhaps I should warn you that you may find one labeled with his name in some secondary sources. The story of this portrait is that in the 19th century, a publisher took one of the heads from Rembrandt's famous picture of Nicholas Tulp's *Anatomy Lesson* and put out a lithograph that he labeled with Swammerdam's name. Swammerdam was a schoolboy at the time Tulp was teaching, so this was a stroke of imagination rather than fact.

The second great Dutchman to engage in this problem of neuromuscular action was Antoni van Leeuwenhoek, whose endeavour was to explore the anatomy of the nerve serving the

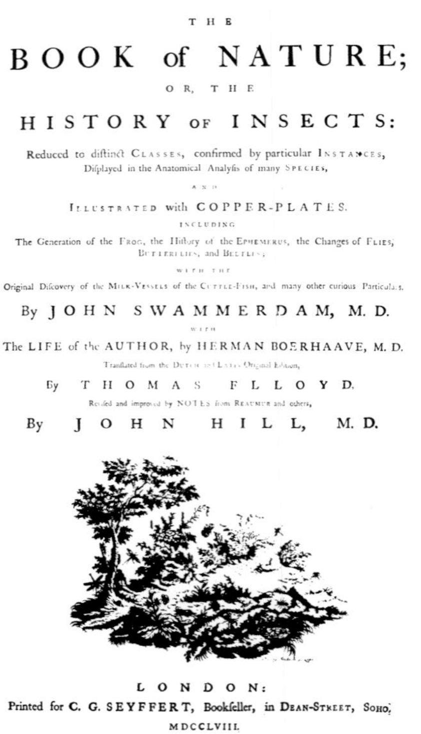

THE

BOOK of NATURE;

OR, THE

HISTORY OF INSECTS:

Reduced to distinct CLASSES, confirmed by particular INSTANCES, Displayed in the Anatomical Analysis of many SPECIES,

AND

ILLUSTRATED with COPPER-PLATES.

INCLUDING

The Generation of the FROG, the History of the EPHEMERUS, the Changes of FLIES, BUTTERFLIES, and BEETLES;

WITH THE

Original Discovery of the MILK-VESSELS of the CUTTLE-FISH, and many other curious Particulars.

By JOHN SWAMMERDAM, M. D.

WITH

The LIFE of the AUTHOR, by HERMAN BOERHAAVE, M. D.

Translated from the DUTCH and LATIN Original Edition,

By THOMAS FLLOYD.

Revised and improved by NOTES from REAUMUR and others,

By JOHN HILL, M. D.

LONDON:

Printed for C. G. SEYFFERT, Bookseller, in DEAN-STREET, SOHO.

MDCCLVIII.

FIG. 2. Title page of the first English translation of the *Biblia Naturae*, giving a comprehensive list of its contents.

muscle. Leeuwenhoek, born in the same decade as Swammerdam, also came from entomology but as an amateur, for he had no university education, could not read or write any language other than his native Dutch, and earned his living as a tradesman, though he rose high in the town affairs of his native city, Delft. He was, however, an ingenious craftsman, spending much effort to make the technical step from the single magnifying glass to the primitive microscope.

With his simple instrument, Leeuwenhoek unveiled the microscopic structure of insects, seeds, and the "little animals" he found in ditchwater, sweat, and spittle (Fig. 3). The existence of these little animals was unsuspected in the medical world. At the famous Paris hospital, the Hôtel Dieu, situated as it is on the island in the Seine, the sheets from the beds of the patients were still being washed by novitiates in the river (Fig. 4), which contained these little animals.

By then, Leeuwenhoek's little microscope made a critical addition to the general use of magnifying glasses. It consisted of a biconvex lens mounted between two plates (Fig. 5). His specimen was glued onto a silver point and viewed through a pin hole. An almost similar device, making use of a pinhole, had been designed by Torricelli in the 1640s (Fig. 6), but with Leeuwenhoek's lack of knowledge of Latin, it is unlikely that he knew of Torricelli's microscope. In fact, the scientific world might never have learned of Leeuwenhoek's discoveries had they not attracted the attention of his fellow townsman in Delft, Regnier de Graaf.

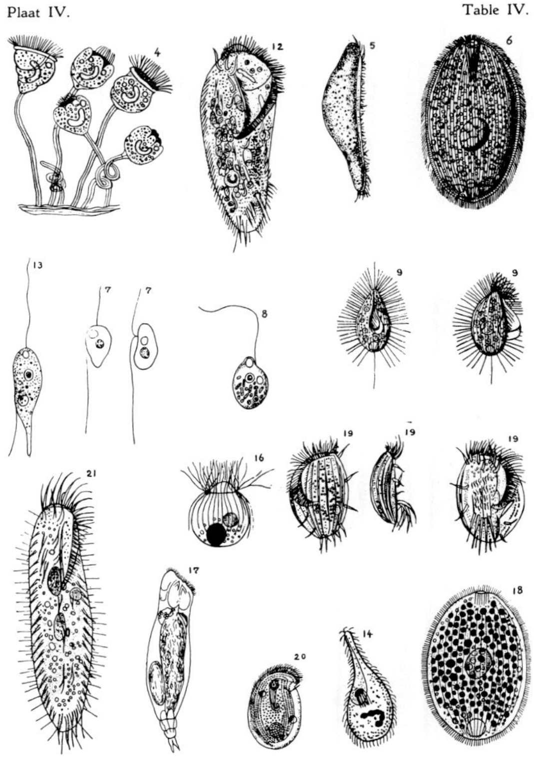

FIG. 3. The "little animals" found by Leeuwenhoek in rain water. (From Letter to Oldenburg, October 9, 1676. In: *The Collected Letters of Antony Leeuwenhoek*, Vol. 2, Swets and Zeitlinger, Amsterdam, 1939.)

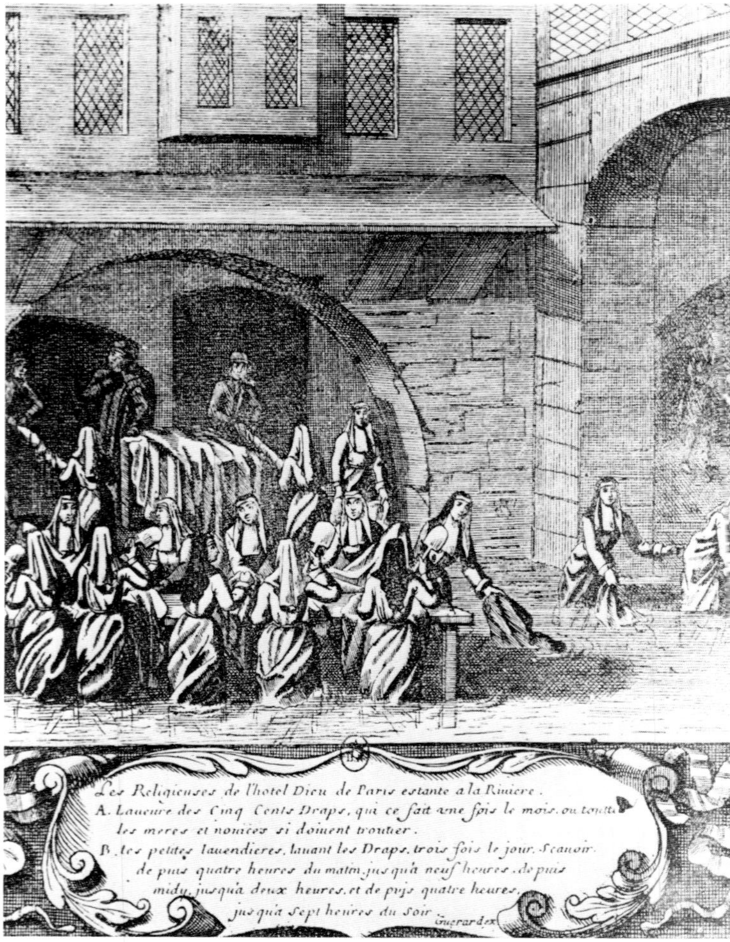

FIG. 4. Religious novitiates washing in the Seine the sheets of the patients at the Hôtel Dieu. (17th-century print, courtesy of the Hôtel Dieu.)

De Graaf, a physician and a Corresponding Member of the Royal Society, was so impressed with these discoveries that he offered to introduce Leeuwenhoek to Oldenburg, the Secretary of the Royal Society. He urged Leeuwenhoek to write of his findings for publication in the recently established *Philosophical Transactions*. This introduction resulted in a long series of letters to Oldenburg, which were then translated from the Dutch, beginning in August 1673 (9) and continuing for many years. Only a selection is quoted in this chapter. These letters reached a very great number, for Leeuwenhoek reported every finding in this publication, his only outlet to the scientific world, but all of his findings were not printed. They were, however, preserved and are in the archives of the Royal Society.

In the letters dating from 1674, we find the reports that concern mammalian nerves. Leeuwenhoek corresponded with Swammerdam and with the great Danish anatomist Stensen, both of whom were open opponents to the accepted concept of canals within the nerves through which animal spirits were said to flow. Here then, with Leeuwenhoek's microscope, was an opportunity to check whether or not canals could be seen in a cross section of nerve.

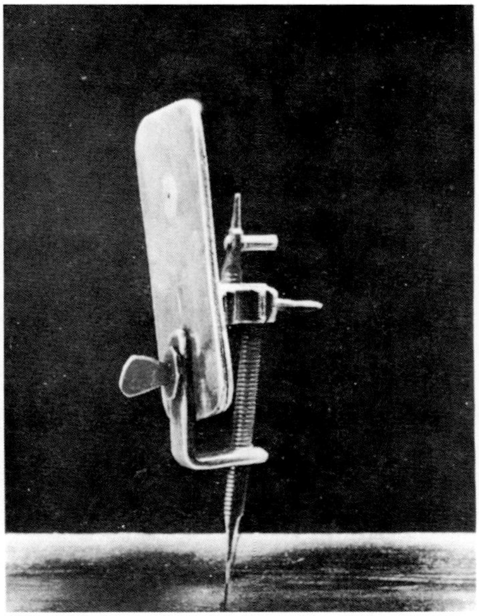

FIG. 5. The microscope of Leeuwenhoek. (Courtesy of Dr. P. H. Kylstra, Director of the Universiteitsmuseum, Utrecht.)

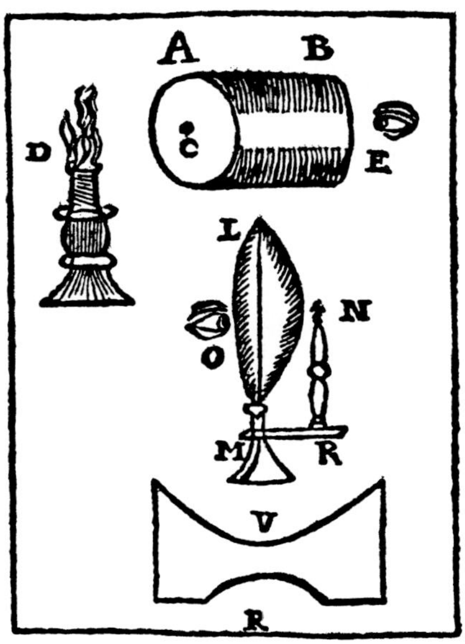

FIG. 6. Included in this picture is the microscope invented by Torricelli in 1644, illustrated in the *Ars Magna Lucis et Umbrae* of Athanasius Kircher, Rome (1646). (Biblioteca Accademia dei Lincei, Rome.)

We find the first report on this search in a letter to Oldenburg, written in September 1674 (10). Leeuwenhoek had obtained calves' heads from the slaughterhouse and it was their optic nerves that he put to the test. In his first letter on this subject, he wrote that he "could find no hollowness" in these nerves nor was he more successful with the vagus nerve.

Galenists were unwilling to accept these observations. One of them, a fellow Dutchman named Dr. Schravesande, told him that "Galen had on a clear Sun-shiny day seen a hollowness therein" and he encouraged Leeuwenhoek to "view that Nerve again with more attention." This Leeuwenhoek did and his report (11) is of interest. It reads as follows:

> I took therefore, afresh, eight distinct Optic Nerves, and observed that after those nerves had been but a little while cut off from the Eye, the filaments, of which they are made up, did shrink up, which shrinking cannot be so much on the external surface or coat of the Nerve, as 'tis of the filaments that lie within the same; And upon this shrinking up, a little pit comes to appear about the middle of the Nerve; and 'tis this pit in all probability, that Galen took as a cavity . . .

But in the same letter he goes on to say: "Having then dried such a Nerve, and made a transverse segment thereof, I not only saw in it a hole, but very many, which made it resemble a Leathern Sieve . . ." When one remembers the "silver point" to which the specimens were fixed and the fact that he spread them on "a little plate of talc or excessively thin-blown glass," one can easily understand the danger of the specimen drying out (Fig. 7).

Leeuwenhoek clearly hoped to confirm Galen's dicta and he was disappointed that he was never able to demonstrate any cavities to observers (12):

> I have been unfortunate in this procedure, for no sooner did I move them to my eyes for examination than almost immediately in less than a minute, they dried out and contracted so that this astonishing sight wholely vanished beyond recall . . .

Leeuwenhoek sent Oldenburg a very crude sketch (he was no artist) of what he saw in this disappearing trick. A draftsman at the Royal Society improved upon it, but it is not

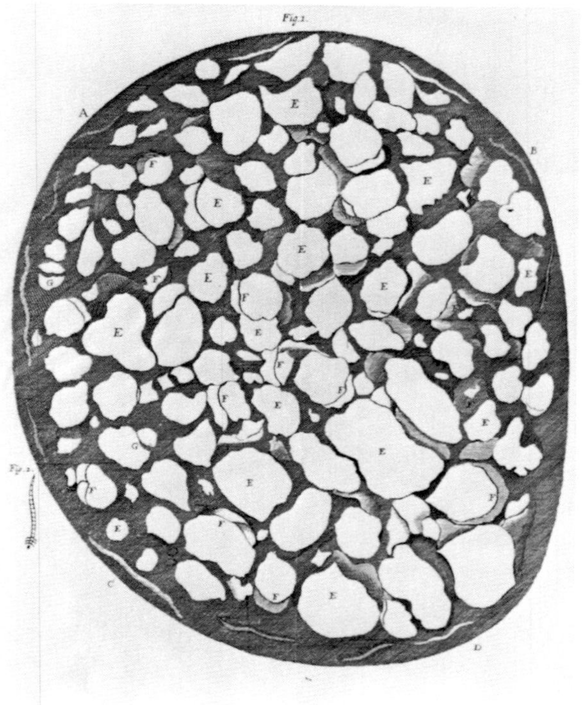

FIG. 7. Cross section of the optic nerve of the calf, redrawn for *Philosophical Transactions* from a rougher sketch sent to the Royal Society by Leeuwenhoek. [*Phil. Trans. Roy. Soc.*, (1675): 10:378–385.]

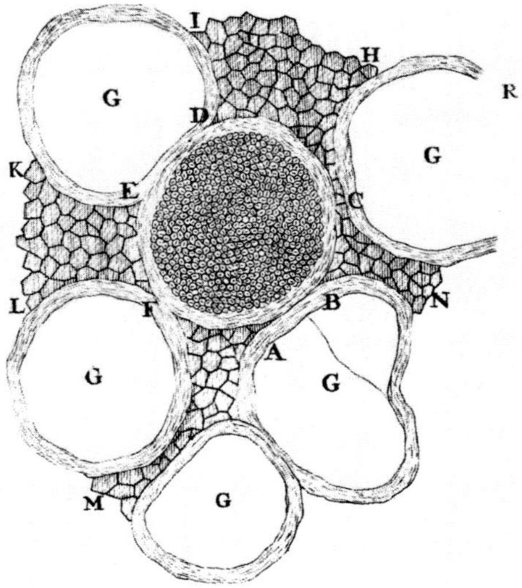

FIG. 8. Cross section of the nerve drawn by an artist by the direction of Leeuwenhoek (from memory) at the age of 84. (From Letter to Abrahamo van Bleiswyk, March 2, 1717. Published in *Epistolae Physiologicae Super Compluribus Naturae Arcanis.* Beman, Delft, 1719.)

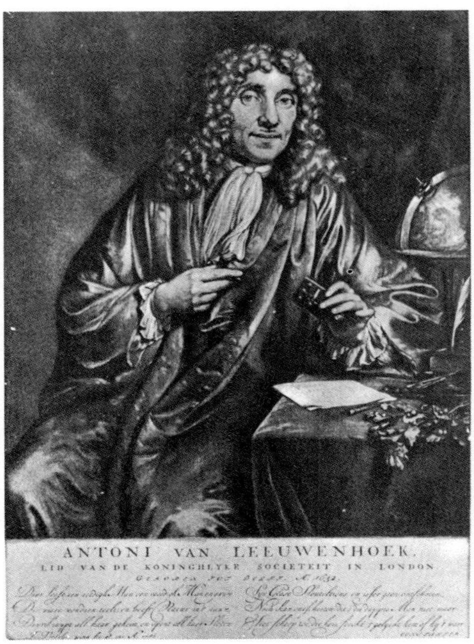

FIG. 9. Portrait of Leeuwenhoek holding his microscope. The artist has enlarged the microscope which, in fact, was much smaller in comparison with the hand. [From the portrait by J. Verkolje, 1686 (Gabb Collection).]

until the end of his long life, at 84, that the delicate drawing with which we are familiar (Fig. 8), was made by an artist, at the request of Leeuwenhoek.

This drawing was enclosed in a letter (13) to a fellow citizen of Delft, in which he stated that he "very distinctly recognized the canals" and remarked that, as the specimens were drying out, he found "little hills raised on them." His interpretation was that "what humor was in them is driven out and rises up like little hills." The letter ends with the credo of a convinced Galenist: "What material is that was enclosed in them I was never able to determine with certainty, although I believe that it was a very fluid humor which passed off as vapor." This letter was written in 1717. Galen had died in 200 A.D. The first use of microscopy in this field had failed to revoke his concepts. One hundred years later the issue was still unresolved.

Therefore, we have to admit rather sadly that it is not to our knowledge of the nerve that this industrious experimenter made any critical contribution, but to opening the eyes of scientists to the swarming life that could be seen through his primitive microscope, for the science of microbiology was as yet unborn.

Leeuwenhoek received recognition during his lifetime, being made a Fellow of the Royal Society in 1680. There are several portraits of him, but the one in Fig. 9 is chosen because it shows him holding his microscope. Leeuwenhoek made very many of his little microscopes, and on his death in 1723 he bequeathed a collection of them, now unfortunately lost, to the Royal Society. One of the few remaining original instruments made by his own hand is preserved in the museum of the University of Utrecht. The magnifying power is 175 times, a range that opened a window on a new world.

REFERENCES

1. Swammerdam, J. (1678): Letter to Thévenot. In: *The Letters of Jan Swammerdam to Melchisadec Thévenot*, edited by G. A. Lindeboom. Swets and Zeitlinger, Amsterdam.
2. Swammerdam, J. (1658): Note dated 1658 found after his death according to Boerhaave. In: *Biblia Naturae*, 2 vols., published by Boerhaave, 1737 and 1738. Severinus, Amsterdam. (A translation into Latin of the original Bybel der Natuure). Translation into English by Th. Flloyd, London (1758).
3. Borelli, Giovanni Alfonso (1680): *De Motu Animalium* (posthumous). Bernado, Rome.
4. Willis, Thomas (1664): *Cerebri Anatome*. Flesher, London.
5. Croone, W. (1664): *De Ratione Motus Muscularum*. Flesher, London.
6. Swammerdam, J. (1737 and 1738): *Biblia Naturae*, published by Boerhaave. Severinus, Amsterdam.
7. Glisson, F. (1677): *Tractatus de Ventriculo et Intestinis*. Henry Brome, London.
8. Goddard, J. (1669): In: *Birch's History of the Royal Society*.
9. Leeuwenhoek, A. (1674): More microscopical observations made by the same Mr. Leeuwenhoeck (sic) and promised in Number 97 of these Tracts communicated in his letters of August 15, 1673 and of April 7, 1674. *Phil. Trans. Roy. Soc.*, 6:23.
10. Leeuwenhoek, A. (1674): More observations from Mr. Leeuwenhook (sic) in a letter of Sept. 7, 1674 sent to the publisher. *Phil. Trans. Roy. Soc.*, 9:178. (More generally, cf. Edwin Clarke (1968): The doctrine of the hollow nerve in the seventeenth & eighteenth centuries. In: *Medicine, Science and Culture*, edited by L. G. Stevenson and R. P. Multhauf, pp. 123–141. Johns Hopkins Press, Baltimore.)
11. Leeuwenhoeck, A. (1675): Microscopical observations of Mr. Leeuwenhoeck (sic) concerning the optic nerve in a letter of Dec. 7, 1675. *Phil. Trans. Roy. Soc.*, 10:378.
12. Leeuwenhoek, A. (1693): An extract of a letter from Mr. Anthony van Leeuwenhoek to the Royal Society containing his observations of the optic nerves. *Phil. Trans. Roy. Soc.*, 17:949.
13. Leeuwenhoek, A. (1719): *Epistolae Physiologicae super Compluribus Naturae Arcanis*. Beman, Delft. (Letter No. 32 in Latin addressed to Domino Abrahamo van Bleiswyk, March 2, 1717.)

Historical Aspects of the Neurosciences,
edited by F. Clifford Rose and W.F. Bynum.
Raven Press, New York ©

The Evolution of the Concepts of Peripheral Paralysis and of Sensory Ataxia in the 19th Century

J. D. Spillane

Prescelly, Newport, Pembrokeshire, Wales

During the first half of the 19th century, progress was slower in the field of diseases of the nervous system than in those of the heart and lungs. No Laënnec or Auenbrugger had arrived at the bedside of the paralyzed patient. Very little was known about motor and sensory paralysis. It was appreciated that paralyzed muscles could be soft and limp or hard and stiff. Some paralyzed limbs were observed to waste rapidly, others scarcely at all. Pain and numbness were variable accompaniments. Paralysis was sometimes accompanied by reflex "excitement," "agitation," or "convulsion." These might be spontaneous or they might require elicitation. Moreover, a patient might have paralyzed muscles showing some of these features and others which might not, or which might show signs of an opposite kind. Lastly, it was confusing to note that the physical signs in a paralyzed limb could alter with the passage of time, even though the disease itself appeared not to be progressing.

It was only in the second half of the century that paralysis arising in the periphery of the nervous system came to be distinguished from that of central origin, and that the features of spinal ataxia and paralysis were differentiated. But in both multiple neuritis and locomotor ataxia, the "idea" was there for some years before clinical recognition was achieved.

Graves (1), writing of the possibility of a lesion in the periphery of the nervous system in some cases of paralysis, wrote in 1848 that "In a word, may not the decay and withering of the nervous tree commence occasionally in its extreme branches? and may not a blighting influence affect the latter, while the main trunk remains sound and unharmed?"

In 1826 Bell (2) wrote that "Between the brain and the muscles there is a circle of nerves; one nerve conveys the influence from the brain to the muscle, another gives the sense of the condition of the muscle to the brain." And Bell (3) wrote in 1833:

> When a blind man, or man with his eyes shut, stands upright . . . by what means is it that he maintains the erect position? . . . he touches nothing . . . he sees nothing . . . it can only be by the adjustment of muscles . . . it must be a property internal to the frame by which we thus know the position of the members of our body.

MULTIPLE NEURITIS

When Graves made his suggestion, he said that "pathologists have neglected the nerves as, in the vascular system, they have neglected the capillaries," and he referred to an obscure epidemic of a nervous disorder that he had seen in Paris in 1828. He wrote (1):

> One of the most remarkable examples of disease of the nervous system commencing in the extremities, and having no connection with lesions of the brain or spinal marrow, was the curious *epidémie de Paris*, which occurred in the spring of 1828. Chomel has described this epidemic in the 9th number of the *Journal Hebdomadaire*, and having witnessed it myself in the months of July and August of the same year, I can bear testimony to the ability and accuracy of his description. It began (frequently in persons of good constitution) with sensations of pricking and severe pain in the integuments of the hands and feet, accompanied by so acute a degree of sensibility, that the patients could not bear these parts to be touched by the bedclothes. After some time, a few days, or even a few hours, a diminution, or even abolition of sensation took place in the affected members, they became incapable of distinguishing the shape, texture, or temperature of bodies, the power of motion declined, and finally they were observed to become altogether paralytic. The injury was not confined to the hands and feet alone, but, advancing with progressive pace, extended over the whole of both extremities. Persons lay in bed powerless and helpless, and continued in this state for weeks and even months. . . .
>
> At last, at some period of the disease, motion and sensation gradually returned, and a recovery generally took place, although in some instances, the paralysis was very capricious, vanishing and again reappearing.
>
> The French pathologists, you may be sure, searched anxiously in the nervous centres for the cause of this strange disorder, and could find none; there was no evident lesion, functional or organic, discoverable in the brain, cerebellum, or spinal marrow.

Graves thought this was an "instance of paralysis creeping from the extremities towards the centre . . . can anyone . . . hesitate to believe that paralysis . . . may arise from disease commencing and originating in the nervous extremities alone?" He did not mention, however, that in one autopsy "the nerves were dissected and followed to the tips of the fingers and toes" and no lesions were seen (4). This was recorded in the account by Chomel to which he referred.

There is no record of the number of cases that were seen nor of the sex incidence nor of the mortality rate. But infants, it seems, were spared. There appeared to have been acute, subacute, and relapsing varieties, but on the whole, the majority recovered. There were only two autopsies. One patient died of respiratory paralysis. The general condition of the patients remained satisfactory. There was no evidence of ergotism or plumbism. The motor and sensory paralysis was usually, but not always, symmetrically distributed. Pains were sharp, intermittent, worse at night, and often provoked by touch or pressure. Tenderness of the feet caused some to discard their shoes or boots and wear sabots or woollen socks. Sensibility of the feet was sometimes so impaired that a shoe might fall off without the wearer's knowledge; a cold pavement was not felt. The steps of a staircase sometimes felt as if they were giving way; they felt "soft." Involvement of the fingers and hands caused difficulties in dressing, eating, and in identifying objects. One patient could not tell the difference between a key and a pair of scissors, by touch. Objects might be dropped because touching them was so disagreeable. Gait was clumsy, and feet were lifted up and put down in a flat-footed manner. Some patients walked with their legs separated "as if they had some affection of the genital organs." The hands and feet were erythematous in some cases; there was sweating and desquamation at times. The digits appeared swollen and the skin, glossy. The toes and fingers drooped.

Chomel did not actually discuss the possibility of peripheral neuritis, although presumably he suspected it. Graves was convinced that that was the explanation and he was no doubt quite correct. It was an epidemic of polyneuritis. The paralysis, numbness, and skin changes in the hands and feet of alcoholics had, of course, been noted by Lettsom (5) in 1787 and by Jackson (6) in 1822, but the neuritic nature of the illness had not been suspected.

Before Duchenne began to show in the 1850s how vital it was to examine carefully a paralyzed limb, physical examination was a cursory procedure. There was little attempt to identify which muscles were affected and to what degree. The tendon reflexes did not appear on the scene until 1875. As for sensory testing, it was in its infancy. An important early contribution was that of Landry.

Landry on "Physiological and Pathological Researches into Tactile Sensations"

Landry (7) was only 26 when he published his study with the above title in 1852. He followed it with a second contribution, which we shall consider when we turn to ataxia, entitled *On the Paralysis of Feeling of Muscular Activity* in 1855 (8). His famous account of *Acute Ascending Paralysis* came in 1859 (9).

In 1852 Landry thought that there had been too many "theoretical dissertations" on tactile sensibility, few careful clinical observations, and little critical analysis. The word "sensation," he thought, had been ill-defined and used in a variety of ways. It should only be employed to mean "the perception by the brain of peripheral impressions and not the appreciation which entailed a judgement." An intellectual operation was involved in the latter, whereas "sensation" itself occurred passively. He had been impressed by the many different ways in which sensation could be altered by disease of the nervous system. Nature provided, as it were, valuable experiments to study. "I have seen many disorders of cutaneous sensibility in which the tactile phenomena have been, as it were, *dissected*."

Landry recorded the degree and distribution of sensory alterations on the head, trunk, and limbs in patients with and without motor paralysis, and in organic and hysterical illnesses. There were many cases of paraplegia and hemiplegia in his collection. Naturally, the nature of many of his cases is not known, but one can recognize syringomyelia in the case of the patient with analgesia of both upper limbs, in which he found that tactile sensation was normal. Another patient presented with a Brown-Séquard syndrome: paraplegia with analgesia of the right lower limb and retained tactile sensibility in that limb. There were patients in whom there were various combinations of tactile anesthesia and hyperesthesia, analgesia and hyperalgesia, and perversions of feeling. Delay in the recognition of pain or temperature were recorded.

Landry thought that clinicians were using too many terms to signify types of sensation: temperature, pain, contact, rustling, vibration, tickling, weight, resistance, consistency, form, dryness, humidity, thickness, size, movement, and many others. He felt that there essentially were a small number of actual cutaneous modes of sensation. "There really exist only three primitive cutaneous sensations: those of temperature, pain, and contact, to which must be added the three secondary ones of pressure, vibration and tickling, which are modified sensations of contact." In addition, there was the special sensation of muscular activity. The combined use of these four modalities enabled one to judge shape, size, surface, dryness and wetness, weight, position,and movement. He wondered whether or not "these diverse sensations have different nerves" and thought that they probably did. There were "four special sensations, based on four orders of nerves whose functions are quite distinct."

Five categories of cutaneous sensory abnormality were found in neurological patients: (a) Touch is altered but pain is normal; (b) Pain is altered but touch is normal; (c) Pain and touch are altered, but perhaps in different ways; (d) Only temperature appreciation is unaltered; and (e) Only temperature appreciation is altered. Tactile impressions could be exaggerated or suppressed independently of the sensation of pain. Touch and pain must be essentially distinct modalities, but hot and cold were not "absolutes." In a given cutaneous zone, touch and pain could be altered in a variety of ways, at the same time. With regard to the interpretation of delay in feeling a stimulus, Landry thought that "it is impossible to suppose a slowing down of the peripheral impressions to the brain"; it was more likely that the delay occurred in the superficial tissues involved. He stressed the "passive" and "active" nature of the processes concerned in general sensibility. We can see without "looking, hear without listening." Touch could be passive or "attentive."

Despite the title of his paper, Landry did not consider the possibility that certain types of sensory loss might be the result of lesions in the peripheral nerves. The nature of the loss commanded his attention. There is no mention of the areas affected by particular nerves and no hint that he glimpsed the "glove-and-stocking" pattern of multiple involvement of the peripheral nerves.

In 1859, when he described "acute ascending paralysis," he did not consider the possibility of a lesion ascending the peripheral nervous system. The illness began with "formications in the tips of his fingers and toes," and the sensory loss, which felt "like a band around the affected parts," spread upwards. But even when his patient was virtually paralyzed, after three weeks, there was only slight sensory impairment on the soles of his feet. On the day he died, touch was lost in the feet and impaired only in the lower third of the legs and in the finger tips. Over the trunk there were areas where the differences between "touching" and "rubbing," and between "light touch and pressure," were poorly distinguished. "Pain and temperature sensation were not altered anywhere." Appreciation of passive movements was completely lost in the fingers and toes.

Yet Landry had recognized that the motor paralysis was unusual. It had begun in the toes, which were soon totally paralyzed; the fingers were soon similarly affected. The paralyzed limbs remained painless and "supple," the muscles did not waste, and there were no "cramps," "convulsive movements," "involuntary spasms," or "contractures," which characterized most forms of paraplegia. His failure to induce "reflexes" refers no doubt to the superficial ones commonly tested at that time, like the plantar and withdrawal movements of the lower limbs. In addition, the spine was not painful, and the sphincters continued to function normally. Indeed, because of the gross nature of the paralysis, the flaccidity and the paucity of signs, Landry's chief suspected that the patient might have been malingering.

The nerves were not examined at autopsy, but a careful microscopic examination of the spinal cord revealed nothing abnormal. Landry mentioned that he had personally seen four similar cases and had read of four others. There had been three deaths, and in one autopsy the cord had been normal but the nerves were not examined.

Many years were to elapse before Landry's syndrome was considered to be a multiple symmetrical peripheral neuritis and before the term "multiple neuritis" was introduced by Leyden (1832–1910) in 1880. Neither Gull (10) in 1858 nor Wilks (11) 20 years later examined the nerves in cases that were "peripheral" forms of paraplegia. Gull quoted Graves and suggested that the nerves should be examined; his cases 8,10,17, and 20 were almost certainly examples of polyneuritis in which he found that the spinal cords were microscopically normal. Wilks spoke of "alcohol paraplegia," "diphtheritic paralysis," "peripheral paralysis," "acute ascending paralysis," and "recoverable paraplegia" in cases in which the spinal cord was normal.

It is to a physician of a humbler status, working in Rouen, that we are indebted for the first proof that diffuse paralysis could result from disease of the peripheral nerves.

Duménil on "Motor and Sensory Peripheral Paralysis Affecting the Four Limbs"

This crucial communication by Duménil (12) was published in 1864 in the same journal that had carried Landry's paper. One is left wondering whether or not Landry realized that it contained the clue to his own case. Duménil's patient with polyneuritis did not, it is true, present with such an acute and symmetrically ascending paralysis, but the similarities were obvious enough. The illness began with peripheral paresthesia, followed by a flaccid, distal paralysis with muscular wasting and loss of faradic responses. The sensory loss was first observed largely in the distribution of the left ulnar and right median nerves and on the outer side of the legs. Death occurred after five months, and at autopsy no evidence of a lesion was found in the brain, spinal cord, or spinal nerve roots. But a microscopic examination of the nerves was undertaken, even though on inspection nothing abnormal had been found except some questionable "transparency" of terminal nerve elements in the toes. The microscope revealed that in preserved, but unstained, specimens of nerve from each limb, there was "a genuine atrophy of the medullary substance of the peripheral nerve tubes." This change was most obvious where muscle wasting and sensory loss had been most pronounced.

In a second paper two years later, Duménil (13) described three other cases with peripheral motor and sensory paralysis due to "Neuritis," and he summarized six published case reports, some of which, however, were clearly not examples of multiple neuritis. One of his patients died, and the microscope again revealed atrophy of the peripheral nerves. He realized that in his two autopsies he had not actually shown that the lesion began in the extremities of the nerves, but he thought it most likely. He considered that there were "acute" and "chronic" forms of "neuritis." He concluded:

> There is a class of spontaneous peripheral paralyses due to an atrophy of the nerves. In a certain number of cases, if not in all, the responsible morbid process is inflammatory. These paralyses can affect sensation and motion with equal intensity, either simultaneously or successively, and in the latter case motion appears to be affected by reflex action. They are often limited to one portion of the branches of one or several nerves, and do not necessarily correspond to the anatomical distribution of the trunks. They may be accompanied by alterations in the nutrition, not only of the muscles, but also of the skin and joints, as in paralyses from nerve injury. The responsible morbid process may follow an ascending course and extend to the spinal cord, leaving unquestionable, substantial traces. Pathological anatomy amply confirms Graves' opinion.

Graves, he considered, had originated the concept of peripheral neuritis, and he commented that Todd had been one of the first to point out the neuritic nature of lead paralysis. He did not mention Landry.

In the English-speaking world, recognition of the syndrome came after the introduction of the term "multiple neuritis" (14) and the publication in 1881 of a paper by Stewart (15), entitled *On paralysis of hands and feet from disease of the nerves*. In France, meanwhile, various forms of "neuritis" were being recognized—"febrile," "convalescent," "diphtheritic," and "alcoholic" (16)—and in Germany, Westphal was the first to observe loss of the knee jerk. The examination of the tendon reflexes starting from 1875 certainly assisted in diagnosis. Stewart observed that in his three cases sensory symptoms preceded the motor, the tendon reflexes progressively subsided, distal muscles were the first to waste, and the skin of the extremities became glossy and thin. In his autopsied case, the peripheral nerves were normal to the naked eye, but the microscope showed a striking "breaking up of the axis cylinders," especially "in the lower stretches of the nerves."

By 1893, when Ross and Bury (17) published their monograph on *Peripheral Neuritis*, they found that there were 90 published case reports of acute ascending paralysis, with 52 deaths and 42 autopsies. The spinal cord had been examined microscopically in 26 and reported as normal in 14. The nerves had been examined in only nine, with signs of neuritis in six. They concluded that Landry's paralysis was "an acute form of multiple neuritis." The state of the knee jerk had been reported in 16 cases and in all of them it was lost.

THE "MUSCLE SENSE"

It is now generally recognized that when Bell (18) printed his *Idea of a New Anatomy of the Brain* in 1811, he had not set out to establish the functions of the spinal nerve roots. He was concerned with refuting the "prevailing doctrine of the anatomical schools . . . that the whole brain is a common sensorium . . . that impressions . . . differing in kind, are carried along the nerves to the sensorium, and presented to the mind; and that the mind, by the same nerves which receive sensation, sends out the mandate of the will to the moving parts of the body."

Bell had three ideas about nervous function: "That the cerebrum and cerebellum are different in function as in form; that the parts of the cerebrum have different functions; and that the nerves which we trace in the body are not single nerves possessing various powers, but bundles of different nerves, whose filaments are united for the convenience of distribution, but which are distinct in office, as they are in origin from the brain." In all this he was proved right despite the incompleteness of his observations and deductions about the spinal nerve roots and the subsequent falsity of his later claims.

Bell conceived of three categories of nerves, motor, sensory, and vital, each distinctive in course and function. In the last sentence of the *Idea*, he said that the vital nerves were concerned with "the secret operations of the bodily frame, and the connections which unite the parts of the body into a system . . . through the cerebellum and nerves proceeding from it."

But it transpires that Bell was not thinking about coordination of movement but about the "instinctive motions" and the "secret operations of the vital organs." The cerebrum was the source of the motor and sensory fibers that traversed the anterior half of the medulla and spinal cord; cerebellar fibers were in the posterior columns and "especially govern the operation of the viscera necessary to the continuance of life." He was not then thinking in terms of the "Nervous Circle" between brain and muscle, although Walker (19) in 1809 had spoken of a "circle" in his own *New Anatomy and Physiology of the Brain*. Walker said that "the medullary matter may be traced" upward from the anterior columns of the cord, to the medulla, peduncles, corpora striata, and hemispheres, and thence, via the thalami, corpora quadrigemina, and superior cerebellar peduncles, into the cerebellum. From there fibers descended in the posterior columns of the cord. "Thus," Walker said, "the medullary fibres form a most remarkable circle, of which this is the direct course." It was then that he became the first to suggest that the anterior and posterior spinal nerve roots had different functions and he ascribed sensation to the former and motion to the latter.

It is evident, therefore, that neither Walker's "circle" nor Bell's "secret operations" amounted to glimpses of the feedback mechanism of locomotion. Walker's notion was really a development of the ancient Galenic teaching that sensory nerves were "soft" and motor nerves were "hard" and that the cerebrum, being softer than the cerebellum, was thus the sensory center of the brain, and the cerebellum was the motor. Bell's concept of vital nerves was little different from Willis's. Both believed that the cerebral hemispheres were concerned with voluntary, and the cerebellar, with involuntary innervation.

By this time, anatomists had finally agreed that the pyramidal tracts decussated in the medulla, but the course of the fibers in the posterior columns had not been established. After Magendie's publications in 1822, and 1823, Bell's statements concerning the function of the posterior columns underwent several changes. In 1826 (20) Bell was saying that "the anterior column is for motion, and the posterior for sensibility . . . we should say that the cerebrum had power over the motions of the body, and the cerebellum over its sensibility." The posterior columns were still linked to the cerebellum. Bell was, of course, an expert dissector (he once said he was "A Captain of Anatomists"), but by 1834 (21), his dissections of the posterior columns were taking him into the brain stem and hemispheres, where they could be "seen descending continuously in their whole length, from the back of the pons to the spinal nerves." He added, "it is easy to trace their filaments into the posterior roots of the spinal nerves." This widely accepted view, that the posterior columns were the continuation of the posterior spinal roots, which conveyed sensation to the brain, was questioned by the young Brown-Séquard and it led him to his experiments on the spinal cord.

Meanwhile, Bell's studies of the innervation of the face and orbit and the mechanism of the hand had provided him with ideas concerning the existence of "a muscle sense." He wrote in 1821 that "It is in the face that we have the best opportunity of observing the subservience of the nerves to the uses of the parts" in the acts of speaking, chewing, and breathing (22). Although he erred in defining the actual distribution of the branches of the fifth and seventh cranial nerves and in some of his interpretations, he did succeed in showing that the muscles of the face and orbit were innervated by both motor and sensory nerves.

In 1823, in his essay *On the Motions of the Eye* (23), Bell said, "It is to the muscular apparatus, and to the conclusions we are enabled to draw from the consciousness of muscular effort, that we owe that geometrical sense, by which we become acquainted with the form, and magnitude, and distance of objects . . . it is by the consciousness of the degree of effort put upon the voluntary muscles, that we know the relative position of an object to ourselves . . . if the sense of muscular activity be excluded," such judgments would be difficult to explain. "How minute and delicate," he said, "the sense of muscular motion is by which we balance the body, and by which we judge of the position of the limbs, whether during activity or rest."

By 1826, Bell felt able to entitle one of his papers before the Royal Society (24), *On the Nervous Circle which connects the voluntary muscles with the Brain*. It was here that he wrote, "I called this consciousness of muscular exertion a sixth sense." He cited examples such as the blind man, the tight-rope walker, and the power of weighing in the hand, to illustrate his theme. Later (25), he referred to the army captain, with locomotor ataxy, "who could feel the touch of a lady's petticoat on the calf of his legs," but who "could not tell the position of his feet without looking at them." In his treatise on the hand (3), a largely philosophical work, he again referred to this "sixth sense," "the muscle sense." We can stand upright with our feet together and eyes closed, we can differentiate a shilling from a sovereign with eyes closed, we can feel fatigue in muscles, and pain, and we can judge resistance and movement. "Muscle sense" thus came to be regarded rather loosely, meaning different qualities to different observers.

Landry "On the Paralysis of the Sensation of Muscular Activity"

In his paper of 1852 (7), Landry referred to the "sensation of muscular activity," which he concluded must "reside in the muscular tissue itself, that is to say, it is a perception by the brain of the state of the nervous terminations in the muscles." He quoted three cases, two of which could not walk unassisted; the third had a paralyzed left upper limb. If she actually watched her feet, the first patient could manage to walk a little, but in bed she could not direct a foot at an object and judge the latter's position when her eyes were closed, even after she had first visually estimated what movement would be necessary. In the second case, walking was impossible without vision, and in bed he was totally unaware of any passive movements of his feet made by Landry. Electrically induced movements caused pain but no sensation of movement. Neither could he estimate weights hung on his legs nor the force used by Landry in attempting to flex his extended leg against resistance. In the third case, in which superficial sensation in the affected hand was normal, the patient said a heavy "pewter goblet" felt as "light as a feather" in that hand.

There was, of course, great confusion about what was actually being tested in many of these cases at this time. Judging weights (introduced by Weber) and observing the effects of visual deprivation on the execution of voluntary movements were popular, but tests of coordination, of sense of position, and of appreciation of passive movement had yet to be developed. Landry was one of the first to study these aspects of the neurological examination. He returned to the subject in 1855 (8) and concluded that when there was "paralysis of the sensation of muscular activity," superficial sensation could be normal, but there was impairment of the appreciation of "the dimensions of objects," of "form," "consistency," "weight," and "resistance," and of the "sense of position" and of "passive movement." On the motor side, in consequence, movements became "clumsy and uncoordinated" but could be assisted by vision; the limbs did not feel "heavy" as in "ordinary paralysis"; and the muscles retained their electrical irritability.

He asked whether this type of deep sensory loss arose centrally or peripherally. He did not think his own observations supported the concept of Müller and others of "the idea of the force used" in muscular contraction, but that it "depended on local trouble." Normally, Landry thought, the actual movement of the limb provided the brain with the appropriate sensory information. It was not a by-product, as it were, of the willed effort, coming from the brain.

Duchenne on "Paralysis of the Muscular and Articular Sensibility"

Duchenne (26) had read Bell's book on *The Hand* and lamented the fact that it had not been translated into French because it contained a chapter on the "muscular sense," which he considered to be "the pearl of the book." Duchenne believed muscles were endowed with sensibility because they were supplied by mixed nerves and because faradization could cause pain that persisted after muscle contraction. But he thought that Bell's "sixth sense" was "a myth." It was just common muscular sensibility. It was "articular sensibility," which provided awareness of the "attitude and movement of the limbs," which was so important in locomotion:

> I have shown that articular insensibility is sometimes partial, and may be limited to one or more of the little joints of the fingers whose movements are no longer perceived. I have on the other hand discovered that, in certain cases of locomotor ataxy, patients who have preserved to a fair extent the sensibility of the skin and muscles of a limb could no longer perceive in the dark the movements given to the joints of the limb, nor the various attitudes given to it.

Duchenne said that "Before I studied locomotor ataxy deeply I attributed the loss of coordination to loss of muscle and joint sensibility," but he came to the conclusion that coordination also required "harmony" of action between opposing groups of muscle and "instinctive association" between muscles. He was surprised that Galen had not appreciated this, but, in fact, he had in *De Moto Musculorum* (27), where he explained that in many movements there was contraction of some muscles with relaxation of others. Duchenne looked upon coordination as a "faculty" of the central nervous system, influenced by, but largely independent of, sensory impressions. In locomotor ataxy, movements became "dissociated"; eventually, there was an "anarchy of the movements," so that visual guidance failed to compensate. He reexamined one of Landry's patients and thought that there had been some faulty interpretation of signs. Duchenne concluded that "There seems to exist a kind of sense which resides in the muscle . . . which . . . in the absence of sight, enlightens the brain as it were, before the latter, stimulated by the will, provokes muscular contraction."

Bastian on the "Muscular Sense"

The nature of the "muscular sense" remained a subject of speculation and controversy among clinicians, physiologists, and philosophers for the rest of the century. Bastian's paper of 1869 (28), for example, occupied 12 closely printed pages of the *British Medical Journal*, whereas the debate organized by the Neurological Society in London in 1886 took up 137 pages of *Brain*, with Bastian's opening contribution of 89 pages (29). Clinical and pathological observations in locomotor ataxy and the effects on motion of sections of posterior spinal nerve roots in animals provided most of the background for the discussions. Bastian concluded in 1869 that

> Although there is no evidence to lead us to believe that we derive any conscious impressions through the intervention of this so-called "muscular sense," there is evidence to show that the brain is assisted in the execution of voluntary movements by guiding impressions of some kind, which, whilst they differ from the impressions producible by means of the ordinary cutaneous and deep sensibility, may differ still further from these, owing to the fact of their not being revealed in consciousness to all. . . . These *unconscious* impressions of the "muscular sense," travelling to the cerebellum or the cerebrum would be almost exactly comparable with other unconscious impressions which pass from one point of the spinal cord to another . . . as in all reflex acts depending on the spinal cord.[1]

Jones (30) has pointed out that this was the only mention of the cerebellum made by Bastian as the possible terminus for "unfelt impressions." He came to regard the sensorimotor cortical centers of the cerebrum as being their final destination. One agrees with Jones when he says that if Bastian had related his unconscious "muscle sense" to the cerebellum, he would have been expressing a modern view that information from special muscle receptors does, in fact, pass to the cerebellum. But although the difference between cerebellar and sensory ataxia was emerging, no one mentioned the cerebellum in the 1886 debate.

The debate turned out to be largely an argument between Bastian and Ferrier. Bastian saw that in loss of "muscular sense," there were three distinct but related defects. He described them as

> Defective knowledge of the extent of movements executed, either actively or passively, as well as of the position of the limbs, when the eyes are closed.
> Difficulty in discriminating differences in weight or degrees of resistance when muscles are

[1]Hall, Marshall (1850): *Synopsis of the Diastaltic Nervous System*, p. 27, J. Mallet, London. Hall had said, "We have no consciousness of the condition of individual muscles . . . the muscular sense is not in the muscle . . . but in the nerve of touch or of vision; and volition is not directed to any muscle, or set of muscles, but to the aim, object and purpose of their contraction."

called into play.
Difficulty in accurately performing given movements when the eyes are closed.

But Ferrier could not agree with Bastian that there might be "unfelt" muscle impressions, for "the sense of movement is an act of conscious discrimination, and I am unable to understand how unfelt impressions can affect the sum of this consciousness." Ferrier stressed that coordination of movement and the sensation of movement were totally different things. A patient could lose one and not the other. In locomotor ataxy, he said, the sense of movement could be retained notwithstanding profound disorder of coordination.

ATAXIA AND THE POSTERIOR COLUMNS OF THE SPINAL CORD

During Bell's lifetime (1774–1842), incoordination of voluntary movements was noted in various nervous illnesses; experimentalists such as Rolando and Flourens had observed it after cerebellar ablations, and pathologists had recorded lesions of the posterior columns of the spinal cord. But it was not until 1840 that disturbance of gait was actually associated with a lesion of those tracts. Stanley's paper (31) was entitled *A case of disease in the posterior columns of the spinal cord.* The disturbance of gait in his patient was quite marked, yet "there was no discoverable impairment of sensation in any part of either limb; on scratching, pricking, and pinching the skin, nowhere was any defect of feeling acknowledged by the patient." At autopsy the disease was restricted to the posterior columns, and "the roots of the spinal nerves were unaltered." Bell had long since abandoned his view that the posterior roots directly entered the posterior columns, and there had been no suggestion that his muscle sense was connected with them. But in 1847 Todd (32) had some crucial observations to make.

Todd and "The Office of the Columns of the Cord"

Todd did not think that "the posterior or sensitive roots were implanted solely in the posterior, and the anterior solely in the anterior columns." In lesions of the anterolateral columns, the paralysis affected motion and sensation. With regard to the function of the posterior columns, "there was great difficulty." He agreed with Bell's later view that the posterior columns were not just a continuation of the posterior nerve roots. He thought that if the posterior columns were sensory, they would expand at levels "which correspond to the origins of the largest sensitive nerves," and this was not the case. Lastly he had personally noted and had read in the literature that cases of degeneration confined to the posterior columns were not characterized by loss of superficial sensation in the lower limbs. He quoted the report by Stanley. But Todd thought that although sensation had not been "*destroyed*" in that case, it might be impaired "in some way or other." He went on to say that

> I have long been strongly impressed with the opinion that the office of the posterior columns of the spinal cord is very different from any yet assigned to them. They may be in part commissural between the several segments of the cord, serving to unite them and harmonising them in their different actions, and in part subservient to the function of the cerebellum in regulating and coordinating the movements necessary for perfect locomotion.
>
> If the cerebellum be the regulator of these locomotive actions, it seems reasonable to suppose that these columns, which are so largely connected with it, each forming a large proportion of the fibrous matter of each crus cerebelli, should enjoy a similar function, and that, as they are the principal medium through which the cerebellum is brought into connection with the cord, it must be through their constituent fibres that the cerebellum exerts its influence

> on the centre of innervation to the lower extremities and other parts concerned in the locomotive function . . .
>
> Now, an analysis of the locomotive actions shows, with great probability, that they are partly of a voluntary character, and partly dependent on the influence of physical impressions upon that segment of the cord from which the nerves of the lower extremities are derived. There are two objects to be attained in progression, namely, to support the centre of gravity of the body, and to propel it onward. . . . The support of the centre of gravity of the body requires that the muscles of the lower extremities, the pillars of support to the trunk, should be well contracted in a degree proportioned to the weight they have to sustain. . . . The stimulus is afforded by the application of the soles of the feet to the ground; it is therefore proportionate to the weight which presses them downwards. It is well known that reflex actions are more developed in the lower than in the upper extremities, and the surface of the sole of the foot is well adapted for the reception of sensitive impressions. . . . All the structural arrangements necessary for this purpose are found in the antero-lateral columns. The posterior columns come into exercise in balancing the trunk and in harmonising its movements with those of the lower extremities.

As a clinician, Todd had noted that

> In many cases, in which the principal symptom has been a gradually increasing difficulty in walking, the posterior columns have been the seat of disease. Two kinds of paralysis of motion may be noticed in the lower extremities, the one consisting simply in the impairment or loss of the voluntary motion, the other distinguished by a diminution or total loss of the power of coordinating movements. In the latter form, while considerable voluntary power remains, the patient finds great difficulty in walking, and his gait is so tottering and uncertain that his centre of gravity is easily displaced.
>
> In two examples of this variety of paralysis I ventured to predict disease of the posterior columns . . . and this was found to exist on a post-mortem inspection.

In all this we can readily see how important a role Todd played in the separation of the paraplegias and in the concept of ataxia of locomotion.

Romberg on "Anaesthesia of the Muscular Sense"

Romberg had translated Bell's *Nervous System of the Human Body* in 1832. He thought Bell was the "Harvey of our century." In his *Manual* (33), Romberg described his well-known sign in a chapter entitled "Anaesthesia of the Muscular Sense":

> I have observed that anaesthesia of the muscles alone without loss of tactile power, invariably accompanies tabes dorsalis. A simple experiment suffices to determine the fact. If the patient is told to shut his eyes while in the erect posture, he immediately begins to move from side to side, and the oscillations soon attain such a pitch that unless supported he falls to the ground. Even if the trunk is supported, if the patient be sitting and leaning against the back of the chair, the phenomenon takes place to the same extent, and he will slip off the chair. From the commencement of the tabes dorsalis, as soon as the muscular power becomes diminished, this anaesthesia manifests itself; it becomes evident as the disease progresses; and it is only towards its termination, when the muscular debility approaches to paralysis, that it can no longer be clearly distinguished. The eyes of such patients are their regulators, or feelers; consequently, in the dark, and when amaurosis supervenes as is not infrequently the case, their helplessness is extreme. Except during the last stage the skin remains sensitive; the complaints of the patient that they feel when they walk or stand as if a soft body, such as a layer of wool, intervened between the ground and the soles of their feet, must consequently be referred to the diminished muscular sense.

Romberg's description of the clinical features of tabes dorsalis comes later in the book, in a chapter dealing with "spinal paralysis" and "neuroses of motility." Of the incoordination, he then said (34):

> Early in the disease we find the sense of touch and the muscular sense diminished, while the sensibility of the skin is unaltered in reference to the temperature and painful impressions. . . . The feet feel numbed in standing, walking or lying down. . . . The rider no longer feels the resistance of the stirrup, and has the strap put up a hole or two. The gait begins to be insecure, and the patient attempts to improve it by making a greater effort of the will; as he does not feel the tread to be firm he puts down his heel with greater force. From the commencement of the disease the individual keeps his eyes on his feet . . . the insecurity of the gait also exhibits itself more in the dark . . .

As Duchenne was to point out, Romberg did not sufficiently distinguish between weakness and incoordination despite his observations on the numbness of the feet and the help afforded by visual guidance. Duchenne said that he always made his own observations first, before consulting others, to avert, he said, "looking at my facts with another man's spectacles." But Romberg did note what Duchenne first missed—the "partial atrophy of the spinal cord" with the naked eye. It was most evident in the lower dorsal and lumbar regions, and there were cases where the atrophy was practically confined to the posterior nerve roots and the posterior columns of the cord. In Duchenne's first cases, this was missed; Duchenne commented that the ataxia was then (1858) attributed to cerebellar disease. But it was not long before Romberg's pathological observations were confirmed, and established by the Charcot School.

Reynolds on "Anaesthesia Muscularis"

In 1855 Reynolds (35), in his book on diseases of the nervous system, described a disease he termed "Anaesthesia Muscularis." The description comprised only two pages. He viewed the disease as "a distinct morbid condition," which was "liable to be confounded with paraplegia." The patient suffered "not absolute loss of power, but a diminution in the faculty of controlling movements." Cutaneous sensation was unimpaired, "reflective functions are not interfered with," but motility was in "a peculiar condition." The disability, clumsiness, was most marked in the lower limbs, which caused a drunken gait. This clumsiness was aggravated by eye closure. Reynolds therefore concluded that there was no primary defect of coordination, but that "sensational guidance" being corrective, there must be an impairment of "the muscular sense, or the intuitional perception of the muscular states." This could not be attributed to "any particular organic change of a special organ," but as affected patients subsequently become paraplegic, he thought that "the centripetal tract of fibres is affected." He recognized that the cerebellum was "the organ by which motorial impulses from volition are combined, and rendered effectual . . . ," and that it appeared possible that it was not receiving "one class of sensorial impressions." He did not actually say that this disease was one of the spinal cord, and it is not placed in that section of his book. But Reynolds does seem to have implied this, and also to have felt that the disease was a lesion affecting a sensory pathway to the cerebellum. Surprisingly, he made no reference to the similar accounts of Todd and Romberg on ataxia, although he did refer to them on other topics. He was only 27 when his book was published.

Gull on "Cases of Paraplegia"

Gull (36,37) in 1856 and 1858 analyzed 32 cases of paraplegia in some detail, describing the autopsy findings in the 29 fatal ones. There were cases of compression, inflammation, softening, induration, tuberculosis, etc. He thought a cord lesion could be "partial" in two senses. You could have a lesion confined to a segment of the cord or to one of its columns. "There was evidently a tendency in lesions to spread longitudinally in the cord rather than transversely through it."

Particularly striking was the way a degenerative lesion could be seemingly limited to the posterior columns. He noted Brown-Séquard's suggestion that sensory loss depended on whether or not there was a considerable diseased "length" of these columns. He was struck by one of his cases (Case 19), in which incoordination, and not paralysis, of the lower limbs was the presenting feature, and how the disease was confined to the posterior columns. He said that his experience confirmed the concept of Todd in relation to the function of the posterior columns, but he did not discuss the question of "muscle sense" and its significance in relation to the posterior columns. The slight nature of the superficial sensory loss puzzled him.

The cause of incoordination in locomotor ataxia continued to be debated for many years. In 1868 Allbutt (38), in a meeting at Oxford attended by Duchenne, asserted that it was the result of "loss of tactile sensibility", a conclusion vigorously contested by Duchenne.

By the end of the century, with the discovery of the muscle spindles and the demonstration of their sensory nature, the old "muscle sense" became unnecessary. It was displaced by Sherrington's concept of "proprio-ceptors," deep receptors which supplied information "of our own motion."

REFERENCES

1. Graves, R. J. (1848): *Clinical Lectures on the Practice of Medicine*, 2nd ed., reprinted by New Sydenham Soc., p. 574. London, 1884.
2. Bell, C. (1826): *Phil. Trans.*, 116:163.
3. Bell, C. (1833): *The Hand, its Mechanism and Vital Endowments, as Evincing Design*, p. 197. Pickering, London.
4. Chomel, A. F. (1828): *J. Hebd. de Méd.*, 1:333.
5. Lettsom, J. C. (1787): *Mem. Med. Soc. London*, 1:128.
6. Jackson, J. (1822): *New Eng. J. Med. Surg.*, 11:351.
7. Landry, J. B. O. (1852):Physical and pathological researches into tactile sensations. *Arch. Gen. Méd.*, 29:257; 30:28.
8. Landry, J. B. O. (1855): On the paralysis of feeling of muscular activity. *Gaz. Hôpitaux*, 28:262,269,282,318,334.
9. Landry, J. B. O. (1859): Acute ascending paralysis. *Gaz. Hebd. Méd. Chir.*, 6:472, 486.
10. Gull, Sir W. W. (1858): In: *A Collection of the Writings of W. W. Gull, MD, FRS*, edited and arranged by T. D. Acland, 2 vols., 1894 and 1896, Vol. 1, p. 109.
11. Wilks, Sir S. (1878): *Lectures in Diseases of the Nervous System Delivered at Guy's Hospital*, Churchill, London.
12. Duménil, L. (1864): Motor and sensory peripheral paralysis affecting the four limbs. *Gaz. Hebd. Méd. Chir.*, 1:203.
13. Duménil, L. (1866): *Gaz. Hebd. Méd. Chir.*, 3:51, 67, 84.
14. Leyden, E. von (1880): quoted by H. R. Viets (1934), *Arch. Neurol. Psych.*, 32:337.
15. Stewart, T. G. (1881): On paralysis of hands and feet from disease of the nerves. *Edin. Med. J.*, 26:865.
16. Viets, H. R. (1934): *Arch. Neurol. Psych.*, 32:337.
17. Ross, J., and Bury, J. S. (1893): *On Peripheral Neuritis; A Treatise*. Griffin, London.
18. Bell, C. (1811): *Idea of a New Anatomy of the Brain*. In: Documents and Dates of Modern Discoveries in the Nervous System, by Alexander Walker (1839); facsimile of the original edition of 1839, with an introduction by Paul F. Cranefield (1973), p. 37. Scarecrow Reprint Corp., Metuchen, N.J.
19. Walker, A. (1809): New anatomy and physiology of the brain. *Arch. Univ. Sci.*, 3:172; reprinted in 1817, p. 30.
20. Bell, C. (1826): *Anatomy and Physiology of the Human Body*, 6th ed., p. 29. Longmans, London.
21. Bell, C. (1834): *London Medical Gaz.*, 15:626.
22. Bell, C. (1821): *Phil. Trans. Roy. Soc. London*, 111:398.
23. Bell, C. (1823): On the motions of the eye. *Phil. Trans. Roy. Soc. London*, 113:166.
24. Bell, C. (1824): On the nervous circle which connects the voluntary muscles with the brain. *Phil. Trans. Roy. Soc. London*, 116:163.

25. Bell, C. (1836): *The Nervous System of the Human Body*, 3rd ed., p. 338. Longmans, London.
26. Duchenne, G. B. A. (1883): Selections from the clinical works of Duchenne (De Boulogne), translated and edited by G. V. Poore, chap. XXIII, p. 378. New Sydenham Soc., London.
27. Fulton, J. F. (1930): *Selected Readings in the History of Physiology*, 1st ed., p. 184. Charles C. Thomas, Springfield, Ill.
28. Bastian, H. C. (1869): On the muscular sense. *Br. Med. J.*, 1:394.
29. Bastian, H. C. (1887): *Brain*, 10:1.
30. Jones, E. G. (1972): *J. Hist. Med.*, 27:298.
31. Stanley, E. (1839–1940): A case of disease in the posterior columns of the spinal cord. *Med. Chir. Trans.*, 23:80.
32. Todd, R. B. (1847): *The Cyclopaedia of Anatomy and Physiology*, Vol. 3, p. 721.
33. Romberg, M. H. (1853): *A Manual of the Nervous Diseases of Man*, translated and edited by E. H. Sieveking, M. D., 2 vols., New Sydenham Soc., London, Vol. 1, p. 226.
34. Romberg, E. H. (1853): *A Manual of the Nervous Diseases of Man*, translated and edited by E. H. Sieveking, M. D., Vol. 1, p. 226; Vol. 2, p. 395, New Sydenham Soc., London.
35. Reynolds, J. R. (1855): *The Diagnosis of Diseases of the Brain, Spinal Cord, Nerves and their Appendages*, p. 165. Churchill, London.
36. Gull, W. (1856): *Guy's Hosp. Rep.*, 2:143.
37. Gull, W. (1858): *Guy's Hosp. Rep.*, 4:169.
38. Allbutt, T. C. (1869): *Br. Med. J.*, 1:157.

Historical Aspects of the Neurosciences,
edited by F. Clifford Rose and W. F. Bynum.
Raven Press, New York ©

Development of the Concept of Supraspinal Control

T. J. Steiner

Department of Neurology, Charing Cross Hospital, Fulham Palace Road, London W6, England

> For the sole cause of all the movements of the members is that certain muscles contract, and that those opposite to them elongate; and the sole cause of one muscle contracting rather than that set against it, is that there comes from the brain some additional amount of animal spirits, however little it may be, to it rather than to the other. Not that the spirits which proceed immediately from the brain suffice in themselves to move the muscles, but they determine the other spirits which are already in these two muscles, all to issue very quickly from the one of them and to pass into the other.

In these terms, expressed in 1649 and recognizably based on the 2nd century postulates of Galen (48), the concept of supraspinal control was understood by René Descartes (15). Although considerably predating classical neurology, it nonetheless propounded from the outset that movement in a muscle, supraspinally initiated, was achieved by potentiation of its subsistent activity at the expense of the antagonist.

However, it was the prerogative of the philosophers to philosophize: to proffer theories that were the product of reasoning and not of factual basis. With the neurologist, who evolved much later, lay the onus of experimental proof, the acquisition of knowledge rather than merely of an understanding. The story is suspended then for nearly 200 years.

Awareness of areas within the brain having anatomical definition and specific physiological roles dates from the early 19th century. Localization and description of these areas occupied physiologists from that time. Their efforts at first, inevitably imprecise, depended on experimental progressive ablation (by slicing) of the brain in the otherwise intact animal and observation of residual or newly acquired behavior. Lesions of the nervous system presenting in the clinic were a source of additional, fortuitous aid, from which observers soon learned to benefit. By the year 1875, Hughlings Jackson was able to state clearly the concept of integration at various levels of the central nervous system, up to the cerebral cortex (29).

Neurologists, however, were rapidly giving way to neurophysiologists, with Sir David Ferrier the acknowledged link. In 1870 Fritsch and Hitzig (20) had demonstrated that electrical irritation of the anterior parts of the brain gave rise to movements on the opposite side of the body. With the door thereby opened for electrophysiological investigation of the brain, Ferrier (19) soon published many of his researches. Probably the first mapping experiments to be carried out, with stimulation mainly on the surface, they covered most of the brain, including the cerebrum, basal ganglia, corpora quadrigemina, and cerebellum. He watched for induced movement and readily obtained it: in cats, dogs, and rabbits partially narcotized with ether, his reported results included backward somersaults head over heels off the table, evoked merely by touching the corpora quadrigemina with the electrodes.

Stimulation in the living animal at first required dissection, so that electrodes might be positioned under direct vision. Despite all their disadvantages, these methods enabled the idea of discrete "centres" in the brain to be formulated. In 1908 experimental techniques were revolutionized by the stereotaxic method developed by Horsley and Clarke (28), at once making possible not only localized stimulation, but also localized ablation, so that anatomical boundaries of brain centers might be precisely determined. As the ability to record neural signals later developed in company with advances in instrumentation, the same methods facilitated placement in the brain of recording electrodes.

Although researchers at the time showed little apparent haste in applying these methods, subsequently, such zeal was demonstrated that the literature bulges with their endeavors. In consequence, the search to understand the manner and mechanism of supraspinal control over the skeletal muscular system is a wandering tale of great length and complexity, fragmentary, contradictory, and inconclusive. In this short account of descending control of transmission in reflex pathways, occasional themes are adopted from the literature to the commencement of the last decade.

THE FOREBRAIN

Voluntary control of movement is within everybody's experience, but Tower (57) noted in 1940 that corticospinal influence was not limited to voluntary acts: it included all motor activity at any level. The extensive involvement of the cerebral cortex in reflex control was well developed in Lundberg's review (37). "There is now strong evidence that the reflex is the unit reaction upon which the corticospinal tract operates in the cat," he concluded, so confirming the prediction of Sherrington (49) early in this century.

Subcortical control of reflexes was also demonstrated at that time by comparison of reflex actions in decerebrate and spinal animals (26). In Sherrington's laboratory, for example (50), the flexor reflex was more easily obtained in spinal than in decerebrate cats, in which decerebrate rigidity was present.

In 1948 Hess (24) elicited a variety of actions, frequently purposive, by stimulating the diencephalon in the cat. Austin (3) found no evidence of a homogeneous undifferentiated system for facilitation or inhibition in the diencephalon or in the upper mesencephalon. On the contrary, he reported a number of specific nuclei and fiber tracts, with definite effects on the motor system and spinal reflexes. These might be facilitatory or inhibitory, depending on the specific structure activated, its degree of activation, and the "balance of other systems converging upon the common segmental neuronal pool." Hinsey (25) later believed that evidence supported "levels of integration for somatic as well as autonomic activity" in the hypothalamus and subthalamus.

THE MIDBRAIN

Historically always of interest, the red nucleus enjoyed rapidly developing attention in the 1930s. At the same time, interest centered on integration, supraspinally, of reflex activity into movement patterns. The red nucleus had been considered the focal point of the so-called tegmental response, chiefly a curving of the back and neck to make a concavity on the stimulated side, and flexion of the ipsilateral forelimb. However, Ingram's experiments with others in 1932 (30,31), obtaining this response pattern from most of the tegmentum, but not the red nucleus itself, largely relieved it of such a role. Mussen (43) believed this nucleus was concerned with flexion of the head and body and rotation toward the ipsilateral side and therefore could govern complex but integrated movements involving all parts of the body. Bilateral destruction of the red nucleus in Ingram's laboratory (32) disturbed gait and increased extensor tone. These authors, however, admitted possible involvement of the "premier cerebellar-efferent pathway" in their experiments, and perhaps this equally applied to Mussen's stimulations (43).

Later, a somatotopic organization within the nucleus was demonstrated in kittens by Pompeiano and Brodal (44), and it became generally agreed that the rubrospinal pathway led mostly to facilitation of flexor and inhibition of extensor motor nuclei (18,27,39,47,56). This finding was not without exception. For instance, dominating excitation was reported in the motor nuclei of toe extensors (27). Following repetitive stimulation of the red nucleus in cats, Burke et al. (6) discovered predominantly inhibitory postsynaptic potentials in slow twitch units and mixed or predominantly excitatory postsynaptic potentials in fast twitch units.

Bradley et al. (4) found that cervical motoneurons could be affected from the magnocellular part of the red nucleus in cats by using very weak stimuli. To influence lumbar motoneurons, much stronger stimuli were required, so involving, the authors thought, structures adjacent to the nucleus. They suggested that this correlated with the relatively greater number of rubrospinal fibers terminating at cervical levels (44) and the possible involvement of the nucleus in righting reflexes for neck and forelimb.

THE RETICULAR FORMATION

Much of the experimental work of the 1950s and 1960s concerned the reticular areas of the mid- and hindbrains. Sprague and Chambers (55), for instance, in 1954 studied the medullary reticular formation in anesthetized, unanesthetized, and decerebrate cats, and its effects on postural tonus. Clear-cut reciprocal effects were demonstrated: of ipsilateral flexion and extensor inhibition, contralateral extension and flexor inhibition from the medial reticular formation; of a similar but opposite pattern from the lateral reticular formation. Reciprocal effects on reflexes were shown by Gernandt and Thulin (21), with medial and lateral areas again giving opposite responses. In their experiments, stimulation of the medial reticular formation inhibited the ventral root reflex response evoked by gastrocnemius nerve stimulation and facilitated the reflex from the peroneal nerve. The reverse could be obtained from the lateral reticular formation. Brooks et al. (5) investigated bulbar and suprabulbar reticular formations. Although effects were sometimes reciprocal, they found more usually a generalized inhibition that, incidentally, persisted for a period of 2 to 3 minutes in a high percentage of cases. Shimamura and Fujimori (51) also found generalized effects more usual. In decerebrate cats, monosynaptic and polysynaptic flexor and extensor reflexes were inhibited from most points in the medial medulla oblongata, inhibited or facilitated from the lateral medulla, facilitated from the pons (especially the ventromedial pons), and facilitated or inhibited (though not very markedly) from the midbrain. Differences between ipsilateral and contralateral sides were mainly insignificant.

Lindblom and Ottosson (35) found inhibition or facilitation of flexor reflex activity. The pattern of responses changed "practically from point to point." The type of response could not be predicted from the location of the point stimulated. Shimamura and Fujimori (51) noted that the threshold of facilitatory effects was generally lower than that of inhibitory effects; in some instances, facilitation by weak stimuli changed into inhibition when stronger stimulation was applied.

Mandell and Bach (38) inhibited the patellar reflex in cats under sodium pentobarbital (Nembutal) or ether anesthesia by stimulating the medullary reticular formation, but they were never able to do so in unanesthetized animals. They concluded that removal of supraspinal influences (by surgery or anesthesia) was necessary to demonstrate bulbar reticular inhibition of this reflex. Downman and Hussain (16), by brain-stem sectioning, showed tonic inhibition of thoracic reflex arcs in the decerebrate cat, descending from the medullary reticular formation. The inhibition was absent in anesthetized cats with intact central nervous systems (2).

Prout remarked in 1963 (45): "The occurrence of opposite effects on somatic reflexes consequent upon activation of reticular formation is evidence that this structure does not exert mass effects." He added that caution should be applied in labeling any part of the reticular formation "facilitatory" or "inhibitory."

Long sustained responses from the reticular formation, for several minutes into the poststimulation period, were described by Brooks, Koizumi and others (5,33). Effects of such length were not unknown from other brain areas: the diencephalon, which readily produced prolonged autonomic responses, also, for instance, inhibited the jaw-opening reflex for 2 to 3 minutes (1).

Lettvin had suggested that inhibition of somatic reflexes by stimulation of the bulbar reticular formation was mediated through the interneuron pool (34). Subsequent studies, such as those of Eccles and Lundberg (17) and Alderson and Downman (2), tended to confirm this, but it was certain that depolarization of primary afferents was also a mechanism available to the brain stem (8,13,14), as it was to the cerebral cortex (9,36) and cerebellum (7,8). Furthermore, the possibility became apparent of primary afferent hyperpolarization (12,40,41). It was also understood that reflex arcs, though having both receptor and effector at spinal levels, might nonetheless pursue a route ascending to and returning from supraspinal levels. The spino-bulbo-spinal reflex system, for instance, relaying in the bulbar reticular formation, was thought to be a pathway through which the integrative influences of that area might affect all ascending and descending interlimb reflexes (52).

THE CEREBELLUM

Snider et al. stimulated the cerebellum in 1949 (53,54). Reflexly or cortically induced movements were suppressed by electrical stimulation of the anterior lobe, paramedian lobules, and the nearby folia, but facilitation could be elicited from a nearly coextensive area. Snider and Magoun (54) suggested that differing responses might have been the result of different stimulus frequencies. Moruzzi (42) inhibited decerebrate rigidity and myotatic reflexes by stimulating the anterior lobe at 50 to 300/sec and facilitated them using frequencies of 2 to 30/sec; intermediate responses occurred when frequencies of 30 to 50/sec were used. Such effects were not without analogue in other parts of the brain [e.g., hypothalamus (23)].

Chambers and Sprague (10,11) proposed that the mammalian cerebellum was organized functionally into three longitudinal, corticonuclear zones: a medial (vermal cortex and fastigial nucleus), an intermediate (paravermal cortex and interpositus nucleus), and a lateral (most of the hemispheral cortex and dentate nucleus). Later experiments achieved a fairly precise localization of function in the cerebellum of the rat. Goodman and Simpson (22) elicited ipsilateral flexion and adduction and contralateral extension and abduction from the vermis on either side of the midline; a limb posture the mirror image of this from the paravermal area; and movements from the hemispheral cortex lateral to this area which were similar, in general, to those from the vermis. These results seemed to support the proposals of Chambers and Sprague (10,11).

CONCLUSION

"Classical neurology," wrote Oliver Sacks a few years ago (46), "is atomistic, mechanistic and hierarchic. It divides brain function and behaviour into an enormous number of isolated functions or faculties; it lodges each of these in a special unit of some type—a 'centre' or 'system'; it sees these centres or systems as being integrated by a network of connections (as in a computer or telephone exchange), and as being disposed at various levels, so that 'higher' centres can command or constrain 'lower' centres."

The bid to define the concept of supraspinal control occupied laboratories throughout the world. This depiction in place of a central nervous system of an accumulation of nervous centers of diverse, separate functions may have been the major hindrance. In those laboratories today, the need is still largely outstanding to reconstitute the entire system from its component parts. As Wall and Dubner (58) said, success will depend on selection of the correct elemental categories.

REFERENCES

1. Achari, N. K., and Thexton, A. J. (1972): Diencephalic influences on the jaw opening reflex in the cat. *Arch. Oral Biol.*, 17:1073–1080.
2. Alderson, A. M., and Downman, C. B. B. (1966): Supraspinal inhibition of thoracic reflexes of somatic and visceral origin. *Arch. Ital. Biol.*, 104:309–327.
3. Austin, G. M. (1952): Suprabulbar mechanisms of facilitation and inhibition of cord reflexes. *Res. Publ. Assoc. Res. Nerv. Ment. Dis.*, 30:196–222.
4. Bradley, D. J., Fox, M., and Williams, T. D. (1971): A comparison of the effects of stimulation of the red nucleus on the monosynaptic reflex in the forelimb and hindlimb of the cat. *Brain Res.*, 29:151–154.
5. Brooks, C. M., Koizumi, K., and Siebens, A. A. (1956): Inhibitory action of bulbar and suprabulbar reticular formation on the spinal reflex pathway. *Am. J. Physiol.*, 184:497–504.
6. Burke, R. E., Jankowska, E., and Bruggencate, G. ten (1970): A comparison of peripheral and rubrospinal synaptic input to slow and fast twitch motor units of triceps surae. *J. Physiol. (London)*, 207:709–732.
7. Cangiano, A., Cook, W. A., Jr., and Pompeiano, O. (1969): Primary afferent depolarization in the lumbar cord evoked from the fastigial nucleus. *Arch. Ital. Biol.*, 107:321–340.
8. Carpenter, D., Engberg, I., and Lundberg, A. (1966): Primary afferent depolarization evoked from the brain stem and the cerebellum. *Arch. Ital. Biol.*, 104:73–85.
9. Carpenter, D., Lundberg, A., and Norrsell, U. (1963): Primary afferent depolarization evoked from the sensorimotor cortex. *Acta Physiol. Scand.*, 59:126–142.
10. Chambers, W. W., and Sprague, J. M. (1955): Functional localization in the cerebellum. I. Organization in longitudinal cortico-nuclear zones and their contribution to the control of posture, both extrapyramidal and pyramidal. *J. Comp. Neurol.*, 103:105–129.
11. Chambers, W. W., and Sprague, J. M. (1955): Functional localization in the cerebellum. II. Somatotopic organization in cortex and nuclei. *Arch. Neurol. Psychiat.* (*Chicago*), 74:653–680.
12. Chan, S. H. H., and Barnes, C. D. (1971): Presynaptic facilitation: positive dorsal root potentials evoked from brain stem reticular formation in lumbar cord. *Brain Res.*, 28:176–179.
13. Cook, W. A., Jr., Cangiano, A., and Pompeiano, O. (1969): Dorsal root potentials in the lumbar cord evoked from the vestibular system. *Arch. Ital. Biol.*, 107:275–295.
14. Cook, W. A., Jr., Cangiano, A., and Pompeiano, O. (1969): Vestibular control of transmission in primary afferents to the lumbar spinal cord. *Arch. Ital. Biol.*, 107:296–320.
15. Descartes, R. (1649): *Passions de l'Ame.* Henry le Gras, Paris. English translation in: Haldane, E. S., and Ross, G. R. T. (1969): *The Philosophical Works of Descartes*, Vol. 1. Cambridge University Press, London.
16. Downman, C. B. B., and Hussain, A. (1958): Spinal tracts and supraspinal centres influencing visceromotor and allied reflexes in cats. *J. Physiol.* (*London*), 141:489–499.

17. Eccles, R. M., and Lundberg, A. (1959): Supraspinal control of interneurones mediating spinal reflexes. *J. Physiol., (London)*, 147:565–584.
18. Erbel, F., Brehm, K. H., and Bruggencate, G. ten (1970): Recording of spinal reflexes evoked by dorsal root stimulation in unanesthetized free moving cats. *Pflügers Arch. Ges. Physiol.*, 316:208–212.
19. Ferrier, D. (1873): Experimental researches in cerebral physiology and pathology. *W. Riding Lunat. Asyl. Med. Rep.*, 3:30–96.
20. Fritsch, G., and Hitzig, E. (1870): Ueber die elektrische Erregbarkeit des Grosshirns. *Arch. Anat. Physiol.*, 300–332.
21. Gernandt, B. E., and Thulin, C. -A. (1955): Reciprocal effects upon spinal motoneurons from stimulation of bulbar reticular formation. *J. Neurophysiol.*, 18:113–129.
22. Goodman, D. C., and Simpson, J. T., Jr. (1961): Functional localization in the cerebellum of the albino rat. *Exp. Neurol.*, 3:174–188.
23. Hare, K., and Geohegan, W. A. (1941): Influence of frequency of stimulus upon response to hypothalamic stimulation. *J. Neurophysiol.*, 4:266–273.
24. Hess, W. R. (1948): Zwischenhirn und Motorik. *Helvet. Physiol. Pharmacol. Acta*, 6(Suppl. 5).
25. Hinsey, J. C. (1966): The hypothalamus and somatic responses. In: *The Hypothalamus and Central Levels of Autonomic Function*, Chap. 25, *Proc. Assoc. Res. Nerv. Ment. Dis.*, 20:657–685. Facsimile of 1940 edition. Hafner Publishing Co., New York.
26. Holmqvist, B. (1961): Crossed spinal reflex actions evoked by volleys in somatic afferents. *Acta Physiol. Scand.*, 52(Suppl. 181): 1–67.
27. Hongo, T., Jankowska, E., and Lundberg, A. (1969): The rubrospinal tract. I. Effects on alpha-motoneurones innervating hindlimb muscles in cats. *Exp. Brain Res.*, 7:344–364.
28. Horsley, V., and Clarke, R. H. (1908): The structure and functions of the cerebellum examined by a new method. *Brain*, 31:45–124.
29. Hughlings Jackson, J. (1875): On the anatomical and physiological localisation of movements in the brain. Reprinted in: *Selected Writings of John Hughlings Jackson*, edited by S. Taylor, Vol. 1, pp. 37–76 (1931). Hodder and Stoughton, London.
30. Ingram, W. R., Ranson, S. W., and Hannett, F. I. (1932): The direct stimulation of the red nucleus in cats. *J. Neurol. Psychopathol.*, 12:219–230.
31. Ingram, W. R., Ranson, S. W., Hannett, F. I., Zeiss, F. R., and Terwilliger, E. H. (1932): Results of stimulation of the tegmentum with the Horsley-Clarke stereotaxic apparatus. *Arch. Neurol. Psychiat., (Chicago)*, 28:513–541.
32. Ingram, W. R., Ranson, S. W., and Barris, R. W. (1934): The red nucleus. Its relation to postural tonus and righting reactions. *Arch. Neurol. Psychiat., (Chicago)*, 31:768–786.
33. Kleyntjens, F., Koizumi, K., and Brooks, C. McC. (1955): Stimulation of suprabulbar reticular formation. Effect on elements of spinal reflex pathways. *Arch. Neurol. Psychiat., (Chicago)*, 73:425–438.
34. Lettvin, J. Y. (1948): The path of suppression in the spinal gray matter. *Fed. Proc. Fed. Am. Socs. Exp. Biol.*, 7:71.
35. Lindblom, U. F., and Ottosson, J. O. (1956): Bulbar influence on spinal cord dorsum potentials and ventral root reflexes. *Acta Physiol. Scand.*, 35:203–214.
36. Lindblom, U. F., and Ottosson, J. O. (1957): Influence of pyramidal stimulation upon the relay of coarse cutaneous afferents in the dorsal horn. *Acta Physiol. Scand.*, 38:309–318.
37. Lundberg, A. (1964): Supraspinal control of transmission in reflex paths to motoneurones and primary afferents. *Prog. Brain Res.*, 12:197–221.
38. Mandell, A. J., and Bach, L. M. N. (1957): Failure of the bulbar inhibitory reticular formation to affect somatic reflex activity in the unanesthetized cat. *Am. J. Physiol.*, 190:330–332.
39. Massion, J. (1967): The mammalian red nucleus. *Physiol. Rev.*, 47:383–436.
40. Mendell, L. (1970): Positive dorsal root potentials produced by stimulation of small diameter muscle afferents. *Brain Res.*, 18:375–379.
41. Mendell, L. M., and Wall, P. D. (1964): Presynaptic hyperpolarization: a role for fine afferent fibres. *J. Physiol., (London)*, 172:274–294.
42. Moruzzi, G. (1950): Effects at different frequencies of cerebellar stimulation upon postural tonus and myotatic reflexes. *Electroenceph. Clin. Neurophysiol.*, 2:463–469.
43. Mussen, A. T. (1934): Cerebellum and red nucleus. A preliminary report on a new method of physiologic investigation. *Arch. Neurol. Psychiat., (Chicago)*, 31:110–126.
44. Pompeiano, O., and Brodal, A. (1957): Experimental demonstration of a somatotopical origin of rubrospinal fibers in the cat. *J. Comp. Neurol.*, 108:225–251.
45. Prout, B. J. (1963): Supraspinal control of direct and reflex actions of the autonomic nervous system. Ph.D. thesis, University of London.
46. Sacks, O. (1972): The great awakening. *Listener*, 88:521–524.
47. Sasaki, K., Namikawa, A., and Hashiramoto, S. (1960): The effect of midbrain stimulation upon alpha motoneurons in lumbar spinal cord of the cat. *Japn. J. Physiol.*, 10:303–316.
48. Sheer, D. E. (1961): Brain and behaviour: the background of interdisciplinary research. In: *Electrical Stimulation of the Brain*, edited by D. E. Sheer, Chap. 1, pp. 3–21. University of Texas Press, Austin, Tex.

49. Sherrington, C. S. (1906): *The Integrative Action of the Nervous System*. Yale University Press, New Haven.
50. Sherrington, C. S., and Sowton, S. C. M. (1915): Observations on reflex responses to single break-shocks. *J. Physiol., (London)*, 49:331–348.
51. Shimamura, M., and Fujimori, B. (1961): Studies on effects of brain stem stimulation upon motor and autonomic reflexes, with special references to interrelationships between effects. *Japn. J. Physiol.*, 11:238–251.
52. Shimamura, M., and Livingston, R. B. (1963): Longitudinal conduction systems serving spinal and brain-stem coordination. *J. Neurophysiol.*, 26:258–272.
53. Snider, R. S., McCulloch, W. S., and Magoun, H. W. (1949): A cerebello-bulbo-reticular pathway for suppression. *J. Neurophysiol.*, 12:325–334.
54. Snider, R. S., and Magoun, H. W. (1949): Facilitation produced by cerebellar stimulation. *J. Neurophysiol.*, 12:335–345.
55. Sprague, J. M., and Chambers, W. W. (1954): Control of posture by reticular formation and cerebellum in the intact, anesthetized and unanesthetized and in the decerebrated cat. *Am. J. Physiol.*, 176:52–64.
56. Thulin, C. -A. (1963): Effects of electrical stimulation of the red nucleus on the alpha motor system. *Exp. Neurol.*, 7:464–480.
57. Tower, S. S. (1940): Pyramidal lesion in the monkey. *Brain*, 63:36–90.
58. Wall, P. D., and Dubner, R. (1972): Somatosensory pathways. *Ann. Rev. Physiol.*, 34:315–336.

Historical Aspects of the Neurosciences,
edited by F. Clifford Rose and W. F. Bynum.
Raven Press, New York ©

History of Binocular Movements

Morris B. Bender and *Stefan Shanzer

*Department of Neurology, The Mount Sinai Medical Center, New York, New York 10029; and *Departments of Neurology, The Mount Sinai Medical Center and Beth Israel Medical Center, New York, New York 10003*

Observations on conjugate eye movements were described in cases of what appeared to be epilepsy or "falling sickness" hundreds of years ago (1). One of the earliest written medical contributions on eye movements other than in epilepsy was in the 16th century (2). At that time, the chief interest was to determine whether individual eyes moved upward or downward or "on the side." Most of the observations were on monocular strabismus, with little, if any, reference to binocular or conjugate movements. During the next two centuries, monographs were written on strabismus and its treatment (3,4), but there were no publications on binocular movements.

The earliest reports appeared in the beginning of the 19th century, and most of these were descriptions of what appeared to be nystagmus. Erasmus Darwin, in his studies on vertigo, noted "rolling movements" of both eyes, which must have been nystagmus (5). He also observed that at the same time the subject saw apparent movement of objects in a direction "contrary to previous rotation" in the horizontal or vertical plane, thus linking eye movements with the sense of vision. About 25 years later, Purkinje observed that repetitive visual stimuli induced what is now known as optokinetic nystagmus (6). The other sensory function linked with eye movements was vestibular. The vertigo elicited on rotation was, according to Purkinje, caused by the "associated to and fro rolling of the eyes" or nystagmus (7). He thought that a lesion of the cerebellum caused nystagmus, which in turn resulted in vertigo. Purkinje also observed vertigo and binocular nystagmus on galvanic stimulation of the mastoid region in man, but he did not realize that he was stimulating the semicircular canals. Subsequently, he attributed both vertigo and nystagmus to irritation of the semicircular canals rather than a cerebellar lesion.

During the same period, effects of experimental lesions of the labyrinth were studied by one of Purkinje's contemporaries. This was Flourens, who destroyed parts of the horizontal or vertical canals and noted rolling of the head instead of the eyes in pigeons (8). Another investigator, Hertwig, found that stimulation or section of either the cerebellar hemispheres, the vermis, or the middle cerebellar peduncle resulted in skew deviations of the eyes (9). The eye on the side of the lesion deviated downward while the opposite eye looked upward. This was known as the "Hertwig-Magendie eye position." Similar results were reported by Hertwig after pontine cuts.

Accounts of binocular movements other than nystagmus appeared somewhat later, and contemporaries of Purkinje, such as Johannes Müller and Magendie, made scientific contributions on conjugate movements of the eyes (10,11), pointing out that the ocular globes turned about a center of rotation, a concept derived from the astronomer Kepler 200 years previously (12). These investigators speculated as to anatomical and physiological correlations for the mechanisms that are involved in conjugate eye movements. The earliest experimental research on smooth binocular movements was by Müller (13). His investigations were concerned with the position of the center of rotation and with the rolling movements of the eyes. He conducted experiments where horizontal or vertical eye movements were executed around a fixed center of rotation in man.

Experimental lesions were made systematically in the nervous system of animals during the same period. Flourens described the effects of serial bilateral ablations of the cerebrum, cerebellum, colliculi, and section through the medulla in pigeons (8). At first he thought the functional deficits produced by the bilateral lesions did not correlate with the part of the brain removed. In later investigations, when Flourens found that unilateral lesions, e.g., of the colliculus, resulted in abnormalities in the contralateral eye, he conceded that the side of the lesion influenced the resultant behavior.

Although localization of function dates from Herophilus and Galen (14), specific body activities were not localized to any region of the brain until the turn of the 18th century, when Gall introduced the concept that different regions of the cerebral cortex acted as centers for specific function (15). His "phrenology," which included over 30 different faculties, was severely criticized by many of his contemporaries. Bell stated that Gall described the brain as being composed of "many particles and independent organs" and that Gall tended to assign each of the "residents" some special faculty (16). Nevertheless, Gall's hypothesis stimulated investigation of brain functions by experimental lesioning and stimulations of the cerebrum. These studies led to a trend away from Flourens' hypothesis and ultimately evolved into the modern concept of "centers." Bell, who was so critical of Gall, initiated refined dissection of the spinal cord and brain to make localization of function scientifically respectable (17). Among his investigations, he made important observations on binocular movements; Bell described the occurrence of upward rolling of the eyes on bilateral eyelid closure in patients with facial paralysis (18), an observation now known as Bell's phenomenon. Between 1823 and 1833, Bell published his findings on other types of eye movements and on various cranial nerve dysfunctions, including that of facial palsy (Bell's palsy). Besides upward vertical eye movements associated with lid closure, he described rotatory nystagmus, which was either congenital in origin or associated with amblyopia. Nystagmus due to disease of the nervous system was not recognized until 50 years later. In another instance, Bell described a case of inability to move the eyes downward. He wrote, "they rolled upward and they could move from right to left but not down." It is not clear whether or not this description was an instance of paralysis of downward gaze.

During the second half of the 19th century, there were further reports of researches on vestibular functions and coordination of eye movements. A Russian-born physiologist, von Cyon, observed that horizontal or vertical eye movement occurred on mechanical stimulation of a particular semicircular canal (19). A similar effect was previously noted by Flourens when he "pricked" the semicircular canals in pigeons. Later investigations by others showed that besides rotational, mechanical, and electrical stimulation, the canals could be activated thermally and chemically and that each canal influenced binocular movements in a specific direction (20). Bárány, a Viennese otologist, was the first to demonstrate that caloric stimulations of individual canals evoked specific eye movements (21). For his numerous clinical and experimental anatomic studies of the vestibular system, he was awarded the Nobel Prize in Medicine in 1914. His works became the foundation of modern vestibulo-ocular physiology. Historical development of knowledge on vestibular functions during the

19th and early 20th centuries may be found in the monograph by Camis (22). During the middle of the 19th century, Helmholtz started his meticulous investigations in vision and coordination or conjugacy of binocular movement, and these were published in three installments between 1856 and 1866, translated and amply annotated by Southall (23). Bárány's numerous articles on researches into the motion of the eyes, the direction of gaze, and the role of vision in binocular movement are discussed in detail in his third volume.

Helmholtz propagated the idea that coordination of eye movements is a learned skill. It was Hering, a contemporary of Helmholtz, who suggested that the two eyes were "yoked," like a team of horses, and moved as a unit (24,25), a concept previously suggested in 1858 by Foville (26). The movements of the "double eye" were for conjugate deviation and for vergence. Hering also made accurate experiments concerning the relations between the head and binocular movements (24). Laws for torsional and fusional movements of the eyes, as described by Franz Donders and Johann Listing in the mid-19th century, may be found in Helmholtz's third volume. Clinically, the concept of coordinated eye movements was reaffirmed by Jackson (27), who wrote on lateral binocular deviation in hemiplegia and in epileptiform seizures.

Investigations on the speed of eye movements were started in 1846 by Volkmann (28). He gauged the speed of binocular movements by counting the number of times a subject could look back and forth between two points for a given time interval. Later, the velocity of movements was measured by Lamanski (29), a student of Helmholtz, with different methods. Binocular movements were known to be slow, smooth, or quick. The latter was found in nystagmus. Detailed studies of saccadic eye movements were begun in 1891 by the Swiss ophthalmologist Landolt (30), and this trend to investigate saccades extended into the 20th century. Stratton in 1902 recorded jerky binocular movements while viewing moving patterns on film (31). Our eyes were said to move like the second hand of a watch—a jerk and a little pull, then another jerk. During the jerks, we practically do not see at all (32). A great step forward in analysis of eye movements began with the American psychologist Dodge (33), who published his study of five types of binocular movements. As for the recording of eye movements, numerous techniques were developed, but the electrical method, which was introduced by Schott in 1922 (34), was the most reliable. Ultimately, with various improvements, this method evolved into modern electro-oculography and nystagmography.

As noted previously, prior to the 19th century, most descriptions of defective eye movements were of individual ocular muscles, and there was little information on impairments of conjugate gaze. Andral (35) was one of the first to describe a case of defective horizontal gaze, associated with ipsilateral hemiplegia, but it was not clear whether the ocular deficit was a strabismus or an impairment of conjugate gaze. After the middle of the 19th century, many descriptions and reports of paralysis of horizontal conjugate gaze appeared, especially by the French school (36). By that time, two clinical entities were recognized, namely, the conjugate eye palsy associated with ipsilateral hemiplegia (35) and that associated with contralateral hemiplegia (26). Prévost (37) simplified these gaze palsies as follows: The patient looks with eyes turned away from the hemiplegia in a cerebral lesion and with eyes turned toward the hemiplegia in a pontine lesion.

The years 1858 to 1859 were a particularly productive period for reporting abnormal eye movements, again primarily as the result of careful observation in the Paris clinics. Gubler (38) described a number of crossed syndromes associated with brain-stem lesions in a series of papers in the 1850s, which was finally gathered in a single volume; this volume consisted of reprints from the *Gazette Hebdomadaire*, where so many of the French clinicians published their findings (39). It appears that the *Gazette*, which served both French and German scientists, usually followed an original presentation at the Anatomical Society, where, incidentally, Millard (40) presented his case of abducens palsy with contralateral hemiplegia in 1856. However, this was not the first description of a crossed syndrome since Yelloly (41) presented a similar case to the Royal Society in 1808. Yelloly's case was due to a tuberculoma involving the pons, which in those days was the most common lesion in the brain. Reviewing his report, one gets the impression that the concept of a crossing of descending cerebral pathways, even for movement, was not yet firmly established and was considered by some scientists with amazement.

While Gubler (39) described a number of crossed syndromes, including those involving the third (medial rectus), sixth and seventh cranial nerves, the concept of conjugate gaze palsy essentially eluded him, although he was familiar with Foville's case. During those days, a number of authors were searching for a "single nerve" that would move both eyes conjugately in one direction. Some believed that the economy of the nervous system seemed to demand the existence of such a nerve.

Foville's case deserves special consideration. His patient was a man who was born with or developed an early atrophy of the right arm. All his other limbs were well muscled and strong. He had a marked inclination toward alcohol but not to "venereal excesses." At age 43, he suddenly lost consciousness. This was followed by vomiting and an inability to speak. The diagnosis of cerebral apoplexy was made, and the patient was treated with "blood letting and a bottle of Seidlitz water," resulting in a marked improvement of his general condition. Examined six days later by Foville, he showed a complete left facial paralysis of the lower motor neuron type. The tongue was deviated to the right. There was a right hemiplegia with "beginnings" of return of function in the right leg. The detailed description of the eye phenomena is of importance: the patient was able to look up, down, and to the right normally, but he could not look to the left at all, either with one or with both eyes; neither eye moved across the midline to the left. On inclining the head to the left side, the eyes moved normally in the direction opposite to the head or to the right side (oculocephalic reflex). There was no mention of convergence and no report of any later examination. Subsequently, the patient showed a rapid improvement in his right hemiparesis but not in the left facial palsy nor in the paralysis of conjugate gaze to the left. Since the patient survived, there was obviously no anatomical confirmation of the site of the lesion.

With the anatomical knowledge available at the time, Foville deduced that the site of the lesion was in the left pons. He devoted considerable thought to the paralysis of the right internal rectus, and reasoned that, since the right internal rectus was the only muscle paralyzed on "the right side of the face," it must be due to a lesion in the left pons, where the posterior rootlets of the III nerve originate and cross to the other side "as all oculomotor fibers do," according to his knowledge. Whereas this anatomical explanation is no longer acceptable and was replaced by others within a few years of Foville's description, another concept of his deserves a note. Foville stated that in order to direct the two eyes in the same direction, nature has employed means which are similar to those of a man who has to drive a pair of horses together and knows how to hold in each hand the reins that with one single motion will direct both of them to the right or to the left. This concept of yoked movements of the eye was later developed by Hering (24). Foville also warned that the "synergistic fibers," i.e., innervation of the two eyes, cannot exist in a "single nerve trunk" since no crossing is seen once the ocular nerves leave the brain stem. Thus, the crossing must occur within the stem, with the fibers directed to the adductor crossing the midline on their way from the pons. Foville's concept was the foundation of subsequent clinical (42), anatomical (43–45), and electrophysiological (46,47) interpretations of the role of the posterior longitudinal bundle or the median longitudinal fasciculus in conjugate gaze or associated lateral movements. In later years, more careful observations were made in cases of associated lateral gaze palsy, and it was noted that the paralyzed eyes could move under certain conditions. Féréol (48) reported a patient with a pontine left lateral gaze palsy, who could move the right eye to the left beyond the median plane when the left eye was covered. Thereafter, there were many other reports of such observations, including preservation of convergence in cases of bilateral paralysis of conjugate horizontal gaze (36), where it was felt that the medial rectus was paralyzed for lateral gaze and not for convergence. Based on Foville's theory, many authors reasoned that this dissociation in conjugate gaze had something to do with the functions transmitted by the median longitudinal fasciculus. Later it was learned that this fasciculus indeed transmitted two types of function, one for contralateral horizontal gaze and the other for convergence, as verified by Spiller in 1924. He was the first to report a patient with paralysis of adduction for lateral gaze, but with preserved convergence, who at autopsy showed destruction of the posterior longitudinal bundle (43).

A topic of special interest, mostly to the French neurologists of that time, was head and eye deviations. Prévost, working in Vulpian's clinic as well as with Charcot, quoted the latter as being tempted to admit that a head and eye rotation exists to a greater or lesser degree in every attack of apoplexy or stroke. Prevost's observations, both clinical and experimental, were assembled as a monograph in 1868 (37). The first part consisted of case reports of impairment of horizontal conjugate gaze, and these reports were divided into nine groups, the first eight referring to different anatomical loci of the lesion and the ninth to nonautopsied cases. There was detailed compartmentalization of conjugate (horizontal) eye movements, which could be grouped as follows: the horizontal eye deviation was always to the side opposite of the hemiplegia when caused by (a) lesions of the cerebral gray matter; (b) lesions of the meninges, including pachymeningitis hemorrhagica or subdural hematoma, which compressed the cerebral cortex; (c) lesions of the centrum ovale; (d) lesions of the striatum, thalamus, and centrum ovale; (e) hemorrhage with rupture into the lateral ventricle; (f) lesions limited to the striatum; (g) lesions limited to the thalamus or extending to the cerebral peduncle; and (h) encompassed lesions of the pons and cerebellum. Of the four cases described in the latter group, only one had a pure left pontine lesion with a crossed syndrome, in which the head and eyes were deviated to the right (paralysis of conjugate gaze to the left) with left facial weakness and a right hemiplegia. The other three patients had a gaze paralysis or paresis in the direction of a cerebellar lesion, presumably with secondary pontine compression.

Following the above description by Prévost, one finds references in the literature to the "Prévost rule," which stated: "the patient looks toward the lesion in cases with cerebral involvement and away from the lesion in cases with lesions of the brainstem." In his discussion of the clinical phenomenon, Prévost made a number of points that are as substantial today as they were over 100 years ago. He emphasized the close relationship of head and eye movements and noted that on bringing a forcefully deviated head to the midline, one enhances the eye deviation. He was fully aware of a variability in the intensity of the phenomenon and pointed out that at times it is inconspicuous and that special maneuvers may be needed to elicit the ocular deviation. He thought on the whole that the forced eye deviation tended to be more persistent than the abnormal head posturing, and he noted that both the head and eye deviation tended to be transient in patients with strokes. Importantly, Prévost pointed out that there were cases of stroke without abnormal head and eye posturing and that there were means of distinguishing those without eye and head deviation from those with the deviation. In attempts to correlate the finding of head and eye deviation with the site of the pathology, Prévost concluded that the lesions were usually, but not invariably, located deep in the brain. He speculated whether or not the "superficial" lesions, such as pachymeningitis hemorrhagica or subdural hematoma, might not act by exerting an "influence" on deeper cerebral structures. During the 1870s, there were notes on the effect of coma and anesthesia on conjugate gaze (49), where again, these authors spoke of specific centers in the brain that kept the eyes together.

At the time of Prévost's writings, some knowledge was available from previous experimental studies on animals and specifically on circling behavior following cerebral lesions. This circling, attributed at first to the eye deviation, was shown to persist after ocular ablation. Prevost's discussion of the animal experiments is detailed and instructive. He distinguished the turning or circling movement after lesions from "rolling" movements, and he tried to reconcile the direction of the two types of movements by defining the observer's position in relation to the subject. On the whole, he found from writings of others, which described experiments on frogs, rabbits, dogs, and even sheep, that cerebral lesions result in turning to the side of the lesion. His own experiments on dogs consisted of direct cerebral incisions and, in some instances, injection of tobacco grains suspended in water into the carotid artery. Studies of lesions of the brain stem and cerebellum date back to the 18th and early 19th centuries (11,50,51), and all described a rotating eye and head movement in the same direction as the lesion. Longet (52), on the other hand, noted a rotation in the opposite direction, explaining the divergent results by involvement of uncrossed and crossed systems, respectively. Many other authors appeared to be interested in this problem, with conflicting results, possibly because of the rather gross nature of the lesions inflicted with a knife.

Although Prévost was unable to outline the actual cephalo-oculomotor pathways, his general conclusions are still sound and valuable. It remained for his successors to try a more detailed anatomical analysis of the observable phenomena. Graux (53) devoted his doctoral thesis to a similar problem and concluded that there must be in the floor of the fourth ventricle a structure that connects the abducens and oculomotor nuclei and that plays a crucial role in transmitting impulses from one to the other, thus making conjugate gaze possible. He was able to demonstrate this structure (apparently the median longitudinal fasciculus) in cats, but his slides on human brain were not satisfactory. This may have been an elaboration of Foville's hypothesis, implying the median longitudinal fasciculus or the posterior longitudinal bundle as a crucial structure in conjugate or associated horizontal gaze. Subsequently, there were reports stressing the importance of this bundle and its connections with the abducens nucleus (54–56). The latter was considered as a center for horizontal gaze, particularly when a lesion confined to this nucleus resulted in ipsilateral paralysis for horizontal conjugate gaze (57). The latter theory is no longer tenable in the light of recent investigations on the pontine reticular formation (58).

Although stimulation experiments were virtually nonexistent prior to 1870, we do get hints of eye deviations due to cerebral irritation with seizures. Jackson (27) described a case of ocular deviation as part of a seizure, and Prévost (59) quotes a case of a man who was seen to turn around several times prior to a generalized seizure and who knew that this turning would be followed by a grand mal fit. Similarly, in one of Prévost's experiments with intracarotid injections of tobacco, there appeared a circling with the eye turning in the direction opposite to the injected side. In later years, cerebral centers for horizontal eye movements were postulated.

As for vertical gaze, the first description of paralysis for "upward" movement was in 1864 by Henoch (60), for both "upward and downward" gaze by Wernicke (61), and for "downward gaze" by Gee (62). Each of the case reports included gross autopsy findings, and the responsible lesion was usually a large tuberculoma located in the "quadrigeminal region." The clinical descriptions were sketchy and inadequate, and there was no indication whether or not the remaining binocular movements were intact. Thus, Gee (62) described a patient with presumed paralysis of downward gaze because the eyes "appeared to be rolled upward." Better descriptions of defects in vertical eye movements were made by Parinaud (63), an ophthalmologist in Charcot's clinic and probably the first and only neuro-ophthalmologist for many years. He described the syndrome of difficulty in upward and downward gaze and included the state of the pupils and of defects in binocular vergence, but there were no postmortem examinations of his patients. About this time, more articles on paralysis of vertical gaze were published with autopsies that revealed a lesion in the quadrigeminal plate. Thereafter, Parinaud (64) claimed that the "center" for vertical gaze was located in the colliculi; still later, he thought that this "center" must be situated in the frontal lobe (65). This notion was in accord with the conclusions of Munk (66) and Mott and Schaefer (67), whose stimulation experiments of both sides of the brain in dogs and in monkeys led them to postulate that the inferior part of the "frontal eye center" controlled upward movements of the eyes and the superior part controlled binocular downward movements. More recent experiments have shown that bilateral stimulations in many regions of the brain will result in vertical gaze and that specific bilateral small lesions in the mesodiencephalic region will cause paralysis of either upward or downward movements (58,68,69). Although Parinaud's concept for vertical gaze was incorrect, credit should be given for his excellent observations. He was the first to describe impairments of convergence and divergence in conjunction with paralysis of upward gaze (63). Thereafter, a center for convergence was sought and localized to a group of cells or nucleus of Perlia situated in the midbrain (70), but this hypothetical center could not be linked with certainty to the act of convergence. As for a center of divergence, there is still controversy and doubt as to its existence, even in modern times (71). Impaired convergence is frequently observed in conjunction with paralysis of upward gaze. In addition, a so-called convergence nystagmus may occur. Fragments of this syndrome were noted in cases described by Smith (72) before Parinaud. After Parinaud, an additional phenomenon that was found in cases of paralysis of upward gaze was retractory nystagmus, as first described by Koerber (73).

Parinaud's localization for vertical eye movements was challenged by Spiller (74). In his presidential address to the American Neurological Association, Spiller reviewed the French, German, and English literature on paralysis of vertical gaze and, based on his own additional 19 autopsied cases, concluded that the lesion responsible for paralysis of vertical gaze was situated in the vicinity of the "aqueduct of Sylvius." Even though Spiller was an excellent and meticulous pathologist, the clinical descriptions in those days were sketchy and the pathological lesions were gross, extending over many critical areas in the brain. It should be noted that in his clinical description of paralysis of upward gaze, Spiller demonstrated a marked eyelid retraction in three of his patients, but he did not comment on this phenomenon, which is a frequent occurrence in this type of lesion.

Despite these inaccuracies, clinicians continued to believe that localization of normal oculomotor functions was provided by the study of brain lesions that caused defects in ocular gaze. With this in mind, they prodded the experimentalist to search for a "physiological" interpretation of eye movements. It was known that an "irritative" lesion of the cerebrum resulted in a contralateral horizontal or oblique "associated eye movement" (27,75), but the precise localization of the lesion that caused a particular defect in movement could not be ascertained without comparative investigations in experimental animals. About that time, more careful investigations on the excitability of the cerebral cortex in the monkey and other animals were begun (76,77), and it was learned that electric stimulation of the cerebral cortex evoked body, head, and eye movement. The eyes almost always moved conjugately to the contralateral side (78–80). With the innovation of the stereotaxic instrument in the first quarter of this century (81), electric stimulation and discrete focal lesioning in the brain stem provided more precise additional information on binocular movements (82–84). Sherrington's (85) contributions on reciprocal innervation in eye movements and, later, anatomical and physiological studies on neuronal models, within the pontine reticular formation, by Lorente de Nó (87), became the basis of modern physiology of oculomotor functions. Electrical recording of eye movement, a method first intoduced by Schott (34) and later improved (86), contributed immensely to more precise measurement of eye movements. As more sophisticated and better technical equipment became available, there followed an ever increasing number of investigations, which led to a tremendous dissemination of information on eye movements in the experimental and clinical literature. Since the mid-20th century, there have appeared many journals, texts, monographs, reviews, and symposia devoted to neurology and physiology of the oculomotor system. Generally, texts and reviews tended to assign specific functions to specific areas of the cerebrum and brain stem and then proceeded to stress pathways connecting these "centers," but morphological as well as physiological evidence of these presumed pathways is still incomplete (58).

The concept of brain centers for eye movements originated many years ago, and this most besetting of all studies of the central nervous system continues to be the principle of localization of function in a specific part of the brain. The concept of the brain as a composite of suborgans dates back hundreds of years. The literature of the Middle Ages and Renaissance, identified "the seat of the soul" in various parts of the brain (see Chapter 6 of this volume). This concept was emphasized in the last century by Gall's anatomical studies in the years from 1822 to 1835 and by Broca's inferences in 1861 that the neural apparatus for speech was in a particular convolution of the left frontal lobe (88,89). Still later, the classic experiments of Fritsch and Hitzig (77) and those of Ferrier (78) emphasized specific cortical functions. This naive formulation of the phrenologist, as well as minute cytoarchitectural anatomical parcellations into functional units, has hampered progress. Haste in assigning specific functions to specific areas or "centers" has often caused neuroscientists and clinical neurologists to overlook many aspects of the overall organization of the oculomotor system. In modern neurobiology, the trend has been to determine the geographical boundaries of neuronal aggregates or assemblies of neurons acting as functional units in behavior rather than centers for eye movements.

REFERENCES

1. Temkin, O. (1945): *The Falling Sickness*. Johns Hopkins Press, Baltimore, Md.
2. Bartisch, G. (1583): *Augendienst*. Feyrabend, Frankurt an Main.
3. Porterfield, W. (1735): *Med. Essays and Obs. Soc.*, Vol. III, 160 (1737): Vol. IV, 124.
4. Hunter, J. (1786): *Observations on Certain Parts of the Animal Oeconomy*, p. 225.
5. Darwin, E. (1794): *Zoonomia or the Laws of Organic Life*, Vol. I, pp. 227 and 569, London (3rd ed., corrected, London, 1801).
6. Purkinje, J. (1819): Beobachtungen und Versuche zur Physiologie der Sinne. In: *Beiträge zur Kentniss des Sehens in subjektiver Hinsicht*; Vol. 1, p. 50. J. Calve, Prague.
7. Purkinje, J. (1820): *Beyträge zur naheren Kenntnis des Schwindels aus heautognostischen Daten*, p. 79. der k.k. Österreichen Staates, VI, Band II, Stück, Vienna.
8. Flourens, P. (1824), (1842): *Recherches Expérimentales sur les Propriétés et les Fonctions du Système Nerveux dans les Animaux Vertrès*. Crevot, Bailliere, Paris.
9. Hertwig, K. W. (1826): *Experimenta Qaedem De Effectibus Laesionum in Partibus Encephali Singularibus Et De Verosimili Illarum Partium Functionne*, Berlin.
10. Müller, J. (1826): *Zur vergleichenden Physiologie des Gesichtssinne*, p. 254. Leipzig.

11. Magendie, F. (1824): *J. de Physiol. Exp.*, 4:399. (1843): In: *An Elementary Treatise on Human Physiology*, 5th ed., translated by J. Revere. Harper, New York.
12. Kepler, J., cited by Helmholtz, H. von (1924): *Handbuch der Physiologischen Optik*, 3rd ed., translated by J. P. C. Southall, Vol. III, p. 120. Dover, New York.
13. Müller, J. (1834): *Handbuch der Physiologie des Menschen für Vorlesungen*. Coblenz & Berlin. English translation, W. Baly, *Elements of Physiology*. Taylor & Walton, London.
14. Herophilus and Galen, cited by Prochaska, G. (1784): *Dissertation on the Functions of the Nervous System*, translated by Thomas Laycock, p. 446. Sydenham Society, London (1851).
15. Gall, F. J. (1851): *Sur les fonctions du cerveau et sur celle de chacune de ses parties*. Balliere, Paris.
16. Bell, C. (1833): *The Nervous System of the Human Body*. Duff Green, Washington.
17. Bell, C. (1811): *Idea of a New Anatomy of the Brain*. Straham & Preston, London. (1830): *The Nervous System of the Human Body*, 2nd ed. Longmans, London.
18. Bell, C. (1823): *Phil. Trans. Roy. Soc., London*, 166.
19. Cyon, E. von (1876): *C. R. Acad. Sci.*, 82:856.
20. Ewald, J. R. (1887): *Arch. f. d. ges. Physiol.*, 41:463.
21. Barany, R. (1906): *Monatschr. für Ohrenheilkd.*, 43:191.
22. Camis, M. (1930): *The Physiology of the Vestibular Apparatus*, p. 144. Clarendon Press, Oxford.
23. Helmholtz, H. von (1909): In: *Handbuch der Physiologischen Optik*, Voss, Hamburg. Edited and translated by J. P. Southall for The Optical Soc. of America (1924).
24. Hering, E. (1868): *Die Lehre vom Binocularen Sehen*, Engelmann, Leipzig.
25. Hering, E. (1879): *Über Muskelgerausche des Auges*. Sitzungsber. Akad. Wiss. Wien Math Naturwiss. Kl. Abt., p. 137.
26. Foville, A. L. (1859): *Gazette Hebdomadaire*, 6:146. (1858): *Bull. Soc. Anatomique*.
27. Jackson, J. H. (1866): *Lancet*, 1:311.
28. Volkmann, A. W. (1846): *Sehen in Wagner Handwörter-buch der Physiologie*, p. 265. Vieweg & Sohn, Braunschweig.
29. Lamanski, S. (1869): *Pflüg. Arch. ges. Physiol.*, 2:418.
30. Landolt, E. (1891): *Arch. Ophthal. Paris*, 11:385.
31. Stratton, G. M. (1902): *Wundt's philosophische Studien*, XX Band, p. 336. Engelman, Leipzig.
32. Brown, A. C. (1895): *Nature*, 52:184.
33. Dodge, R. (1903): *Am. J. Physiol.*, 8:307.
34. Schott, E. (1922): *Deutsches Arch. klin. Med.*, 140:179.
35. Andral, G. (1834): *Clinique Médicale ou Choix d'Observations*, p. 359. Paris.
36. Freeman, W. (1922): *Arch. Neurol. Psychiat.*, 7:454.
37. Prévost, J. L. (1868): *De la deviation conjuguée des yeux et de la rotation de la tête dans certain cas d'hemiplegie*. V. Masson, Paris.
38. Gubler, A. (1856): *Gazette Hebdomadaire de medicine et Chirurgie*, 3:749.
39. Gubler, A. (1859): *Mémoire sur les paralysies alternes en général, et particulièrement sur l hemiplégie alterne avec lésion de la protruberance annulaire*, p. 1. V. Masson, Paris.
40. Millard, A. L. (1856): *Bull. Soc. Anat.*, 31:206.
41. Yelloly, J. (1812): *Medico-Chirurgical Trans.*, 1:181.
42. Potts, C. S., and Spiller, W. G. (1903): *Univ. of Penn. Med. Bull.*, 16:362.
43. Spiller, W. G. (1924): *Brain*, 47:345.
44. Bender, M. B., and Weinstein, E. A. (1944): *Arch. Neurol. Psychiat.*, 52:106.
45. Graybiel, A. M., and Hartweig, E. A. (1974): *Brain Res.*, 91:551.
46. Baker, R., and Highstein, S. M. (1975): *Brain Res.*, 91:292.
47. Highstein, S. M. (1977): In: *Eye Movements*, Assoc. for Research in Vision and Ophthalmol. Symposium, edited by B. A. Brooks and F. J. Bajandas, p. 127. Plenum Press, New York.
48. Féréol, L. H. F. (1874): *Bull. et mem. de la Soc. Méd. des Hopit. de Paris*, 10:124.
49. Mercier, C. (1877): *Br. Med. J.*, 1:292.
50. Pourfour Du Petit, F. (1710): *Nouveau Système De Cervau*, Namur.
51. Serres, A. E. (1823): *J. Phys. Exp. de Magendie*, III.
52. Longet, F. A. (1842): *Anat. et Physiol. du Système Nerveux*, Paris.
53. Graux, G. (1878): *De la paralysie du moteur oculaire externe avec deviation conjugée*. Thesis 383, Paris.
54. Hunnius, M. (1881): *Zur Symptomotologie der Brückenerkrankungen und über die conjugirte Deviation der Augen bei Hirnkrankheiten*. Cohen & Sohn, Bonn, p. 1.
55. Bleuler, P. E. (1885): In: *Zur Casuistik der Herderkrankungen der Brücke Mit Besonderer Berucksichtigung der Störungen der Combinirten Seitlichen Augenbewegungen*. edited by J. B. Hirschfeld. Leipzig.
56. Monakow, C. von (1895): *Arch. Psychiat. Nerv. Krankh.*, 27:1, 386.
57. Bennett, H., and Savill, T. (1889): *Brain*, 12:102.
58. Bender, M. B. (1980): *Brain*, 103:23.
59. Prévost, J. L., and Cotard, J. (1866): *Etudes Physiologiques et Pathologiques sur le Ramollissement Cérébral*. A. Delamaye, Paris.
60. Henoch, E. H. (1864): *Berliner Klin. Wochenschrift*, No. 13 (March 21), p. 125.

61. Wernicke, C. (1876): *Berliner Medizinisch-psychologische Gesellschaft*, Sitzung, vom F. (Feb. 1876). *Berliner Klin. Wochenschrift* (July 3), p. 394.
62. Gee, S. (1890): *Saint Bartholomew's Hosp. Rep.*, 26:106.
63. Parinaud, H. (1883): *Arch. Neurol.*, 5:145.
64. Parinaud, H. (1886): *Brain*, 9:330.
65. Parinaud, H. (1892): *Ann. d'Oculistique*, 197:283.
66. Munk, H. (1890): *Brain*, 13:45.
67. Mott, F. W., and Schaefer, E. A. (1890): *Brain*, 13:165.
68. Pasik, P., Pasik, T., and Bender, M. B. (1969): *Brain*, 92:521.
69. Kömpf, D., Pasik, T., Pasik, P., and Bender, M. B. (1979): *Brain*, 102:527.
70. Brouwer, B. (1918): *Z. f. Neurol. Psychiat.*, 40:152.
71. Jampolsky, A. (1970): *Trans. Am. Ophthal. Soc.*, 68:730.
72. Smith, P. (1879): *Ophthal. Hosp. Rep. and J. Roy. London Ophthal. Hosp.*, 9:22.
73. Koerber, H. (1903): *Die Ophthalmologische Klinik Internationales Helbmonatsblatt fur Pathologie und Therapie der Augenkrankheiten*, Vol. 7, p. 65. Stuttgart.
74. Spiller, W. G. (1905): *J. Nerv. Ment. Dis.*, 32:417.
75. Jackson, J. H. (1870): *"St. Andrews Med. Graduates" Assoc. Trans.*, 3:162.
76. Adamük, E. (1870): *Zentr. med. Wiss*, 8:65.
77. Fritsch, G., and Hitzig, E. (1870): *Arch. Anat. Physiol. Wissensch. Med.*, 300.
78. Ferrier, D. (1875): *Proc. Roy. Soc. Lond.*, 23:409.
79. Schaefer, E. A. (1888): *Brain*, 11:1.
80. Beevor, C. E., and Horsley, V. (1888): *Phil. Trans. Roy. Soc., Lond.*, 179:205.
81. Horsley, V., and Clarke, R. H. (1908): *Brain*, 31:45.
82. Hess, W. R. (1932): *Die Methodik Lokalieserten Reizung und Auschallung Subcorticaler Hirnabschnitte UN Vol.* George Theime, Leipzig.
83. Monnier, M. (1946): *Rev. Neurol.*, 78:422.
84. Bender, M. B., and Shanzer, S. (1964): In: *The Oculomotor System*, edited by M. B. Bender, p. 81. Hoeber, New York.
85. Sherrington, C. S. (1893): *Proc. Roy. Soc. London*, 53:407.
86. Mowrer, O. H., Ruch, T. C., and Miller, N. G. (1936): *Am. J. Physiol.*, 114:423.
87. Lorente de Nó, R. (1933): *Arch. Neurol. Psychiat., Chicago*, 30:245.
88. Broca, P. (1861): *Bull. Soc. Anat.*, VI:398.
89. Critchley, M. (1970): *Aphasiology*, p. 53. E. Arnold, London.

Historical Aspects of the Neurosciences,
edited by F. Clifford Rose and W. F. Bynum.
Raven Press, New York ©

The Seat of the Soul

G. W. Bruyn

Department of Neurology, Academic Hospital, State University, Leyden, The Netherlands

Where is the place of understanding?
Job 28:12, 20, 28

In a *livre jubilaire* honoring the Nestor of neuropsychology, it seems only appropriate to fashion one's contribution so as to fit the frame determined by the recipient's life and work. If a tree is known by its fruit, then Dr. Critchley's *Opera Omnia* indicate his lifelong occupation with the intriguing relationship of the mind and the brain. He approached this relationship from a neurological study of deranged psychological states and functions occasioned by (or at least associated with) deranged states of the physicochemical matrix we denote with the word "brain." This, of course, is a legitimate and empirically heuristic procedure, because the basic, if tacit, tenet of such a method is that the major function of the brain is the organism's adaptative coordination of transients between the *milieu extérieur et intérieur*, among which figures mental activity. Basic physiological processes often become known and hermeneutically ordered upon their being deranged by either experimental intrusion or pathological disruption. As such, a lesion of the brain may entail a disturbance of its functions (among which are the mental), and the conditions are then met for scientific analysis and synthesis.

The philosophers, of course, will point out that during such a procedure, there remains the *petitio principii* of the snake biting its tail: To explain (= mental activity) a function (e.g., mental activity) of an organ (e.g., the brain) in terms of the same function (= mental activity) is essentially equivalent to von Münchhausen's trick of lifting himself and his horse by the horse's hair. Epistemologically, the proposition is undecidable, and comparable to Gödel's theorem in formal logic, which shows that the consistency of a logic-mathematical system can never be proven with the aid of that system's methods unless one accepts its incompleteness, resulting in the paradox that mathematics is either incomplete if it is consistent or complete if inconsistent. Gödel's shattering theorem added quasi-insult to the injury sustained by classic Newtonian physics when quantum mechanics showed that Determinism's scepter wields no power in the fundamental realm of physical reality, namely, elementary particulate matter, an injury fatally inflicted by Heisenberg's uncertainty principle of the irreconcilability of the measurements of a particle's place and speed. Statistics instead of Determinism turned out to be matter's tyrant.

In spite of this, a review of man's thoughts upon the mind's *domicilium* may still appeal to Dr. Critchley, if one recalls his own 1966 Harveian Oration (1) reference to the slightly pornographic novel *Les Bijoux Indiscrets* by Diderot (2), which stated that the soul resides in the feet of the baby, in the legs of the child, ascends to the thighs in adolescence, and that there are persons in whom the soul "n'a jamais remonté plus haut."

This presentation will not deal at length with the many great men in neurological history: After all, the greatness of a man is solely to be measured by the length of time his ideas impede progress. For instance, the ancients held nerves to be hollow (ποροι). Dr. Mary Brazier has outlined in this volume the effort of two of my 17th century countrymen, Jan van Swammerdam and Antoni van Leeuwenhoek, to falsify this notion, an effort crowned with success lasting 300 years. Only in the past few decades has neuroscience proved the ancients' superior sophisticated speculation by revealing that nerve fibers are indeed hollow tubes with a lively axoplasmic flow. Be this as it may, this presentation reflects a personal opinion (δοξα); I feel assured that Dr. Critchley would rather have me doing the wrong thing for the right reasons than vice versa.

> And he said unto man, behold, the fear of the Lord, that is wisdom; and to depart from evil is understanding.
>
> *Job 28: 28*

We will leave Job's reproachful and diplomatic interlocution with Jahwè, the παντων δεσποτησ, whom Job called to book on His breach of Treaty and so-called Justice, ending with Job's silence (3), aside for the moment. It is the Pythagorean physician Alkmeon of Kroton (5th century B.C.) who may be considered as the initiator of our story. As a Descartes *avant-la-lettre*, he distinguished between the senses and the thoughts, and postulated that each sensation occupied a certain territory in the brain. Like his teacher Pythagoras, he held the immortal soul to reside in the brain.

Theophrastus Eresius (327–287 B.C.) (4) concurred with this point of view, ascribing disturbed sensation and intelligence to imbalance in the brain produced by blockage of the hollow nerves carrying the sense organs' impressions to the brain. Leukippos, the *auctor intellectualis* of Determinism, his pupil Demokritos of Abdera (460–370 B.C.), as well as Plato (5), emphasized the brain as the primary center of control of the soma. The corpus of Hippokrates of Kos and the work of Aetius Amideni (6) testify to this, as does the work of Aristotle (7).

Plato rendered the primacy to the brain because in its rounded part of the medulla (made out of the right proportions of Pythagoras/Empedokles' four elements—fire, water, air and earth—derived from straight and smooth primary triangles), God planted and enclosed the soul. The *Corpus Hippocraticum*, being more physiological than philosophical, while holding onto the concept of cerebral primacy, acknowledged the vulnerability of the brain due to its afferent influences of air, water, and the venous phlegm. The passage of air to the brain in particular is considered crucial:

> When a man draws breath into himself, the air first reaches the brain and so is dispersed through the rest of the body, leaving however its quintessence, and all it has of intelligence or sense, in the brain.(8)

The brain ("a tapering hollow") attracts water and also has to be purged from its impurities, and when that goes awry, hydrocephalus, phlegmasia, or epilepsy results. The brain accordingly might deviate from its optimal moistness (or dryness) and coldness (or warmth) (Fig. 1).

All the Greek Natural Philosophers subscribed to the doctrine of the spirit, which taught that the *spiritus naturalis* originates in the liver, is transported to the heart and lungs, where it is converted to the essential principle of life, the *spiritus vitalis* (πνεῦμα ζωτικόν) through the admixture of air. It finally becomes, by distillation in the brain, the *spiritus animalis*

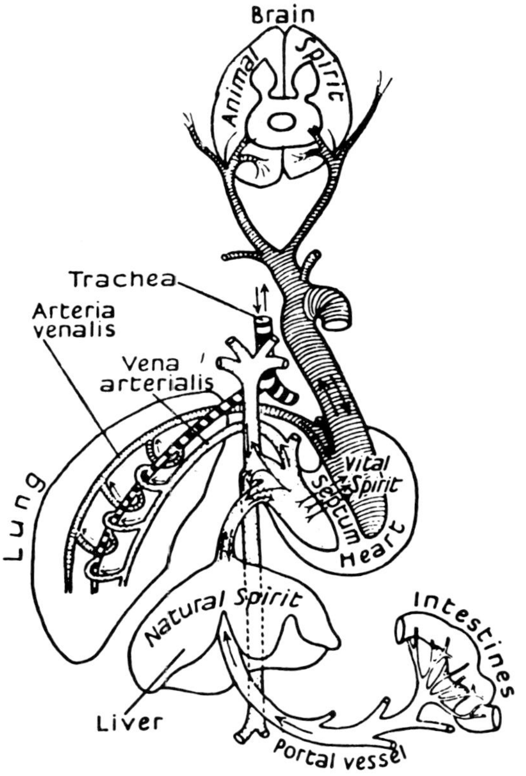

FIG. 1. Spiritus Doctrine. [From Florkin, M. (1972): *History of Biochemistry*, Elsevier, New York, with permission.]

(πνευμα ψυχικον), which is the carrier of thought (το φανταστικον), judgment (διανουτικον), and memory (μνημονευτικον). The Natural Philosophers considered the brain as the residence of the soul, mind, and emotion, be it that the relationship between the soul (ηγεμονικον ψυχησ), of which the *pneuma animale* is the most important instrument (πρωτον οργανον), and the δυναμεισ ψυχησ remains hierarchically much less clear, as did the precise habitat (cerebral parenchyma or cerebral ventricles?) of the hegemonikon. A δυναμισ is a faculty, a potentiality, with an aspect of future, of teleology, an 'ενεργεια is the faculty in operation with the present tense aspect of a function in action, an 'εργον is the effect of the 'ενεργεια with the past tense.

The great Stagyrite, Aristotle (384–322 B.C.), set himself apart from the Natural Philosophers by postulating the primacy of the heart. He held on to the Hippokratic notion of a hollow tapering brain and considered, not unreasonably, that this "kettle" regulated the body's temperature by refrigerating (through aspired air?) the vertical bloodstream and chilling the waste products (phlegm) of the serum. He compared this to the development of rain, from vapor rising up and condensing in the air. His shadow was to loom ahead 15 centuries, and he became alive again when the Occident became acquainted with his works in the 12th century A.D.

Although Artistotle may have detected the middle cerebral ventricle (9), the first actual description of the cerebral cavity system of lateral, third, and cerebellar ventricles, and interventricular foramen, was provided by Herophilos of Chalcedon (320–250 A.D.), who taught at the Alexandrian School. The contention by Celsus (10) and Tertullianus that Herophilus (and his colleague Erasistratus of Chios, in age his junior, in professional status his equal) dissected human brains derived from executed criminals (something that would yield controversy with notions based on animal dissection by the older corypheans) is most doubtful. Nonetheless, even if these Alexandrinian Masters only dissected animal material, they did establish the existence of the cerebral ventricular system, thereby converting the previous hazy ideas on a hollow organ into a defined concept; together, they cooked up a different kettle of fish, probably under the impression of the importance of their own discovery. Herophilus, noticing the fourth ventricle situated in close proximity to the spinal cord and motor nerves, went on to contend that the forces (the soul) responsible for all animal activities reside in the ventricular system. Herophilus may well have been prepared by the Stagyrite's comment on Demokritos that "the body is moved by the soul" (11).

In the meantime, two streams of thought appear to have developed: Aristotle held that the tripartite soul (φαντασια, μνημη, and αναμνησισ), a concept in which he was influentially followed by Posidonius of Apamea (12) (280–180 B.C.), perished with the body, whereas Plato (and, later, the influential Plotinus) emphatically argued the immortality of the soul.

At this point, the query underlying this chapter should transpire. οι αρχαιοι located the mental faculties in the brain, an organ provided with afferent tubes from the sense organs (through which air is aspired into it and upon evaporation leaves its *quinta essentia*, Aristotle's fifth and purest element) and from the veins (through which water and serum reach it). The brain was seen as an organ of necessity, conceptualized as hollow because the vapors are refrigerated by it and from which the impure refuse, the *pituita*, is purged. This concept leaves Herophilus no choice: He is the first in history to propose that the soul resides in the *caves* of the brain.

The status of the Alexandrian School, flourishing from the third century B.C., with a library containing approximately 650,000 volumes, was such that the impact and consequences of Herophilus' postulate cannot be passed over lightly, even if one considers that Erasistratus appears to have had his doubts with respect to his senior's opinion on the seat of the soul. We must infer these doubts from the fact that Erasistratus postulated a relationship between the degree of cerebral cortical convolution, i.e., parenchyma, and animal intelligence; this he based upon his observation that fast cursorial animals, such as the deer, have more numerous and intricate cerebellar folia than slow ones. The Erasistrateans emphasized, perhaps out of sheer oedipal antipathy against the Herophilian School, the importance of tissue (yes, if not the cortex, then the meninges) for the soul's residence, which led to bitter strife between the two giants.

It should be kept in mind that Hellenic medicine was embedded in Attic culture, of which *Naturphilosophie* was a dominant feature. Even as early as the ninth century B.C., the Homeric songs contain hints of later humoral and pneuma doctrines. During the Natural Philosophers' epoch (600–450 B.C.), initiated by Pythagoras, it was Alkmeon who taught that health was to be based on the balance of the dry, the moist, the cold, and the warmth in the body, to which Empedokles of Agrigentum (495–435 B.C.) added the protochemical doctrine of the four elements—fire, water, earth, and air—and the theory of sensory perception. Leukippos and Demokritos of Abdera, on the basis of their atomistic-mechanistic *Weltanschauung*, founded protophysical thought in medicine, and Diogenes of Apollonia (450 B.C.) studied the anatomy of blood vessels. The theurgic Asklepiades Schools of Kos, Knidos,and Sicily constituted the transition to the classic Hippokratic medicine, of which the basis was purely natural and not supernatural. It is no coincidence that this period (450–300 B.C.) witnessed Protagoras' doubt with respect to the existence of Gods ("man is the measure of all things"). In this period, humoral pathology ("dyscrasia") became firmly rooted as well as the πνευμα theory, which holds that in the φυσισ, the embedded warmth (το εμφυτον θερμον) of the heart influences metabolism by the action of inspired air. Under the influence of Aristotle's Nature Philosophy (384–322 B.C.), a nosological turn was taken on the basis of advances made in knowledge of hygiene, plants and drugs, and constitution.

Theophrastus Eresius (372–287 B.C.), Menon, and Mnesitheos of Athena were the leading physicians. Plato's idealistic doctrine together with Sokrates' teaching clearly separated body and soul, and prepared the Alexandrian blossoming that melted together sceptic, Hellenic, Western, and Eastern elements of medicine, with the founding of large libraries under the rulers of Pergamon and the Ptolemeans.

Gradually, the vaporous humoral pathology was abandoned in favor of the solidity pathology, which stressed the significance of the solid parts (walls of the pores) of the body, as is evident by the writings of the Methodists Themison of Laodicea (± 50 B.C.), Cornelius Celsus, Thessalos of Tralles, Plinius Senior [24–79 A.D., "The brain is the citadel of sense-perception, the crowning pinnacle, the seat of government of the mind" (13)], and Soranos, the colleagues who were the progenitors of Asklepiadic medicine in Rome (14). On the Roman scene, the humoral and solidity pathologies were subsequently abandoned for the pneumatic doctrine (Athenaios from Attaleia during the reign of Emperor Claudius), culminating in the work of Galen of Pergamum (129–199 A.D.) during the reigns of Emperor Antoninus Pius (138–161 A.D.) and Marcus Aurelius (161–180 A.D.). The preoccupation with the pneumatic doctrine explains why Galen attributed the *soul functions to the cerebral parenchyma, while locating the pneuma in the cerebral ventricles.*

Hellenic medicine bifurcated to Rome (Asklepiadic Schools in Sicily) and Alexandria, where Plato's philosophy became a dominant root, and to Antioch, where the Aristotelian philosophy was dominant. This appears to be an important (if incomplete) dichotomy in view of later developments.

The latent equivocality of the parenchymal versus ventricular cerebral residence of the soul constitutes a *pendant* of the two avenues of thought that determine the maze of streets and (blind) alleys that pattern the philosophical and religious deliberations on the *commercium animae cum corpore*: (a) the Platonic immortal soul temporarily receiving board and lodging in the prison of the mortal brain; and (b) the Aristotelian soul residing in the heart and perishing with it. These two irreconcilable concepts flared up again in medieval scholasticism one and a half millennia later.

The Christian religion spread within the Roman Empire, and in its neonatal stages, it met with the Platonic thesis of the immortal soul imprisoned in the mortal body. The second and third century Gnosticism flourished on the premise that man, part of God (μοῖρα Θεοῦ), after the Fall remains essentially able to move under his own steam toward his Creator: The Christian belief (πιστισ) and intellectual knowledge (γνωσισ) can be united. The Platonic philosophy, handed down by such men as Plotinus, Poseidonius, and Proclus, became partly known in the occidental world and remained there, if latent, during the Dark and Iron Ages following the decline of the western Roman Empire; for example, Plato's *Timaeus*, *Alcibiades*, and perhaps *Meno* were known. Although Aristotelian tripartite soul functions conformed elegantly with the divisions of the temple (*vestibulum*, *consistorium*, and *apotheca*), Christian religion vouchsafed the viability of Platonic concepts over those of the Stagyrite in the patristic and early medieval ages.

In the Levantine part of the Roman Empire, Byzantium, the study of Greek philosophy and medicine was granted some repose. Following Saracen conquests, the Hellenic treasure was translated under the aegis of the Baghdad caliphs and spread, with Islam, eastward to Persia and westward to Egypt, North Africa, and Spain. Aristotelian philosophy was compiled (if not altogether meticulously commented upon) by the Arabian philosophers and physicians Al-Kindi, Al-Gazali, Al-Farabi, Ibn Roschd (Averroës), Al-Razi (Rhazes), and Ibn-Sina (Avicenna). Charles Martel overcame the Moors at the battle of Poitiers (732 A.D.), and the Carolingian Renaissance of the ninth century was not an accidental sequel. Culturally,

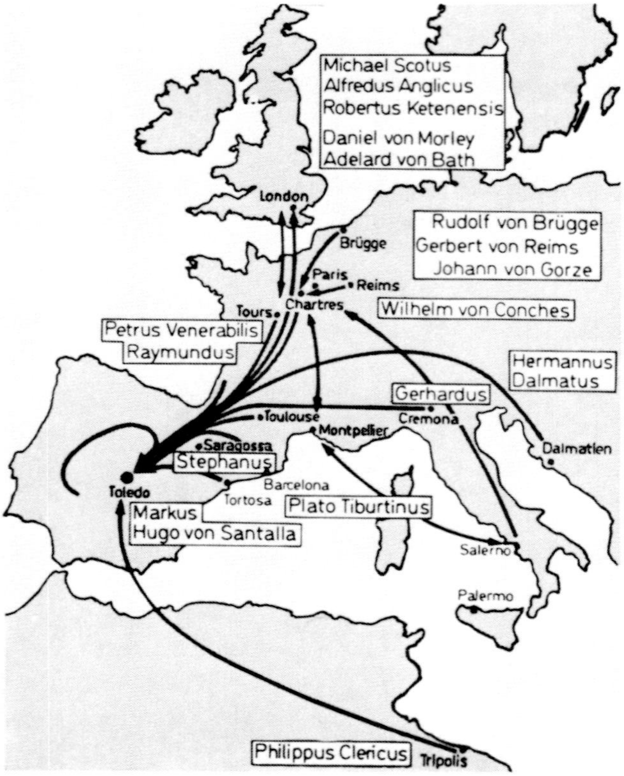

FIG. 2. Spread of Hellenic medicine and philosophy with the Moors. [From Schipperges, H. (1976): *Arabische Medizin im Lateinischen Mittelalter*, Springer, Berlin, with permission.]

barbaric Europe came into contact with the lavish riches of the Moors in Spain and with the cultural treasures (often translated by Jews) of Hellenic antiquity. Without the Moors, Western Europe would not at that time have inherited the fruits of Hellenic civilization. The Renaissance of the 12th century, known by such features as the Crusades, urbanization, the switch from Roman to Gothic, revival of Latin classics, and birth of vernacular prose, received a decisive impetus from the influx of Arabic-Aristotelian rationalism and metaphysics (15–17). The firm and broad base of the Hellenic third pillar was added to the Judeo-Christian and Latin-Roman pillars of subsequent Western civilization in the 12th and 13th centuries A.D., thanks to the instrumental Moors, who stayed in southern Spain. Medieval scholasticism as a rationalistic method cannot be fully appreciated if the Western indebtedness to the Arabic world is not recognized (Fig. 2).

> Hanc habet sensus arcem . . . , hoc culmen altissimum, hic mentis est regimen.
> *Plinius Senior (10)*

Questions concerning the soul in particular preoccupied the Christian mind *ab ovo*. In the patristic era (the first three or four centuries A.D.), both the Stoic distinction between soma, nous (=pneuma), and psyche (soul), and the Gnostic elements of man's capacity to acquire

M E D I E V A L   E N C Y C L O P Æ D I S M

1100/25	HONORIUS AUGUSTODENSIS	De Imagine Mundi	platonic christian
1125/35	GUILLAUME DE CONCHES	De Philosophia Mundi	platonic christian
1145	" "	Dragmaticon Philosophiae	
1150	ALEXANDER NECKAM	De Naturis Rerum	
1159	JEAN DE SALISBURY	Policraticus	humanistic christian
± 1175	RAOUL DE LONGCHAMP	Summa Philosophiae	1st Aristotelic infl.
1211	GERVAIS DE TILBURY	Otia Imperialia	
1235	BARTHÉLEMY DE GLANVILLE	De rerum proprietat.bs	
1240	PHILIPPE DE VITRY?	Compendium Philosophiae	Aristotelian Exhaustive
± 1250	VINCENT DE BEAUVAIS	Speculum Naturale	Dominican
1266/7	ROGER BACON	Opus Maius	

FIG. 3. Medieval Encyclopedists and their main Opera.

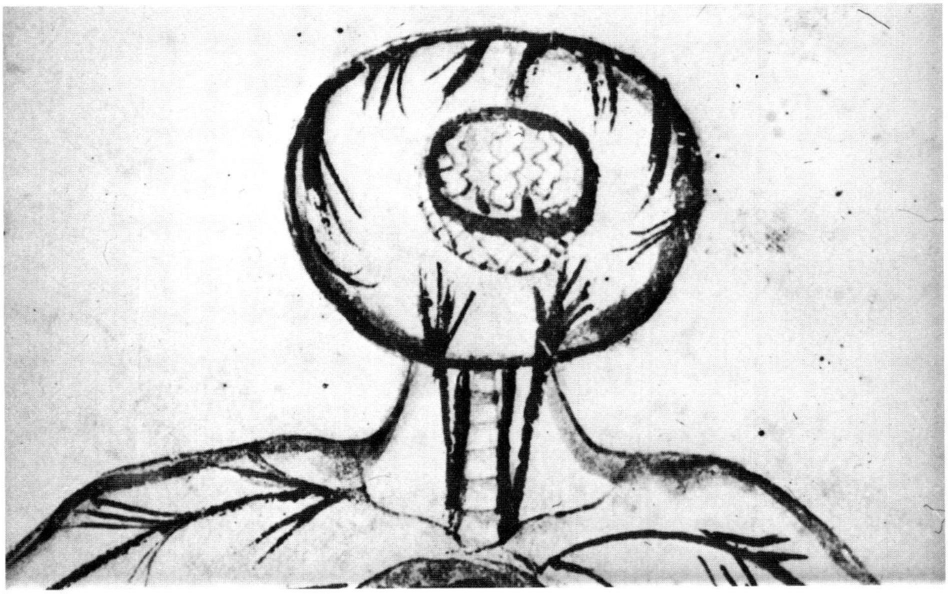

FIG. 4. Öffentl. Biblioth. Universität Basel, Ms. DII, 11, fol. 170r, written ca. 1250 A.D. in the provençal tongue of the Langue d'Oc, textually derived from Salernitan teaching, referring to Aristotle. The pertinent text (lines 116ff) states that the brain has three chambers: the first is called imaginativa, the second logistica, and the third memoria.

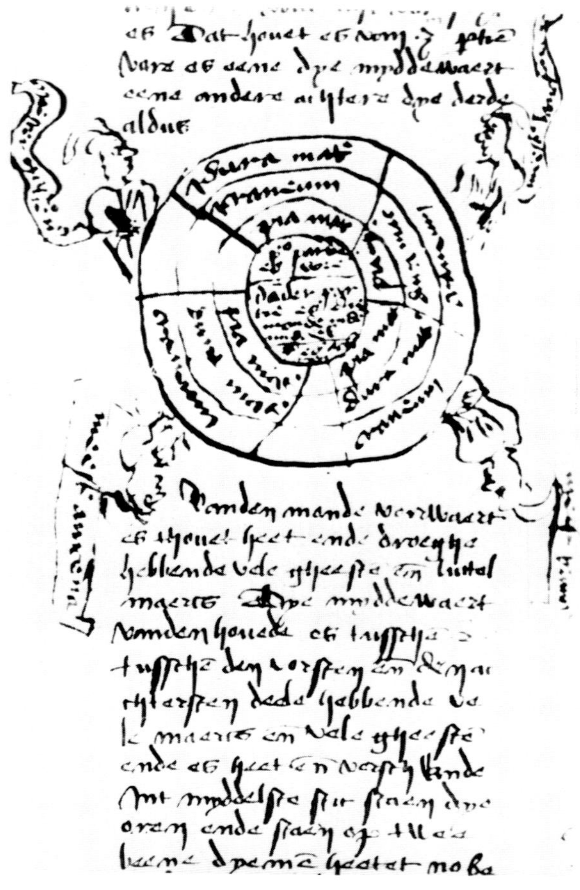

FIG. 5. Univ. Library Gent, Ms. 1273, title: "Cyrurgie" by Meester Jan Yperman, 1328 A.D., fol. 3ᵛ. Jan Yperman was born at Yperen in 1275, studied with Lanfranc in Paris, from 1297 to 1303, returned to Yperen as practicing physician, and died there ca. 1330. The head shows the cranium, dura mater, pia mater, with the brain divided schematically into three horizontal parts, "cells," in which from above downward is written: "prima partie es vore, dander partie es die monde in den middel, tertia es achter," meaning "the first part is in front, the other part is the mouth in the middle, the third is behind." The figurines surrounding the illustration are Meester (= Magister) Galen, Avicenna, Lanfranc and Bruun (= Bruno de Longoburno). The Flemish text (written out *in extenso* by van Leersum, Leiden, 1912) states that the forward part contains the knowledge (cognitiva) as well as visus, gustus, and olfactus; in the middle part reasoning and hearing, surrounded by thinking; and it the hinder part memory: "thus say Rogerus and Roelandinus in Latin": "in prima cellula sit ymago, in media ratio, in posteriori memoria". (Roger and his pupil Rolando, both of the Salerno School, were independent of influences of Constantinus Africanus; their work appeared ca. 1180–1220).

a certain measure of knowledge of God were fairly common money (cf. Romans 1:19–21; I Thessalon. 5:23; Proverbs 1:5–9). The early church fathers, notably those of the active Christian community at Alexandria, who were well versed in Greek philosophy, were hard put to marry the Stoic and the Pauline teaching of the immortal soul with Aristotelian teaching. The απολογεισϑαι of antiquity (meeting the Gnosis) and of the Middle Ages had to reconcile the "reasons of the heart which Reason knoweth not" with reason itself.

Here I submit my thesis that Christianity's stroke of Gordian genius came to bear: The Christian doctrine contains an Aristotelian element, i.e., the soul is an essential part of the

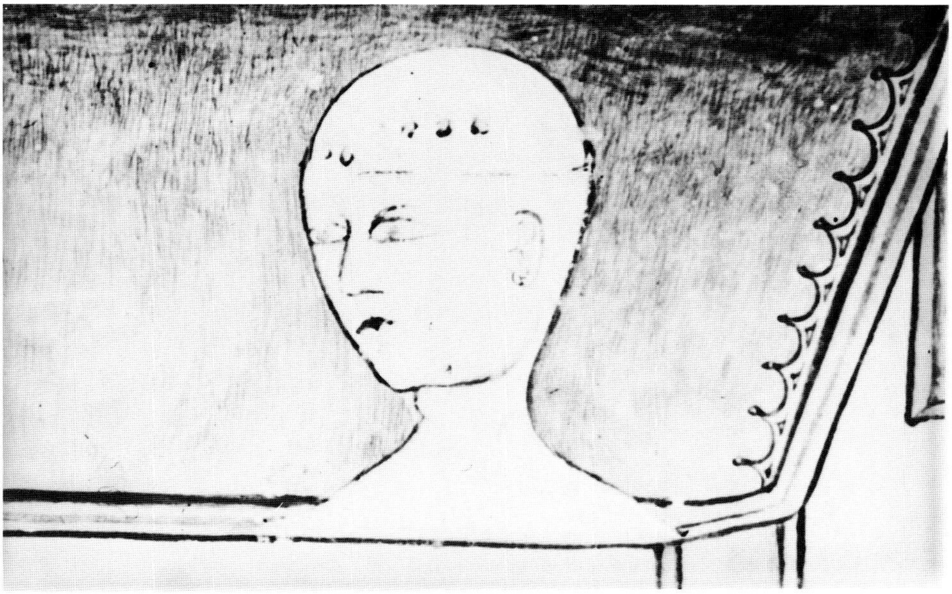

FIG. 6. Librairie Chateau de Chantilly, Musée Condé nr. (334) 560, an "Anatomy" of Guido de Papia, better known as Guido de Vigevano, Vigevano being a small Lombardian town belonging to the diocese of Pavia. Guido was physician to Queen Jeanne de Bourgogne and of the French King Philippe VI de Valois. This work was written in 1345 A.D., mainly based upon Galen and Avicenna.

human nature as is the body, and the two, substantially united, will perish but ultimately be resurrected,[1] thereby acquiring immortality, satisfying and transcending Plato's element.

It is worthwhile to mention here Bishop Nemesios Emesenus (340–396? A.D.). Knowledge of his work *Premnon Physikon* (περι φυσεωφ ανθρωπον) (18) was a medieval must. Although a Christian and a Platonist, he accepted the doctrine of the Aristotelian elements and qualities and postulated that the soul possesses three faculties: *imaginativa* (irrational), *memorativa* (retains and reproduces the recollections), and the cognitive *intellectus*. In particular, Nemesios Emesenus stated that the anterior cerebral ventricle contains the instruments of *imaginativa*, the five senses, and the *spiritus animalis*, that reason (το διανοητικόν) is in the middle ventricle, and that *memorativa* resides in the posterior ventricle, a lesion of which entails loss of memory. Nemesios is not quite consistent, however; in the third chapter ("On the union of body and soul") of his book, he stated that the soul cannot be localized or contained in any specific place. St. Augustine maintained essentially the same thesis, lending it all the weight of his authority. Nemesios' influence thus reached the Middle Ages through St. Augustine, having both Costa ben Luca (Constabulus), and Constantinus Africanus (± 1050) as intermediaries for scholastic medieval anthropology.

Oreibasios of Pergamon (325–403 A.D.) went a step further in stating that both anterior ventricles see to the respiration of the brain and cook up the πνευμα ψυχικον, excreting

[1]My friend, Prof. F. F. Blok from Amsterdam, pointed out to me that, in spite of the fact that any idea of spiritualization of Man was foreign to the Jews of the Old Testament holding on (like the Sadducaeans) to the Torah, the idea of Resurrection spread from the Babylonian Exile to become common coin at the time of Christ (cf. Job 19:25,26; Ezech. 37:1–4; Dan. 12:2; 2 Maccab. 7:11,14; 2 Maccab. 12:39–46).

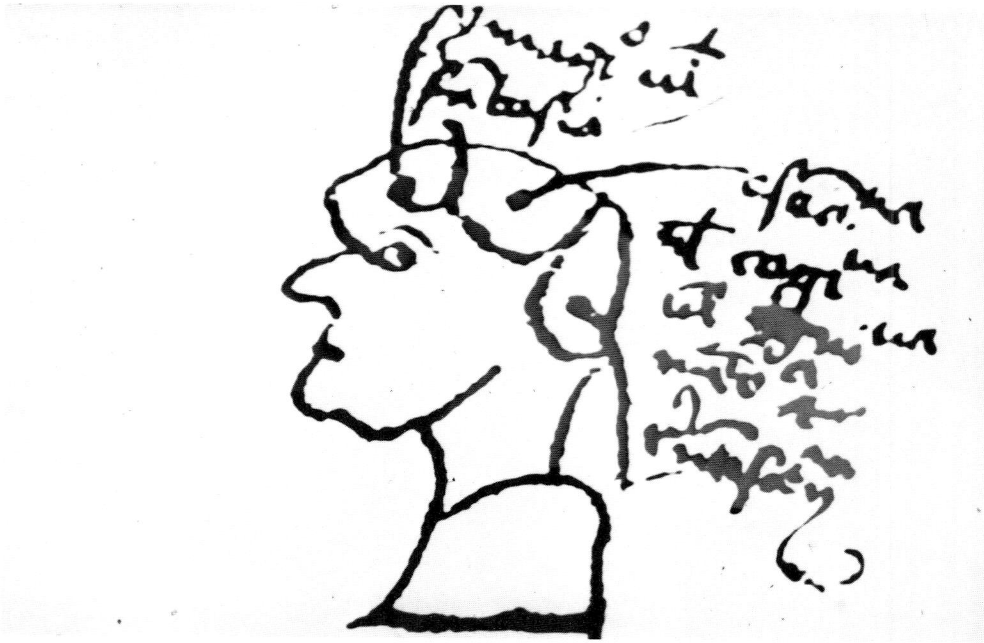

FIG. 7. Bayer. Statsbiblioth., Cod. Lat. Monacensis 73, ca. 1413 A.D. A crude sketch on the frontispiece of a "Liber Doctoris Hartmanni Schedel" of Nuremberg, written by the Viennese Prof. Martin Guldeln. The diagram of a triad of "cells" states: "ymaginatio vel fantasia, aestimativa vel cogitativa, memorativa vel reminiscentia."

this down the line to the other ventricles. The bishop Poseidonius of Epirus in Byzantium (350–420 A.D.) localized phantasy in the anterior part of the brain, reason in the middle ventricle, and memory in the posterior part of the brain (19,20).

The intriguing problem of the medieval concept of ventricular residence of mental faculties, such as expertly studied by Pagel (21), is, under this tissue versus cavity ambiguity, illuminated by the fact that the Aristotelian "line" of philosophy adheres to attributing the divine and immortal soul to the cerebral parenchyma.

This explicitly follows from Galen's passus (22 a,b,c) that the ventricles cannot be the seat of the soul (ϵγϵμονικὸν ψυχῆσ), although the soul's πρῶτον ὄργανον (= the pneuma) resides there. The soul's forces, according to Galen, are: φανταστικόν, διανοητικόν, and μνημονευτκον (22b), thus following Aristotle. His contemporary, the pagan Theodorus Macrobius, is of the same opinion that the soul inhabits the cerebral parenchyma, which produces the spirits that are excreted into the ventricles.

The Holy Aurelius Augustinus (345–430), only later in life converting to Christianity, remains nebulous; he attributes to parts of the brain certain mental faculties (23a) and, in his earlier work, he attributes senses, phantasy, and imagination to the anterior, rationality to the third, and memory to the posterior ventricles, or memory to the middle and motion to the posterior ventricle (23b).

With the passing of the centuries, a gradual simplification (or choice) seems to crystallize in favor of a ventricular habitat of the soul. The monk Johannes Damaskenos (756 A.D.), not to be confused with Janus Damascenus (= Mesuë Sr.), localized phantasy in the anterior

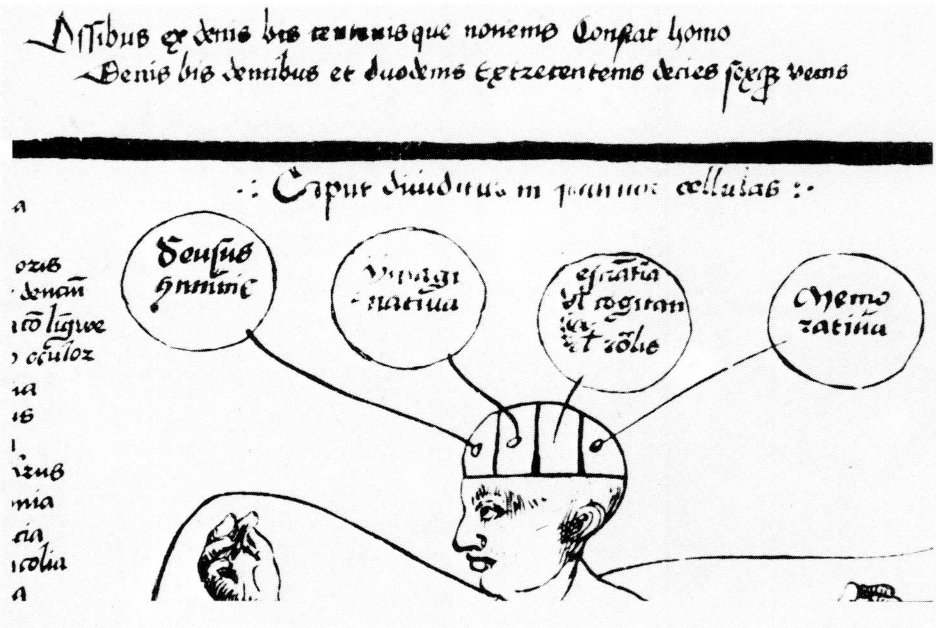

FIG. 8. Example of four-cell doctrine. Ms. 84b, 2°, folio 5r, Kongelige Bibliothek, København, a "Ketham" Ms. of ca. 1491. A facsimile was made by R. Nier, Milano, 1924 (plate 13). The text above the disease-man states: "Caput dividitur in quattuor cellulas: (in the four circles) sensus communis; ymaginativa; aestimativa vel cogitativa vel rationalis; memorativa."

ventricle and διανοητικόν (the πνευμα ψυχικον itself) in the middle, and mnemoneutikon in the posterior ventricle (24).

Constabulus (864–923 A.D.) (25), also known as Costa ben Luca, explicitly stated that intelligence, cogitation, cognition, and providence are executed by the spirit that is in the ventricles and operates the five senses: "*. . . et cum his operator, quem Graeci phantasiam vocant, et quod spiritus, qui est in ventriculo medio, operatur cogitationem et cognitionem atque providentiam, et spiritus, qui est in posteriori ventriculo, operatur memoriam et motum.*"

It would appear that pagan and Arabic-Aristotelian rationalistic philosophy, which did not fully reach the Occident before approximately 1150 A.D., opts for localization in the cerebral tissue, and that Christian/Neoplatonic thought would favor the ventricles as the soul's residence.

Major determinants for 12th- and 13th-century medieval thought, next to Nemesios, whose works were often wrongly assumed as having been written by Gregory of Nyssa, were the following early encyclopedic sources: Flavius Magnus Aurelius Cassiodorus (485–575 A.D.) from Calabria; Isidorus of Sevilla (565–636 A.D.), for whom the supernatural was more real and substantial than the evidence of the senses and whose iron logic presaged the fight between Universals and Nominals, and finally, the *Corpus Areopagiticum of Pseudo-Dionysios*, translated by Johannus Scotus Eriugena (810–860).

Scholasticism testifies to the attempts of the Ratio to systematically account for the irrational, even absurd, matters of religious revelation. This basic issue remained unchanged,

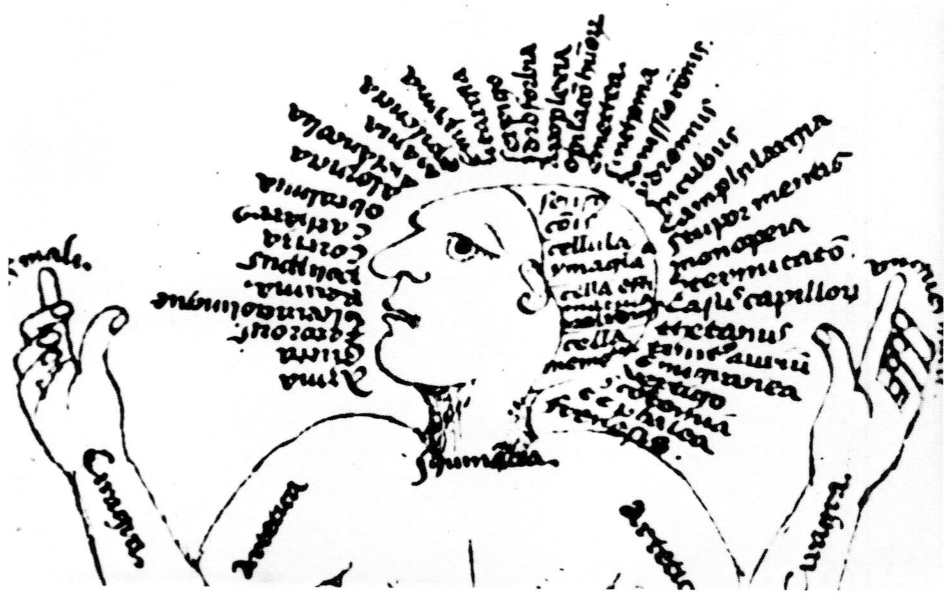

FIG. 9. Another four-cell doctrine example, from a "Ketham" Ms., Biblioth. Nationale, Paris, Ms. Latinus, No. 11229, tabula IV. In the head, from frontal to occipital is written: (a) sensus communis, (b) cellula ymaginativa, (c) cella aestimativa rationis, and (d) cella memorativa.

from the "Credo quia absurdum," the "Credo ut intelligam," the "Fides quaerens intellectum," to the Faustian "Zwei Seelen wohnen, ach, in meiner Brust . . .". In the 12th- and 13th-century *Scholasticus*, this issue is crystallized in sharp, yes, acute, relief as rational systematic Aristotelian influx reaches Occidental shores. The 12th- and 13th-century Encyclopedists (Adelard of Bath, Guillaume de Conches, John of Salisbury, Alexander Neckam, Gervais of Tilbury, Vincent de Beauvois) in their "Specula," "Summae," and "De rerum . . . ," rigidly reiterate natural philosophical and medical concepts (Fig. 3).

The Latin feeder-line from St. Augustine and Boëthius and the Neoplatonic feeder-line from Plotinus-Porphyrius-pseudo-Dionysios end with St. Thomas Aquinas, whereas the systematic Aristotelian logic culminates via Poseidonius and Avicenna in Albertus Magnus. Medical concepts were governed by the religious and philosophical preemptions, notwithstanding the influx of Salernitan-Greco-Arabic medicine: (a) Jehan Hebes Mesuë Senior (Masawaih-al-Mardini) (777–837), Christian physician; (b) Johannes Damaskenos, the greatest Syrian theologist of the Greek Orthodox Church; (c) the superior intellectual Hunain-ibn-Ishaq (Johanitius, son of Isaac) (809–873), famous collector and translator of Greek into Arabic, the "Erasmus of Arabic Renaissance" and employee of the "Three Brothers," Bana Musa, sons of Musa ibn Shakir; (d) Constantinus Africanus of Salerno (ca. 1050), founder of Scholastic medicine, who was secretary of Robert Guiscard, duke of Salerno, and who became the major translator of Arabic medicine into Latin, localizing, like Galen, the soul in the parenchyma and the pneuma in the ventricles, and influencing Avicenna; (e) Costa ben Luca; (f) Bartholomaeus Anglicus (1240), "De Rerum proprietatibus"; and (g) the eminent Guy de Chauliac (1300–1368).

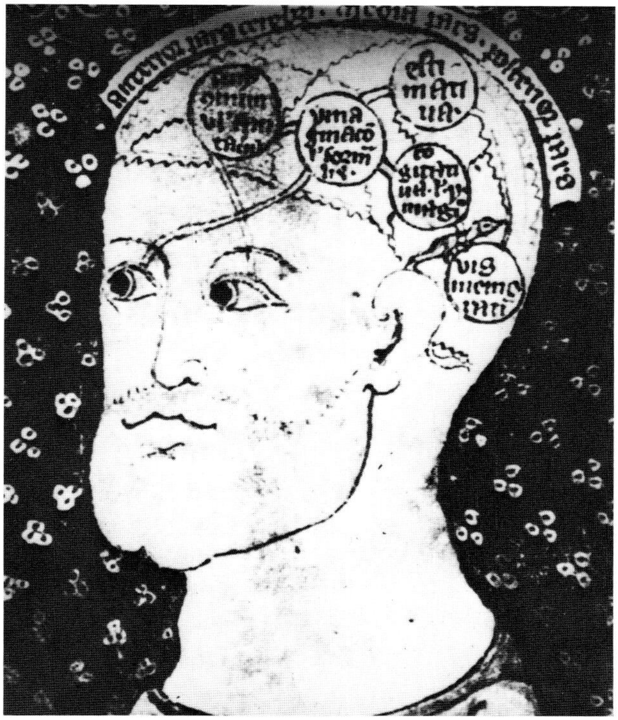

FIG. 10. Cambridge Univ. Libr. Ms. G.g.1, 1310 A.D., fol. 490^r–491^r. The extensive text is based on Galen's 8th book of *De usu partium*, with the addition by Costa ben Luca (864–923 A.D.) on the dynamic element of the vermis (worm) between the fourth and fifth cell. The text above the head mentions three *parts* (anterior pars cerebri, media pars, posterior pars) of the *brain*, but the five cells are prominent, with the worm between the cogitativa vel ymaginativa and the vis memorativa.

The iron systematic of the medieval age, caught in its own rigid corset of rational method, reiterated Nemesios', Poseidonius', and Oreibasios' concept of ventricular residence of the mental faculties, as is evidenced by Sudhoff's fundamental paper (26).

As has been argued convincingly by Leyacker (27), the medieval localization theory of the soul's powers (ψυχικαι δυναμεισ) in the brain cavities appears to be built upon Galen's teachings. This, however, with the qualifications that (a) both Nemesios' and Poseidonius' statements rest on Porphyrius' *Timaeus* commentary and do not directly derive from Galen; (b) Porphyrius amalgamated Galenic and Poseidonian doctrine and is to be regarded as the real initiating *auctor intellectualis* of the ventricular residence of the soul; (c) St. Augustine's teaching, which places in the last ventricle *motus* (motiva) instead of the dianoetikon, rests, via Marius Victorinus, upon the *Origines*; (4) the mystic Hugo of St. Victor (1096–1141) of the Parisian Abbey clearly confounded the Nemesian-Poseidonian and the Augustinian opinions as to the localization by putting memory where *motus* had its place; (5) the localization theory shows an Eastern mode of empirical tradition (Porphyrius, Nemesios, Gregory of Nyssa, Basileios) and a Latin-Western mode (*Origines*, St. Augustine).

It was mainly Constantinus Africanus from the Salernitan School, who mediated by way of his translations of the Arabic sources these views in the 11th century to the Western medieval Encyclopedists for further vulgarization (28). This influence was augmented by

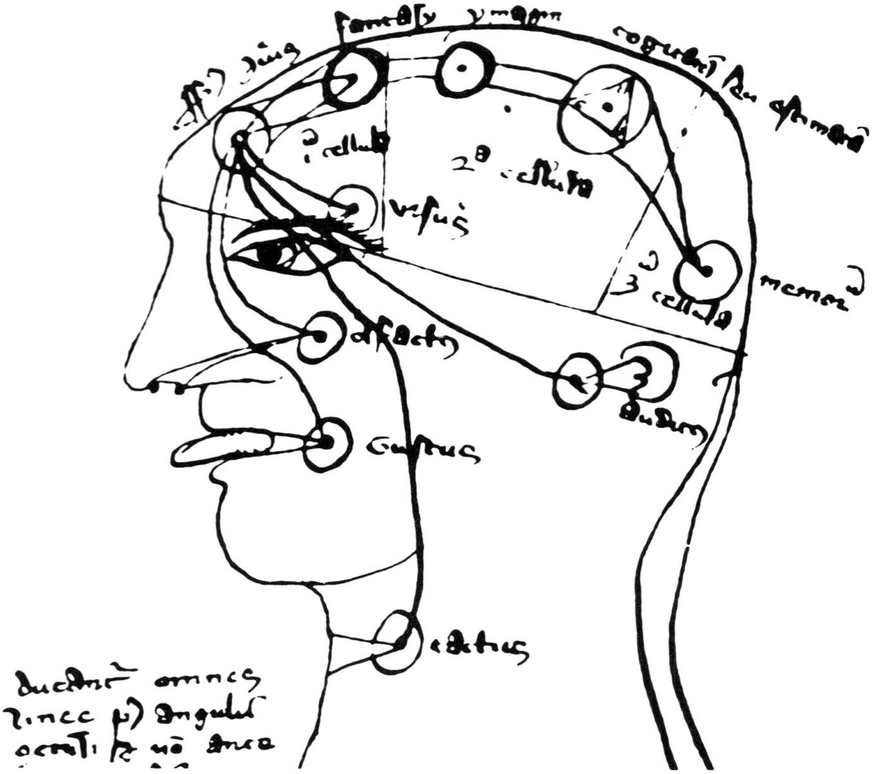

FIG. 11. Bayerische Statsbibl., Munich, Codes Lat. 527, fol. 64ᵛ. A treatise by Avicenna, on the anatomy of the head for physicians. The head contains three cellulae and five encircled faculties: sensus communis, fantasy, imaginativa, cogitativa seu estimativa, and memorativa.

the identical views of the Baghdad physician Al-Gazzali (1059–1111), the Spaniard Ibn-Zuhr (Avenzoar, ca. 1162) in his "Al-Teisir" (29), and Ibn-Roshd (Averroës, 1126–1198) in his "Canon" and "Colliget" (30). It was at the Chartres School that Guillaume de Conches (1080–1150) developed the thesis further, stating that vision and phantasy are in the dry and warm first ventricle, logic and discerning *ratio* in the warm and moist middle ventricle, and memory in the dry and cool posterior ventricle, and that things well defined by logic are transferred through the foramen to memory: *"Ergo antiqui merito discebant in capite esse sedem sapientiae. . . ."* The idea was clinched by Richard of Salerno (1130–1180) and, ultimately, as far as the 15th century, by the "Universal Mind and Aristoteles of the Middle Ages," Albertus Magnus, who, *in professo*, refers to Costa ben Luca, while St. Thomas Aquinas refers to Avicenna. Albertus Magnus, epitomizing late medieval anthropology, localized, in his *Philosophia Naturalis*, the *sensus communis* and *vis* (virtus) *imaginativa* in the first two ventricles, the *vires extimativa, imaginativa, cogitativa*, and *formativa* in the middle, and the *vis memorativa* and *membrorum motiva* (the Aristotelian element) in the posterior ventricle.

Scholastic anthropology came to a head when most of Aristotle's works (part of which had been transmitted by Boëthius) reached the Occident in the final third of the 12th century, to be followed by the bulk of the work by Plato and the Neoplatonists in the late 13th century

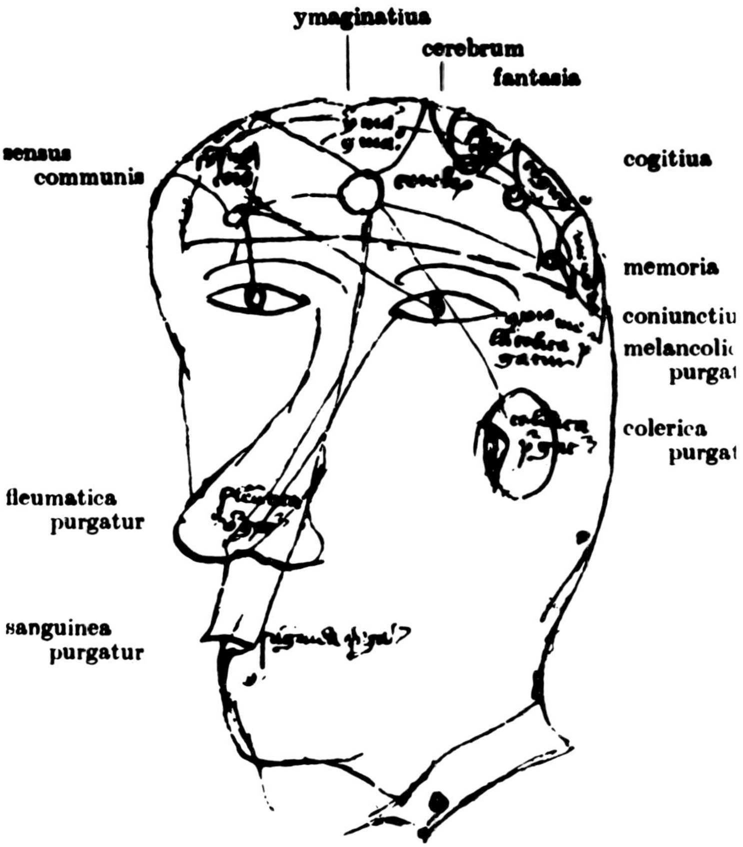

FIG. 12. British Museum, Ms. Sloane 2156, fol. 11^r. An "Anathomia of Hieronymo Manfredi," based on Avicenna in Roger Bacon's "De Scientia Perspectiva," A.D. 1428. There are five faculties or cells (and no tripartite brain cells) called sensus communis, ymaginativa, fantasia, cogitativa, and memoria.

through Willem van Moerbeke's translations of Proclus (31). Although the Latin heritage was such that one customarily distinguishes in these ages an *Aetas Ovidiana*, an *Aetas Horatiana*, and an *Aetas Vergiliana*, the indebtedness of the West for its "12th century Renaissance" to the Arabic-mediating influx of Hellenic philosophy cannot be passed over lightly.

Gradually, a cellular doctrine of psychical function, not of brain function, emerged. Those writers, who interpret the medieval doctrine of the *virtus animae* as a doctrine of cerebral physiology or of cerebral ventricular physiology, project their modern bias into an epoch of which the *Zeitgeist* was dominated by the ecclesia. Christianity inculcated the medieval community not only with an ontological basis of the Universe (God as Being), with the notion of man as a creature of the Creator, of man as a *Homo Viator* in need of grace and salvation, but also with the powerful essence of the *potestas clavium* of *Matthew 18:18*—only via the ecclesia may man be saved from eternal perdition. The antinomy between the Christian and Greek philosophies, between reason and dominating, even terrorizing, faith, was the birth and death of scholasticism. For instance, when a triune Deity may correspond with Plato's triad of the soul (λογιστικον, ϑυμοειδεσ, and 'επιϑυμητικον), the brain

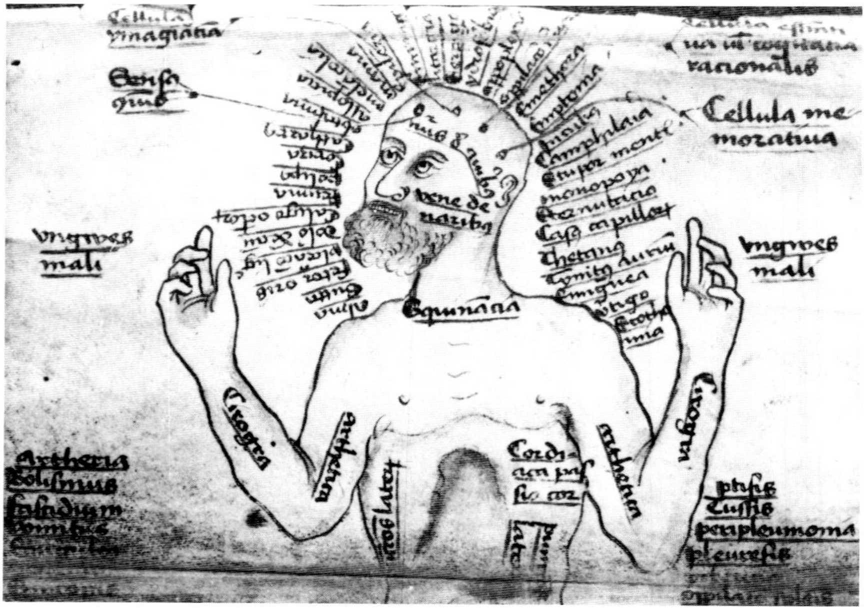

FIG. 13. Univ. Biblioth., Heidelberg, Codex Pal. Germ. 644, fol. 1, ca. 1430 A.D., a "Ketham"; a translation in German of an unknown exactatus latinus. The *four-celled* brain, from left to right, accomodates sensus communis; cellula imaginativa; cellula aestimativa vel cogitativa rationalis; and cellula memorativa.

doctrine finds its pictorial expression in tricellular fashion (Figs. 4–7). When more inner faculties were decided upon by the scholastic clerus as inner senses in addition to the sensorium commune, four or five cells are posed to accomodate them (Figs. 8–12).

In the Ketham manuscripts (e.g., Bodleian Library Ms. Canon Misc. 366, fol., 1ᵛ, ca. 1380 A.D. and the Heidelberg University Bibl., Codex Pat Germ. 644, fol. 2, ca. 1470 A.D.), the functions are allocated to cells: "memory cell," "cellula ymaginativa," etc. (Fig. 13). One of the most eloquent illustrations is found in the "Epitomata" of Gerardus de Harderwijk, where an illustration preceding the "De Sensu" contains, at the top of the page, left side, a four-celled brain (representing the teachings of Galen and Avicenna) and on the right side, a five-celled brain, said to derive from St. Thomas Aquinas and Albertus Magnus (Fig. 14). Anatomical concepts were dictated by the clergy. Schneider's monograph systematically deals with the confusion arising out of Averroëstic-Aristotelian determinants and Neoplatonic-Augustinian roots in Albertus Magnus' psychology (32). Roger Bacon, William of Saliceto, Lanfranc of Bec, Henry of Mondeville, Raymondo de Lucci ("Mondino"), Guy de Chauliac, and Guy de Vegevano, all rigidly and slavishly reiterate the systematic classification of the mental faculties and their ventricular allocations.

Sudhoff synthesized the confused matter in Table 1, modified by the present author in the knowledge that study of all original sources is certain to make further modification necessary.

The measure to which the subject of the seat of the soul in those days was alive among medical, theological, and philosophical savants, even as late as the 15th century, has recently been highlighted by the Leiden medievalist, Dr. J. R. Smeets, in his study on the final verses of François Villon, "Le Lais" (33):[2]

36. Ce faisant, je m'entroublié
non pas par force de vin boire
mon esperit comme lié;
Lors je sentis dame *mémoire*
reprendre et mettre en son aumoire
ses especes collateralles,
oppinative faulce et voire
et autres intellectualles
37. Et mesmement *l'estimative*
par quoy *prospective* nous vient
similative, *formative*,
desquelles souvent il advient
fol et lunatique par mois:
je l'ay leu, se bien m'en souvient
en *Aristote* aucunes fois
38. Dont le *sensitif* s'esveilla
es esvertua *Fantasie*
qui tous organes resveilla
et tint la souvraine partie.

Smeets argued that François Villon derived his data from Bartholomaeus Anglicus (34), who (erroneously) refers to Aristotle (35). Smeets also showed that the term "formative" is equivalent to "imaginative" by Vincentius of Beauvais (36), the medieval Encyclopedist indubitably known to this rogue-poet who lived close to the Sorbonne. The term "formative" is encountered as "formalis" in the Munich Codex Lat. 5961. The term "prospective" may have been used by Villon in poetic liberty on the basis of Constabulus' term "providentia," with which Villon must have been familiar. This leaves only the term "similative" to remain a *corpus alienum* within the medieval context. It may be a contraction for "assimilative," which conceptually conforms to *virtus incorporativa* found in the illustration of the Cod. Lat. Monac. 5961 (Fig. 15), of which the text refers to Avicenna and follows verbatim the text of the Cambridge Ms.0.25:40 (Fig 16). Smeets considered Villon's reference to Aristotle a tongue-in-cheek "espièglerie estudiante."

In the present writer's opinion, the alternative and at least equally feasible explanation may be forwarded, that Villon in the Plato-Aristotle controversy takes sides with Aristotle in this philosopher's postulate of the heart's primacy: The κηρυγμα that the bell of the Sorbonne's chapel foretells each evening at 9 o'clock makes him "prier comme le *coeur* dit," and, focusing in prayer on his soul's relation with its Creator, memory ("les neiges d'antan . . .") aids in this act by excluding all things of the common senses, phantasy, ratiocination, and logic. Being a poet well past the age of 50, Villon now yields the realm of reason's disputes to the serenity of memory's prayer. Is it coincidence that he termed these verses "Le Lais," i.e., the denuded terrain the sea, upon its retiring, yields to the "domaine public"?

[2]The author has italicized certain words in François Villon's poem.

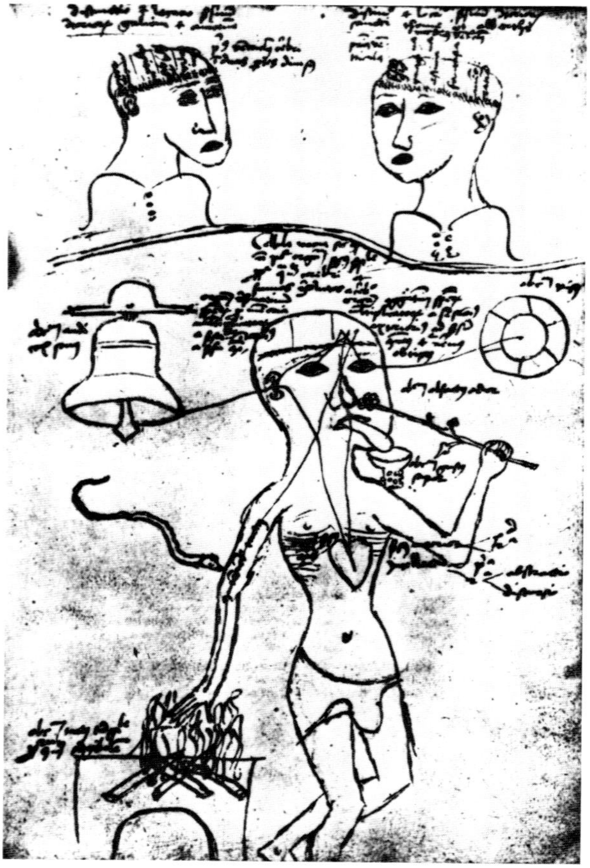

FIG. 14. Wellcome Historical Museum, Library. Illustration on blank leaf (KKb) in copy of Gerard de Harderwijck's "Epitomata seu reparationis totius philosphia naturalis Aristotelis," 1496 A.D. The Aristotelian *heart* figures prominently. At top left, a *four-celled* head (description according to Galen and Avicenna); at top right, a *five-celled* head (description according to Thomas Aquinas and Albertus Magnus). In the heads is written: *left*, fantasia, sens. comm., cogitativa, and memorativa; *right*, sens. comm., ymaginativa, estimativa, fantasia, and memorativa.

If one turns from literature to psychiatry, it should cause no wonder that amentia, mania, melancholy, phrenesis, sleep, and vigilance are explained on the frame of this scholastic conception of the soul's seat and the pneumatic theory of natural, vital, and animal spirits. The Salernitan school (40) teaches that phrenesis is due to a warm *apostema* (swelling) of the anterior cellula migrated to the meninges. Constantinus Africanus, Arnaldus of Villanova, and Bartholomeus the Englishman postulate that mania is localized in the anterior and melancholy in the middle ventricle and that mania essentially is a poisoning or infection of the anterior cellula, with loss of imagination, just as melancholy is caused by depression of the middle cellula with loss of the *ratio*. Mania and melancholy are diseases of the brain leading to *disturbatio* or *corruptio* of the *imaginatio* or *estimatio* [H. H. Beek, 1969 (41)].

I submit the thesis (which may explain the apparent confusion with respect to tri-, quarto-, or quintapartite brain cells) that in the late medieval era the brain cells are not conceptually identical with brain ventricles. Not only did the clerus experience difficulties in reconciling

TABLE 1.

	I. cellula	II. cellula	III. cellula
Posidonios	φανταστικον	λογιστικον	μνημονευτικον
Nemesios	αισθησις	διανοητικον	μνημονευτικον
Augustine	*sensus communis phantastica imaginaria*	*rationalis*	*motus omnis*
Johannes Damaskenos	φανταστικον	διανοητικον	μνημονευτικον
Costa ben Luca	*sensus, phantasia*	*intellectus cogitatio providentia cognitio*	*memoria motus*
Razes	*imaginatio*	*cogitatio*	*memoria*
Haly Abbas	*phantasia*	*cogitatio*	*memoria*
The pure brothers	*phantasia*	*cogitatio*	*memoria*
Avicenna	*sensus communis phantasia*	*cogitativa imaginativa existimatio*	*conservativa memorialis*
Constantinus Africanus	*sensus phantasia*	*intellectus ratio*	*motus memoria*
Copho	*phantasia*	*ratio*	*memoria*
Adelard of Bath	*phantasia*	*ratio*	*memoria*
Avenzoar Averroës	*imaginativa*	*cogitativa extimativa*	*reminiscibilis conservativa*
Algazel	*sensus communis imaginativa*	*imaginativa cogitativa*	*aestimativa memoria*
Guillaume de Conches	*cellula phantastica*	*cellula logistica sive rationalis*	*cellula memorialis*
Richardus Salernitanus	*cellula phantastica, imaginatio*	*cellula logistica ratio*	*cellula memorialis memoria*
Albertus Magnus	*sensus communis, imaginatio, phantasia et estimativa*	*existamativa (imaginativa) cogitativa formativa*	*memorativa, virtus motiva*
Bartholom. Anglicus	*imaginatio*	*ratio*	*memoria, recordatio*
Thomas Aquinas	*sensus communis phantasia sive imaginatio*	*existimativa cogitativa*	*memorativa*
Ricardus Anglicus	*operationes sensibiles*	*ymaginationes cogitationes*	
William of Saliceto	*sensus communis phantasio imaginatio*	*cogitatio existimatio*	*memoria*
Lanfranc	*sensus communis ymaginativa phantasia*	*aestimativa*	*conservat. sententias pronuntiatas (memoria)*
Henri de Mondeville	*sensus communis ymaginativa*	*aestimativa*	*secreta thesaurizat (memoria)*
Mondino	*fantasia sensus communis imaginativa*	*cogitativa et rationalis*	*motiva memorativa*
Guy de Chauliac	*sensus communis imaginativa*	*cogitativa et rationalis*	*conservativa, memorativa*
Guido de Vigevano de Pavia	*apresensiva fantastica*	*raciocinativa*	*memorativa*
Roger Bacon	*sensus communis imaginatio aestimatio*	*cogitativa logistica rationalis*	*memorativa*

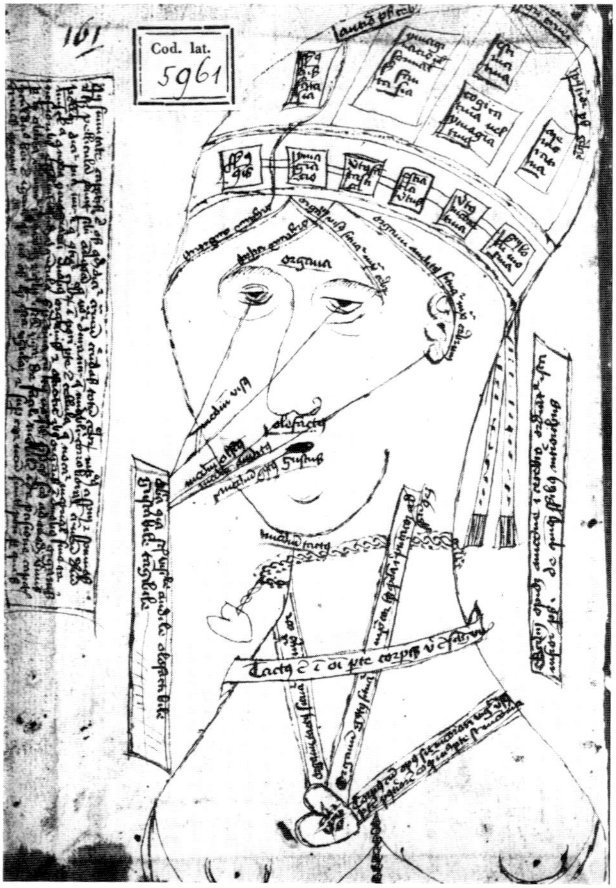

FIG. 15. Bayer. Statsbibl. München, Cod. Lat. Monac. 5961, 1441 A.D. Truly remarkable. Not a man is depicted, but a woman. The text is based on Aristotle and Avicenna (the heart is emphasized twice, and is said to constitute the sensory center; the heart is connected with touch and taste. The three parts of the brain show four divisions with five different faculties (sens. comm., fant., ymaginativa vel formalis, estimativa, cogitativa, memorativa), among which in a series of quadrangles from left to right are listed sens. comm., ymag., virtus phant., estimativa virtus, *virtus incorporativa*, and secundam locum motiva.

authoritative pagan (Greek and Arabic) philosophy with the Christian teaching, not only were they hampered by their medical-anatomical incompetence, but the prevalent medical data mainly derived from Galen and Avicenna were not inherently consistent.

Galen was too much of a medical pragmatist to allow philosophical consideration to tie him down. His text (27) leaves room for equivocal interpretations: The pneuma psychicon, the πρῶτον ὄργαυον of the soul, fills the ventricles, but it also pervades the σῶμα τοῦ 'εγκεθαλου. The Codex Augustanis 42 of the Library at Wolfenbüttel, an *Anathomia Mundini* of Padua ("factus est in mense Januario A.D. 1315") contains an illustration of the soul's faculties on fol. 264^{v} with the telling legend, "Avicenna dissents from Galen and Aristotle" (Fig. 17).

In view of the importance of the subject to the scholastic mind, it is not unlikely, and highly probable that the soul's powers were not exclusively tied to the ventricles. At any rate, one cannot, without further qualifications, equate the cellulae with the ventricles.

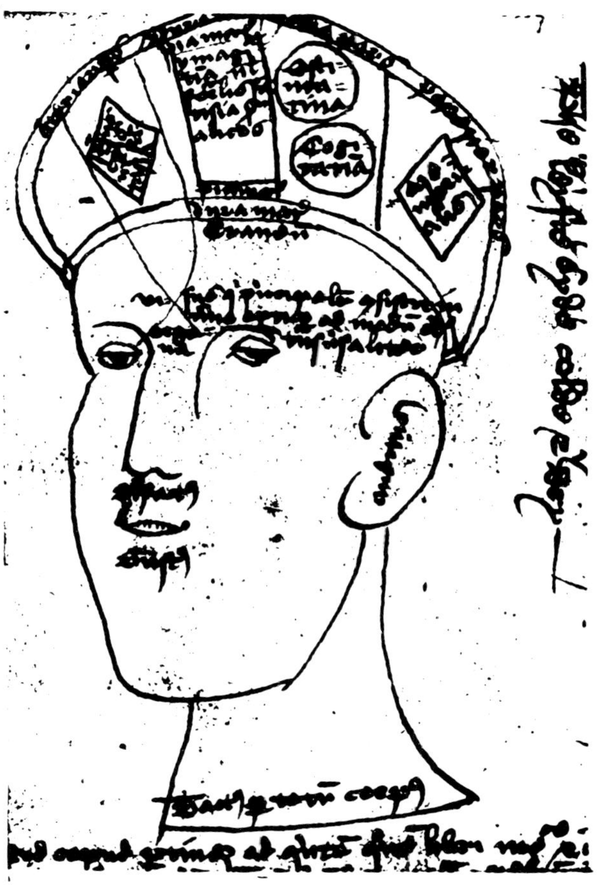

FIG. 16. Cambridge Univ. Libr. Ms. 0.2.40, fol. 57v, 1410 A.D. The medieval English text to the right of the head needs no comment. Based on Avicenna, there are depicted five cells or compartments (sens. comm. vel fant.; ymag. vel formalis, front. secundo Avicenna; estimativa; cogitat.; memorialis).

Theodorus Macrobius and Johannes Damaskenos appear quite explicit on this point, and it is apparently only Constabulus who explicitly accords the spirits, operating the faculties, a ventricular domicile. This view is reflected by the illustration of fol. 1v of Ms. Canon Misc. 366, written ca. 1390 A.D. (Oxonian Bodleian Library), which shows a *quinta*partite division of mental faculties, a *quarto*partite ventricular system, and a *tri*partite division of the brain (Fig. 18). The same is illustrated in the Cod. Lat. 5961 (ca. 1440 A.D.) of the Munich Bayerische Statsbibliothek, postulating a *quarto*partite division of the seat of the soul and a *tri*partite brain division. Dürer also illustrated these divisions (Fig. 19).

Over two millenia, the question of the seat of the soul has intrigued thinking man. Stratos of Lampsakos placed the soul between the eyebrows (37). Shakespeare echoed the opinion of Erasistratus (who oscillated between the meninges and the cortex as tissues of choice to house intelligence) when, in *Love's Labour Lost*, Act 4, Scene 2, he has Holofernes state that ideas are nourished in the womb of the "pia mater," and when, in *Troilus and Cressida*, Act 2, Scene 1, he puts the pejorative remark about Ajax in Thersites' mouth: "his pia mater

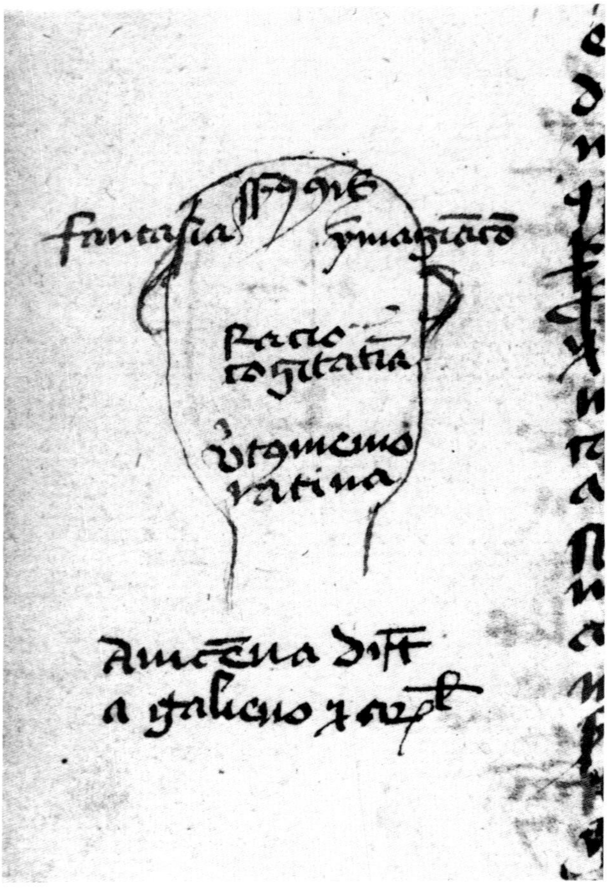

FIG. 17. Herzogl. Bibl. Wolfenbüttel; Codex Guelf 42 (Cod. August. 42), fol. 264^{r}, an "Anathomia Domini et Magistri Mundini" (=Mondino de Luzzi), 1315 A.D. The caption underneath stresses the divergence between Avicenna on one side and Galen and Aristotle on the other.

is not worth the ninth part of a sparrow." Sir Kenelm Digby preferred for the soul the septum pellucidum, Henry More placed the purer animal spirits in the fourth ventricle of the brain, the mystic alchemist Fludd accorded the soul a triad of places in the cerebrum (Fig. 20), and Descartes accorded the pineal gland the honor of housing the soul. With regard to his contemporaries, Thomas Willis allocated the *sensus communis* to the corpus striatum, the *imaginatio* to the corpus callosum, and memory to either cortex or corpus cinereum. Lancisi (1654–1720) placed the soul in the corpus callosum, von Haller (1708–1777) in the medulla oblongata, Vieussens (1641–1730) in both corpora striata, van Steenbergen in the centrum semiovale, and van Helmondt, running true to gourmet inclinations, in the stomach.

The Swedish mystic and philosopher Emanuel Swedenborg (38) housed the soul first in the cortex and subsequently in all cerebral parts (Figs. 21 and 22). The discoverer of the substantia nigra, Soemmering, as recently as 200 years ago, reverted to the revival of medieval times by voicing his conviction that the ventricular fluid is the immediate organ, the repository of the soul (39).

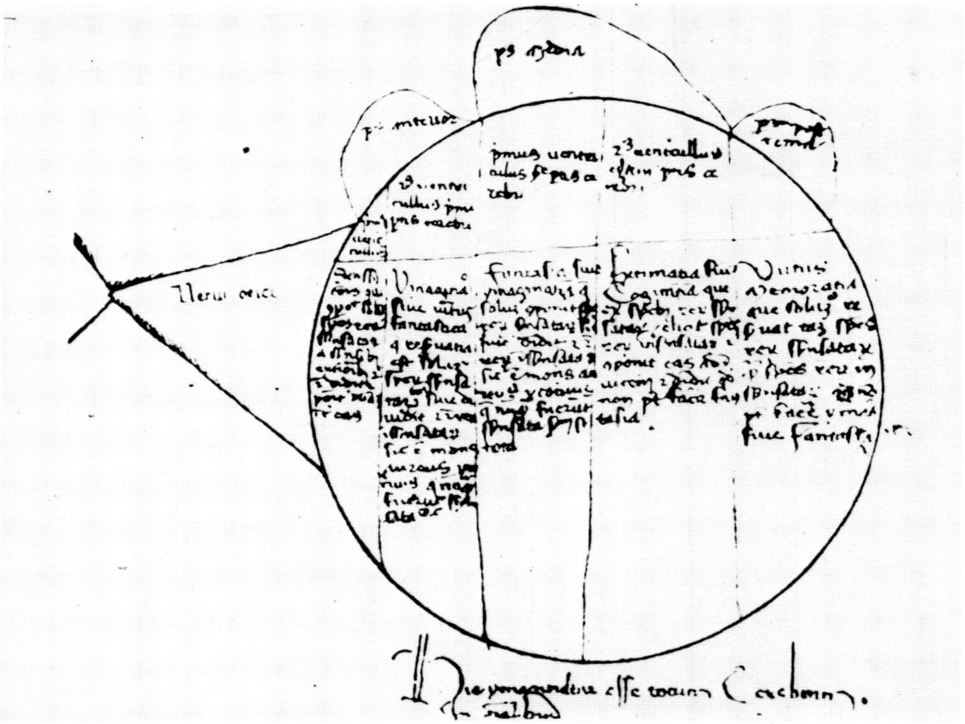

FIG. 18. Bodleian Libr. Ms. Canon. Misc. 366, fol. I, 1390 A.D. "Hic ymaginatur esse totum cerebrum in animalibus." The first part of the brain has two ventricles, so has the second part; the posterior part has one ventrical; a three part, five-celled brain.

The *commercium animae cum corpore* is not, however, any more a question of anatomy rigidly controlled by the clerus. It is a question of physiology insofar as the mental phenomena figure among the functions by which an organ, the living brain, manifests. In the natural sciences, a function stochastically describes the covariant changing relationship between entities, and as such, the neuropsychologist studies phenomena of energy transfer.

Cartesian conflict between *res cogitans* and *res extensa*, the two disparate platonic worlds that have nothing in common, has been destroyed, first by Kant, who showed the epistemological *a priori* parameters of time and space, then by Freud, who showed the activity of the "unconscious" mind (a conceptual *contradictio in terminis* for the scholastic), and ultimately by Einstein, who showed the Kantian *a priori*'s to be relative rather than absolute.

As a representative κατ'εξοχην of English neurology, Macdonald Critchley appears, if one peels off his many cloaks of artful actor, delicate diplomat, dignified doctor, lordly linguist, keen connoisseur, fastidious philosopher, and astute clinician, fundamentally as a physiologist, studying the fleeting phenomena of the Word.

In the beginning was the Word. The Logos is Critchley's fascination. Even its form of silent phrase, Gesture, has not escaped his attention, because precisely there, most delicately yet eloquently in soundless movement or posture, the mind-matter union is given expression.

Now it turns out that the various courses of what he called "The divine banquet of the brain," such as perception, cognition, emotion, and volition, need nectar for a full appre-

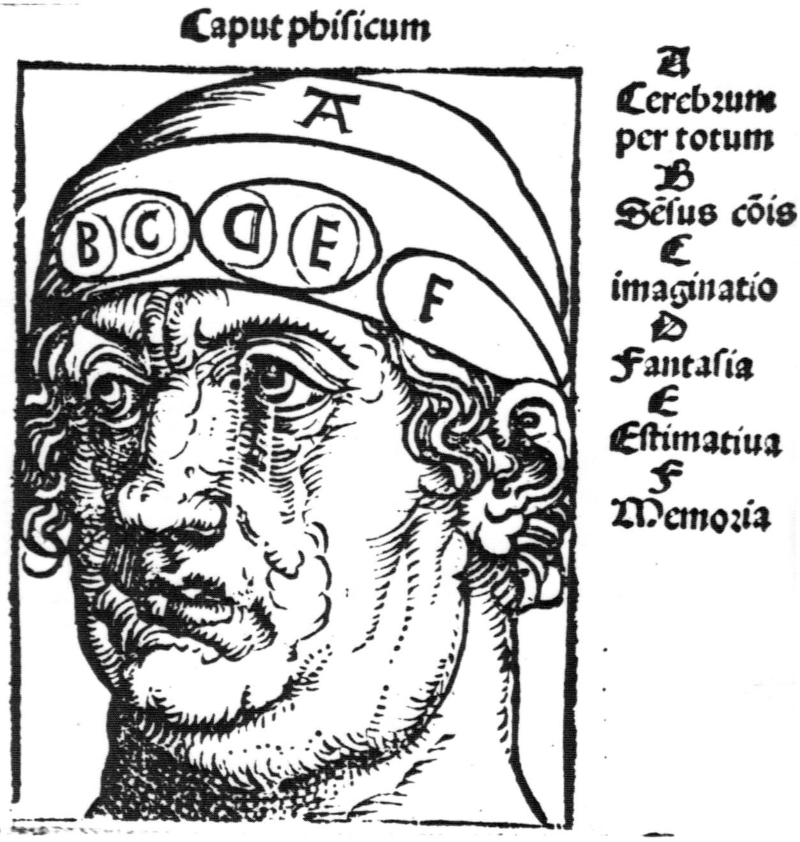

FIG. 19. Utrecht, Univ. Bibl., Ms. F-4^6.11^6, vol. 77^r, 1498 A. D., Ludovicus de Prussia "Trilogium Animae." Albrecht Dürer's friend Willibald Pirkheimer served as a model for this pearl of a woodcut by the artist, to illustrate the 17th chapter, "De potentiis apprehensivis animae."

ciation of the parenchymal solids. Should it not be therefore appropriate that Nature, at this Banquet, provides the CSF in elegantly shaped ventricular tumblers? Should it not be judged fair that recent work appears to rehabilitate the Ancients' conjectures by showing that the CSF transports a neuropeptide such as vasopressin to its proper sites as to enable an event to be consolidated in the "stores of memory"? Should not vasopressin be properly called the *vis memorativa*?

Would it—in view of the recent data on β- and γ-endorphins—be too farfetched to credit destyrosine-γ-endorphin with the *epitheton ornans* "virtus cogitativa vel imaginativa"? Might not a hallucinogen-like fragment circulate there as *vis phantastica*, disturbing the *sensus communis*? After all, the tanycytes of the ventricular ependyma do secrete their "quintessence" into the CSF, not gratuitously. Does this not seem a fair tribute to old Galen's views on the involvement of both parenchyma and ventricular fluid in the *commercium animae cum corpore*?

The untold quantity of treatises titled "De Anima," "De Spiritu," reflects, since Pythagorean times up to the present day, man's preoccupation with his own nature, experienced as split in soma and spirit with a flagrant discongruity of physical and mental reality.

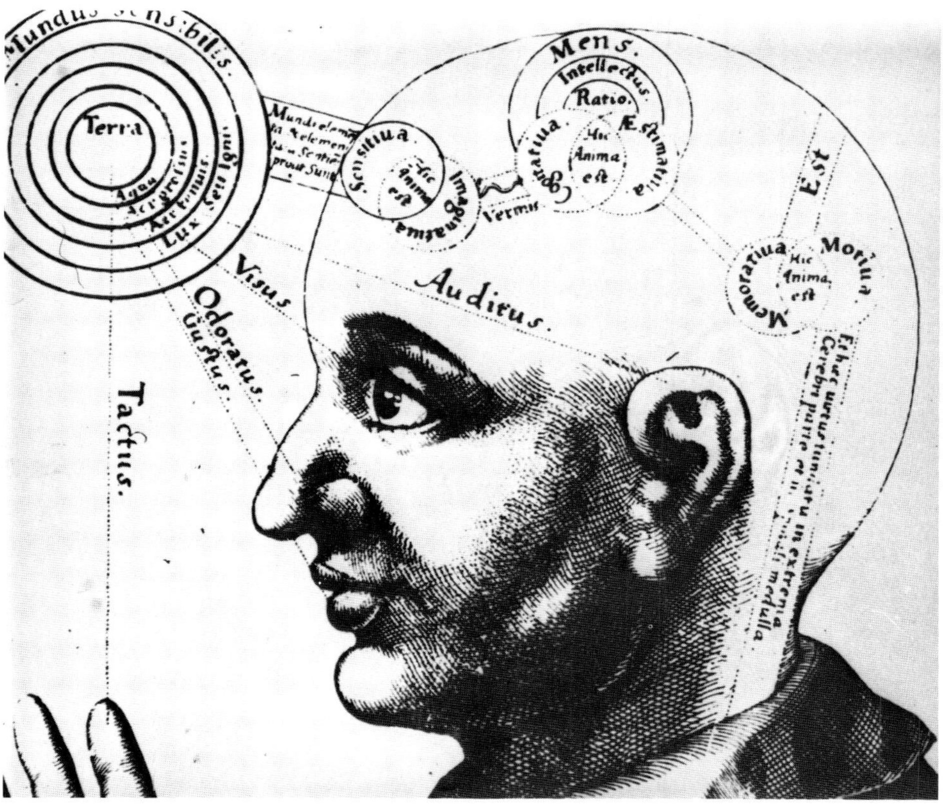

FIG. 20. R. Fludd, "Utriusque cosmi maioris scilicet et minors, metaphysica, physica atque technica historia." Tom II, de Brij, Frankf., 1619–21 A.D.

I submit that present-day neuroscience strongly indicates that the living brain is a crystal-grid of myriads of binary elements, spatially organized, processing myriads of energy transients, and being in what Dr. Christopher Game, the gifted son of one of Critchley's dear friends, calls a critical state. The integral of it is an emergent field force denoted as "mind," comparable to the field force "gravity" emerging in the presence of sufficient matter. Mind and matter are two sides of a coin. Very recent quantum physics experiments, carried out to test the famous 1935 Einstein–Podolsky-Rosen dilemma, appear to offer the choice that either speeds in excess of that of light occur (which violates Einstein's separability axiom and the Bell inequality axiom) (42), or that no reality exists independently of consciousness and that elementary matter seems to carry "mental" aspects (43). Quantum theory indeed seems closer to the truth than the realistic theory of nature. Rather than an abysmal split between spirit and soma, mind and matter do show duality's union, like light manifests itself, according to the methodology of inquiry, as either a wave or a particle. Reality's tissue is a parable, a 'ομοιωμα, perceptively phrased by Goethe, when he sang "Alles Vergängliche ist nur ein Gleichnis" and "... deinen höchsten Feuerflug, hat schon am Gleichnis, schon am Bild, genug." Macdonald Critchley's *Opus* testifies to his conviction that, in spite of Shakespeare's desperate cry, "life ... is a tale told by an idiot, full of sound and fury, signifying nothing," a cry presaging our century's cynical barbarism that rids itself

lam oblongatam, hinc concludere ve-
lim, ipſam animam præcipue reſidere
in ſubſtantia cerebri corticali & ad par-
tem etiam in medullari, ubi nexus ta-
lium ſubtiliſſimarum membranarum a
particula ad particulam eſſe queat, &
pariter ſupra, circum & intra quamli-
bet particulam illius ſubſtantiæ : ſub-
ſtantia corticalis vel cineritia, prout
vocatur, immediate & arcte ſubſtrata
eſt meningibus, & quidem in cerebro
ad craſſitiem circiter 2 linearum in ſer-
pentinos flexus quaſi repens, & ſæpe
ipſum cerebrum penetrans; in cere-
bello vero adhuc copioſior adeſt per
formam vegetantium arbuſculorum
R 2 pulchre

FIG. 21. E. Swedenborg, *Prodromus Philosphiae*, Part II, p. 259, Hekel, Dresdae (1734).

Poſito, quod jam per omnem illam
ſubſtantiam ſit diffuſa, ſequitur, quod
anima non ſit in uno loco ſed ubique
quaſi præſens in cerebri partibus, &

FIG. 22. E. Swedenborg, loc. cit., p. 25; 260–1.

of the soul under the motto "never *mind*, it doesn't *matter*," clinical neurology and its priests shall live by the physician's dictum: Mind! Man *does* matter!

REFERENCES

1. Critchley, D. (1966): *The Divine Banquet of the Brain*. The Harveian Oration. Harrison & Sons, London.
2. Diderot, D. (1923): *Les Bijoux Indiscrets*, pp. 159–165. Edit. Garnier, Paris.
3. Jung, C. G. (1973): *Antwort auf Hiob*. Walter-Verlag, Olten.
4. Theophrastus Eresios: "De Sensibus." In: Stratton, G. M. (1963): *Theophrastus and Greek Physiological Psychology Before Aristotle*, Bonset, Amsterdam. Also in: Hippokrates: *De Morbu Sacer*, 14, 17.
5. Plato, *Phaedon*, cap. 45, Loeb Classical Library, Vol. 36, Harvard/Heinemann, London (1914).
6. Aetius Amideni (1534): *Medici Clarissime*, Lib. IV, 3, 4, 5, 7; IV, 17/1, Venice.
7. Aristotle: *De Anima* I, 3: 405/406, Loeb Classical Library, Vol. 288, Heinemann, London (1975).

8. Hippokrates: *On Ancient Medicine*, Vol. I, Loeb Classical Library, Vol. 147, Heinemann, London.
9. Aristotle: *Hist. Animal.*, Lib. I, cap. XVL, Loeb Classical Library, Vols. 9–10, Harvard/Heinemann, London.
10. Celsus: *On Medicine*, edited by W. G. Spencer, Loeb Classical Library, Harvard/Heinemann, London.
11. Aristotle: *De Anima* I, 2:405, I, 5:409.
12. Posidonius of Apamea. See Galen: De Hipp. et Platon. Placitis, Liber IV, cap. 5, *Corp. Medic. Graec.*, Vol. 5, edited by P. De Lacy.
13. Plinius Senior, C. D.: *De Hist. Nat.* Lib. XI, cap. 49, 135, Loeb Classical Library, Vol. 353, Harvard/Heinemann, London.
14. Brook, A. J.: Introduction to Galen's "On the Natural Faculties," pp. XII, XIV, Loeb Classical Library no. 71. Harvard/Heinemann, London (1979).
15. Haskins, C. H. (1976): *The Renaissance of the Twelfth Century*, 6th ed., Harvard Univ. Press, Cambridge, Mass.
16. Knowles, D. (1962): *The Evolution of Medieval Thought*. Vintage Brooks, Random House, New York.
17. Gilson, E. (1947): *La Philosophie au Moyen Age*. Payot, Paris.
18. Nemesios Emesenus: *Premnon Physikon* (Peri physeos anthroopon), cap. 3. Also in: Koch, H. A. (1921): *Quellenuntersuchungen zu Nemesios*, Weidmann, Berlin. Also in: Jaeger, W. W. (1914): *Nemesios von Emesa*. Berlin.
19. Aëtios of Amida: *Tetrabiblos*, Lib. VI, cap. 2.
20. Aetius Amideni (1534): *Medici Clarissime Libri Sedecim*. Venetië.
21. Pagel, W. (1958): Medieval and Renaissance contribution to knowledge of the brain and its functions. In: *The Brain and Its Functions*, edited by F. N. L. Poynter, pp. 95–114. Oxford Univ. Press, New York.
22. Galen: (a) *De Placitis*, Lib. VII, cap. 3. (b) *De Symptom. Differ.*, cap. 3. (c) *De Locis Affect.*, Lib. III, cap. 9.
23. Aurelius Augustinus: (a) *De Spiritu et Anima. Opera Omnia*, Vol. VI; see J. P. Migne, (1884): 40,782ff. Paris. (b) *De Genesi ad Litteram*, Lib. XII.
24. Johannes Damaskenos: *De Fide Orthodoxa*, Liber II, cap. 17, 19, 20; see J. P. Migne, (1864): *Patr. Gr.*, Vol. 94. Paris.
25. Constabulus (Costa ben Luca): *De Differentia Animae et Spiritu Liber*, cap. 2; see Sigm. Barach, Innsbrück (1878).
26. Sudhoff, W. (1813): Die Lehre von den Hirnventrikeln in textlicher und graphischer Tradition des Altertums und Mittelalters. *Arch. Gesch. Med.*, 7:149–205.
27. Leyacker, J. (1927): Zur Entstehung der Lehre von den Hirnventrikeln als Sitz psychischer Vermögen. *Arch. Gesch. Med.*, 19:253–286.
28. Constantinus Africanus: Lib. IV, cap. 19; Lib. VI, cap. 11.
29. Ibn-Zuhr: "Al-Teisir", Lib. IX, tract. 9, cap. 4.
30. Ibn-Roshd: (a) "Colliget," Lib. II, cap. 20. (b) "Canon," Lib. I, fla. 1, doctr. 6, cap. 6.
31. Leff, G. A. (1980): *Medieval Thought*. Merlin Press, London.
32. Schneider, A. (1903): *Die Psychologie Alberts des Grossen nach den Quellen dargestellt*, Vol. I. Aschendorff, München.
33. Smeets, J. R. (1971): *François Villon: De Laatste Strophen van Le Lais*; *Lyriek en Wetenschap*, pp. 63–96. Servire, Wassenaar.
34. Bartholomaeus Anglicus: *Liber de Proprietatibus Rerum*, Liv. V, cap. 3.
35. Aristotle: *De Hist. Animal.*, XII, cap. 3.
36. Vincentius of Beauvais: De sensu communi et phantasia. In: *Speculum Naturale*, Lib. XXV, cap. 86B.
37. Aetius: *Placita Philos.*, IV, 5.
38. Swedenborg, E. (1734): De mechanisma operationis animae et corporis. In: *Prodromus Philosophiae*, Cap. II, Hekel, Dresdae.
39. Soemmering, S. I. (1796): *Uber das Organ der Seele*. Friedrich Nikolovius, Königsberg.
40. Collect. Salernit. II:96; IV:374.
41. Beek, H. H. (1969): *De Geestesgestoorde in de Middeleeuwen: Beeld en Bemoeienis*. Thesis, Fac. Med., Leiden.
42. d'Espagnat, B. (1979): The quantum theory and reality. *Sci. Am.*, 241(5):128–140.
43. Jammer, M. (1980): Le paradoxe d'Einstein–Podolsky–Rosen. *Recherche*, 11:510–519.

Historical Aspects of the Neurosciences,
edited by F. Clifford Rose and W. F. Bynum.
Raven Press, New York ©

The Relationship Between the Soul and the Brain

Andrew Peacock

Nuffield Department of Clinical Medicine, John Radcliffe Hospital, Headington, Oxford OX3 9DU, England

This chapter examines the shifts in opinion concerning the neurophysiology of mind from the early 19th century to the early 20th century.

At the beginning of the 19th century, a dispute developed between two scientists, Pierre Flourens (1794–1867) and Franz Josef Gall (1758–1828). Gall, who founded phrenology, believed that the mental "higher" faculties could be localized to discrete areas of the cortex, whereas Flourens, defending a widely held view, believed the opposite, that the cortex was "equipotential" in its operation, i.e., all parts were equally capable of performing all functions. The balance of physiological opinion at that time favored the views of Flourens, but later in the 19th century, opinion swung toward the "localizationist" view. In the early 20th century, many influential neurologists and neurophysiologists felt that such an analytic approach was insufficient, that the mental faculties had to be looked at differently, in order to account for the special features of the highly developed nervous system of the living organism. Neurologists and psychologists talked in terms of the "holistic" approach to mental functions, an approach that regarded the performance of the whole as being different from the sum of the performances of its individual parts.

We begin by looking very briefly at (a) the problem of mind up until the 17th century, (b) the influence of Descartes in the 17th century, and (c) the way the Cartesian view was disturbed by Lockean "sensationalism" in the 18th century. We then examine in detail the dispute in the early 19th century between Flourens and Gall, and see whether or not this dispute can be correlated with a further dispute in neurophysiology a century later between the "holists" and the "localizationists."

THE LOCALIZATION OF THE SOUL: THE EMERGENCE OF NEUROPHYSIOLOGY FROM ANTIQUITY TO DESCARTES

Aristotle considered that the function of the brain was to cool the blood, and he placed the soul in the heart; however, other philosophers followed Plato's lead and placed the soul in the brain. Although disagreeing with Aristotle, these philosophers held the conviction that there could be no relation between the structure of an organ of such homogeneous character as the brain and the extraordinary faculties of the soul. Galen remained faithful to Plato, and he was followed by most of the medieval writers, although the controversy was not completely dead, even as late as the 16th century, as one can see from Shakespeare's *Merchant of Venice* (1596):

> Tell me where is fancie bred
> Or in the heart or in the head.

The early writers may have agreed that the brain was the seat of the soul, but there was further controversy about whether the soul should be localized in the ventricles of the brain or in the substance of the brain itself. Galen had no doubt, as he indicates in *De Locis Affectis* (1), that the soul was located in the substance of the brain. Galen was, of course, one of the earliest of what we would now call neurophysiologists. He experimented with the cutting of the motor and sensory nerves of the pig, and he speculated that the sensory nerves traveled to the front part of the brain, which was soft and able to receive impressions, whereas the motor nerves were derived from the back part of the brain, which was composed of harder substance. This localization of "lower" (motor and sensory) functions to specific areas of the brain was important, because it was just such localization, which was achieved experimentally by neurophysiologists in the 19th century, that led to a similar localization of "higher" functions.

The search for the seat of the soul was the earliest and a most important stimulus to attempts at cerebral localization. Galen had located motor and sensory ("lower") functions in specific areas of the brain, but no real attempt had been made to connect these "lower" functions with their corresponding "higher" functions of volition and conscious perception. In other words, the "will" that initiates movement of the limbs and the conscious appreciation that accompanies stimulation of the sensory nerves were not considered to be on the same level of understanding as those "lower" functions. By implication, the functions of the mind were separate from the functions of the body. Descartes was the first to make this mind-body dualism explicit.

RENÉ DESCARTES (1596–1650)

Descartes' philosophy was an all-embracing one, encompassing a mechanical view of all physiological processes. By reducing these physiological processes to the action of machines, Descartes eliminated the tripartite soul of Plato and replaced it with a single indivisible soul, which was the agent of thought, i.e., conscious perception, memory, imagination, and reason. He rejected the belief that the senses provided accurate and valid information. Moreover, by restricting himself to the fundamental belief, *cogito, ergo sum*, he was led to the concept that all "ideas" were innate. This isolation of the self from its physical surroundings and Descartes' restricted definition of the soul—for he had transferred the other two parts of Plato's soul, namely, the appetite and the emotions, to the "machine"—produced the separation of mind and body usually known as Cartesian dualism.

In attempting to find a seat for the soul, Descartes rejected any anatomical relationship between its functions and its situation, but there were, for him, two reasons to find a single location of the soul. The first was the need to find a single location for a unitary soul (or at least for its function since, for Descartes, the soul was an unextended substance), and the second was the need to find a single common area for the duplicated senses to be registered. The pineal gland satisfied both these demands because of its unique and solitary central position in the brain. Its smallness did not matter, because Descartes was localizing not a relationship between structure and function, but a philosophical relationship between mind and body.

It might appear that Descartes was the supreme example of a localizer of brain function, but this is not the case. He had in no way related structure to function; the soul and its functions remained unextended and indivisible. His localization of the soul's activities in the pineal gland solved the philosophical problems he set himself, but it was not a localization of physiological function so much as a localization of an infinitely small area of contact (analogous to a mathematical point) between each motor and sensory stimulus and the "higher" functions of the mind. The term "localization of brain function" had become irrelevant in Cartesian terms, because it provided no basis for investigation of the workings of the mind in physiological terms.

The Cartesian concept of the soul and its mode of action was important in the dispute between Flourens and Gall at the beginning of the 19th century. The "equipotentiality" theory of Flourens can be considered a physiological reformulation of the *a priori* philosophical concept of soul proclaimed by Descartes. Some historians (2) have also argued that Gall, in opposition to Flourens, was strongly influenced by Lockean "sensationalism," and it is the development of this school of thought that will now be discussed very briefly.

LOCKEAN SENSATIONALISM AND THE 18TH CENTURY

The 18th century, for physiology, can be seen as a transitional period, between the Cartesian belief in the incommensurability of mind and body and the 19th-century faith that all the attributes of the soul would one day be reduced to anatomicophysiological correlates. This transition was marked by the philosophical inheritance of Locke in the form of French "sensationalism" and the practice of physicians such as Morgagni and surgeons such as La Peyronie.

John Locke (1632–1704), in his *Essay Concerning Human Understanding* (1690), rejected the "innate ideas" of Descartes and substituted the concept of the mind as a *tabula rasa* (literally, a blank tablet). Locke believed that although ideas existed only in the mind, they had their origins from two sources: from sensations imparted by external bodies and from "internal observations of our minds perceived and reflected on by ourselves." Ultimately, therefore, the content of the mind depended on external phenomena; this implied a close relation between the mind and the world. This view was maintained by the French "sensationalists" who followed Locke in the 18th century. They believed that nothing stood between the mind and the world, between knowledge and the experience of the external world on which it was founded. Hence, in the transition from 17th-century Cartesianism to 18th-century "sensationalism," one can perceive a softening of the rigid separation of mind and body. "Sensationalism" allowed a degree of proportionality between the brain and the mind that, it could be argued, allowed anatomists and physiologists at least to consider a connection between the structure of the brain and its functions. Certainly, there is some evidence that such a connection was being made by men such as Morgagni and La Peyronie.

Morgagni worked in the early 18th century, publishing the results of his case histories and postmortems in 1761 as *De Sedibus et Causis Morborum*. Morgagni correlated the symptoms experienced in life by his patients with the findings at autopsy after their death. He was cautious about making too strong a link between mental function and damage to the brain, as can be seen from the passage with which he opens the chapter "On Diseases of the Head" (3):

> there may be some incongruity in associating inflammation of the membrane, or of the substance of the brain, with a state of the mental faculties.

However, he went on to say that insanity, loss of mental rather than physical capacity, could result from "induration" (hardening of the brain) and that apoplexy (stroke) or head injury could result in loss of speech (which Morgagni considered to be a "higher" function) as well as paralysis of the limbs. The importance of this assertion was that by saying that the same agent, in this case stroke or head injury, can simultaneously lead to loss of both "higher" and "lower" functions, Morgagni had provided a structural link between the mental and the physical.

La Peyronie (1678–1747) was part of a tradition of French surgery well used to the examination and treatment of head wounds, usually from war injuries. The surgeons were often faced with localized injuries to the brain associated with some functional deficit. Their observations of the changes in human behavior that accompanied discrete brain injury thus encouraged them to localize function to certain areas of the brain. However, they formulated no association between specific "higher" mental functions and areas of the brain, but they did localize areas of "stupefaction" or "insensibility," conditions that often resulted from head injury.

La Peyronie was surgeon to the King and one of the founders of the Académie Royale de Chirurgie. In a paper, "Observations par lesquelles on tache de decouvrir la partie du cerveau ou l'ame exerce ses fonctions," delivered in Paris in 1741, La Peyronie described an experiment that became famous in French medical circles. He had a patient with a very severe wound of the head that extended to the depth of the corpus callosum (the connecting part between the two great cerebral hemispheres of the brain). Into this wound La Peyronie injected water, which rendered the patient unconscious. Removal of the water restored consciousness, leading La Peyronie to suggest that he had found the place where the soul "exerts its functions." This paper became a classic, being taken, particularly by the surgeons, as evidence for a primary seat of action of the soul.

During the 18th century, one can see a shift, in both philosophy and psychology, away from the idea that mental functions were constituent of an unextended—and therefore unapproachable—soul, toward a belief that the mental faculties could be localized in discrete areas of the brain and that the content of mind was intimately related to external events. Some historians (4) have argued that the philosophical traditions of both Descartes and Locke persisted in the beginning of the 19th century and that the dispute between Flourens and Gall, which is the first well-known dispute between those who were localizers of brain function and those who were not, can be seen as a confrontation between these two traditions.

THE 19TH CENTURY: THE ERA OF LOCALIZATION

The Flourens/Gall Dispute

On September 13, 1848, a group of men were building part of a railway line near Cavendish, Vermont. Their foreman, Phineas Gage, by all accounts a trusted and well-liked man, took charge of the operation of pouring gunpowder into a hole drilled in a rock that was to be blasted out of the way of the line. As Gage was tamping down the powder, it ignited, and the tamping rod, three and a half feet long, and an inch and a quarter in diameter, was fired out of the hole, entering Gage's head via the left orbit. It passed through the frontal lobes of his brain and exited through the top of his skull. Gage fell to the ground, convulsed briefly, but was soon conscious, speaking and moving all his limbs. Within a few weeks, he was out of bed and suffering no apparent deficit of mind or limbs, but he had developed a new personality. He was, as one of his workmates said, "no longer Gage."

J. M. Harlow, one of the doctors who attended him, wrote:

> His physical health is good and I am inclined to say he has recovered . . . (but) . . . The equilibrium or balance, so to speak, between his intellectual faculties and animal propensities, seems to have been destroyed. He is fitful, irreverent, indulging at times in the grossest profanity (which was not previously his custom), manifesting but little deference for his fellows, impatient of restraint or advice when it conflicts with his desires, at times pertinaciously obstinate, yet capricious and vacillating, devising many plans for future operation, which are no sooner arranged than they are abandoned.(5)

Gage became unemployable; he eked out an existence traveling around the country exhibiting himself and the tamping rod that had changed him, and his case became well known in medical circles in the United States and Europe. His case was extraordinary, not simply because it was remarkable that a man with such a terrible injury should survive, but also, more importantly, because the injury had affected Gage's "higher" mental functions, his personality, rather than the movement of his limbs or his ability to receive sensations.

For the historian, the dispute between Flourens and Gall, between "equipotentiality" and the "organs of the mind," could be crystallized around a discussion of the case of Gage. Flourens is reported to have stated that Gage was unaffected by his injury. The comments of the followers of Gall are unrecorded, but there is little doubt that they would have considered the case of Gage as good evidence for the localization of higher mental functions.

Franz Josef Gall published with Spurzheim their *Recherches sur le Système Nerveux* in 1808 as a memoir for their candidacy of the Institut de France. This was followed by Gall's *Anatomie et Physiologie du Système Nerveux* (1819). Gall's work quickly achieved notoriety (and much interest from the lay public), using as it did evidence from "new" sources, comparative anatomy and psychology. In asserting that the brain was an expansion of lower and less complex arrangements of the nervous system, he was predicting the hierarchical view of the function of the nervous system that so influenced Herbert Spencer and, following him, Hughlings Jackson. Above all, he was the first since Willis (6) to recognize the importance of the cortex and to give man the dignity of significant anatomical development (especially in the frontal lobes of the brain) over animals. He believed that the brain was the seat of all mental functions (both intellectual and emotional), and he divided them into 27 separate faculties that were associated with discrete organs in the brain. As Gall wrote in 1810: "Chaque intelligence a son organe propre" (7). These organs, he claimed, could be palpated through the cranium (cranioscopy). The analysis of "bumps" on the cranium—the "science" of phrenology—excited much popular interest, but simultaneously it drew criticism from the scientific establishment, especially when followers of Gall increased the number of faculties to 50 or more, each with its individual organ.

Pierre Flourens praised the anatomical work of Gall, but he maintained that Gall's theory of phrenology had not been based in anatomy. In *Examen de la Phrénologie* (1842), Flourens wrote (8): "(Gall) commence par imaginer une hypothese et puis il imagine une anatomie pour son hypothese."

Flourens was a powerful figure in French medicine: a protegé of Cuvier (the head of a committee from the Institut that examined Gall's work), a member of the Académie des Sciences, and a professor of medicine at the Collège de France. He pioneered the technique of precise extirpation of the cortex in such animals as pigeons, dogs, and rabbits; the evidence gained from this empirical work supported his "equipotential" theory of the action of the nervous system. He peeled off successive layers of the cortex of his animals and found little relation between the area of cortex removed and the reduction in the animal's capabilities. In an 1823 memoir, Flourens stated his position on the workings of the mental faculties (9):

> all perceptions, all volitions occupy the same seat in these (cerebral) organs . . . the faculty of perceiving, of willing merely constitute a faculty which is essentially one.

Some historians (10) argue that Flourens, though purporting to attack Gall on scientific methodological grounds, was in fact defending the then current establishment view that, in the tradition of Cartesian philosophy, there was no equation between mind and brain, and that the soul was a unitary and indivisible phenomenon. They further argue that Gall's work was strongly influenced by the Lockean tradition found in French "sensationalism." In his works, Gall often respectfully cited such sensationalists as Condillac (1715–1780), Bonnet (1720–1790), and Cabanis (1757–1808). Sensationalism gave rise to the concept of the content of the mind as an association of ideas created from sense impressions by the brain, and one can argue that Gall extended this concept of the "transforming and integrating" functions of the brain to that of the brain having distinct higher faculties which, because function elucidates structure, could be discretely localized in organs of the mind.

Bynum (11) has pointed out that there was an important link between the work of Flourens and Gall: They shared a doctrine of psychological continuity between man and animals in that they believed that the minds of both were equally dependent on neurological development. Both Flourens and Gall did of course use comparative anatomy as evidence. Flourens' use of this method would tend to refute the argument that he was defending the Cartesian line, for Descartes made an absolute separation between rational man and animal-machines. Furthermore, as Young (12) has shown, the two men, while coming to opposite conclusions concerning the operation of the mental faculties, shared a belief in the innateness of those faculties. Now, if Gall believed in the innateness of the faculties, surely this would not be compatible with the argument that he was a follower of Lockean sensationalism?

Notwithstanding these two objections, there is evidence that Flourens and other biologists were defending the commonly held belief that the soul cannot be divided or linked with discrete structure. In *Examen de la Phrénologie*, Flourens reacted to the philosophical consequence of phrenology in his charge to Gall (13):

> Vous ne dites rien de l'unité de l'intelligence, de l'unité du moi, ou vous la niez. Mais l'unité de l'intelligence, l'unité du moi est un fait sens intime . . . Gall renverse la philosophie ordinaire, et puis il veut que toutes les consequences de la philosophie subsistent. Il suprime le moi, et il veut qu'il ait une ame. Il suprime le libre arbitre, et il veut qu'il ait une morale.

The committee of the Institut (chaired by Cuvier), reporting on Gall's and Spurzheim's *Anatomie du Cerveau*, commended their anatomical achievement, but the committee stated that there could be no real link between anatomy and mental function (14):

> The functions of the brain are of a different order from those of other viscera . . . (and) suppose an eternally incomprehensible mutual influence between divisible matter and the indivisible "moi."

Overall, it would appear that although the dispute between Flourens and Gall was not conducted solely in philosophical terms, as a battle between the Cartesian and Lockean traditions, there is evidence that Flourens was defending an indivisible soul. At that time his defense was successful, though later in the 19th century, the paradigm shifted to a localizationist view.

French and British Neurology in the 19th Century

The "equipotentiality" theory was soon challenged even within the scientific establishment. In a lecture in 1825, Bouillaud (1796–1875), a professor of medicine in Paris, challenged

Flourens, and as an example of his belief in the localization of "higher" function, he postulated the possibility of an organ of speech. The possibility became reality when, in 1861, the anatomist and anthropologist Paul Broca, in a paper to the Société d'Anthropologie, described the clinical and postmortem findings on one of his patients (15).

Broca had examined and followed for many years a patient with an isolated aphasia (inability to speak); he was called Tan, which was the only word he could utter. This patient appeared normal in all other respects right up until his death. Broca conducted the postmortem and found an isolated defect of the third frontal convolution of the cerebrum, an area that became known as Broca's speech area.

Broca's faith in cerebral localization was supported by the experimental work (published in 1870) of Fritsch and Hitzig. These German physiologists showed that specific movements could be elicited by electrical stimulation of the cortex of dogs and that those movements were lost if that area of the cortex was removed.

In the *Lancet* of January 18 and February 1, 1873, the eminent neurologist John Hughlings Jackson (1835–1911) published his clinical findings. He studied the causes of palsies (paralysis) and focal epileptic seizures (later known as Jacksonian epilepsy), making a correlation between the clinical syndrome and the pathology that he observed postmortem. This correlation appears to be a significant step in the crossing of the mind-body divide, because Jackson stated that higher functions such as volition could be upset by brain damage (16):

> In cerebral damage the parts suffer as much in voluntary operation as they do in automatic operation, in other words, the will is affected.

He went as far as to equate all mental functions with the workings of a "sensory-motor" machine. In other words, not only was he localizing brain function to anatomical areas, but he was proposing the reductionist line that the workings of the mind were simply motor responses to sensory stimuli. In a paper of 1870, he said (17):

> Surely the conclusion is irresistible that mental symptoms from disease of the hemisphere are fundamentally like hemiplegia, chorea, and convulsions. They must all be due to lack, or the disorderly development of, the sensory-motor processes.

Following Jackson, David Ferrier (1843–1928), cofounder of the Journal *Brain*, attempted to confirm Jackson's clinical conclusions by experiments on apes. He used cortical stimulation and ablations (removal of parts of the brain) to mimic the "discharging" and "destroying" lesions of Jackson, being led by his results to the concept of discrete motor and sensory regions of the brain adjacent to the central fissure.

The experimental work of Fritsch, Hitzig, and Ferrier corresponded with the clinical work of Broca and Jackson. There remained only the necessity of anatomical confirmation (something which Gall could never provide) to complete the scientific "picture." This was provided by the work of P. E. Fleschig and K. Brodman. Fleschig (1847–1929) studied the myelinization of the cortex (the growth of fatty sheaths that enclose nerve fibers), and on this basis, he divided the cortex into motor and sensory areas. Brodman (1868–1918), working at the same time (the end of the 19th century), studied the cytoarchitectonics (morphology of brain tissue) of the gray matter, as well as the white matter (to which Fleschig had restricted himself), dividing the cortex up into what are known as "Brodman's areas."

These 19th-century "localizationalists" received considerable support from other scientific and nonscientific sources. Herbert Spencer, the philosopher, whom Jackson acknowledged as a significant influence on his own work, published a new edition of *Principles of Psychology* in 1881. In a chapter on the scope of psychology, Spencer stated his belief that localization of function was a natural law and no less applicable to the cerebrum than any other organ (18):

> Localisation of function is the law of all organisation whatever, thus distinct psychical activities must occur in distinct anatomical areas of the cerebrum.

Also in *Principles of Psychology*, Spencer spelled out his psychological theory of evolutionary associationism. Associationist psychology was the inheritance via Hartley of Lockean sensationalism. This school of psychology believed that ideas were discrete units (atoms) and that their association occurred in the brain. The importance of such an atomistic-associationist view of psychology was that if mental functions could occur in such discrete units, then surely these units could be localized to discrete structures. The theory of evolution proposed by Darwin in the mid-19th century had a dramatic effect on psychology, because it led to the abandonment of the separation between animal and human modes of behavior. This allowed the extrapolation of observations of animal behavior (usually rats) to humans. The behaviorists founded their psychology on these studies, and by continuing to believe that the mind was composed of a series of units of consciousness (in this case stimulus-response units), they maintained a tradition of atomistic associationism that was important as support for the localizationists in their explanation of brain function. It was not until the development of the Gestalt school of psychology (which I deal with later) that associationism was seriously challenged.

An examination of the clinical and experimental evidence from within the discipline of neurophysiology may, when coupled with the support from psychology, appear adequate reason for the attachment of 19th-century physiologists to the "localizationist" view, but a similar reductionist approach can be found in other scientific fields. In 1858 Virchow proposed his "cell theory," showing that the tissues of organisms were composed of individual discrete subunits. This theory proved particularly fruitful for neurophysiology when, in the 1890s, Cajal elaborated it into his "neurone theory." Cajal (1852–1934), a Spanish histologist, showed that the nervous system was not a continuous network as had been previously supposed, but was composed of discrete cells that he called "neurones." The analogy is obvious to the historian: There is a simple parallel between the concepts of brain cells and their connections, and ideas and their associations. Outside biology, in other sciences, a reductionist analysis to single quality bearing units also seemed possible; examples were physics and chemistry, where particle physics and the atomic theory were both components of late 19th-century thinking. This fact may not be important in itself, but the changes in physics that occurred in the early 20th century were significant, at least to such men as A. N. Whitehead, as discussed later. During the 19th century, a "localizationist" and reductionist view of the "higher" functions of the brain accorded with prevailing philosophical, psychological, and scientific ideas. As an example of the supreme confidence with which neurologists supported the localization of even "higher" functions to defined areas of the brain, one only has to look at the startling increase in the number of surgical operations for derangement of those functions that occurred in the late 19th and early 20th centuries.

Surgery for Mental Disease

The first "psychosurgical" operation was performed by Burckhardt, a Swiss surgeon, who did an ablation for schizophrenia in 1890. His results are unrecorded, but in 1935, two scientists, Jacobsen and Fulton (19), reported that they had cured one of their chimpanzees of its particularly temperamental behavior by frontal lobectomy (removal of part of the frontal lobes of the brain). A Portuguese neuropsychiatrist, Egas Moniz, was at the meeting, and within a year he had commenced operating on psychiatric patients. He was followed by several other surgeons, but the operations were, to say the least, not always successful; Moniz himself was shot in the spine by one of his lobectomized patients. The largest series of cases was published in the 1930s by two enterprising gentlemen at George Washington University, Freeman (a neurologist) and Watts (a neurosurgeon) (20). The two men performed more than 600 lobectomies and frontal lobotomies (section of the lobes rather than their removal) with, they claimed, a 60% success rate. Indeed, such was Freeman's enthusiasm for the operation that he invented an instrument like an ice pick, which he knocked with a hammer through the orbits of his temporarily anesthetized patients and to which he gave a quick twist in order to lobotomize them. "A keen neurologist," said Freeman, "ought to be able to treat 15 of such patients during a morning session in the office."

The rationale behind this surgical assault on the frontal lobes as treatment for mental disease was that neurologists believed that the frontal lobes were the site of location of the "higher" functions, such as intelligence, memory, and emotions. There are a number of reasons for this. First, these lobes are silent to experimentation, there being no motor or sensory effect with stimulation or ablation. Second, they are larger in man and in the higher animals, which corresponded to man's greater mental capabilities. Finally, and not least, the old phrenological doctrine persisted—that people with bulging foreheads were more intelligent.

The use of psychosurgery could be considered to represent the pinnacle of confidence in the localizationist view, and the decline in its use in the early 20th century could, equally, be considered to indicate the waning of that confidence. Certainly, much of the experimental evidence on which the localizationist view was based was not as unequivocal as its proponents claimed and, in addition, there were, for many doctors and laymen, philosophical objections to the reduction of mental function to a series of structurally defined organs of the mind. Ablation experiments were fraught with the technical difficulties of sepsis, edema, and overly enthusiastic surgery. For instance, Munk claimed that extirpation of the frontal lobes resulted in paralysis of the trunk, whereas Ferrier claimed that the same operation led to loss of head and eye movements, and Schafer maintained that it had no effect whatsoever (21). Electrical stimulation experiments could also be misleading, as it was shown that the motor and sensory regions of the cortex had not been as well mapped as previously thought. Although a useful research tool, electrical stimulation was not really equivalent to any physiological process, and loss of function with the removal of parts of the brain does not mean that the part of brain removed subserves the function lost. Behaviorism as a mode of understanding mental function entailed the abandonment of the idea of an indivisible soul and the loss of "free will," with the consequence that there could be no such thing as moral constraint on behavior: Behavior was simply controlled by programmed response.

These objections to localization of "higher" functions are well demonstrated in the writing of Sherrington. Sir Charles Sherrington (1857–1952) is perhaps the best-known neurophysiologist in the history of the discipline. He was brought up in the best mechanistic tradition, studying under Virchow and Koch in Berlin and Foster at Cambridge, but he was to pioneer the idea of "integration" in the nervous system, a concept that was only a short step from the theories of "equilibrium" and "interrelationship," which were the hallmarks of the "holists" in the 1920s and 1930s. Sherrington was aware that, although his experiments had been particularly fruitful in the analysis of "lower" motor functions, they pointed to the fact that, for the "higher" functions, a far more complex system must be at work. In *Integrative*

Action of the Nervous System, Sherrington wrote (22):

> a step is reached where the physical situation leads to the psychical . . . How is it that the brain achieves such powers of integrative control over the function of the human body . . . resulting in the complete organism we call the individual?

Later, in a lecture in 1933, he said (23):

> but indeed what right have we to conjoin mental experience with the physiological? No scientific right, only the right of busy commonsense. To many of us, a mere juxtaposition of the two sets of happenings proclaims their disparity . . . As mental events, I should suppose them aloof.

The Emergence of Holism

Sherrington appears to have doubted whether or not there was any validity at all to a scientific approach to the study of the functions of the brain, but his extreme views were not totally shared by other 20th-century physiologists, whether "localizationist" or "holist" in inclination. "Busy commonsense" had been a very useful approach in both the 19th and 20th centuries. Knowledge of neurophysiology had been greatly advanced by the analytic approach to biological phenomena: The traditional line of demarcation between mind and body had been pushed further and further back, and there was no longer much dispute that there were discrete areas of the brain representing "lower" motor and sensory functions. For the "higher" functions, there was no such agreement. Here the "localizationists" believed that all "higher" functions would eventually be localized, while the "holists" maintained that such functions were the product only of the integral brain. Thus, both parties agreed that a structure-function relationship existed; they merely disagreed about the interpretation of this relationship.

Some historians (24) have argued that this early 20th-century dispute between "holists" and "localizationists" was a continuation of the dispute between Flourens and Gall one century earlier. But this seems questionable. The similarity is merely superficial; an analysis of the writings of the 20th-century thinkers reveals quite different objectives. "Equipotentiality" was not the same as "holism." "Equipotentiality" meant, in the sense that Flourens used it, that all areas of the brain had equal potential for producing what were the indivisible functions of the soul. "Holism," on the other hand, involved a belief that all areas of the brain worked synchronously in the production of the "higher" functions. The "holists," unlike Flourens, were materialists in the sense that they rejected any unknowable source of mental function. While rejecting a mechanical approach, they espoused the materialist view of mental function that had developed during the 19th century. The arguments between the "holists" and "localizationists" were on a completely different level from those between Gall and the French scientific establishment, a level that was very much related to the 20th-century view of biological problems in general and unrelated to the problems posed by Cartesian dualism. I am not arguing that Cartesian dualism was no longer relevant in 20th-century neurophysiology, but simply that it was not relevant to the dispute between the "holists" and the "localizationists" in the 1930s. The important point as far as "holism" was concerned was not whether a structure-function relationship existed or not, but that this relationship could not be analyzable to isolated organs of the mind. The analytic method, while useful for the understanding of very simple processes, led to the disintegration of the individual; it denied the very organization that was so special to living organisms.

There is evidence that "holism" was gaining popularity among neurologists quite early in the 20th century. Kurt Goldstein, a professor of neurology at Tufts Medical College, studied patients suffering from brain damage in World War I and published widely in journals as well as three major books (25). In these works, Goldstein developed the theme that living organisms in general, and the human organism in particular, always functioned as a whole. Damage to the nervous system did not therefore simply result in the loss of that function associated with the structure injured, but it led to "isolation" of the functions remaining.

Goldstein was not alone in holding these anti-localizationist views. Judson Herrick, a professor of neurology at the University of Chicago, wrote (26) in 1924:

> beyond these fields (motor and sensory areas) mosaic localisation (discrete localisation) of cortical functions is of very doubtful validity.

Henry Head, a physician at the National Hospital for Nervous Diseases in London, said (27) in 1926:

> no function is localised strictly to any part of the cortex and no form of activity, somatic or psychical is built into a mosaic of elementary processes.

Nor were these opinions confined to neurologists. The psychologist Karl Lashley (28) wrote in 1937:

> the trace of any activity is not an isolated connection between sensory and motor elements. It is tied in with the whole complex of spatial and temporal axes of nervous activity which form a constant substratum of behaviour.

It was the work of Karl Lashley that provided powerful experimental evidence for a "holist" view of "higher" function, in this case the function of memory. Lashley's book *Brain Mechanisms and Intelligence* (29), published in 1929, was the first important direct challenge to the localizationists, because not only did he use similar experimental techniques (cortical ablation), but he applied similar psychological methods (maze learning) to assess the effects of such ablation and analyzed the results by statistical methods. If Goldstein's work on humans could be criticized for being anecdotal, Lashley's work on rats was rigorously "scientific" and could only be criticized for being limited to rats!

Lashley analyzed the effect of the removal of parts of the cortex, varying in both loci and extent, on the ability of his rats to form and retain memory of mazes. His results indicated that formation and retention of maze habits varied with the extent of the lesion but not its locus, and that the defect in performance occurring after a lesion was directly proportional to the complexity of the task. Hence, for Lashley, all the cortex was involved in the performance of at least one "higher" function, namely, memory.

Lashley and Goldstein were friends and referred to each other's work in their writings. They also both admitted to being influenced by the Gestalt school of psychology; Goldstein wrote in *Human Nature* (30): "We are not trying to build the organism brick by brick, we are trying to discover the Gestalt." Gestalt (literally, pattern or configuration) psychology was a significant departure from the atomistic-associationist psychology of the 19th century, being the first system of psychology to make "organization" its cornerstone. The Gestalt movement was founded in Berlin about 1910 by Wertheimer, Kohler, and Koffa, becoming widely known and controversial after its three founders emigrated to the United States in 1930. Their purpose was the discovery of the whole and, in their belief, this was possible. They rejected the philosophical dualism of mind and body as opposed to Flourens who had espoused such dualism.

While there were unique influences on 20th-century neurophysiology to be found in the writings of Lashley, but more especially in those of the Gestalt psychologists, there were other influences, perhaps less obvious, that one should take into account, other areas where a "holist" view prevailed. These areas include biological fields such as embryology and biochemistry; the physical sciences, particularly physics and chemistry; the social sciences, including politics and economics; and even philosophy. All these areas showed significant changes in direction at the same time men such as Goldstein were formulating their "holist" neurophysiology.

Social science became a recognized discipline only in the 20th century, though its origins can be traced back to the work of Auguste Comte and Herbert Spencer. It is useful to consider the possible influence of social science, because one of the principal thinkers at the beginning of its recognized stage of development was the Gestalt psychologist, Kurt Lewin. In *A Dynamic Theory of Personality* (1933), Lewin applied the concept of "field" to the motivation of behavior. He conceived of the mind as a tension system and behavior as an attempt by an individual to be relieved of those tensions in order to return to his equilibrium. However, Lewin was aware that the individual was part of, and subject to, a wider environment (both physical and social) than merely his internal tensions. He consequently broadened his "field" (a term borrowed from magnetism and gravity) to consider these influences. In his *Field Theory and Social Science* (1951) (31), Lewin argued that, for an individual, the scientist had to deal with that individual's life space, i.e., the personal and psychological environment as it existed for him; for a group, he had to extend the same approach, so that a wider and wider realm of determinants had to be treated as part of a single interdependent field. The idea of interdependence was what also drove Goldstein: It was Gestalt, it was "holism," and it was, simultaneously, a concept that achieved prominence in biology and physiology.

The "holist" biologists of the 1920s and 1930s believed in a materialist philosophy,but one that refused to limit the organism by imposing an explanation of its function in terms of the laws of physics and chemistry. L. J. Henderson was such a man; although he worked on the chemistry of the blood, he did so with the belief that there existed a system of internal control that oversaw the functions of those individual chemical processes.

Henderson was a professor of biochemistry at Harvard until 1942. During the period from 1904 to 1912, he did his famous work on the inorganic "buffers" present in the blood. He discovered that tissue fluids and blood contained complex "buffer" systems that integrated with respiratory control of blood CO_2 to maintain very fine control over blood acidity and alkalinity. Henderson admitted that his work bore a major intellectual debt to Claude Bernard. Claude Bernard's concept of "milieu interieur," which he formulated in the mid-19th century, was a brilliant philosophical stimulus to the sort of control that Henderson had found experimentally. Henderson personally arranged the publication of Bernard's work *Introduction to the Study of Experimental Medicine* in the United States.

The concept of internal control was further expanded by W. B. Cannon, a colleague of Henderson at Harvard in the 1920s, to include not only the chemistry of the blood, but also the interaction of the nervous and endocrine systems. He did work on "shock" in World War I and maintained the conviction that this devastating state, which was an accompaniment to many serious medical conditions, was due to a breakdown of the internal equilibrium of the body; this equilibrium he termed "homeostasis."

J. S. Haldane, the English physiologist, whose principal work was on the regulation of respiration, was the first man to call himself an "organicist" (someone who believes that some or all complex wholes have the kind of systemic unity characteristic of what are literally organisms). He had been trained as a philosopher before taking up biology, and he had contributed, while still a medical student, to a volume entitled *Essay on Philosophical Criticism* (1883) that was dedicated to the influence of post-Kantian philosophy. With his "organicist" stance and his belief that "philosophy enabled us to frame a working conception, not merely of part, but of the whole of our experience," it was perhaps no coincidence that his views were related to those of the philosopher A. N. Whitehead (1861–1947).

Whitehead, who, incidentally, was teaching at Harvard at the same time as Henderson, was explicit in his formulation of the new view of organicism. In *Philosophical Interpretation of Nature* (1921), he wrote that living organisms should be treated not as parts, but as combinations of processes, and in *Philosophy of Organism*, he wrote (32):

> The concrete enduring entities are organisms, so that the plan of the whole influences the very character of the various subordinate organisms that enter into it.

Surely, this view was not far from the "holism" of Goldstein or the "field" theory of Lewin?

Biologists were unhappy about reducing the laws of the living to the laws of physics and chemistry, but even within these disciplines ideas had changed. If particle physics had been a useful analogical model for atomistic physiology, then the loss of the particle was much more important. Whitehead, in *Science and the Modern World*, outlined the events of physics and their importance for 20th-century biology. The quantum theory and the theory of relativity had, he argued, broken the machine analogy for physics; thus they had also liberated biology from the constraints of mechanism. In chemistry too the change was important; Loeb had written in 1890 (33):

> the development of the "atomic theory" (of chemistry) has put science (all science) for a long time and probably irrevocably on a mechanistic basis.

However, in the 1840s, Pasteur had discovered that there were two optical isomers (forms of the same compound) of tartaric acid, but in the early 20th century, workers had found that, while one was biologically active, the other was not. Thus, even chemical compounds did not have immutable qualities; their character depended on their form.

In politics too, it is possible to argue that the "organismal" view was taking hold after the "social Darwinism" of the 19th century. Already in 1889 a form of the "organismal" view in socialist thinking was being propounded by Sidney Webb in his *Fabian Essays*:

> We must take even more care to improve the social organism of which we form a part, than to perfect our own individual developments. Or rather, the perfect and fitting development of each individual is not necessarily the utmost and highest cultivation of his own personality, but the filling, in the best possible way, of his humble function in the great social machine

If "social Darwinism"—literally the "survival of the fittest" in society—was the hallmark of Victorian conservatism, perhaps the "social organism" was the best interpretation of the complete subjection of the individual to the state in socialist thinking.

In economics, the laissez-faire capitalism of Adam Smith was replaced by the "homeostatic" control of Keynes. Keynes' system proposed the novel approach of deficit spending to maintain the equilibrium of the nation's economic forces. Indeed, Henderson himself described the Keynesian system as a superb example of the nonmechanist but still materialist economy.

One could no doubt find many other examples, both "internal" to neurophysiology, and "external" in biology, in the physical sciences, and in society, of a movement away from the "atomism" of the 19th century to the "holism" of the 20th century. Some of these examples may seem more distant than others from the core of the problem, but all are indicative that neither physiology nor any other science works in a vacuum. The work of the "holist" neurophysiologists was a product of 20th-century thinking. The changes in outlook that were proposed for neurology were changes occurring within the much larger framework of the 20th-century social and scientific milieu.

CONCLUSIONS

In this chapter, I have attempted to document shifts in opinion during the 19th and early 20th centuries concerning the neurophysiological basis of the "higher" cerebral functions. From the time of the Greeks until the present day, philosophers, physiologists, psychologists, and neurologists have attempted to provide a rational explanation for the workings of the mind. The Greeks and the medieval writers largely ascribed these functions to the brain but postulated no precise localization. The mind-body dualism of Descartes had sought to prevent the possibility of any structure-function relationship being proposed for what Descartes believed were the functions of an unextended soul. Lockean "sensationalism," by deposing the innate ideas of Descartes, appeared to have at least allowed some proportionality between brain and mind.

In the early 19th century appeared the first well-known example of a dispute about the brain's function between those who localized brain function and those who did not. When looked at superficially, this dispute seems to have recurred in the early 20th century. That early dispute between Flourens and Gall was "won" by Flourens, who represented the French scientific establishment, and Gall's theories were dismissed as merely popular. However, during the 19th century, views changed, and localization of brain function became accepted. It was not until the early 20th century that physiologists were to show any signs of a change in opinion. These men, who have been called the "holists," came to diametrically opposed conclusions concerning the workings of the brain, and I started work on this chapter hoping to find out why they did so.

Some historians believe that similar criteria could be applied to the 19th-century dispute between Flourens and Gall and the 20th-century dispute between the "holists" and the "localizationists." It became evident to me during my research, however, that the similarities were only superficial. Flourens was defending the indivisible soul against the fragmentation proposed by Gall. He proposed his theory of "equipotentiality" to contradict Gall's "organs of the mind." In the 20th century, the dispute was on a different level. Both parties believed in a materialist neurophysiology, but the "holists" were convinced that the brain acted as one, at least for "higher" functions, whereas the "localizationists" asserted that even these functions could be placed in discrete areas in the brain.

Since there appeared to be so little correlation between the two disputes, it seemed necessary to try to find out what kind of evidence was used, first by those 19th-century physiologists who favored localization, and second by those in the early 20th century who espoused "holism." Why, for instance, did neurologists such as Goldstein come to the conclusions they did when British and French surveys of the same type of injuries during the same war came to opposite (traditional) conclusions? Why had psychologists such as Lashley, doing similar work to the 19th-century localizationists, come to such different conclusions? Furthermore, why did such a "paradigm switch" not occur until the 1920s and 1930s, when Claude Bernard had formulated his concept of "milieu interieur"—so similar to the ideas of the "holists"—in the mid-19th century?

For the "holists," the brain worked synchronously and interdependently with its local and external environment to produce mental functions that fully reflected that "organization" and interdependence. But as the "holists" believed that views on mental functions had to take into account all possible impinging factors, so the historian could not fail to be aware that the "holists" themselves were working within an environment. They were not "isolated" figures either inside or outside neurology, and I have tried to show that one can find a change in views compatible with the neurophysiological shift in opinion from "localization" to "holism" right across the spectrum of early 20th-century thought. It is no coincidence that views in psychology, biology, physics, chemistry, and even economics, politics, and philosophy also changed from a reductionistic approach to one more sympathetic to "organization." Therefore, it is not sufficient to analyze in isolation the change in direction of a single scientific theory such as that concerning brain function; the change must be considered in the light of shifts in thought that occurred in all other areas which impinged on those who developed that theory.

REFERENCES

1. Clarke, E., and O'Malley, C. D. (1968): *The Human Brain and Spinal Cord*, p. 491. University of California Press, Berkeley, Calif.
2. Swazey, J. (1970): Action propre and action commune. *J. Hist. Biol.*, 3 (No. 2):213–235.
3. Morgagni, J. B. (1761): *Seats and Causes of Diseases*, annotated by Cooke, London (1822): Chapter on diseases on the head.
4. Swazey, J. (1970): Action propre and action commune. *J. Hist. Biol.* 3(No. 2):213–235.
5. Harlow, J. M. (1868): Recovery from the passage of an iron bar through the head. *Mass. Med. Soc. Pub.*
6. Blakemore, C. (1977): *Mechanics of the Mind.* Cambridge University Press, Cambridge, England.
7. Swazey, J. (1970): Action propre and action commune. *J. Hist. Biol.*, 3(No. 2):221.
8. Swazey, J. (1970): Action propre and action commune. *J. Hist. Biol.*, 3(No. 2):220.
9. Swazey, J. (1970): Action propre and action commune. *J. Hist. Biol.*, 3(No. 2):227.
10. Swazey, J. (1970): Action propre and action commune. *J. Hist. Biol.*, 3(No. 2):213–235.
11. Bynum, W. (1976): Varieties of Cartesian experience. In: *Philosophical Dimensions of the Neuro-medical Sciences*, edited by J. F. Spicker and H. T. Engelhardt, Jr., Boston.
12. Young, R. M. (1973): Animal Soul. In: *Dictionary of the History of Ideas*, edited by P. P. Weiner, Scribner's, New York.
13. Swazey, J. (1970): Action propre and action commune. *J. Hist. Biol.*, 3(No. 2):222.
14. Figlio, K. (1975): Theories of perception and the physiology of mind in the late eighteenth century. *Hist. Sci.*, 12:177–212.
15. Clarke, E., and O'Malley, C. D. (1968): *The Human Brain and Spinal Cord*, p. 494. University of California Press, Berkeley, Calif.
16. Cranefield, P. (1957): Organic physics of 1847 and the biophysics of today. *J. Hist. Med. Allied Sci.*, 12:407–423.
17. Clarke, E., and O'Malley, C. D. (1968): *The Human Brain and Spinal Cord.*, p. 502. University of California Press, Berkeley, Calif.
18. Spencer, H. (1881): *Principles of Psychology*, London.
19. Blakemore, C. (1977): *Mechanics of the Mind.* Cambridge University Press, Cambridge, England.
20. Fulton, J. (1948): *Functional Localisation in Frontal Lobes and Cerebellum*, Chap. 3. Oxford University Press, Oxford, England.
21. Tizard, B. (1959): Theories of brain localisation from Flourens to Lashley. *Med. Hist.*, 3:132–145.
22. Sherrington, C. S. (1947): *Integrative Action of the Nervous System*, Preface. Cambridge University Press, Cambridge, England.
23. Fulton, J. (1948): *Functional Localisation in Frontal Lobes and Cerebellum*, Preface. Oxford University Press, Oxford, England.
24. Swazey, J. (1970): Action propre and action commune. *J. Hist. Biol.*, 3(No. 2):213–235.
25. Goldstein, K. (1940): *Human Nature in the Light of Psychopathology.* Harvard University Press, Cambridge, Mass. Idem (1942): *After Effects of Brain Injury in War.* Heinemann, London.
26. Herrick, C. J. (1920): *Brains of Rats and Men*, p. 247, University of Chicago Press, Chicago.
27. Lashley, K. (1929): *Brain Mechanisms and Intelligence*, p. 154. New York.
28. Clarke, E., and O'Malley, C. D. (1968): *The Human Brain and Spinal Cord*, p. 573. University of California Press, Berkeley, Calif.
29. Lashley, K. (1929): *Brain Mechanisms and Intelligence*, New York.

30. Goldstein, K. (1940): *Human Nature in the Light of Psychopathology*. Harvard University Press, Cambridge, Mass. Idem (1942): *After Effects of Brain Injury in War*. Heinemann, London.
31. Lewin, K. (1951): Field theory and social science. In: *Selected Papers of K. Lewin*, edited by D. Cartwright, Harper, New York.
32. Emmett, D. (1966): *Whitehead's Philosophy of Organism*, p. 185. Macmillan, London.
33. Allen, G. (1978): *Life Sciences in the Twentieth Century*, p. 77. Cambridge University Press, Cambridge, England.

Historical Aspects of the Neurosciences,
edited by F. Clifford Rose and W.F. Bynum.
Raven Press, New York ©

The Great Confrontation: The Meeting Between Broca and Jackson in 1868

Robert J. Joynt

Department of Neurology, University of Rochester, Rochester, New York 14642

It was noted in the Medical Annotation section of the Lancet of July 25, 1868, that Professor Broca would be attending the meeting of the British Association for the Advancement of Science to be held at Norwich from August 19 to 25 of that year (1). This was followed by an item in the same section which read (2):

> M. Broca at Norwich
>
> A very interesting discussion on Aphasia is likely to take place at The British Association Meeting at Norwich. M. Broca, whose anatomical researches in connexion on aphasia have done so much to clear up that difficult subject, will be present and will doubtless speak in the discussion on Dr. Hughlings Jackson's paper on the same topic. It will be no small attraction to the meeting that visitors will thus have the opportunity of immediately comparing the best English and the best French views on the pathology of this remarkable disease.

It is obvious that the writer of this item thought that the meeting of these two scientists was of special interest. It is also suggested that there may be some chauvinistic appeal and, indeed, a confrontation. Judging from the numbers of entries around that time in the English and French journals, the topic of aphasia and the related problem of cerebral localization of speech function were very popular. Interestingly, the two individuals involved were not greatly interested at that time in "the pathology of this remarkable disease." It is safe to say that Broca had largely lost interest or had at least turned to other things, having published his last paper on the subject two years before (3). His paper at the meeting was published (4) in 1869, but it represented nothing more than a summary of previously expressed views. His bibliography for the preceding few years was devoted to his primary interests of surgery and anthropology (5). Jackson was much more interested in the mechanisms underlying speech and its loss, although he had already extended Broca's notions about cerebral dominance by suggesting that the right hemisphere had functions peculiar to itself (6).

The background to the meeting is well known regarding Broca's contributions, but less so of Jackson's. Broca was hailed as the founder of cerebral localization, although his priority had been questioned after the republication of the paper by Marc Dax (7). Broca had described two patients in 1861 with loss of speech (8,9), and in 1863 he reported on eight patients (10), noting that all had lesions in the left third frontal convolution. Broca noted this as a peculiar fact and awaited more proof. In 1865 (11), he stated that we speak with the left hemisphere. By this time, the work of Marc Dax written in 1836 was well known, although it had probably not been reported or publicly distributed at that time (12).

The principal points on which Jackson came to differ with Broca arose when Broca suggested a classification for speech loss and when Broca speculated on the reasons for cerebral dominance. These attempts were made in the 1861 and 1865 discussions (3,8) and formed much of the basis for Broca's presentation at Norwich (4). Broca used his term "aphemia" to designate that condition where one lost the faculty to coordinate the movements for articulation. But, he pointed out, the "memory" for words was still intact. In verbal amnesia, "amnésie verbale," the patient has lost the association between the idea and the word, so that he can no longer express his ideas by speaking or writing. In regard to the thorny and still elusive question of the reason for left hemisphere localization of language function, Broca believed that this hemisphere was more advanced in its development than the right hemisphere. He cited the anatomical work of Gratiolet, and he pointed out that with this lead in anatomical development, not only is the left hemisphere earlier constituted to direct the complicated motor acts with the right hand, but also the complicated act of speaking. In a sense, Broca suggested that it is the left hemisphere that is educated for language. He excluded the simple act of articulation, which depends on both hemispheres to an equal degree.

Broca's ideas on classification arose prior to Jackson's first paper on the subject, but Broca's speculation on the reason for cerebral lateralization of speech came after Jackson's early papers. It is unlikely that Broca was ignorant of Jackson's views. Although Jackson often published his work in rather obscure journals and in a difficult style, two points made by Henry Head (13), Jackson's work had been singled out and summarized in a French editorial (14). Fritz, the summarist, had noted the intensive discussions about language and its loss, and so believed that the views of Jackson, which had been published in the *Lancet* (6), would be pertinent.

Jackson by 1868 had already published several papers on language and its disturbances. In the early papers, he had buttressed Broca's notions on the unique role of the left hemisphere in speech. In the correspondence section of the *British Medical Journal* on May 21, 1864, he reported 31 cases with right hemiplegia (15). He also noted that he had not seen any cases with left hemiplegia with loss of speech, but two had been reported to him. He stated, "M. Broca believes that disease of the brain *on the left side only* produces loss of speech; and, if I were to judge from the cases under my own care, I should think so too." Jackson had certain reservations, however, by stating that he agreed with Broca regarding the importance of the left hemisphere, but only in a general way with the notion that speech is in a circumscribed area of that hemisphere (16). He noted that his cases were clinical observations, so that exact localization was not possible.

Jackson by 1866 had developed his views further, both on classification of speech disorders and the contributory role of the individual hemispheres. Summarizing his views in an article in the *Medical Times and Gazette* (17), he now said. "I must here say that I believe less in some of the views propounded by Broca than I did, although I think the scientific world is under vast obligation to him for giving precision to an important inquiry." In this paper, he reiterated his earlier view that voluntary speech is located on the left and automatic on the right, and it is not just the left side that is educated: "I think that both sides are probably educated but the left one is the one that begins to act, and that those educated utterances, which are in a sense involuntary, have become so by habit—i.e. frequent education—and may be the result of action of the right side only." Jackson said that the left hemisphere in speech is "the elder brother." He had already suggested a classification of speech defects different from Broca (16).

This was the background leading up to the Norwich meeting of 1868. It was in the report of the meeting in the *Lancet* (18) that it was "perhaps unfortunate" that the International

Congress of Prehistoric Archeology was held at the same time. Knowing Broca's consuming interest in anthropology and his waning interest in aphasia, it is likely that the archeological meeting was of more interest to him. The President of Section D of the British Association was Reverend M. J. Berkeley, who gave a long address on the contributions of Darwin. He also mentioned some noteworthy biological experiments by Herbert Spencer, which should have pleased Jackson if he were in the audience. While many of the papers were reported *in extenso* in the transactions (19), there was only the listing of titles for Broca's and Jackson's contributions, and there were no details of the discussion. Broca published his talk later (4); Jackson's remained only in summary form, but it formed the basis for many of his later papers. The discussion was briefly summarized in the *Lancet* (18) and the *British Medical Journal* (20), and more extensively in the *Medical Times and Gazette* (21).

Jackson's paper, "The Physiology of Language," was first. In this paper, he made the following points: In healthy language there are two kinds, intellectual and emotional; in disease it is usually the latter which is affected. Both halves of the brain are educated and the left half leads, but automatic speech may arise from the undamaged right half. Although there are some exceptional cases, such as when hemiplegia occurs with loss of speech, it is almost always on the right; the language function cannot be localized to any one spot, but the nearness of a lesion to the left corpus striatum determined the degree of intellectual defect in expression.

Broca followed and used a diagram and plaster cast to illustrate his ideas on localization. He reiterated his view on the left third frontal convolution being the center for articulate language, and he suggested that the corpus striatum was merely the "medium of expression." He demonstrated circumscribed lesions of the left third frontal convolution with loss of articulate speech. Finally, Broca suggested that there was an original organic force that directed speech and other results of education which were confined to the left hemisphere.

There was a third paper on the program by R. Dunn. Dunn argued against the thesis of exclusive left cerebral hemisphere localization for speech function, and he referred to the contributions of Gall, who had localized speech in both anterior lobes.

It was noted in the three summaries that there was "a most interesting and animated discussion" (21), "very spirited" (20), and "very animated" (18). The discussants expressed their views for and against Broca's theory of localization, but there was no evidence that the points made by Jackson were discussed at all. Most remarkably, the record contains no mention of any comments or questions by Broca regarding Jackson's presentation, nor comments or questions by Jackson for Broca's. The confrontation did not take place in the public forum. Perhaps, in the corridors . . . ? We will never know.

How has time dealt with these two early pioneers? Has it settled the confrontation? It is fair to say that both have been vindicated. There is little doubt that the language disturbance described by Broca is situated more anteriorly as he suggested. Also, Jackson's view on the contribution of the right hemisphere is correct in that lower order language is represented there. The fundamental question as to why one hemisphere is dominant for speech remains an enigma. Broca's idea that it is more developed is borne out by the facts now known about anatomical asymmetries of the two hemispheres (22). But why the functions of the two are different still puzzles us. Benton and Joynt (23) point out that the association has been established by empirical observations, but "its basic psychoneurologic significance still eludes us."

ACKNOWLEDGMENT

Supported by a Senior International Fogarty Fellowship and The Commonwealth Fund.

REFERENCES

1. Medical Annotations (1868): *Lancet*, ii:121. See also Francis Schiller (1979): *Paul Broca: Founder of French Anthropology, Explorer of the Brain*, pp. 203ff. Univ. of California Press, Berkeley, Calif.
2. Medical Annotations (1868): *Lancet*, ii:226.
3. Broca, P. (1866): Noveau cas d'aphémie traumatique. *Bull. Soc. Anth.*, (2 série) 1:396.
4. Broca, P. (1869): Sur le siege de la faculté du langage articule. *Trib. Méd.*, 74:254; 75:265.
5. Unsigned (1880): Paul Broca. *Rev. d'Anth.* (2 série) 2:577.
6. Jackson, J. H. (1864): Clinical remarks on cases of defects of expression (by words, writing, signs, etc.) in diseases of the nervous system. *Lancet*, ii:604.
7. Dax, M. (1865): Lesions de la moitie gauche de l'encéphale coincident, avec l'oubli des signes de la pensee: *Gaz. Hebdom. Med. Chir.*, 2:259.
8. Broca, P. (1861): Remarques sur le siège de la faculté du langage articulé, suives d'une observation d'aphémie. *Bull. Soc. Anat.*, 36:330.
9. Broca, P. (1861): Nouvelle observation d'aphémie produite par une lesion de la moitie posterieure des deuxieme et troisieme circonvolutions frontales gauche. *Bull. Soc. Anat.*, 36:398.
10. Broca, P. (1863): Localisation des fonctions cerebrales. Siège du langage articulé. *Bull. Soc. Anth.*, 4:200.
11. Broca, P. (1865): Sur le siège de la faculté du langage articulé. *Bull. Soc. Anth.*, 6:377.
12. Joynt, R. J., and Benton, A. L. (1964): The memoir of Marc Dax on aphasia. *Neurology*, 14:851.
13. Head, H. (1926): *Aphasia and Kindred Disorders of Speech*, Vol. I, p. 30. Cambridge University Press, London.
14. Fritz, E. (1864): Troubles du langage. *Gaz. Hebdom. Med. Chir.*, 1:873.
15. Jackson, J. H. (1864): Hemiplegia on the right side with loss of speech (correspondence). *Br. Med. J.*, 1:572.
16. Jackson, J. H. (1864): Loss of speech: its association with valvular disease of the heart and with hemiplegia of the right side. *Cl. Lect. and Rep., London Hosp.*, 1:388.
17. Jackson, J. H. (1866): Notes on the physiology and pathology of language. *Med. Times and Gaz.*, 1:659.
18. Medical Annotations (1868): British Association for the Advancement of Science. *Lancet*, ii:291.
19. Report on the 38th Meeting of the British Association for the Advancement of Science (1869). Held at Norwich in August 1868. John Murray, London.
20. Reports of Societies (1868): British Association for the Advancement of Science. *Br. Med. J.*, 2:259.
21. British Association for the Advancement of Science (1868): *Med. Times and Gaz.*, 11:273.
22. Geschwind, N., and Levitsky, W. (1968): Human brain: Left-right asymmetries in temporal speech regions. *Science*, 161:186.
23. Benton, A. L., and Joynt, R. J. (1960): Early descriptions of aphasia. *Arch. Neurol.*, 3:205.

Historical Aspects of the Neurosciences,
edited by F. Clifford Rose and W. F. Bynum.
Raven Press, New York ©

Sigmund Freud's Contribution to the Early History of Aphasiology

E. Bay

Moorenstrasse 70, D-4000 Düsseldorf, Federal Republic of Germany

Sigmund Freud is world famous as the father of psychoanalysis. Far less known is the fact that he was an outstanding neuroanatomist and neurologist, who made valuable contributions to the developing science of neurology during the last decades of the 19th century. The most interesting and important of Freud's neurological writings is a small monograph entitled "Zur Auffassung der Aphasien" (1), in which he dealt with the then topical problem of aphasiology. This article remained largely unnoticed by Freud's contemporaries in Germany and even more so in England. According to Stengel (2), only 257 copies of the original book had been sold, and there seemingly did not exist a single copy in Great Britain. Only in 1953 did Stengel (2) make this work known in Great Britain in an English translation. (The quotations in the present chapter are from Stengel's translation.) What was the aim and implication of this sole contribution of Freud to the problem of aphasia?

The papers of Broca (3) aroused a vivid interest in aphasia throughout the medical world, inciting in the last decades of the 19th century a flood of clinical observations and an even greater number of theoretical interpretations. From the numerous discussions, the so-called classical doctrine of aphasia finally emerged, contrived by Wernicke (4), and brought to completion by Lichtheim (5) with the famous Wernicke-Lichtheim scheme of aphasia (Fig. 1), explaining in a single homogeneous theory the various types of disordered speech. This theory includes in essence two simplifying factors of high didactic value, which is why it has remained so convincing up to the present day.

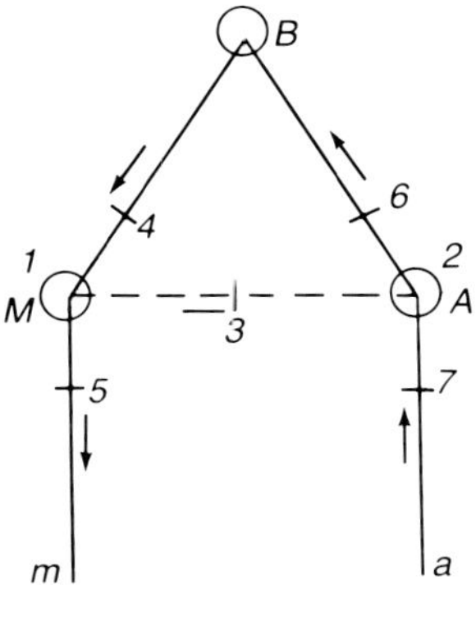

FIG. 1. The Wernicke-Lichtheim scheme of aphasia.

The first is the essentially static nature of this "psychological study on anatomical base" (4), comprising the cerebral speech apparatus of two independent (motor and sensory) speech centers connected by "association fibres." In this system, the different types of disordered speech depend exclusively on the site of a given lesion interrupting the speech circuit in one or another center or tract of association fibers. The other suggestive quality of the Wernicke-Lichtheim scheme is the strict symmetry of the speech circuit with its ingoing "sensory" and outgoing "motor" branch. Both correspond fully in their connections with the periphery, with each other, and with the symbolic "center of concepts" (B), representing the numerous parts of the cortex from which the speech apparatus can be stimulated to action. This symmetry of the scheme infers that the "word-sound-images" (in A) and the "kinesthetic word impressions" (in M) are of equal importance for the speech mechanism and that the corresponding disorders (sensory and motor aphasia, respectively) are of equal pathological importance (6).

By virtue of its ingenious simplicity, this "classical" scheme slowly but steadily found general consent, while more sophisticated theories, e.g., the concepts of Jackson or Kussmaul (7), which were undoubtedly more adequate to the extremely complex problem of speech and speech disorders, did not find contemporary approval. This is a fascinating, though not comforting, chapter of the early history of aphasiology.

In this scientific scenery, Freud launched his monograph on aphasia. Contrary to most papers of the time, it was not based on some more or less cursory and biased examinations of selected patients (8) but exclusively on a critical analysis of the theory, its premises and inferences. Although accepting the current concepts of association psychology and its anatomical representations in circumscribed cortical centers and subcortical association fibers, respectively, Freud rejects the fundamental concepts of the classical doctrine one by one with brilliant and astute reasoning, which one can still read with pleasure today despite its time-dependent errors.

Right from the beginning, the fascinating simplicity and uniformity of the classical doctrine presented difficulties in one point, i.e., in explaining the common occurrence of paraphasic distortions in the speech of patients with sensory aphasia. According to the theory, sensory aphasia is caused by an isolated destruction of center A. Therefore, the whole motor tract being intact, spontaneous speech should be undisturbed. To explain this discrepancy, Wernicke was compelled to introduce, in a rather weak argumentation, functional aspects into his otherwise strictly static theory. Demonstrating the fallacy of Wernicke's arguments, Freud at the same time stressed the necessity to consider, for a full comprehension of aphasic speech, functional as well as anatomical aspects.

Functional aspects in this context mean that damage to a "center" does not necessarily produce complete destruction with full loss of function, but less severe damage may produce functional deterioration with different involvement of functionally different activities as, for instance, reactions to "volitional stimulation," to "associative stimulation," and to "direct sensory stimuli" (9).

Freud writes (2):

> Furthermore, the impact of an only partly destructive lesion on the whole apparatus must be taken into consideration. Two possibilities are conceivable, both of which do in fact occur. Either some parts of the apparatus are put out of action . . . while the intact parts continue to function as usual; or it reacts to the lesion as a unitary whole, in which case there is no loss of part functions but a lowering of function in general. (p. 30)

He remarks "that the speech apparatus shows in all its parts the latter kind of reaction to incomplete lesions. . . . For instance, a small lesion in the motor speech area would never cause the loss of a hundred words, the type of which would depend only on the site of the lesion" (p. 31).

The impairment of a function in general may be due to an incomplete lesion or to a purely functional disorder without an anatomical lesion. Freud explicitly mentions "that the paraphasias observed in aphasic patients do not differ from the incorrect use and the distortion of words which the healthy person can observe in himself in states of fatigue or divided attention under the influence of disturbing affects" (p. 13). This, indeed, is a remarkable precursor of later psychoanalytic ideas.

Another target of Freud's criticism is the differentiation of aphasic syndromes in cortical aphasias (due to a lesion of a center) and subcortical ones (due to a lesion of connecting fibers only). Here, too, the clinical facts did not correspond with the pattern derived from the theory. The differences between syndromes are better explained by partial deterioration of function due to incomplete lesions which, in Freud's opinion, are always cortical. Therefore, in this respect, too, the purely anatomical consideration of the Wernicke-Lichtheim scheme must be replaced by a partially functional one.

Finally, Freud advocated an organization of the speech apparatus essentially different from the classical one. He illustrated his concept by the scheme shown in Fig. 2, anxiously making clear that this figure was only a "psychological schema of the word concept" and was not meant to represent anatomical structures in the same sense as Fig. 1. Apart from this difference in meaning, the difference in structure is evident. The cortical apparatus for speech no longer has the fascinating symmetry between input and output. Rather, the area of the "word-sound-images" (corresponding to center A in Fig. 1) is the cardinal point of the speech apparatus to which the other (kinesthetic, visual) verbal images are only secondary.

Still more important, however, is the fact that the word-sound-image provides the sole connection of the speech apparatus with the "object associations" that, in Freud's symbolic figure, are represented by their visual, tactile, and auditory components rather widely distributed over the cortex in an "open complex." Freud writes (2):

> In the light of observations in speech disorders we have formed the view that the word concept (the idea of the word) is linked with its sensory part, in particular through its sound impressions, to the object concept. In consequence, we have arrived at a division of speech disorders into two classes: (1) verbal aphasia, in which only the associations between the single elements of the word concept are disturbed; and (2) asymbolic aphasia, in which the association between word concepts and object concepts are disturbed. (p. 78)

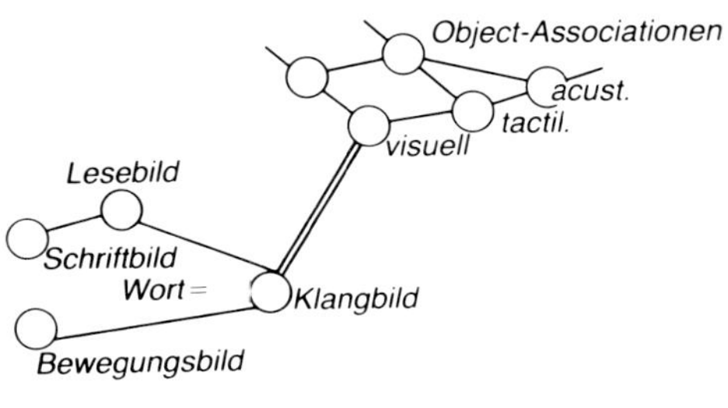

FIG. 2. Freud's concept of an organization of the speech apparatus. Translations of the German words are as follows: *Object-Associationen* = Object Associations; *acust.* = auditory; *tactil.* = tactile; *visuell* = visual; *Lesebild* = visual image for print; *Schriftbild* = visual image for script; *Wort-Klangbild* = word-sound-image; and *Bewegungsbild* = Kinesthetic image.

Freud is less certain about a third, hypothetical type of aphasia, which he termed "agnostic aphasia." Here, his evidence is not based on his own experience but on poorly described cases in the literature; correctly, however, he did not ascribe these to lesions in the speech area. The fact that in this paragraph, Freud incidentally coined the term "agnosia" without making any substantial contribution to the problem of agnosia, paradoxically produced the only lasting effect of his book on contemporary medicine.

For an understanding of aphasic symptoms and syndromes, both anatomical and functional aspects must be taken into account. Anatomically, Freud suggests a large, in its extent and location not sufficiently known, cortical speech association area with the auditory area as nodal point. What we know as "speech centers" are the connections of this speech area with the centers for the peripheral (motor, visual, acoustic) instruments of speech. Lesions in these "speech centers" disrupt the respective connections and thereby produce motor aphasia, alexia, or auditory (sensory) aphasia. Freud states (2):

> The further the lesion moves towards the centre of the speech region the less likely it is to cut off any single element of the speech associations, and the more the features of the aphasia will depend on functional factors to which the speech apparatus is subject, independently of the site of the lesion. (p. 82)

It is surprising how well Freud's essentially speculative anatomical considerations agree with modern empirical findings (10).

The functional aspects of disordered speech originate from partial destruction of, or incomplete damage to, the speech area, to which the speech apparatus "reacts as a unitary whole . . . with a lowering of function in general" (p. 31). This lowering of function follows the general rule that the highest and most volitional activities are the first and most severely impaired, while the lower, more automatic performances are longer and better preserved. Obviously, these ideas are derived from Hughlings Jackson, "the author on whose views I have based almost all the arguments which I have advanced in refuting the localizatory theory of the aphasias" (p. 61).

Besides this congruence of views, Jackson and Freud have another feature in common, the complete contemporary disregard of their contributions, which deviated so radically from the current "school of thought." Head, in his comprehensive survey of the history of aphasia (11), complained about this neglect with regard to Jackson, but Freud's contribution escaped even his notice. The reason for this neglect is the same in both cases: The complexity of their concepts compared too unfavorably with the ingenious simplicity of the classical doctrine, in which the whole of aphasiology is comprised in a simple schema. For some aphasiologists, this simplicity is tempting even today; they could still read Freud's monograph with profit.

The experienced psychologist Freud well realized this handicap and closed his treatise with the critical remark (2):

> I am well aware that the considerations set out in this book must leave a feeling of dissatisfaction in the reader's mind. I have endeavoured to demolish a convenient and attractive theory of the aphasias, and having succeeded in this, I have been able to put into its place something less obvious and less complete. I only hope that the theory I have proposed will do more jusice to the facts and will expose the real difficulties better than the one I have rejected. (p. 104)

There is nothing to add to this statement.

REFERENCES

1. Freud, S. (1891): *Zur Auffassung der Aphasien*. F. Deuticke, Leipzig.

2. Freud, S. (1953): *On Aphasia*, translated by E. Stengel. Imago Publishing Co., London.
3. Broca, P. (1861): *Bull. Soc. d'Anthrop.* 2:235. *Bull. Soc. Anatom.*, 6:330,398.
4. Wernicke, C. (1874): *Der aphasische Symptomenkomplex. Eine psychologische Studie auf anatomischer Basis.* Cohn & Weigert, Breslau.
5. Lichtheim, L. (1885): *Dtsch. Arch. klin. Med.* 36:204. *Brain* 7:433.
6. Vogel, P. (1954): *Mschr. Psychiat. Neurol.* 128:256.
7. Kussmaul, A. (1881): *Die Störungen der Sprache.* F. C. W. Vogel, Leipzig.
8. Bay, E. (1973): *Nervenarzt* 44:57.
9. Bastian, H. C. (1869): *Br. Foreign Med.-Chi. Rev.* 63:209,470.
10. Hecaen, H., and Angelergues, R. (1964): In: *Ciba Sympos. Disorders of Language*, edited by A. V. S. de Reuck, p. 223. Churchill, London.
11. Head, H. (1926): *Aphasia and Kindred Disorders of Speech.* University Press, Cambridge, U.K.

Historical Aspects of the Neurosciences,
edited by F. Clifford Rose and W. F. Bynum.
Raven Press, New York ©

Some British Contributors to Cortical Localization

William C. Gibson

Department of the History of Medicine and Science, University of British Columbia, Vancouver, British Columbia, Canada

Macdonald Critchley's predecessors at King's College Hospital, R. Bentley Todd and Sir David Ferrier, left to British neurology a great heritage. Thirty years before Fritsch and Hitzig (1) reported, in 1870, that electrical stimulation of the cerebral cortex in animals produced discrete movements of the opposite side of the body, Todd (2) was driving "fine bradawls into the cranium" of rabbits. By energizing these short metal electrodes by means of a "magneto-electric rotating machine," he was able to observe "general convulsions." In 1840, Todd summarized his work with this succinct statement:

> These experiments, which I repeated several times, and each time with like results, seem to denote that convulsions are modified according to the part of the cerebro-spinal axis which is primarily excited.

However, in March of 1873, Ferrier, while visiting Dr. James Crichton-Browne, the Director of the West Riding Asylum in Wakefield, Yorkshire, began to lay his plans to advance the Fritsch and Hitzig investigations much further. Crichton-Browne, a fellow Edinburgh graduate, invited Ferrier to work out his ideas on cerebral localization in the newly opened laboratories in the asylum.

Thus, we find the 30-year-old Ferrier, who had taken his M. A. in philosophy and classics at Edinburgh with Alexander Bain, prior to his M.D. degree, now embarking on pioneer research in Wakefield. Ferrier was already Professor of Forensic Medicine at King's College Hospital in London, and he condensed into the next few years a program of research that would have defeated any ordinary physician.

After faradic stimulation of brains of the vertebrate series, Ferrier, with the help of a grant from the Royal Society, undertook the study of the ape brain. Such were his results, first published in the Reports of the West Riding Asylum, that he was invited by the Royal Society to give its Croonian Lectures, not only in 1874 (3) but also in 1875. By 1876, Ferrier's mapping of the cortex in animals was virtually complete (4). Clearly, he had learned how to work with great intensity once he had the laboratory he required.

Osler noted in one of his little notebooks, now at McGill University, "Experience is not to be measured by time served, but by the use which a man makes of his opportunities." If ever a man made good use of his opportunities, it was David Ferrier. Soon after graduation in medicine at Edinburgh in 1868, he became an assistant to a busy and cultured general practitioner in Suffolk. There in the garden, over a two-year period, Ferrier carried on his first research on "the comparative anatomy and intimate structure of the Corpora Quadrigemina" of the brain. This work was embodied in his M.D. thesis for Edinburgh, and it brought Ferrier great distinction and a gold medal.

While Ferrier in England was mapping the ape cortex, Dr. Roberts Bartholow (5), a professor of medicine in Cincinnati, Ohio, was stimulating electrically the exposed cerebral cortex of his housemaid, who suffered from an eroding cancer of the scalp and cranium. Weak faradic currents applied to the cortex provoked movements of the limbs of the opposite side and the head turning to that side. The publication of this work, which had been carried on in 1874 by Bartholow, led to his complete ostracism from medical work, so great was the outcry. Cincinnati was not entirely a neurological desert. In 1860, the later-to-be-famous John Shaw Billings was attempting to write his thesis on the value of surgery in the relief of epilepsy. His inability to find books in Cincinnati, or elsewhere, that were helpful in answering his questions led Billings to found the great Surgeon General's Library (now the National Library of Medicine) in Washington, D.C., and to develop the *Index Catalogue* to medical literature.

It should not be imagined that Ferrier's work was well received at first either, for he, like William Harvey, was beleaguered by the theories of the past. Flourens (6) kept shouting: "When one point of the nervous system becomes excited, it excites all others; one point irritated, irritates all." Goltz of Strasbourg was not impressed by the work of those who saw localization of function in the cerebral cortex, and in Goltz we find a forerunner of Lashley's later views.

Actually, the collision between Goltz and Ferrier occurred at the International Medical Congress in London in 1881 (7). Goltz showed that his decorticated dogs, while unable to make purposeful movements, could nevertheless walk. Goltz roared forth: "I will prove beyond the shadow of a doubt that Ferrier's theory is completely false." Ferrier's point was that in the ape, a small ablation in the motor cortex was much more crippling than it would be in a dog. As Ferrier demonstrated hemiplegia in one of his experimental monkeys, before the congress, Charcot cried out, "C'est un malade!" It is of interest that the youthful Charles Sherrington studied the brain of this monkey, under the guidance of J. N. Langley at Cambridge, as his first contribution to neurology (8).

Ferrier's opponents were not only the antilocalization workers. More diligent still were the antivivisectionists (9), who were able to bring Ferrier before the law for his experimental work on animals. The court rejected the allegations made by this ever-strident group, and Ferrier was exonerated. His clinical practice increased, possibly as a result of the trial and his acquittal. Despite his clinical responsibilities, both at King's College Hospital and at the National Hospital, Queen Square, Ferrier kept up his experimental work for many years. Santiago Ramón y Cajal (10) recounts his surprise and pleasure, during his visit to London as Croonian Lecturer in 1894, at finding Ferrier at work in his laboratory. It is little wonder that Ferrier was an active officer of the Research Defence Society.

Ferrier was no mere theoretical neurologist. He foresaw the future for brain surgery that Joseph Lister, his colleague at King's College Hospital, had opened up with his antiseptic surgery, and he urged all his surgeon friends to consider opening the skull to remove what Sherrington has called "certain forms of cerebral tumour and intracranial mischief." Ferrier, through his Marshall Hall Oration in 1883, reiterated his appeal to surgeons to intervene; MacEwen in Glasgow and Rickman Godlee in London heeded the call in that year.

In time, Ferrier's friend Crichton-Browne left Wakefield, and the West Riding Asylum Reports came to an end. It was not long before a new journal, *Brain*, was born, with Ferrier, Crichton-Browne, Hughlings Jackson, and Sir John Bucknell making up its editorial staff.

Another echo of the West Riding Asylum is to be found in the first issue of *Brain*, in the paper by William Bevan-Lewis on the large pyramidal cells of the pre-Rolandic cortex. He was pathologist to the West Riding Asylum and had been an associate of Ferrier, Crichton-Browne, and Clifford Allbutt (of *Middlemarch* fame), who was destined to be the Regius Professor of Physic at Cambridge. It is interesting to note that the distinguished Hughlings Jackson had, in 1873, contributed to the West Riding Asylum Reports his important paper, "On the anatomical, physiological and pathological investigation of epilepsies." In the same volume, one finds Ferrier's first paper, the forerunner of his book (1876). In that paper, Ferrier said:

> The objects I had in view in undertaking the present research were twofold: first to put to experimental proof the views entertained by Dr. Hughlings Jackson on the pathology of epilepsy, chorea and hemiplegia by imitating artificially the destroying and discharging lesions of disease which his writings have defined and differentiated— and secondly, to follow up the path which the researches of Fritsch and Hitzig indicated to me as likely to lead to results of great value in the elucidation of the functions of the cerebral hemispheres, and in the more exact localization and diagnosis of cerebral disease.

Less frequently do we read of Jackson's acknowledged debt to Ferrier. In his "Lectures on the diagnosis of epilepsy," given before the Harveian Society in 1879, Jackson said (11):

> I would take this opportunity of very strongly urging the importance of Ferrier's investigations of the sensory region of the brain . . . Ferrier has, I think, given a new starting-point for the methodical, the scientific investigation of a most important class of paroxysmal affections which are, in scientific regard, epilepsies.

In the introduction to his Lumleian lectures (12), delivered at the Royal College of Physicians in 1890, Jackson paid Ferrier this tribute:

> There are very few men of the day by whom both the art and science have been so greatly helped. It is only since his remarkable researches that medical men in this country have studied convulsions in a thoroughly realistic way. Without further particular acknowledgments I make the general one, that all over the field of neurology I am profoundly indebted to Ferrier.

This is surely high praise coming from one not given to hyperbole.

Ferrier was a founding member of the Physiological Society and for 35 years he served its *Journal*. A member of the council of the Royal Society, he was an ornament of great luster. Honors and medals were heaped upon him but did not change him. Sherrington summed up Ferrier's nature thus (13):

> Slight and erect in figure, genial and alert in bearing, the burden of years long weighed lightly upon him. A reflective quietude of voice and manner tended to veil the underlying energy, no less a part of his nature. Shrewd observer, keenly alive to men and things, and not least to aesthetics and to humour, his talk could exert charm, and owed something to a certain piquant directness and penetrative simplicity enhanced by a remnant of an accent from Aberdeen.

From Jackson to Ferrier to Sherrington, a current of thought and of endeavor "runs deep." Much of it concerns localization of cortical function. Later generations of Sherrington's pupils—Cushing, Penfield, and Fulton, to mention only three—extended and refined the classical work and broke much new ground. Jackson, after his apprenticeship at the York medical establishment, studied at St. Bartholomew's in London. There the ghost of John de Mirfeld (14) was probably at Jackson's elbow. That 14th century "localizer" described epileptic fits in detail, and knew that an injury to the right side of the head could produce paralysis on the left side of the body. Jackson returned to York for three years of work with Thomas Laycock who, in 1857, introduced bromides in the treatment of epilepsy. Laycock, a year earlier, had published "Lectures on the principles and methods of medical observation and research." In turn, Ferrier worked, though briefly, with Laycock later in Edinburgh. Parenthetically, it should be said that it took another Yorkshire man, Jonathan Hutchinson, to persuade Jackson that his future lay in London.

Sherrington has described the reaction of Ferrier to a new atlas on cortical localization; Ferrier said, with a smile, "We know so much now." He may well have been thinking of the classical atlas published by the Australian, A. W. Campbell (15), *Histological Studies on the Localization of Cerebral Function*, in 1905. Campbell had spent 13 years as pathologist to Rainhill Asylum near Liverpool, where he had enjoyed the constant encouragement of the Professor of Physiology at Liverpool, the young Charles Sherrington (16).

We tend to forget the scientific contributions made by physicians in the 19th century working in mental hospitals (17). August Forel, who eventually was the director of the Burgholzi Asylum and who succeeded Hitzig as Professor of Psychiatry at Zurich, made one of his contributions while a medical undergraduate; he wrote a thesis for Meynert on the structure and function of the mammalian thalamus in vision. In 1877, quite independently, he enunciated what Waldeyer later dubbed "the neurone theory." Von Monakow did his best work in the solitude of a mental hospital in Switzerland that had once been a Benedictine cloister. Camillo Golgi developed his silver chromate stain while employed as a resident physician at Abbiategrasso in 1873. Nissl worked out the details of nerve cells and their reaction to injury first in a Munich asylum and later in a similar setting in Frankfurt. However, it was as a medical student that he made a contribution that is appropriate to any discussion of cortical localization. At the age of 24, he produced his prize-winning graduation dissertation: "The pathological changes of the nerve cells of the cerebral cortex." So impressed was Gudden that he took Nissl into his institute immediately upon graduation.

Student contributions to our knowledge of the nervous system generally would have delighted Ferrier the teacher. They are far too numerous to describe in detail, but even a short list of such undergraduates and their work is worth a glance: Rudolph Berlin's classification of cortical nerve cells; Niclas and Spurzheim as assistants to Franz Joseph Gall; Alexander Monro, Secundus, and his ventricular foramen; Domenico Cotugno on sciatica, the cerebrospinal fluid, and the cochlea; Victor Horsley on intervertebral discs; Theodore Billroth on the nerves of electric fish; Robert Remak on the axon as a singular process of vertebrate nerve cells, confirmed by Helmholz in his thesis concerning invertebrate nerve cells; Edouard Brissaud on hemiplegia; Sigmund Freud on the derivation of posterior root ganglion cells; Henry Head on the role of the vagus nerve; Francesco Gennari on the white line in the optic cortex; Marc Dax on epileptic seizures in children followed by hemiplegia; and nostalgically, Christopher Wren, lost to medicine, despite his years of dissecting with Harvey's pupil Sir Charles Scarborough, despite his magnificent drawings for Thomas Willis' *Cerebri Anatome* (1664), and despite his introduction of the method of intravenous injections, notably in dogs, of substances affecting coordination and consciousness.

Finally, as one who has directed our attention forcefully to Huntington's chorea, Macdonald Critchley will be pleased to learn of the flowering of his work in a far distant neurological laboratory in Vancouver. Years ago, he visited the Crease Clinic of the provincial mental hospital in British Columbia, where he was shown by Dr. William Fister no less than 30 Huntington cases. Today in the Kinsmen Laboratory at the University of British Columbia, long associated with the Crease Clinic, Dr. Patrick McGeer and Dr. Edith McGeer are working on the neurochemistry of Huntington's disease, as a sequel to work on another disease, named for another of Dr. Critchley's favorite clinicians, James Parkinson. Few neurologists celebrating their four-score years can claim to have stimulated a whole generation of researchers around the world as can the "compleat teacher," Macdonald Critchley.

REFERENCES

1. Fritsch, T., and Hitzig, E. (1870): *Arch. Anat. Physiol. (Leipzig)*, 300–332.
2. Todd, R. B. In: *Creative Minds in Medicine*, by W. C. Gibson. Charles C. Thomas, Springfield, Illinois, p. 99.
3. Ferrier, D. (1874): (Croonian lecture). *Proc. R. Soc. Lond.* 22:229–232.
4. Ferrier, D. (1876): *The Functions of the Brain.* Smith, Elder, London.
5. Bartholow, R. (1874): *Am. J. Med. Sci.*, 67:305–313.
6. Flourens, P. (1824): *Recherches éxpérimentales sūr les proprietés et les fonctions du système nerveux dans les animaux vertébrés.* Crevot, Paris.
7. (1881): *Trans. Internat. Med. Congr. (London)*, 1:221–228, 234–237.
8. Langley, J. N., and Sherrington, C. S. (1884): *Proc. Soc. J. Physiol. (London)*, 5:vi.
9. French, D. (1975): *Antivivisection and Medical Science in Victorian Society.* Princeton University Press, Princeton, N.J.
10. Craigie, E. H., and Gibson, W. C. (1968): *The World of Ramon y Cajal.* Charles C. Thomas, Springfield, Illinois.
11. Jackson, J. H. (1879): Lectures on the diagnosis of epilepsy. *Med. Times and Gaz.*, 1:29,85,141,223.
12. Jackson, J. H. (1890): Lumleian lectures on convulsive seizures. *Br. Med. J.*, 1:703,765,821.
13. Sherrington, C. S. (1928): Obituary of Ferrier. *Proc. R. Soc. Lond.*, 103:vii-xvi.
14. Moore, N. (1918): *The History of St. Bartholomew's Hospital.* Pearson, London.
15. Campbell, A. W. (1905): *Histological Studies on the Localization of Cerebral Function.* Cambridge University Press, Cambridge, England.
16. Eccles, J. C., and Gibson, W. C. (1979): *Sherrington—His Life and Thought.* Springer, Heidelberg, p. 37.
17. Gibson, W. C. (1958): *Young Endeavour: Contributions to Science by Medical Students.* Charles C. Thomas, Springfield, Illinois.

Historical Aspects of the Neurosciences,
edited by F. Clifford Rose and W. F. Bynum.
Raven Press, New York ©

American Pioneers in the Topic of Word Blindness

Lucius Waites

Texas Scottish Rite Hospital for Crippled Children, Dallas, Texas 75219

Reports of congenital word blindness in America began to appear approximately 10 years following the original descriptions of Hinshelwood, Kerr, and Morgan (1–3). Credit for the original article in America goes to W. E. Bruner, an ophthalmologist of Cleveland, who published "Congenital Word Blindness" in *Ophthalmology*, Volume 1, page 189 (January 1905). He discussed a 9-year-old patient in some detail and stated that visual acuity was not a problem. The concluding remarks of his presentation were interesting as he suggested that training would not be successful in the most severe cases, but the majority of cases would be crowned with ultimate success.

Aloysius Schapringer, an 1872 graduate of the University of Vienna, a German immigrant and an ophthalmologist and otologist of New York City, is credited with the next report, which was read before the Society of Ophthalmology at a meeting of the New York Academy of Medicine on February 19, 1906. Apparently, this report was not published, but recognition was given by Claiborne as described in the next paragraph.

J. Herbert Claiborne, an ophthalmologist of New York City, reported two boys with congenital word blindness. According to his article, "Types of Congenital Symbol Amblyopia," in the *Journal of the American Medical Association*, Volume 47, page 1813 (1906), Claiborne stated that his presentation followed Schapringer's paper at the same New York Academy of Medicine meeting, and he gave credit to Schapringer. Claiborne's article was interesting because he discussed many aspects of the condition, including the possible increased frequency in English-speaking children. He suggested that public school instruction was a factor because of the whole word method teaching. He also discussed left-handedness in his article. In addition, Claiborne discussed difficulty with mathematics and imperfect appreciation of music as analogous to word blindness, but he did not consider these conditions a part of the clinical picture presented by children with congenital reading problems. He made the observation that no postmortem corroboration was available. One of his conclusions was unusual in that he advocated that these children be taught to become left-handed so that speech, symbol, and sound centers on the right side of the brain would be cultivated to the exclusion of those on the left or as a supplementation to the defects on the left.

Next, Edward Jackson, an ophthalmologist of Denver, reported two patients and reviewed the previous cases in "Developmental Alexia (Congenital Word Blindness)" in the *American Journal of Medical Sciences*, Volume 131, page 849 (1906). Jackson was the most eminent of the American physicians who originally reported this condition. He was Professor of Ophthalmology at the University of Colorado School of Medicine and was very active in that speciality. His review of all previously reported cases was well done and his two additional patients brought the total to 21 cases. Jackson discussed the treatment and suggested that congenital word blindness was a question of delayed development.

It is interesting to note that the original reports in America were made by ophthalmologists, and all stated that poor vision was not a factor in congenital word blindness. Claiborne made the observation that the condition had not received the attention it deserved from pediatrics and neurology.

REFERENCES

1. Hinshelwood, J. (1895): Word-blindness and visual memory. *Lancet*, 2: 1564–1570.
2. Kerr, J. (1897): School hygiene, in its mental, moral and physical aspects. Howard Medal Prize Essay. *J. Roy. Stat. Soc.*, 60:613–680.
3. Morgan, W. (1896): A case of congenital word-blindness, *Br. Med. J.*, 2:1378.

Historical Aspects of the Neurosciences,
edited by F. Clifford Rose and W. F. Bynum.
Raven Press, New York ©

The History of the Syndrome of Capgras

John Todd

High Royds Hospital, Menston, Ilkley, Yorkshire, England

> Beware alway of doubleness.
> John Lydgate (1370–1450), English poet

The essential features of the syndrome of Capgras are well described by Critchley (1) as "the non-recognition of familiar persons, with the postulation of imaginary differences and the further expressed belief that the real person has been replaced by a double." This description would be wholly satisfactory even today, some 57 years after Capgras and Reboul-Lachaux (2) presented their classic case entitled "L'illusion des 'Sosies' dans un délire systématisé chronique," if the words "or by an impostor closely resembling the real person" had been added. The source of the word "sosie" is believed to be Molière's play *Amphitryon*, in which Amphitryon's servant, Sosie, is impersonated by Jupiter's herald, Mercury. Molière's play is itself based on a comedy *Amphitruo* by the Roman dramatist, Plautus, which has a similar plot.

In January 1923, Capgras and Reboul-Lachaux (2) presented to the Clinical Society of Psychiatric Medicine (La Société Clinique de Médecine Mentale) the case of a woman patient suffering from a chronic psychosis in which delusions of grandeur were accompanied by the curious conviction that her husband, daughter, and others had been replaced by impersonating doubles ("sosies"). This report of a case in which the patient claims that certain persons have been replaced by impersonating doubles was not the first of its kind, as Magnan (3) had in 1893 described a case showing the essential features of what has come to be known as the "Syndrome of Capgras," since Lévy-Valensi (4) in 1929 suggested that Capgras' contributions to our knowledge of this syndrome had been so great as to merit recognition in this way. It is noteworthy that Capgras and Reboul-Lachaux (2) not only presented one of the two earliest cases of what was later to be called "the syndrome of Capgras," but were the first to draw attention to the probable importance of derealization ("le sentiment d'étrangeté") and of morbid suspiciousness ("une disposition paranoïaque") as factors facilitating the appearance of the syndrome.

The pioneering case of Magnan (3) merits attention and can be summarized as follows: A widow, aged 49 years, the product of an emotionally unstable family, and who was herself of a suspicious and violent disposition, was admitted to a mental hospital in 1888 suffering from a chronic paranoid psychosis (probably schizophrenia). Prior to her admission, her symptoms had included bouts of depression accompanied by suicidal ideas, the suspicion that an attempt had been made to poison her, the conviction that her daughter had been murdered or spirited away by her son-in-law, and the belief that an illegitimate daughter of the patient's husband (doubtless nonexistent) had been substituted for her missing daughter and was living as her son-in-law's mistress. She had perceived imaginary differences of a minor nature in the appearance of her daughter and the woman who had, she supposed, usurped her daughter's place in her son-in-law's household. When shown an identifying mark that her daughter had on her thigh, she expressed the opinion that it was a fake that had been produced by means of silver nitrate. She subsequently challenged the authenticity of a letter written by her daughter, affirming that the handwriting was not hers. In the mental hospital, she remained convinced that her daughter had been replaced by an impostor, with the exception that she had appeared to recognize her daughter on one occasion when the latter had visited her.

In 1903, Janet (5) published the case of a young woman, aged 23 years, who had shown evidence of psychological instability since she was 13 years old. This patient obviously developed a paranoid-depressive psychosis associated with the "illusion of doubles," and the cardinal features of the case are as follows: With the passage of time, she had become increasingly troubled by obsessional symptoms, including an inability to arrive at a decision, interminable doubts, feelings of inadequacy, and intense scrupulosity. Delusions of criminal behavior accompanied by an intense feeling of guilt supervened. She subsequently declared that she was queen of a gang of criminals and that she escaped from her place of confinement during the night in order to carry out criminal activities with the help of her attendants, who were supposedly in collusion with her. She later modified her story by expressing the opinion that she had a double from whom she could hardly be distinguished and who was a member of the gang of criminals previously mentioned. Moreover, she became convinced that one of her attendants had a double, and the only way of distinguishing between the double and the original was that one had an identifiable blemish on the left thumb. She made some serious attempts at suicide.

In 1913, Bessière (6) had recorded a case that was not identical with the Capgras syndrome, but which is in the nature of a close variant of it. In Bessiére's case, a mentally disturbed woman expressed the belief that there was another woman who bore an astonishing resemblance to her and who had taken advantage of this resemblance to perpetrate all kinds of misdeeds. Moreover, the patient stated that there was a second woman who bore a close resemblance to her (the patient's) mother and who likewise took advantage of the resemblance to commit misdemeanors. The patient expressed the conviction that these two women were both in the pay of her husband, whom she accused of persecuting her. This patient inflicted injuries on her skin so that she would not be confused with her double.

A case of this nature differs from a case of the Capgras syndrome in that the doubles or impostors are not actually perceived (they are absent), so that the patient is afflicted by a delusion. In the case of the syndrome of Capgras, the patient is the victim of an illusion when minor, but nonexistent, differences between the appearance of the supposed impostor and the original are perceived, and of a delusional perception when no such differences are perceived to justify the substitution idea. Whether or not the Capgras phenomenon is an illusion or a perception, it is also a delusion, a fact that Capgras did not make clear.

An excellent fictional example of the Capgras syndrome that precedes Magnan's clinical case is that described by the Russian author, Fëdor Dostoevski, who depicted the "syndrome of Capgras" in his novel *The Possessed* (7), which was first published in 1871. In *The Possessed*, the mentally deranged Marya Timofyevna has been secretly married to Stavrogin, but, in their hometown at a social function, he fails to acknowledge her as his wife. Instead, he draws her aside and says: "only think that you are a girl, and that though I'm your devoted friend, I'm an outsider, not your husband, nor your father, nor your betrothed." When Stavrogin comes to visit her a few days later, Marya, her vulnerable mind seared by the bitterness of her recent experience, fails to recognize her husband, but accuses him of impersonating a murdered Stavrogin: "You're like him, very like, perhaps you're a relation—you're a sly lot! Only mine is a bright falcon and a prince, and you're an owl, and a shopman!" And later in the novel, she says: "When I saw your mean face after I'd fallen down and you picked me up—it was like a worm crawling into my heart. It's not *he*, I thought, not *he*! My falcon would never have been ashamed of me before a fashionable lady. Oh heavens! That alone kept me happy for those five years that my falcon was living somewhere beyond the mountains, soaring, gazing at the sun. . . . Tell me, you impostor, have you got much by it? Did you need a big bribe to consent?" (11).

The early writers were careful to distinguish the Capgras delusion from other disorders of recognition such as the illusion of Frégoli described by Courbon and Fail (8) in 1927, the illusion being named after Leopoldo Frégoli, an Italian actor, born in Rome in 1867, who excelled as a mimic (1). In the illusion of Frégoli, the patient believes that his persecutors have the power to incarnate themselves into the bodies of other people and thereby masquerade as (say) a policeman, traffic warden, neighbor, clergyman, etc., in order to further their campaign of harassment. The patient therefore falsely identifies his supposed enemies with ordinary persons going about their daily business.

REVIEW OF THE POSSIBLE ETIOLOGICAL ROLE OF DEREALIZATION IN THE CAPGRAS SYNDROME

When a person has the impression that everything and everybody in his environment is imbued with the attribute of strangeness and unreality, then he is afflicted by the symptom known as derealization. When this feeling of unreality is confined to the self, the symptom is called depersonalization. However, many authorities include the term "derealization" within the purview of the term "depersonalization," which then becomes a composite term. The aura of strangeness experienced by persons afflicted by derealization can be expected to facilitate the occurrence of a simultaneous feeling of familiarity and of nonrecognition when such persons encounter acquaintances, a state of affairs to which Capgras and Reboul-Lachaux (2) attached great importance when discussing factors likely to play a part in the etiology of the "illusion of doubles" (the term used by these authorities in their 1923 paper). Several other authorities have likewise stressed the importance of derealization in the etiology of the syndrome of Capgras. In 1935, Derombies (9) wrote as follows: "The feeling of unreality is encountered as the basis of the 'illusion of doubles' in many cases." With the passing of the years, students of the Capgras syndrome continued to discuss the etiological significance of derealization (10–13). In 1976, Merrin and Silberfarb (14) showed that the importance attached to derealization as an etiological factor in the "illusion of doubles" by the early writers on the subject had stood the test of time when they wrote (when discussing the Capgras syndrome): "As mentioned earlier, a number of cases began with diffuse feelings of unreality or depersonalization, followed by indiscriminate misidentification and finally by the establishment of the Capgras delusion." In 1977, Christodoulou (15) gave cautious support to such a progression with the following observation: "Thus, it seems possible that in certain cases the syndrome of Capgras may represent a delusional evolution of the phenomena of depersonalization and derealization."

HISTORICAL CONFIRMATION OF THE IMPORTANT ETIOLOGICAL ROLE OF PARANOID THINKING IN THE CAPGRAS SYNDROME

The reference made by Capgras and Reboul-Lachaux (2) to their patient's "paranoïac disposition" and strong tendency to be mistrustful had the effect of drawing attention to the possible importance of this factor in producing favorable conditions for the advent of the Capgras delusion, perhaps in association with derealization. The syndrome of Capgras is itself based on mistrustfulness, and it is therefore hardly surprising that patients experiencing the Capgras delusion show evidence of delusions of persecution in addition to the nuclear symptom. The paranoid nature of these patients' thinking is shown by the frequency with which they claim that the missing originals (especially those closest to the patient in kinship) have been kidnapped, imprisoned, or murdered (9,11,12). Other symptoms that are well represented among the ideas of Capgras-syndrome patients and that reflect their morbid mistrustfulness are (a) their complaint that attempts have been made to trick them by means of forged or fake letters purporting to be from the absent person (the original) (10,11,15,16), and (b) their complaint that attempts have been made or would be made to poison them (4,10,11,14,15,17).

The historical significance of this important symptom (morbid suspiciousness) is that students of the Capgras syndrome have continued to draw attention to the morbid suspiciousness of Capgras-delusion patients over half a century after Capgras and Reboul-Lachaux (2) referred to their patients' "paranoïac disposition." Thus, we find Merrin and Silberfarb in 1976 discussing the role of a mistrustful attitude in the production of the Capgras delusion; they wrote (14): "In a setting of increased vigilance and suspicion, a familiar person no longer elicits the same affectual response of recognition in the patient." In 1977, when discussing the "Syndrome of Capgras," Christodoulou (15) wrote: "It is probably worth noting that, irrespective of diagnosis, the clinical picture of almost all patients was dominated by a marked paranoid component."

THE EMERGENCE OF PSYCHOLOGICAL EXPLANATIONS FOR THE OCCURRENCE OF THE CAPGRAS SYNDROME

The first suggestion that the Capgras delusion might be in the nature of a mental mechanism, offering a solution to the patient's intrapsychic conflicts, was made in 1924 by Capgras and Carrette (18). The patient, a young woman displaying the symptoms of a schizophrenic illness, developed the delusion that her mother and father had been replaced by doubles. She had shown evidence of a strong erotic interest in her father, and Capgras and Carrette suggested that the delusion that her father was an impersonating double enabled her to solve the problem of her Electra complex and incestuous desires because "it is not to her father that she has made voluptuous overtures but to his double." However, Lévy-Valensi (4) cast doubt on the credibility of this explanation of the development of the delusion by drawing attention to the fact that the patient also claimed that her brother, uncle, and aunt had likewise been replaced by doubles.

The idea that an impersonating double might be subconsciously created, and have a defensive function, was more convincingly propounded by Dupouy and Montassut (19) in 1924. They recorded the case of a schizophrenic patient who argued that if she was disliked and persecuted by others, it was because she was being mistaken for her (imaginary) double, who lived an evil life, and if her acquaintances and relatives appeared to be insulting her (the patient was hallucinated and heard insulting "voices"), it was because they were not really the prototypes, but impersonating doubles who had replaced the originals.

There is evidence to support the contention that the Capgras theme of an impersonating double is sometimes used to solve the problem of conflicting or ambivalent emotions and to serve the needs of wish fulfillment (11,14). Usually, all the faults of the original are bestowed on the "impostors" (11), the supposedly absent original retaining all his or her virtues in exaggerated form. In this way, a Jekyll prototype and a Hyde double are created. An early example of this Jekyll-and-Hyde dichotomization of ambivalent emotions is that of Brochado (20), who, in 1936, published the case of a patient who had the habit of making invidious comparisons between her attendant nurse and the latter's double ("sosie"), when the nurse had the occasion to induce her to take medication or have her put in a strait waistcoat because of her agitated state. This patient would say, "You are not the nurse; the nurse is kind and she did not make me do that." Although the rule in cases of the Capgras syndrome is for the original to be superior in every way to the imaginary impostor or double, exceptional cases have been recorded in which the reverse has been obtained. For instance, Larrivé and Jasienski (21) in 1931 described the case of a woman who imagined that her poorly endowed, sexually inadequate, mutton-fisted lover had a rich and virile rival closely resembling her lover in appearance but having the small hands and feet of an aristocrat. Moreover, this patient came to the conclusion that she herself had a double, who was a grand lady of some kind or even an Italian princess.

At least two other cases appear in the literature in which the so-called impersonating double is preferred to the "missing" original (11,32). However, powerful emotional links with the object stimulus do not appear to be a *sine qua non* requirement for the Capgras delusion, for patients who exhibited this delusion in regard to people have also had the same delusion of doubling and substitution in regard to inanimate objects. In 1926, Bouvier (10) described the case of a woman who displayed the syndrome of Capgras in regard to persons and who also complained that her trunk had been replaced by a similar one and that some of her garments had been replaced by others with so close a resemblance to the originals that even the creases and wear and tear of the originals had been faithfully reproduced. In 1936, Brochado (20) reported the case of a woman, who in addition to displaying the Capgras syndrome respecting a blood relative, expressed the delusional idea that her spectacles had been replaced by a pair closely resembling the original pair. In 1973, MacCallum (22) described the case of a woman who presented the Capgras syndrome in regard to persons and who also insisted that the hospital had itself been replaced by an "exact replica." Brochado (20) was sufficiently impressed with the involvement of inanimate objects within the purview of the syndrome of Capgras that he referred to "an illusion of doubles of things."

An important milestone in the history of the syndrome of Capgras was the attempt by Coleman (16) in 1933 to offer a psychoanalytical explanation for the occurrence of the Capgras syndrome. His explanation relied on the fact that no male case of the syndrome had so far been reported in the relevant literature. He argued that women developed a distrust of "all subsequent love objects," having been deceived during the "pre-Oedipal phase" by the primary "love object," the mother. Coleman concluded his argument with the words, "The psychotic woman, rather than doubt the genuineness of her feelings, decomposes the object and postulates the existence of doubles." However, subsequent papers by Murray (23), Brochado (20), Davidson (24), and Stern and MacNaughton (25) showed that males could exhibit the syndrome, thus destroying the premise on which Coleman's reasoning had been based.

THE COMPLICATION OF THE ALCMENA COMPLEX

In 1967, Disertori and Piazza (26) drew attention to the "Alcmena complex," which has troubled the mind of some women afflicted by the delusional conviction that their husband or lover has been replaced by an impostor of similar or identical appearance to the original. The term "Alcmena complex" refers to the Greek myth wherein Alcmena, the wife of Amphitryon, is tricked and seduced by the god Jupiter, who successfully impersonates her husband and thereby implicates her in an act of innocent adultery. In the case of the syndrome of Capgras, the wife or mistress may refuse the sexual advances of the supposed impostor so as not to commit the sin of adultery or give way from fear and be in this way saddled with a feeling of guilt. Alcmena was of course an innocent adulterer, and only those Capgras-delusion patients who come to the conclusion that they have innocently been allowing a connubial relationship with an impostor should, strictly speaking, be included under this heading. However, it is convenient to include under the heading "Alcmena complex" all those cases in which difficulties in the sexual sphere have arisen as a result of the patient's conviction that her husband or lover has been replaced by an impostor (15,17,26). A case of special interest is that published by Cenac-Thaly et al. (12), in which a patient, troubled by the delusion that her husband had been replaced by an impersonating double, was convinced that the third of her three children had been fathered by the impostor. Occasionally, the impression given from reading a case report of the Capgras syndrome is that the patient would have been by no means averse to adultery with the double, perhaps tempted by the pleasures and excitement of a forbidden love affair (11).

THE ROLE OF PRIMITIVE THINKING IN THE ETIOLOGY OF THE CAPGRAS SYNDROME

The notion that a reversion to primitive thinking ("une mentalité prélogique") may have a part to play in the development of the "illusion of doubles" was first put forward in 1923 by Halberstadt (27), who was therefore raising the question of a phylogenetic regression as being an important factor underlying the emergence of the double idea in the minds of Capgras-delusion patients. The idea of doubles has undoubtedly had a prominent role in tribal religions, it being held among such tribes as the Nàgas, Karo Bataks, and East Indian Islanders that the soul or ghost of the departed takes the form of an exact replica of the deceased person (28). It is noteworthy that in the Dutch East Indies, the natives believe that spirits may assume the semblance of the husband or lover of a woman, whose death follows the supernatural impregnation (28).

The idea of doubles has also played a part in the religious philosophy of the archaic but advanced culture of the ancient Egyptians (the concept of a *ka*) (29), and in myths or tales of Greek (the Amphitryon and Alcmena myth), Indian (the Nala and Damayanti myth) or British (the monkish anthology of the Emperor Jovinian) origin (30). This idea of a double is necessarily the essential feature of the European folklore respecting the doppelgänger (31). The possibility that a reversion to primitive modes of thought may have a significant part to play in the development of the Capgras delusion has been discussed by Stern and MacNaughton (25) in 1945 and Todd (11) in 1957.

SOME MODERN DATA AND IDEAS RESPECTING THE SYNDROME OF CAPGRAS

In 1976, Merrin and Silberfarb (14) investigated the relative incidence of the Capgras syndrome in the two sexes and in the different psychoses: Of 46 cases reported in the literature, 27 cases have been female and 19 male; in regard to diagnosis, schizophrenia accounted for 28 cases, schizo-affective psychosis for 4, affective psychosis for 7, and an "organic" psychosis for 7.

Students of the Capgras syndrome in the last decade have in general accepted the probable etiological importance of the factors already discussed. However, more attention has been paid to evidence of a concomitant organic disease of the brain, which has been present in some cases (22,32–35), and the part (if any) played by this in the appearance of the Capgras delusion (14,36). For example, Weston and Whitlock (33) and Hayman and Abrams (35) have discussed the possible role of prosopagnosia in producing a handicap favorable to the development of the Capgras delusion. However, convincing evidence of the presence of prosopagnosia [the specific inability to recognize familiar faces (37,38)] has been lacking in the very few cases so far reported in which an attempt has been made to implicate this rare neuropsychological symptom as a contributory factor in the etiology of the Capgras delusion.

In 1977, Christodoulou (15), when discussing the Capgras syndrome, observed: "In certain cases it is doubtful whether the syndrome would have become manifest if this organic component had not existed," and on the evidence, few would challenge this. However, Enoch and Trethowan (36) have, in the present author's opinion, put the part played by organic cerebral disease in the syndrome of Capgras in its right perspective when, in 1979, they made this comment: "We would agree that the Capgras syndrome can occur in the setting of an organic condition, that it can indeed follow the development of organic trauma, but this does not invalidate our description of the essential psychopathology as occurring in the main in the setting of a clear sensorium where there is no evidence of any underlying organic lesion." As the years have passed, students of the Capgras syndrome have emphasized the fact that patients exhibiting the Capgras delusion usually have a clear sensorium (17). Recently, Merrin and Silberfarb (14) have indicated that Capgras-delusion patients may fail to take into account the changes that occur in the appearance of people due to the passage of time and the aging process. This factor does seem to have favored the development of the syndrome in some cases, for the Capgras delusion has occasionally developed when the patient and his or her relatives have met after a period of separation (10,15,25). Moreover, these patients sometimes produce "then" and "now" photographs in an attempt to prove that the originals have been replaced by doubles or by persons of similar appearance (14,39). The patient's confusion of earlier mental pictures of the prototype with his or her current appearance and behavior is doubtless determined by affectual factors such as wish fulfillment. An illustration of this is the case of the patient who had the delusion that she had a man friend who closely resembled her husband and who had all the pleasing traits that her husband formerly possessed but had lost with the passing of the years (11).

RARE ASSOCIATIONS OF THE CAPGRAS DELUSION REPORTED IN THE LITERATURE

In 1962, Cenac-Thaly et al. (12) reported the case of a woman who in 1958 complained that two doctors had broken into her apartment, anesthetized her, and then violated her. These two doctors, she said, had subsequently pursued her to Provence, where she was spending her holidays, and had adopted various disguises by posing as salesmen of trinkets, potato vendors, etc. (illusion of Frégoli). Also in 1958, she complained that her husband had been assassinated and his place in the home usurped by an impersonating double (the Capgras syndrome). In 1966, Bankier (40) described the case of a man suffering from a paranoid psychosis who developed the delusional idea that his wife had been replaced by a double (the Capgras syndrome). Unusual features of this case were that the "double admitted that she was an impostor" and that the patient's brother eventually came to believe the patient's delusional ideas ("folie à deux relationship"). In 1973, Sims and White (41) reported the case of a patient who developed the delusional idea that the woman with the same appearance and name as her mother was an impostor (the Capgras syndrome). She also developed the delusion that a former employer, a man who was much her superior in age and status, had become her lover and was the father of her child. This man had not seen her for 10 years and had no particular interest in her, having only known her in the capacity of employer (the Clérambault-Kandinsky syndrome).

REVIEWS

Outstanding among the early reviews of the Capgras syndrome were the doctoral theses of Bouvier (10) in 1926 and Derombies (9) in 1935. More recent reviews of a detailed nature are those of Merrin and Silberfarb (14) in 1970, Arieti and Brody (42) in 1974, and Enoch and Trethowan (36) in 1979. Although two alienists of exalted fame, Magnan and Janet, described the "illusion of doubles" before Capgras, it is the latter who has justly earned the eponym, for in the words of Lévy-Valensi (4) (referring to the "illusion of doubles"), "... it is to M. Capgras that should go the credit for having clearly defined it and justice would be done were it to be called henceforth 'the syndrome of Capgras.'"

REFERENCES

1. Critchley, M. (1979): *The Divine Banquet of the Brain*, p. 11. Raven Press, New York.
2. Capgras, J., and Reboul-Lachaux, J. (1923): *Bull. Soc. Clin. Méd. Ment.*, 2:6.
3. Magnan, V. (1893): *Leçons Cliniques sur les Maladies Mentales*, Obs. 21, 9e leçon, p. 329. Bataille, Paris.
4. Lévy-Valensi, J. (1929): *Gaz. Hôpitaux*, No. 55 (10th July):1001.
5. Janet, P. (1903): *Les Obsessions et Psychasthenie*. Alcan, Paris.
6. Bessière, A. C. R. (1913): Paranoia et psychose periodique. *Thèse de Paris*, p. 113. Leclerc, Paris.
7. Coleman, S. M. (1934): *Br. J. Med. Psychol.*, 14:3.
8. Courbon, P., and Fail, G. (1927): *Bull. Soc. Clin. Méd. Ment.*, 15:121.
9. Derombies, M. (1935): L'illusion de sosie, forme particulière de la méconnaissance systhematique. *Thése de Paris*, Jouve et Cie, Paris.
10. Bouvier, M. (1926): Le syndrome "Illusion des Sosies." *Thèse de Paris*. Vigné, Paris.
11. Todd, J. (1957): *Psychiat. Quart.*, 31:250.
12. Cenac-Thaly, H., Frelot, C., Guinard, M., Tricot, J. C., and Lacour, M. A. (1962): *Ann. Méd. Psychol.*, 120(Part 2):481.
13. Nilsson, R., and Perris, C. (1971): *Acta Psychiat. Scand.*, 221:53.
14. Merrin, E. L., and Silberfarb, P. M. (1970): *Arch. Gen. Psychiat.*, 33:965.
15. Christodoulou, G. N. (1977): *Br. J. Psychiat.*, 130:556.
16. Coleman, S. M. (1933): *J. Ment. Sci.*, 79:42.
17. Vogel, B. F. (1974): *Am. J. Psychiat.*, 131:922.
18. Capgras, J., and Carrette, P. (1924): *Ann. Méd. Psychol.*, 82 (Part 2):48.
19. Depouy, R., and Montassut, M. (1924): *Ann. Med. Psychol.*, 82(Part 2):341.
20. Brochado, A. (1936): *Ann. Med. Psychol.*, 94(Part 1):706.
21. Larrivé, E., and Jasienski, H. J. (1931): *Ann. Méd. Psychol.*, 89(Part 2):501.
22. MacCallum, W. A. G. (1973): *Br. J. Psychiat.*, 123:639.
23. Murray, J. R. (1936): *J. Ment. Sci.*, 82:63.
24. Davidson, G. M. (1941): *Psychiat. Quart.*, 15:513.
25. Stern, K., and MacNaughton, D. (1945): *Psychiat. Quart.*, 19:139.
26. Disertori, B., and Piazza, M. (1967): *Giorn. Psichiat. Neuropat.*, 95:175.
27. Halberstadt, G. (1923): *J. Psychol. Norm. Pathol.*, 20:728.
28. Crawley, A. E. (1908–1926): In: *Hastings' Encyclopaedia of Religion and Ethics*, Vol. 4, edited by J. Hastings, pp. 853–860. T. and T. Clark, Edinburgh.
29. Mackenzie, D. A. (1913): *Egyptian Myth and Legend*, p. 88. Gresham Publishing Co., London.
30. Tymms, R. (1949): *Doubles in Literary Psychology*, pp. 19–21. Bowes and Bowes, Cambridge, England.

31. Todd, J., and Dewhurst, K. (1962): *Practitioner*, 188:377.
32. Capgras, J., Lucettini, P., and Schiff, P. (1924): *Bull. Soc. Clin. Med. Ment.*, 12:210.
33. Weston, M. J., and Whitlock, F. A. (1971): *Br. J. Psychiat.*, 119:25.
34. Hay, G. C., Jolley, D. J., and Jones, R. G. (1974): *Acta Psychiat. Scand.*, 50:73.
35. Hayman, M. A., and Abrams, R. (1977): *Br. J. Psychiat.*, 130:68.
36. Enoch, M. D., and Trethowan, W. H. (1979): In: *Uncommon Psychiatric Syndromes*, p. 12. John Wright and Sons, Bristol, U.K.
37. Critchley, M. (1953): In: *The Parietal Lobes*, p. 291. Edward Arnold London.
38. Meadows, J. C. (1974): *J. Neurol. Neurosurg. Psychiat.*, 37:489.
39. Bland, R. C. (1971): *Canad. Psychiat. Assoc. J.*, 16:369.
40. Bankier, R. G. (1966): *Canad. Psychiat. Assoc. J.*, 2:425.
41. Sims, A., and White, A. (1973): *Br. J. Psychiat.*, 123:635.
42. Arieti, S., and Brody, E. B. (1974): In: *American Handbook of Psychiatry*, 2nd ed., Vol. 3, pp. 712–714. Basic Books, New York.

Historical Aspects of the Neurosciences,
edited by F. Clifford Rose and W. F. Bynum.
Raven Press, New York ©

The Medical Treatment of Epilepsy: A Historical Review

Ian D. Melville

The Institute of Neurological Sciences, Glasgow, Scotland

The longer you can look back, the further you can look forward.

Winston S. Churchill

It is only fitting in a volume dedicated to a great teacher and neurologist, Macdonald Critchley, that I, who have been his pupil, should discuss Dr. Critchley's teaching on focal sensory epilepsy (1). Considering the quotation at the head of this chapter, Dr. Critchley can look back a long neurological way, and his pupils still take his thoughts and teaching forward to the new neurological generation. I always found the Critchley lectures and demonstrations memorable, and the bedside teaching was even more so, combining education with ingenuity and at times not a little drama.

Dr. Critchley described patients with parietal lesions who reported in their attacks various strange and usually unpleasant cutaneous sensations. He stressed the following criteria, as I do today with my own students:

	Focal (sensory) epilepsy
Simple sensations	Tingling, numbness, pins and needles, cold, warmth, wetness
Sensory absence	"Negative" feelings of affected segments disappearing
Complex sensations	Illusory feelings "as if the limb were moving"
	Telescoping effect, e.g., the hand in the thorax, in "furious agitation"
	Tactile hallucinations
	Complex sensations, usually disagreeable

And so Dr. Critchley insisted on the same clinical and anatomical correlations as his illustrious predecessor at the National Hospital, John Hughlings Jackson (1835–1911) (2). Jackson remains the father figure of British neurology, from whom has come the concept of being a "neurologist," certainly in the United Kingdom and probably also in the United States (Fig. 1). Rolandic, Jacksonian, or Critchleian seizures are dramatic events both to patients and observers, and throughout the centuries, the violence and the drama of epilepsy have gripped medical, religious, and social attention. Here is Raphael's last painting depicting the man who brought his son before Jesus (Fig. 2). Presumably, this is a supplementary motor area seizure with adversion of head and eyes, and along with it we should read Matthew's Gospel, the *cri de coeur* of the parent of the epileptic patient through the human story:

> Lord, have mercy on my son, for he is an epileptic and he suffers terribly; for often he falls into the fire, and often into the water. And I brought him to your disciples, and they could not heal him.
>
> *Matthew 17:15–16*

Aretaeus in the second century said that epilepsy came "in many shapes, and *horrible*," and there can be no other illness that is so repetitively disruptive of ordinary life, creating so much anguish, horror, and distaste. Even today, in a better educated and largely sympathetic society, the flavor of distaste survives. Patients and relatives abhor the label of "epilepsy," for it may weigh across their lives like some malevolent albatross.

So much has been uncovered about epilepsy in the last 100 years and especially in the last 50 years, that the modern neurologist may feel that he knows a lot, if not nearly all, about it. Russell Brain (3) pointed out that it was too easy to minimize Jackson's discoveries in retrospect:

> The discoverer of a substantial thing, such as a bacillus, an extract or a disease, achieves more certain immortality than one who discovers a principle, for permanently valid principles

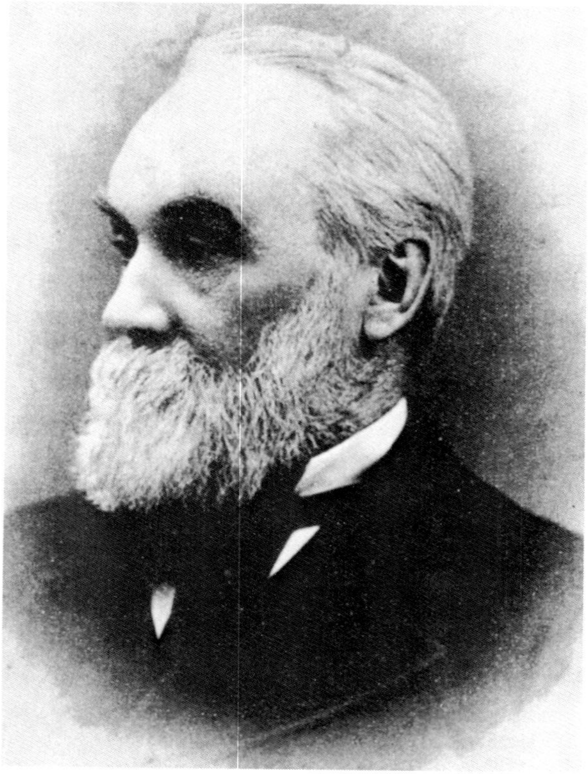

FIG. 1. John Hughlings Jackson (1835–1911). (Reprinted with permission.)

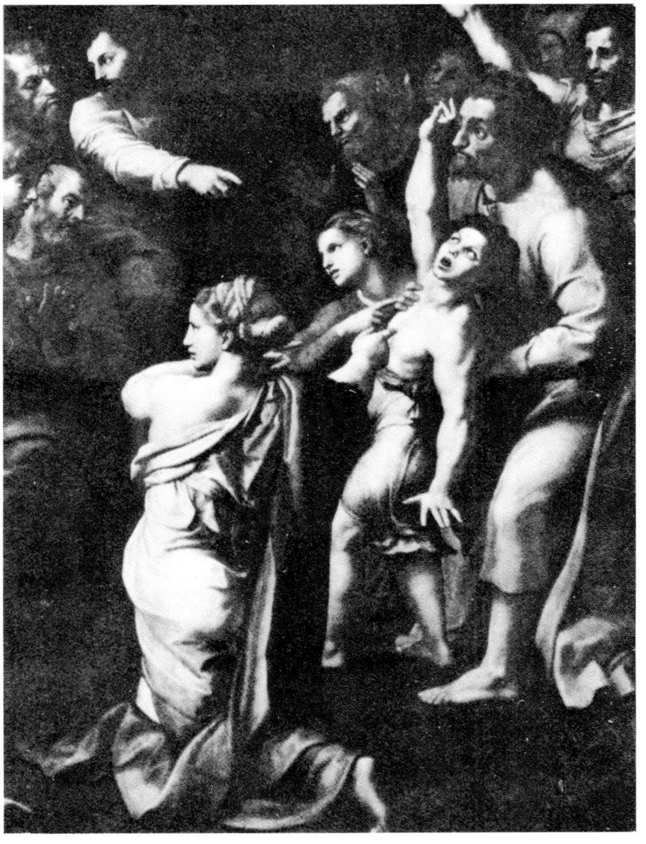

FIG. 2. A detail of "The Transfiguration" by Raphael Sanzio (1438–1520). Vatican Gallery.

soon become part of current thought and in time become so obvious as to have needed no discovery.

He reminded us of a huge debt that we shall continue to owe to Jackson's painstaking clinical observations and brilliant deductions. I suspect that modern neurologists flatter themselves about their knowledge of epilepsy, and we would do well to retain an insight into our ignorance of what seizures really represent in terms of disordered neuronal function. Jackson (4) himself said that "a convulsion is but a symptom, and implies only that there is an occasional, an excessive, and a disorderly discharge of nerve tissue on muscles." Whereas our EEG studies have given ample proof of that, I do not believe that as yet we have uncovered the various reasons at the cellular, synaptic, or genetic level, why orderly discharge becomes disorderly.

Rather than review the general history of epilepsy, which has been done so well by many authors (5–9), I would like to review the medical therapy of epilepsy, which was not at all effective until the late 19th century, which remains rather indifferent, and which shows no great signs of early improvement. The history of epilepsy treatment reflects the history of the understanding and of the attitudes toward the disorder. The great leap forward made by Jackson and Gowers (10) in the 19th century has been followed by pharmacological development from which much is now known of where the molecules of drugs go and of the membranes through which they pass. The next great leap could be pharmacological, which now seems unlikely, or perhaps surgical, probably even less likely, or through electronics or eugenics. Perhaps the leap will be social, toward a society that will take more seriously the prevention of epileptogenic lesions, trauma to the brain, bacterial infections, infant or embryonic anoxia, virus multiplication, and tumor growth.

Drug treatments were mentioned in the Hippocratic writings (11). Measures for general care and personal hygiene were suggested, and so we may presume that the Father of Medicine was familiar with the still current idea of varying seizure liability, and that seizures are not necessarily random, but may be triggered by external observable influences. Many of us, I imagine, are prone to startle, probably a physiological event with orderly discharge of neurons, but very similar to highly disorderly myoclonic attacks. From time to time, we do meet patients who have an identifiable and rather exclusive stimulus for their epilepsy. Dr. Critchley in 1937 (12) reported 20 patients with musicogenic seizures, for which he coined the term "musicolepsia." The stimuli varied among Tchaikovsky, barrel organs, and dance bands. W. G. and M. A. Lennox (6) quoted Gerhard van Sweiten, who in 1754 described a youngster who had a convulsive attack every time he repeated the Lord's Prayer! I have one patient whose telephone is muted as part of her seizure prevention.

Hippocrates would not accept the attribution of epilepsy to the gods. He thought epilepsy was hereditary like other diseases, and he felt that improvement of cerebral functioning could benefit the patient without "illiberal practices like purifications and spells." The records of his treatment are sparse, but some were severe, like complete fasting and fluid deprivation. There are still echoes of these methods in our wards and clinics today.

The Lennoxes (6), in their extensive review of 1960, give a fascinating account of epilepsy management through the post-Hippocratic era and through our Dark Ages. In view of the strange assumptions about the causes of epilepsy, we are not perhaps too surprised by the variety of treatments, sometimes quite literally "cooked up." It has always been the medical man's task or duty to offer a behavior specification for his patient—what he should do, and take, and when, and how often. Just about every aspect of the patient's life has been given direction at some time or another in epilepsy management. Some approaches were aimed at the removal of supernatural influences by gifts and sacrifices. A woodcut (Fig. 3), ca. 1480, from Temkin's monograph (5), depicts a pilgrimage to the Priory of St. Valentine at Rufach in Alsace. We can presume that the patients are in postictal states on the floor, while the devil, in porcine guise, looks on. Another scene of casting out the unclean spirit is shown in Fig. 4. John of Gaddesden, around 1492, advocated scripture reading (13), but was clearly not aware of the dangers of reflex epilepsy when repeating the Lord's Prayer. Every possible method of ridding the body of toxins has been suggested, e.g., trephining, blood-letting, purging, diuresis, diaphoresis, and even coitus, since retained semen was thought epileptogenic.

The use of animal and vegetable materials is readily understood. Kanner (14) in 1930 listed 67 animals with properties inimical to seizures, commencing with ass, bat, and bear, and progressing to weasel, wolf, and woodlouse. Of vegetable materials, elder, garlic, peony, and especially mistletoe were in particular favor. Mistletoe, rooted in the branches of the oak tree, could not fall and was, therefore, in the logic of the time, applicable to the "falling sickness." In Mexico, the Aztecs (15) were using the same perplexed approach. One of their seizure remedies of 1552 gave this prescription:

> ℞In addition to the juice of three shrubs the person with morbus comitialis is to take the

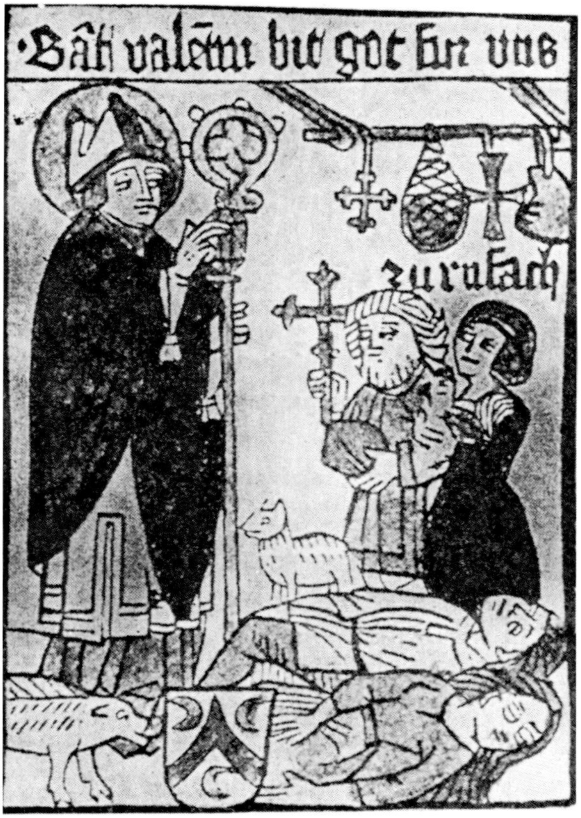

FIG. 3. Woodcut, ca. 1480, depicting a pilgrimage to the Priory of St. Valentine at Rufach in Alsace. (Reprinted with permission; ref.5.)

> stones from the intestines of hawk and rooster, stag's horn, the hair of a corpse, and the burned flesh of a mole shut up in a jar, and well ground in hot water.
> Sig. "The epileptic is to drink this liquor so he will vomit."

This is perhaps an early example of a drug-induced side effect.

The horror continues, for Taxil in 1602 (16) felt that salt water was superior to urine in treatment, since urine "not seldom contains the epileptic virus." But if we regard these medicaments with some amazement, we can also see that what does emerge in the old behavior specifications is an emphasis on the environmental care of the epileptic patient. Aurelius Cornelius Celsus (6), a contemporary of Jesus, Tiberius, and Nero, gave good advice in 25 A.D. that would do for today. The patient should:

> Avoid the sun, the bath, fire and all heating things, likewise cold, wine, venery, the sight of a steep place, vomiting, weariness, anxieties and all business.

Aretaeus the Cappadocian (6) produced a perfect outline for a suburban or rural epilepsy center in the first century A.D.:

> . . . promenades long and straight . . . in a well ventilated place under trees of myrtle and laurel and fragrant herbs . . . advised to cultivate a keen temper without irascibility.

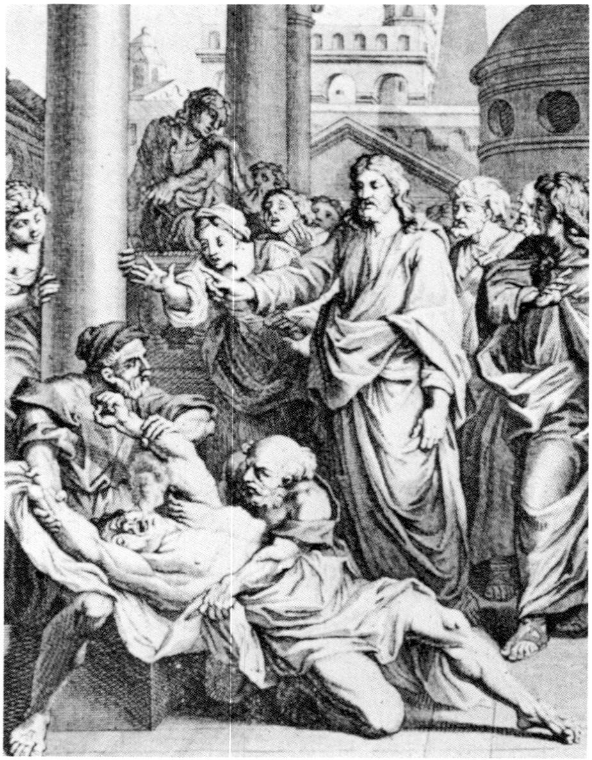

FIG. 4. Another scene of casting out the unclean spirit. (Reprinted with permission.)

The advice to avoid anger is reinforced by Bernard of Gordon in 1305 (17)—no great change over a thousand years! The patient:

> . . . should avoid all vegetables which are difficult to digest, he should avoid long sleep lying on his back with his head inclined; when he is on the top of mountains he should avoid looking downwards; he should avoid the sound of large bells; the roaring of lions, all terrifying things; he should avoid anger and other disturbances of the soul, such as fear, worry, and all those things which make for sudden intake and expulsion of breath.

Here is a behavior specification with a vengeance, with enough interest in it for us, however, to allow the suspicion that Bernard already knew that over-breathing was a seizure stimulus and that anxiety was a factor in sudden and unexpected deterioration of epilepsy control.

We may wonder how our predecessors coped with failures of treatment. How did Galen react when he was told at the follow-up clinic, "the powdered human skull is not working, Dr. Galen." Was this patient not complying with instructions? Should he try a drop of gladiator's blood next or that of an executed criminal? There has always been a tendency to blame the patient for not getting better. In 1974, Neil Gordon (18) asked the question at the Hans Berger Symposium Meeting in Edinburgh: "Why does the medical treatment of epilepsy sometimes fail?" But this question was for doctors and not for patients, pointing out the need for a maintained insight into medical shortcomings.

In passing, we may note that our forebears were familiar with placebo effects in treatment, what I might term the skullduggery of treatment, or even the "kidology." Antonius Guainerius, around 1440, quoted by the Lennoxes (6), wrote:

> Ceremonies are in order that greater confidence be placed in the medicine. The greater the affection with which the sick man takes his medicine, the more eagerly does nature receive it, and the better result is obtained . . . we offer pills in unequal numbers, since the ignorant think that an odd number is much more perfect than an equal number.

Is this the origin of our dosage *ter in die* or *ter die sumendum*, which lingers on at variance with the concept of biological half-life?

Thomas Willis (19), in the 17th century, returned to the Hippocratic view that seizures arise within and not without the brain. Not until the mid-19th century did medicine begin properly to benefit from the Enlightenment that had swept through Europe. In the wake of the stimulus of freedom of thought that Voltaire and others unleashed, traditional ideas were discarded and scientific method and experiment began. Bacteriology, physiology, pathology, and pharmacology as we know them today were founded. Surgery left off the red-hot cautery and turned swiftly to saws and chisels, but under anesthesia and with antisepsis and asepsis. On May 11, 1857, Sir Charles Locock reported to the Royal Medical and Chirurgical Society of London (20) the successful use of bromides in the treatment of epilepsy. Bromide had been previously used for its anaphrodisiac qualities in the treatment of onanism, and there were of course fears that masturbation led to epilepsy as well as visual loss. You will recall that coitus had earlier been recommended as a useful therapy. Perhaps Locock's discovery was a case of being right for the wrong reasons. Subsequently, Charles Édouard Brown-Séquard (1817–1894) was instrumental in widening the use of bromides (21). Samuel Wilks (22) also urged the general use of bromides in epilepsy, and Hughlings Jackson, himself a pupil of Brown-Séquard, commented on their use in 1861 (23). At about this time, Jackson was writing copiously about the convulsive disorders. For example, he wrote (2):

> It is a small matter to me whether a case of convulsions or other paroxysmal nervous seizure is to be called epileptic or not. What I labour to find out is the part of the brain of the functions of which the convulsion is the sudden and brutal development.

With the success of potassium bromide, whose mode of action is still unknown, the scene was set for the onslaught of 20th-century pharmacology, although the momentum was gathered slowly. Bromide is sedative and has a low ratio between effective dosage and toxicity (24,25), but may still be useful in tonic-clonic seizures. In 1912, Hauptmann (26) presented the first use of phenobarbitone in epilepsy, at a time when barbitone was widely used for its sedative properties. Subsequently, more than 2,500 barbiturate compounds were synthesized, only a few reaching therapeutic use in seizure suppression. Thereafter, we had to wait until 1938 for the synthesis of diphenylhydantoin (27), an antiepileptic and nonsedative, or less sedative drug, which still remains in the forefront of treatment. The successful finding of the hydantoinates was the result of a planned search for antiepilepsy agents. Toman et al. (28) tested potentially valuable drugs in patients undergoing electroconvulsive therapy. In 1945, Merritt and Putnam (29) reported their study of 1,000 candidate compounds. Perlstein and Andelman (30) observed the selective action of trimethadione in petit mal or absence seizures, giving a further dimension to the pharmacological push.

In Table 1 are the results of that push, with a fierce momentum between 1947 and 1960, perhaps slowing down a little more recently. The push was probably as much motivated for commercial as well as for scientific reasons. It is interesting that no new drug has emerged since 1973, and it has been interesting to note that each introduction has been followed by a flurry of papers describing the new drug's action and success (31). Later, the Committee

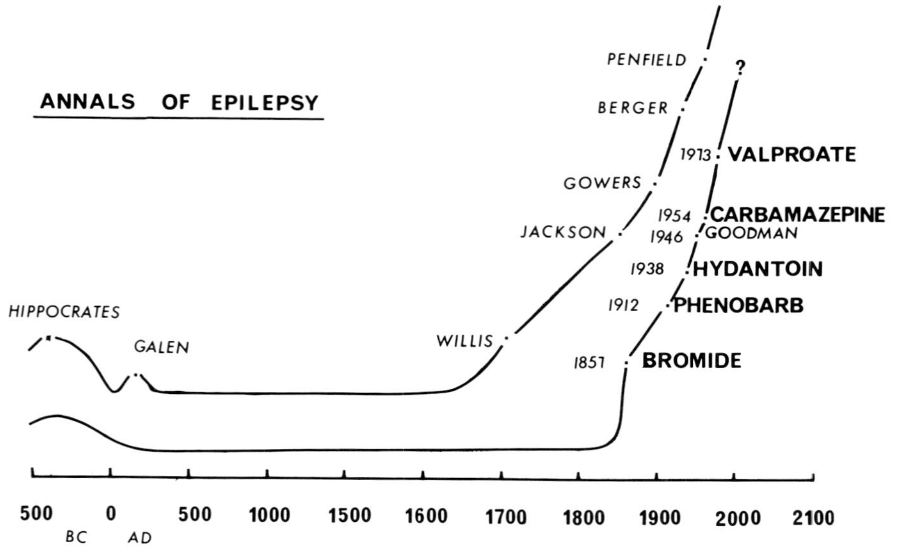

FIG. 5. The annals of epilepsy. (Author's adaptation, from Lennox and Lennox, ref. 6.)

TABLE 1. *Anticonvulsant drugs of the 20th century*

Date	Generic name	Trade name
1912	Phenobarbitone	Luminal
1935	Methylphenobarbitone	Prominal
1938	Diphenylhydantoin	Epanutin, Dilantin
1946	Trimethadione	Tridione
1947	Methylphenytoin	Mesontoin
1949	Paramethadione	Paradione
1949	Phenacemide	Phenurone
1953	Phensuximide	Milontin
1954	Primidone	Mysoline
1954	Carbamazepine	Tegretol
1957	Methsuximide	Celontin
1959	Ethotoin	Peganone
1960	Ethosuximide	Zarontin
1960	Sulthiame	Ospolot
1968	Diazepam	Valium
1973	Sodium valproate	Epilim
1973	Clonazepam	Rivotril

on the Safety of Medicines accumulates the evidence of adverse effects, and in time the new treatment is seen in correct perspective. Of this list, only a few drugs remain in constant use. Many have been dropped because of toxicity, some through ineffectiveness. None approaches the ideal as considered by Goodman (32): "capable of complete suppression of seizures at a dosage level that does not cause sedation or other undesirable central toxicity." The ideal drug should act on the seizure source, be well tolerated, inexpensive, long acting, have a wide safety margin, no systemic toxicity, and no idiosyncratic effects. Clearly there is some way to go. We may recall Polonius' advice to his son:

> Those drugs thou hast, and their adoption tried,
> Grapple them to thy soul with hoops of steel;
> But do not dull thy palm with entertainment
> Of each new hatch'd, unfledged remedy.

Perhaps the final chapter on pharmacology is only beginning, with current neurological practice enjoying the application of pharmacokinetics to the clinical scene. Duration of action, drug interactions, plasma levels, toxicity, and seizure control are under scrutiny, and I can speak for many neurologists who appreciate the huge help in seizure management given by our biochemists.

In conclusion, a presentation of the annals of epilepsy (Fig. 5), adapted from the Lennoxes (6), but brought slightly up to date. Other illustrious names could be added—Woodbury, Penry, Schmidt, Meinardi, Richens, et al.

It seems to me that we can have a long look back on epilepsy treatment, but that we still have a long look forward to the time when we may control by our therapy the Jacksonian "excessive disorderly discharge of nerve tissue upon muscles." We are several steps nearer than poor Galen's powdered human skull and a step nearer than Jackson's and Gower's bromides perhaps, but we are still some way short of Goodman's ideal.

REFERENCES

1. Critchley, M. (1953): *The Parietal Lobes*, p. 86. Edward Arnold, London.
2. Jackson, J. H. (1931): *Selected Writings of John Hughlings Jackson*, Vol. 1. edited by J. Taylor, Hodder & Stoughton, London.
3. Brain, W. R. (1935): *Postgrad. Med. J.*, 11:145.
4. Jackson, J. H. (1870): *Trans. St. And. Med. Grad. Assoc.*, Vol. 3.
5. Temkin, O. (1971): *The Falling Sickness*, 2nd ed. Johns Hopkins Univ. Press, Baltimore.
6. Lennox W. G., and Lennox, M. A. (1960): *Epilepsy and Related Disorders*. Little, Brown & Co., Boston.
7. Penfield, W., and Jasper, H. (1954): *Epilepsy and the Functional Anatomy of the Human Brain*. Little, Brown & Co., Boston.
8. Guthrie, D. (1945): *The History of Medicine*. Nelson, London.
9. McHenry, L. C. (1969): In: *Garrison's History of Neurology*. Charles C. Thomas, Springfield, Illinois.
10. Gowers, W. R. (1901): *Epilepsy and Other Chronic Convulsive Diseases*. Churchill, London.
11. Hippocrates (1849): In: *The Genuine Works of Hippocrates*, Francis Adams translation. Sydenham Society, London.
12. Critchley, M. (1937): *Brain*, 60:13.
13. Gaddesden, John of (1492): In: *Rosa Anglica Practica Medicinae a capite ad pedes*, pp. 157–167. Johannes Antonius Birreta, Pavia.
14. Kanner, L. C. (1930): *Med. Life*, 37:167.
15. The Badianus Manuscript (1940): Johns Hopkins Univ. Press, Baltimore.
16. Taxil, J. (1602): In: *Tracte de L'Epilepsie*. Claude Michelle, Tournon.
17. Bernard of Gordon (1496): In: *Lilium Medicinae*. Joannem & Gregorium de Gregoriis fratres, Venice.
18. Gordon, N. (1974): In: *Epilepsy, Proceedings of the Hans Berger Symposium*, p. 187. Churchill Livingstone, Edinburgh.
19. Willis, T. (1684): *Practice of Physick*. H. Clark, T. Dring, C. Harper, & F. Leigh, London.
20. Locock, C. (1857): *Lancet*, 1:527.
21. Olmsted, J. M. D. (1969): In: *Founders of Neurology*, edited by W. Haymaker and F. Schiller. p. 184. Charles C. Thomas, Springfield, Illinois. See also William Gooddy, this volume.
22. Wilks, S. (1866): *Guy's Hosp. Rep.*, 12:152.
23. Jackson, J. H. (1861): *Med. Times Gaz.*, 1:648; 2:59.
24. Lennox, W. G. (1957): *N. Engl. J. Med.*, 256:887.
25. Woodbury, D. M. (1972): In: *Anti-Epileptic Drugs*, edited by D. M. Woodbury, J. K. Penry, and R. P. Schmidt, p. 519. Raven Press, New York.
26. Hauptmann, A. (1912): *Munch. Med. Wochenschr.*, 59:1907.
27. Merritt, H. H., and Putnam, T. J. (1938): *J. Am. Med. Assoc.*, 111:1068. See also A. P. Friedman, this volume.

28. Toman, J. E. P., Loewe, S., and Goodman, L. S. (1947): *Arch. Neurol.*, 58:312.
29. Merritt, H. H., and Putnam, T. J. (1945): *Epilepsia*, 3:51.
30. Perlstein, M. A., and Andelman, M. B. (1946): *J. Pediat.*, 29:20.
31. Nanda, R. N., Johnson, R. H., Keogh, H., Lambie, D. G., Melville, I. D., and Shakir, R. A. (1977): In: *Epilepsy; the Eighth International Symposium*, p. 163, edited by J. K. Penry. Raven Press, New York.
32. Goodman, L. S., and Gilman, A. (1970): *The Pharmacological Basis of Therapeutics*. p. 206. Macmillan, New York.

Historical Aspects of the Neurosciences,
edited by F. Clifford Rose and W.F. Bynum.
Raven Press, New York ©

The Neurology of Robert Bentley Todd

J. B. Lyons

Department of the History of Medicine, Royal College of Surgeons in Ireland; Mercer's and St. Michael's Hospitals, Dublin, Ireland

From the viewpoint of biography, the bizarre and the dramatic have an irresistible appeal. Nothing in Robert Bentley Todd's practice seems more bizarre today than his prescription of alcohol in gargantuan doses as a remedy for fevers; nothing in his life could have been more dramatic than his death from torrential gastric hemorrhage in his own consulting room on January 30, 1860, presumably the result of overindulgence in his sovereign panacea, for the autopsy disclosed hepatic cirrhosis. Few of his many consultations could have been so fraught with miscalculation as his attendance with Dr. Julius at a bedside in Richmond on April 28, 1859. In due course, they were important prosecution witnesses when their late patient's bigamous husband, Dr. Thomas Smethurst, was tried for murder at the Old Bailey. Though found guilty, Smethurst was subsequently pardoned, a fortunate assertion of justice, for a present-day clinician would suspect Crohn's disease rather than Todd's unlikely diagnosis, poisoning by irritants.

To focus on these salients, however, would destroy perspective, hampering appraisal of a career characterized by sober purpose (using that adjective advisedly), and by unremitting endeavor, directed toward educational and physiological ends. And besides, the space at my disposal must be economically deployed.

My subject was the son of Charles Hawkes Todd (Fig. 1), a professor of anatomy in the Royal College of Surgeons in Ireland and the surgeon to the House of Industry Hospitals, who in the best Hippocratic tradition named his first-born James Henthorn as a gesture of respect to the senior colleague to whom he had been apprenticed. The maternal surname, Bentley, was an equally uncommon given name for the second son, who was born in Dublin on April 9, 1809.

Robert Bentley Todd (Fig. 2) received his early education at a local day school and from a tutor. He entered Dublin University in 1825 to read for the bar, but when his father died unexpectedly in the following year, leaving a large family poorly provided for, Robert was advised to change to medicine. His father's colleagues may have waived their fees at the House of Industry Hospitals and the College of Surgeons, for it was from the latter that he took his professional diploma rather than at the university, where he obtained an arts degree in 1829.

By May 20, 1831, when he became a Licentiate of the Royal College of Surgeons in Ireland (Fig. 3), Todd's address was 5 Charlotte Street, London, but, as he boasted in later years, he was "without a sixpence to help himself." Details of his appointments as lecturer in the Aldersgate Street Medical School and at a school in Dean Street associated with the Westminster Hospital were chronicled by McIntyre (1) and will not be discussed further. It

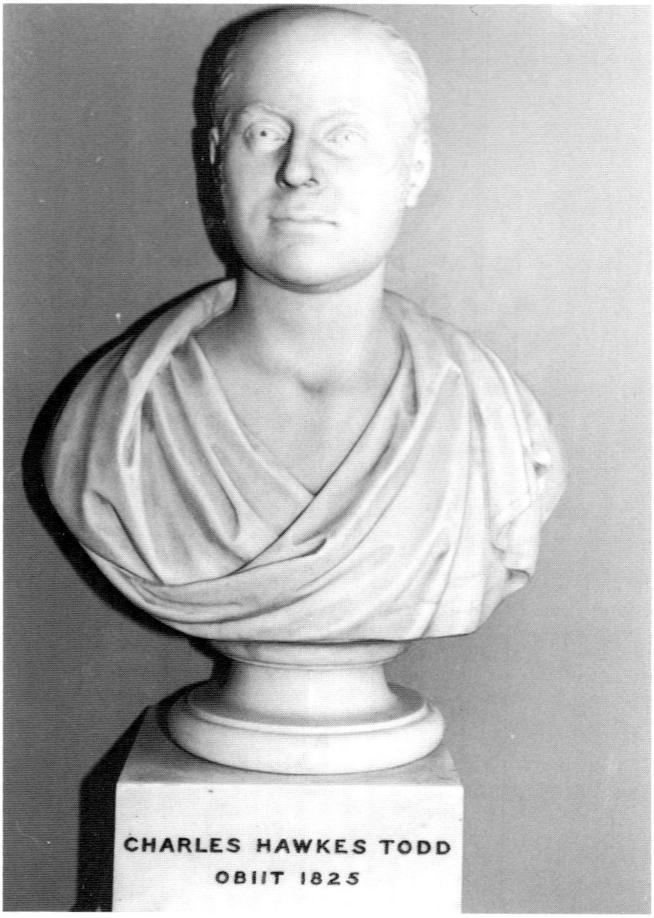

FIG. 1. Charles Hawkes Todd. From the bust in the Royal College of Surgeons in Ireland.

seems appropriate, however, to mention unpublished letters in the British Library (2) relevant to the early years of his career.

Toward the end of 1831, Todd inquired from the Reverend Philip Bliss, University Registrar, regarding the regulations at Oxford for candidates for medical degrees:

> I am a Bachelor of Arts in the University of Dublin—and intend to take the degree of Master of Arts there next February—may I beg to know can I go *ad eundem* to Oxford as M.A.—or can I obtain the degree of M.A. from Oxford without previously taking it from Dublin?
>
> Also what is the earliest period at which I can obtain the degree of M.B. from Oxford and what are the forms etc to be observed . . .

Bliss informed him that a year must elapse between his taking the Oxford M.A. and the M.B.:

> My recommendation to you to incorporate as B.A. and then to proceed regularly in this University was given, because I know that the members of the College of Physicians have complained of graduates in Medicine coming direct from Dublin and obtaining incorporation

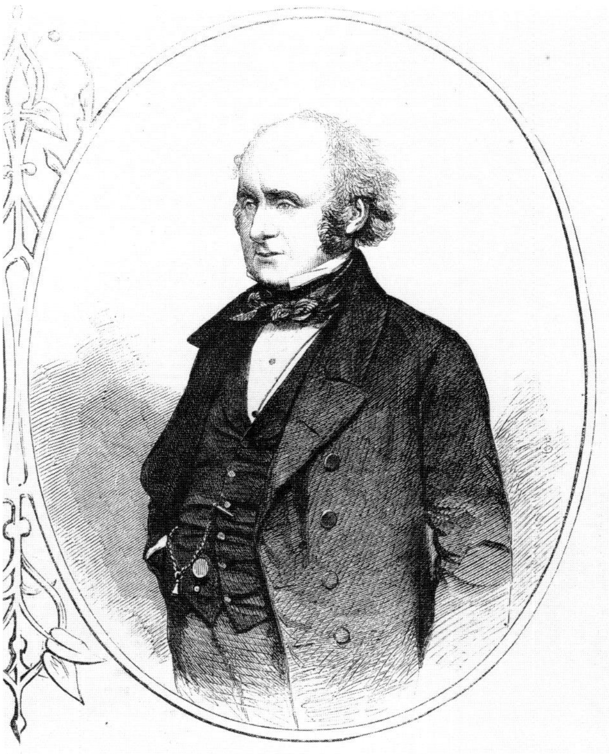

FIG. 2. Robert Bentley Todd. From a photograph by Maull and Polyblank.

> here, and subsequently presenting themselves to the College as graduates of Oxford, without having resided here a single term . . .

Todd managed to keep a couple of terms at Oxford in 1832 and was granted its medical degree in 1833. His brother, the Reverend James Henthorn Todd, Fellow of Trinity College, Dublin, wrote to Charles Babbage, the mathematician, on January 11, 1836:

> My dear friend—the first use I make of your kind permission to write to you sometimes is to ask you a favour—My brother Dr. Todd has been for some time residing in London and has already made some character there in his profession—he is now a Candidate for the place of Physician to the Westminster Hospital, and I believe, with a fair prospect of success—if you could be of any service to him in his Canvass, you would confer upon me a great favour, that he should succeed . . .

He was not to succeed on that occasion, but later in the year he replaced Herbert Mayo as a professor of physiology and morbid anatomy at King's College, where a medical faculty, lacking a clinical department, had been established in 1831. With others, Todd set about supplying the missing clinical amenities; he became secretary of the King's College Hospital fund-raising committee.

When the new institution was opened on April 15, 1840 on the site of the former parish workhouse of St. Clement Danes in Portugal Street, near Lincoln Inn's Fields, the *Medical*

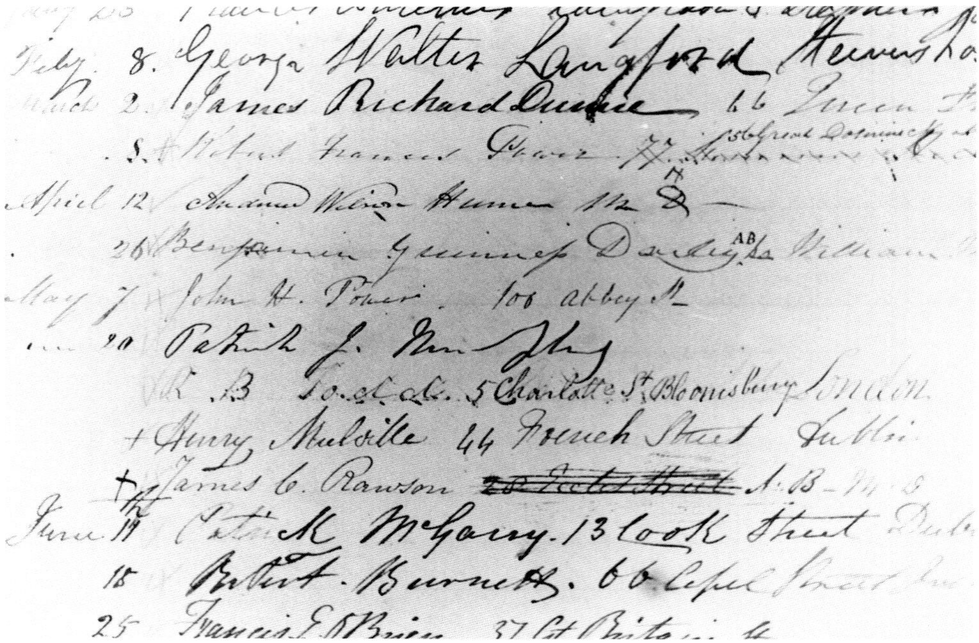

FIG. 3. R. B. Todd's signature in the Register of Graduates, Royal College of Surgeons in Ireland.

Times was less than welcoming: "It's locality is fine—shambles on one side, and a churchyard on the other—butchers within and without—prayers for the living and for the dead . . . Dr. Todd, we understand, intends to gratify the world with a volume of Meditations among the Tombs."

Todd's literary bent was considerable. His most ambitious work, the massive five-volume *Cyclopaedia of Anatomy and Physiology*, which he edited, did more, according to Lionel S. Beale (3), "to encourage and advance the study of physiology and comparative and microscopic anatomy than any book ever published." In the preface to the first volume, which appeared in 1835, Todd explained that his purpose was: "To collect a series of Essays on all of the various subjects of Anatomy and Physiology, by the co-operation of several Authors, who, as far as possible, should be selected in consequence of their special attention to, or interest in, the subject-matter of the articles which each would undertake to furnish. . . ." His aim was to enlist the aid of men whose articles would incorporate the results of contemporary research and of their own investigations.

Sometimes the editor's "most sanguine hopes were fully attained," but now and then he was disappointed when authors failed to fulfill their undertakings "without any assignable reason" or were unavoidably prevented from doing so. Impressed by the authority of many of the contributors, the *Lancet*'s reviewer (4) pointed to the exceptions: "The announcement of some of the 'minora sidera' certainly excited a smile, and some surprise, perhaps. Their light, however, though simply twinkling, and not brilliant, may yet prove useful. As the Scotch say, 'Many mickels make a muckle'." A few years later, the same journal (5) declared the *Cyclopaedia* to be "unquestionably one of the best of the scientific works of the day."

Beale emphasized Todd's warm interest in medical education and referred to his insistence "that the duties which devolve upon the medical profession are such as to render the religious and moral character of its members not less important than their practice and scientific attainments," a principle introduced by the founders of King's College Hospital. He was an effective, clear, and interesting lecturer; his class was well attended, his old students frequently coming back to swell the audience.

His most distinguished pupil, and future colleague, William Bowman, came to King's College in 1837 from the Birmingham General Hospital where he had assisted one of the physicians, Dr. Peyton Blakiston, in research on cardiac muscle. Blakiston, as an expression of gratitude, gave the young man a compound microscope, which he took with him to London, where he carried out the research on the histology of striped muscle for which he was elected FRS in 1841. In the same year, he published a classic paper on the structure of the kidney. Todd's and Bowman's *The Physiological Anatomy and Physiology of Man* was published in 1843.

At St. John's House, Queen Street, Westminster, through the influence of Todd, Bowman, and others, St. John's Training Institution for Nurses was established in 1848. St. John's House supplied Florence Nightingale with some of the ladies who accompanied her to Scutari in October 1855, and through the association with Todd and his colleagues, King's College Hospital became the first London hospital in which the nursing was entrusted to a voluntary sisterhood.

In addition to a large private and consulting practice, Todd served King's College Hospital as honorary physician from 1839 to 1859, having held previous appointments at the Western Dispensary and the Royal Hospital for Children. The breadth of his clinical experience is reflected in the variety of the publications listed in the Appendix, but further comment here is confined to his interest in the nervous system. James Collier (6) expressed the opinion that Robert Bentley Todd was "by far the greatest clinical neurologist Britain had produced until the time of Hughlings Jackson. . . ."

Collier was impressed by Todd's concept of diseases in which the nervous system is "first affected at its periphery in the muscles and nerves and the poisonous influence continuing the contamination gradually advances towards the centre." He may have taken the concept from one of his teachers, Robert J. Graves. This Dublin physician's name is recalled today in the context of hyperthyroidism, but he was the first (7) to describe peripheral neuritis, which he saw in epidemic form in Paris in 1828. Discussing paraplegia, Graves (8) postulated causes which "commencing in the extremities of the nerves, may be propagated towards their centres so as to be finally confounded with diseases originating in the centres themselves."

Convinced of the correctness of his theory, Graves used it to explain cases in which the actual pathology may have been multiple sclerosis or syphilitic meningo-myelitis:

> Of this form of paraplegia I have now witnessed many instances. In most cases I was induced to think that it arose from impressions made by cold and wet on the lower extremities. It is most commonly observed in young gentlemen who are addicted to fishing and shooting, and who in pursuit of their amusements get wet feet repeatedly, from walking over boggy grounds, or wading in the water. It is also observed in labourers whose employment obliges them to stand in water for many hours together, as in draining, pump-sinking, and other similar occupations. In all cases it assumes the creeping form, and generally appears at first in one limb, and afterwards in the other.

Todd's first publication on neurology, an article on paralysis, was included in the third volume of the *Cyclopaedia of Practical Medicine* (9) when he was 25. It was based on wide reading rather than personal experience, though he would have seen many palsied patients in Dublin's House of Industry Hospitals. Twenty years later, he published *Clinical Lectures on Paralysis*, a collection of his lectures at King's College Hospital.

One of the attractions of old texts is the likelihood of finding therein fragments of clinical entities now readily recognizable. The following passage from Todd's article on paralysis is reminiscent of neuralgic amyotrophy: "In some of the cases, the palsy at first occupied the muscles connecting the humerus to the scapula, especially the deltoid, which was wasted; there was therefore, inability to raise the arm, but the power of flexing the forearm remained . . . Considerable pain in the deltoid muscle generally preceded the paralysis. . . ." Another case may have been an example of scapulo-humeral dystrophy: ". . . A young lad aged 14, who had nearly lost the muscular power of the upper part of both his arms, accompanied by a most remarkable diminution of substance of the principal muscles. The deltoid and biceps were reduced to the appearance of mere membranes, and the muscles of the scapula were found nearly in the same state; the affection came on gradually, without any sign of spinal or cerebral disorder."

In explaining the rarity of hemiplegia due to spinal disease by the fact that pathology is seldom restricted exactly to a lateral half of the marrow, Todd anticipated the Brown-Séquard syndrome: ". . . in the *Edinburgh Medical and Surgical Journal* for 1825, a case is related where hemiparesis resulted from concussion of the spine, accompanied by complete anaesthesia of the other side of the body."

The treatment of hemiplegia depends on its cause, the age and general condition of the patient, and other variables. "Bleeding, purging, and other antiphlogistic remedies" are called for when there is evidence of plethora, inflammatory or apoplectic, and mild mercurial treatment may be used. "Abstinence from all stimulating elements, solid or fluid, must be rigidly observed in the great majority of cases." Later, a "change of air and scene are unequivocally of decided advantage and a visit to some watering-place is often made in this stage of the complaint with marked benefit."

Todd supported the application of blisters and tartar-emetic ointment to the head and cited, without any hint of disapproval, Dr. Prichard's advice to make an incision, "completely through the scalp for from four to five inches over the saggital suture, and the edges of the wound to be separated by a row of peas." The paralyzed limbs may be tickled with a feather or stung with nettles; other remedies include dry friction with the hand or by the flesh-brush, blisters, sea-salt, warm baths, and "a hundred strokes from the *gymnotus electricus*, or electric-eel."

Todd's account of paralysis agitans is largely direct quotation, with acknowledgment, from James Parkinson's *Essay* (1817). He remarked that "few cases of this disease are recorded" and regarded the festinating gait as pathognomonic, which may indicate that he was unacquainted with the early stage of the disease when disability is minimal. This would explain his introduction of the term "peripheral hemiplegia" in the *Clinical Lectures on Paralysis* (10) to describe what is clearly the opening phase of akinetic Parkinson's disease. He added the saving rider: "I do not know how far this name is correct, when the whole of the pathology of the affection is taken into consideration; but the appellation is a convenient one, inasmuch as it indicates the most prominent feature of the affection, namely the mode of access of the paralysis." He gave a detailed description of the disease:

> After a time the patient finds that he cannot perform small actions with the diseased arm; he cannot button his clothes, nor pick up a pin with the one hand, as well as with the other; then he notices that he cannot write so well as formerly; his handwriting becomes tremulous, and he has not the same command over his pen. . . . After a longer or shorter period the leg goes through the same series of symptoms . . . the patient drags it after him in walking; his move-

> ments become stumbling; and he speaks slowly and hesitatingly, but yet his mental faculties do not seem to suffer much. This may go on many months, or even years, for these cases are exceedingly chronic; the other side of the body in some instances begins to be affected almost simultaneously with, or very soon after the first; but in others it may be a considerable time before it suffers. . . . The patient begins to stoop; he finds he cannot hold himself erect; and in some instances his gait is apt to pass into that which is known as symptomatic of the disease termed "paralysis agitans" . . .

Todd's *Anatomy of the Brain, Spinal Cord and Ganglions* (1845) presents a scholarly account of neuroanatomy in which the author buttressed his arguments with illustrations from comparative anatomy and quotations from Willis, Vieussens, Santorini, and others. His description of the gross anatomy of the nervous system could be recommended to present-day students but, understandably, his views of functional localization and histology differ greatly from ours.

He doubted (11) the existence of a central canal in the spinal cord: "if such a canal exists, it must be extremely difficult to demonstrate, as I have never, after numberless examinations, been able to see it." He was sceptical, too, of the existence of "the orifice to which Majendie has given the high-sounding title 'Orifice des Cavités Encephaliques'" and envisaged the ventricles as shut off from the subarachnoid space.

This foramen remained controversial until an affirmative decision came through surgical inspection (12). As recently as 1923, Sir John Bland-Sutton (13) said that he had satisfied himself many times that it was an artifact with "such charm for teachers that it maintains a place in textbooks, although sealed up by practical anatomists many years ago." His statement extracted a reply (14) from F. Wood-Jones: "as a teacher I freely admit the charm of this foramen, and as a practical anatomist I also regard it with affection, for of its presence in the undisturbed condition of the roof-plate of the fourth ventricle I have no doubt whatever."

Todd had no conception of the function of the pacchionian bodies, which he regarded as abnormal structures, "the product of a chronic very gradual irritation due to more or less frequent functional excitement of the brain itself." Their true role was suggested by A. Key and G. Retzius of Stockholm in 1875.

When Todd's monograph was published, Schleiden and Schwann's "cell theory" was still a comparative novelty. Von Kolliker, who dealt with the spleen in the *Cyclopaedia of Anatomy and Physiology*, suggested in 1845 that nerve fibers are secondary to nerve cells (15), but confirmation awaited the demonstrations of Wilhelm His and Auguste Forel in 1887. Meanwhile, in the mid-1840s, the orthodox viewpoint was that the "vesicular" or gray nervous matter and the white fibrous matter composed of "nerve-tubes" were independent structures.

Todd (16) accepted this interpretation of microscopic structure, but uneasily, insisting that a major object of anatomical research "should be to find out the precise manner in which the nerve-fibres are united with the nerve-vesicles." He observed that some cells have tail-like "processes," which may be traced a considerable distance and bifurcate and even subdivide again. He remarked: "wherever there is a nerve-vesicle, we find an extremely fine varicose nerve-tube apparently adherent to it." Thus he came close to anticipating Waldeyer's "neurone theory," the consummation in 1891 of the efforts of many workers with the advantage of microtomes and staining techniques unknown to physiologists in the 1840s.

Speculating on the function of the pituitary body, Todd rejected a theory which placed it with the sympathetic system: "It may with more propriety be classed with the glands without efferent ducts. . . ." The importance of the anastomotic function of the "circle of Willis," so well illustrated with modern techniques by Hutchinson and Yates (17), was clear to him: "Thus, a stoppage in either carotid, or in either vertebral would speedily be remedied."

For Todd and his contemporaries, mentation, voluntary movement, and the emotions were functions of the cerebral cortex, the corpus striatum, and the upper midbrain, respectively, a theory of localization that hindered his experimental investigation of epilepsy. The *Anatomy of the Brain* is a reprint of Todd's article "Nervous Centres" in the *Cyclopaedia of Anatomy and Physiology*, but lacks the latter's extensive sections on pathology and physiology. These are included in *Physiology of the Nervous System* (1847).

In a fascinating book, *The Discovery of Reflexes*, Liddell (18) pointed out that the much-needed term "afferent" which "helped to clearer thinking about those sensations which reach consciousness and those sensations (if even they can be called that) which reach only spinal levels," was introduced by Todd in his *Cyclopaedia*. It occurs (19) in the discussion on the two kinds of nerves:

> In the motor nerve the nervous force ordinarily travels from the centre to the periphery, in the sensitive nerve it travels from the periphery to the centre. The former is therefore *efferent*, with reference to the centre . . . the latter is *afferent*.

Liddell also draws attention to a "profound observation of pregnant importance" contributed by Todd. "It was quite simple: posterior columns are not proportionally as large in the upper part of the cord as one would expect them to be if all sensations travel up to the brain."

Gowers (20) credited Todd with "the first really exact account" of tabes dorsalis in the *Cyclopaedia of Anatomy and Physiology* in 1847: "The credit of the discovery of the disease belongs, if to anyone, unquestionably to Todd, and few diseases can with greater truth be said to have been 'discovered'." Gowers referred to the contributions of others: Romberg's description in 1851, and those of Russell Reynolds (1855), Gull (1856), and Duchenne (1858). Duchenne introduced the term "locomotor ataxia," and through Trousseau's *Lectures*, his description of this clinical entity reached a wide readership. In France, the malady came to be known as Duchenne's disease, but Gowers insisted that "if any name is attached to it, that of Todd alone can be right."

Todd himself (21) showed scant respect for eponyms when he suggested that the "absurd name" *torcular herophili* should be discarded. One assumes, nevertheless, that he would not have disowned the term "maladie de Duchenne et de R. B. Todd" used by John Mallet Purser (22). The more important question, however, is his entitlement to such eponymic linkage.

Todd, in the passage (23) referred to by Gowers, made an important distinction between paralysis due to motor weakness and that which results from loss of coordination:

> Two kinds of paralysis of motion may be noticed in the lower extremities, the one consisting simply in the impairment or loss of the voluntary motion, the other distinguished by a diminution or total loss of the power co-ordinating movements. In the latter form, while considerable voluntary power remains, the patient finds great difficulty in walking, and his gait is so tottering and uncertain that his centre of gravity is easily displaced. These cases are generally of the most chronic kind, and many of them go on from day to day without any increase of the disease or improvement of their condition. In two examples of this variety of paralysis I ventured to predict disease of the posterior columns, the diagnosis being founded upon the views of their functions which I now advocate; and this was found to exist on a post-mortem inspection; and in looking through the accounts of recorded cases in which the posterior columns were the seat of lesion, all seem to have commenced by evincing more or less disturbance of the locomotive powers, sensation being affected only when the morbid change of structure extended to and more or less involved the posterior roots of the spinal nerves.

This important observation was a key to understanding the clinical picture of what came to be called locomotor ataxia or tabes dorsalis, yet of itself hardly supplies sufficient data to be regarded as a clinical entity. It lacks the persuasive force of the description (24) that contains an account of what is now called Romberg's sign:

> . . . the resistance of the ground is not felt as usual . . . The rider no longer feels the resistance of the stirrup, and has the strap put up a hole or two. The gait begins to be insecure, and the patient attempts to improve it by making a greater effort of the will; as he does not feel the tread to be firm, he puts down his heels with greater force. From the commencement of the disease the individual keeps his eyes on his feet to prevent his movements from becoming still more unsteady. If he is ordered to close his eyes while in the erect posture, he at once commences to totter and swing from side to side; the insecurity of his gait also exhibits itself more in the dark.

Todd's right to the eponym "Todd's Paralysis" is indisputable. Postictal paralysis is described in the Lumleian Lectures for 1849 (25):

> A paralytic state remains sometimes after the epileptic convulsion. This is more particularly the case when the convulsion has affected only one side or one limb: that limb or limbs will remain paralytic for some hours, or even days, after the cessation of the paroxysm, but it will ultimately perfectly recover.

Meyer and Portnoy's (26) modern study of Todd's paralysis in nine patients with experimental data from monkeys has shown that postictal paralysis results from temporary neuronal anoxia. It may occur in the absence of cerebrovascular disease, but the latter is often the cause of the seizures. If the circulation is normal, longer seizures are required for the increased neuronal demand to outstrip the oxygen supply than when there is vascular insufficiency.

Todd's subject in his Lumleian Lectures was the pathology and treatment of convulsive diseases. Under the term convulsion, he included "all those irregular actions of sets of muscles that are wholly unrestrainable by the influence of the will, and which are excited and kept up by physical irritant." He recognized "three distinct kinds of convulsions"—the jacitating or choreic, tonic or tetanic, and clonic or epileptiform.

Todd recognized two varieties of chorea—general chorea and partial chorea—which occur in both acute and chronic forms. Partial chorea is the more common, and Todd stressed the diagnostic importance of the involuntary protrusion of the tongue: "indeed I would call it pathognomonic." He was aware (27) of the association between chorea and cardiac disease:

> The heart is very frequently morbidly affected in chorea: and this morbid affection shows itself, not in any disturbance of the rhythm of the heart, which, so far as my observation extends, never is disturbed, but in a derangement of its sounds. A bellows sound is frequently present, and is either aortic systolic, when it is almost always an accompaniment of the anaemic state of the patient, but much more frequently it is mitral systolic or regurgitant.
>
> I am surprised that this feature of the clinical history of chorea has not attracted more general attention. It has been well known to me for many years, and I described it in the Croonian lectures on the pathology of rheumatism, which were given by me in this theatre six years ago. But to my friend, Dr. Addison, of Guy's Hospital, is due, so far as I know, the merit of having first made public the frequent occurrence of this bellows sound in chorea.

He attributed the "mitral bellows sound" to a lesion of the valve preventing its closure: "many of the patients who suffer from chorea are of a rheumatic diathesis, and that in consequence of this rheumatic state they experience an insidious endocarditis which generally affects the mitral valves."

The acute general chorea to which Todd referred is likely to have been a very different entity—"these patients literally shake themselves to death"—than the type now called Sydenham's chorea, of which he feels "fully justified in laying it down as a feature of the disease, that its natural tendency is to get well." Todd referred to movements similar to those of chorea occurring in rheumatic or gouty states and also described "a curious affection" that seems a very good example of writer's cramp.

Tetanus, a disease "of extremely fatal tendency," presents an unvarying clinical picture. "If you see a well-developed case of tetanus, you have seen all; variations are only as to the degree of tetanic convulsion: in all you have the tetanic face, the rigid limbs, the locked jaw, the opisthotonos. In the acute form of the disease, indeed, the malady runs its course with much greater, sometimes with extraordinary, rapidity; while in the more chronic form it lasts a fortnight or three weeks, and in a few a much longer period."

Tetanus in infants, trismus nascentium, had become uncommon following improvements in diet, cleanliness, and ventilation. "Dr. Clarke, by means of good ventilation, reduced the mortality from this disease in the Dublin Lying-In Hospital from seventeen per cent to five or six: and in Dr. Collins's mastership of the same hospital, extending from 1826 to 1833, mortality from this disease had fallen to a mere fraction per cent" (28).

Todd remarked that laryngismus stridulus had "many points of resemblance to tetanus" and regarded its pathology as essentially the same. He was familiar with the convulsions caused by strychnine, and he had induced tetanic convulsions in rabbits, subsequently examining the nervous system without finding damage to structures.

Todd presented a very adequate account of epilepsy and mentioned a variety of "precursory symptoms," including those now associated with temporal lobe attacks—"a feeling of terror . . . ," "or smell may be disturbed as in the case mentioned by Heberden, where a smell of musk ushered in the attack"—and a more complicated visual aura, in which "the warning consisted in the phantom of a little old woman in a red cloak coming sharply up to [the patient] and striking him on the head." He described convulsions confined to one side of the body: "I have frequently seen the most intense convulsion of the arm and leg and side of the face on one side, while the corresponding parts on the other side were perfectly quiescent."

Todd was familiar with febrile convulsions, those occurring in uremia and ecclampsia, and seizures associated with poisons. "Epilepsy seldom kills . . . ," but Todd warned that it often led to dementia or other forms of insanity. "Frequent attacks of the epileptic vertigo of Esquirol—the petit mal—are in general pretty certain precursors of a state of dementia or fatuity" (29).

Discussing the etiology of convulsive disorders, Todd argued convincingly that the cause resides in the nervous system rather than in the muscles. His belief that nerve fibers and nerve cells were independent structures led him to draw an ingenious analogy with the generation of galvanic current by the electric battery (30):

> Two dissimilar forms of nervous matter, both bedewed by the same blood, represent the zinc and copper, with the intervening electrolyte of the battery: and as the activity of the battery, and the energy of the galvanic force, depend on the amount of chemical action between the fluid, which is interposed between the metals and one of them, so the activity of the nutrient or chemical changes in the nervous centres determines the degree of development and vigour of the nervous force. And as in the galvanic battery we look to the nature of the metals as well as to that of the interposed fluid, to enable us to judge of the probable quantity and quality of the force generated; so, in the nervous battery, if I may so speak, we must look to the nature of the nervous matter of both kinds, and to the quantity and quality of the blood, to determine the amount of energy of the nervous force developed. Hence we may fairly assume that while the development of the nervous force is much influenced primarily by the nature of the nervous matter, it likewise is greatly dependent on the quantity, but more especially on the *quality* of the blood.

Todd related "the corpora quadrigemina, and the large mass of nervous matter which constitutes the greater part of the mesocephale" to an emotional function, and having observed that fright was a common exciting cause of chorea, he selected this area as involved in chorea, the underlying cause being the disturbance of nutrition or blood which "excites the nervous battery, and causes it to generate its force feebly and irregularly."

The seat of the abnormal process in tetanus Todd placed in the spinal cord and medulla oblongata. He postulated "an exaltation in the generating power of that portion of the great nervous battery in which the chief cerebro-spinal nerves implanted . . ." (31). He further described the nature of tetanus:

> Such then is the pathology of Tetanus. A man receives a wound—this wound occasions an irritated, a polar state of certain nerves—and this polar condition is communicated by a process of induction to the whole spinal cord, which, by some modification of the nutrition of the cord due to some altered state of blood, assumes that state the more readily, and retains it the longer.

He demonstrated that tetanic convulsions induced by strychnine in the guinea pig could be controlled and life prolonged by the use of ether.

Todd advocated two agents in the control of tetanus—cold in the form of ice applied to the spine and chloroform—but "we must take care that the sleep of chloroform does not prove to him the sleep of death by depriving him too long of those supplies which alone can counteract the destructive aesthenia." He had not personally used chloroform on a patient.

In the management of laryngismus stridulus Todd advocated "the plan of dashing cold water in the face, to avert an impending paroxysm, or to shorten an existing one . . ." and mentioned that Sir Henry Marsh "commends the old Tinctura fuliginis" (32).

Todd was familiar with the wide repertoire of epilepsy, its major manifestations in what we today call tonic-clonic seizures, and those instances in which unconsciousness "is accompanied by vacant look" but without convulsive movements. He observed that partial seizures "accompany disease of the hemispheres of the brain or of the cerebellum. I have seen them most frequent in children, associated with the so-called tubercular meningitis. . . ." He referred to a two-year-old who had seizures affecting the left side of the body. The patient died, and the autopsy showed "an extensive deposit of tubercular matter on the surface of the right hemisphere of the brain, opposite to the side on which the convulsions took place. . . ." Unfortunately, he regarded such partial seizures as "essentially distinct from true epilepsy" (33).

Todd argued convincingly to exclude certain areas as sites from which the epileptic paroxysm emanates. He placed this in the cerebral hemispheres and mesencephalon. The latter may seem in accordance with the present-day concept of centrencephalic epilepsy, but Todd's concept was very different from ours (34):

> You will bear in recollection that the complete epileptic paroxysm exhibits two features essentially different from each other: first, the loss of consciousness; secondly, the convulsions. The loss of consciousness and the other mental phenomena are dependent upon a disturbed state of the hemispheric lobes: the convulsions upon a disturbance of the mesocephale, consecutive to, and derived from, the disturbance of the hemispheric lobes.

Todd poses an important question: can a disturbance of the hemisphere cause convulsive movements? His answer was "the fibres are incapable of exciting motion except through their influence on other ganglia," although he had already noted that superficial lesions of the hemisphere had caused convulsive movements. Using the analogy of the battery, he considered that a deposition of tubercle "in the vesicular matter, among the particles of the generating plate," seriously impaired the development of the nervous force.

Todd selected the midbrain at the level of the corpora quadrigemina as an area concerned in epilepsy. He carried out experiments on rabbits, applying galvanic stimulation to the spinal cord and the medulla (35):

> I then tried the corpora quadrigemina and the mesocephale. Having passed fine bradawls into the cranium in such a direction as I had previously satisfied myself would lead to this organ, I subjected it to the influence of the machine; general convulsions were produced, of a character essentially different from those which resulted from stimulating the spinal cord or the medulla oblongata. They were combined movements of alternate contraction and relaxation, flexion and extension, affecting the muscles of all the limbs, of the trunk, and of the eyes, which rolled about just as in epilepsy.
>
> On inserting the awls into the hemispheric lobes, still different effects were produced by the application of the machine. I could observe nothing like true convulsions; but slight convulsive twitchings of the muscles of the face took place, which were no more than what would be caused by the stimulus of galvanism acting upon the nerves of the face.

Referring to these experiments, which were unknown to Hitzig and overlooked by Ferrier, Sir Geoffrey Jefferson wrote (36): "How modern all this is, though it has been eclipsed by much that was discovered later." But Todd failed to see anything novel in the contractions evoked in the facial muscles, nor did he relate it to his observation that an exudate on the surface of the right cerebral hemisphere had been associated with left-sided convulsive movements and adduce, as Jackson was to do later, a sensorimotor cortical function.

Speculating on the causes of epilepsy, he excluded inflammation and congestion but believed that anemia or impoverished blood supply is responsible for epileptic attacks, yet "not in itself the cause of epilepsy." He envisaged a state of abnormal nutrition causing a disturbance of "the nervous force" (37):

> These periodic evolutions of the nervous force which give rise to the complete epileptic paroxysm may be compared to the electrical phenomenon described by Faraday under the name of disruptive discharge.

Here his concept of epilepsy closely resembles the modern concept, and he envisaged rapid discharge in the hemispheres or midbrain "with all the violence of the discharge from a highly charged Leyden jar," spreading to other parts of the brain and the spinal cord.

A conflict between the demands of his practice and his professorial duties caused Todd to resign from King's College in 1853. On the occasion of his farewell lecture on March 20th, he paid a tribute to one of his own teachers, Robert J. Graves of Dublin (38):

> From him I first imbibed a taste for physiological inquiry; and, under his guidance and direction, my first studies upon that subject were pursued. How much more would I have rejoiced to make this public acknowledgement, as I have often done privately, were my friend able to hear it but, alas! this day's post has brought me the sad intelligence of his too early removal—no longer ago than at noon yesterday—from science and from a large circle of sorrowing friends.

The candidates for the vacant chair at King's included T. H. Huxley, but Lionel S. Beale was appointed. The Hippocratic piety shown by Charles Hawkes Todd in naming his eldest son James Henthorn Todd was exceeded by Beale, whose son, born in 1864, was named Peyton Todd Bowman Beale, and he was generally known in King's College Hospital, where he became honorary surgeon, as "Toddles" Beale.

The Todd Ward and the Todd Prize remain as more formal memorials to Robert Bentley Todd. It may be said in conclusion that he made important contributions to the advancement of neurology and neurophysiology but failed in certain instances to reach attainable insights, thus exemplifying an important truism of medical history. Men are simultaneously sustained and fettered by the ideas of their own times. Accustomed to the bracing help of contemporary beliefs, they may strain their shackles, yet fail to walk free toward new perceptions.

APPENDIX: BOOKS AND PAMPHLETS BY R. B. TODD

A Lecture Introductory to the Course of Anatomy and Physiology delivered in the Medical School, Aldersgate Street, London, 21 pp. Adalard, Printers, Bartholomew Close, London (1832).

Pseudo-Morbid Appearances, 14 pp., 8vo. Marchant, London (1833). Reprint from *Cyclopaedia of Practical Medicine* (1834).

The Cyclopaedia of Anatomy and Physiology, edited by R. B. Todd, Vols. I–V. Longman, Brown, Green, Longmans & Roberts, London (1835–1859).

On the Structure of the Mucous Membrane of the Stomach. Goulstonian lectures for 1839, 8 pp., 8^{c}. Wilson & Ogilvy, London (1840).

Practical Remarks on Gout, Rheumatic Fever and Chronic Rheumatism of the Joints, 216 pp., 21cm. Croonian lectures, 1843. J. W. Parker, London (1843).

Anatomy of the Brain, Spinal Cord, and Ganglions. Sherwood, Gilbert and Piper, London (1845).

The Physiological Anatomy and Physiology of Man, R. B. Todd and W. Bowman, 2 vols. Parker, London (1845–1856); Lea & Blanchard, Philadelphia (1850–1857).

Physiology of the Nervous System, 72 pp., 8^{0}. Marchant, Singer & Co., London (1847). Reprint from *Cyclopaedia of Anatomy and Physiology*, Vol. 3.

On the Pathology and Treatment of Convulsive Diseases. The Lumleian lectures for 1850, 72 pp., 8^{0}. Wilson & Ogilvy, London (1850).

On the Resources of King's College, London for Medical Education, 53 pp., 8^{0}. J. W. Parker & Son, London (1852).

Additional Experiments on the Excitability of Paralysed and Healthy Limbs by the Galvanic Current, 23 pp., 12^{0}. C. & J. Adlard, London (1853). Reprint from *Med.-Chir. Tr.* (1853), p. 36.

Farewell Address on his Resignation of the Professorship of Physiology at King's College, March 21, 1853, 12 pp., 12^{0}. W. Tyler, London (1853).

Clinical Lectures on Paralysis, Disease of the Brain and Other Affections of the Nervous System, 311 pp., 23 cm. J. Churchill, London (1854). Lindsay & Blakiston, Philadelphia (1855). 2nd edition with corrections and additions, 474 pp., 16 cm. Churchill, London (1856).

Clinical Lectures on Certain Acute Diseases. J. Churchill, London; Blanchard and Lea, Philadelphia (1860).

Clinical Lectures, 2nd ed., edited by L. S. Beale, XL, 912 pp. Churchill, London (1861). Includes *Clinical Lectures on Paralysis . . . Diseases of the Urinary Organs . . . On Certain Acute Diseases*.

REFERENCES

1. McIntyre, N. (1956): Robert Bentley Todd. *King's Coll. Hosp. Gaz.*, 35:1.

2. Bliss correspondence, BM Add Ms 34570 6484; Babbage correspondence, BM Add Ms 37189 f 269.
3. Beale, L. S. (1870): Lecture on medical progress: In memoriam R. B. Todd.: *Br. Med. J.*, I:485.
4. Anon. (1836): Review of Todd's *Cyclopaedia. Lancet*, I:585.
5. Anon. (1840): Review. *Lancet*, II:855.
6. Collier, J. (1934): Inventions and the outlook in neurology. *Lancet*, II:855.
7. McHenry, L. C. (1969): *Garrison's History of Neurology*, p. 433. Charles C. Thomas, Springfield, Illinois.
8. Graves, R. J. (1848): *Clinical Lectures*, p. 647. Fannin, Dublin.
9. Todd, R. B. (1854): In: *The Cyclopaedia of Practical Medicine*, edited by J. Forbes, A. Tweedie, and J. Conolly, p. 240. Sherwood, Gilbert and Piper, London.
10. Todd, R. B. (1854): *Clinical Lectures on Paralysis*, p. 258. Churchill, London.
11. Todd, R. B. (1845): *Anatomy of the Brain, Spinal Cord and Ganglions*, p. 92. Sherwood, Gilbert & Piper, London.
12. Millen, J. W., and Woollam, D. H. M. (1962): *The Anatomy of the Cerebrospinal Fluid*, p. 56. Oxford Univ. Press, London.
13. Bland-Sutton, J. (1923): On the choroid plexuses and ventricles of the brain. *Lancet*, I:1143.
14. Wood-Jones, F. (1923): A defence of the foramen of Magendie. *Lancet*, II:486.
15. von Bonin, G. (1970): In: *Founders of Neurology*, edited by W. Haymaker and F. Schiller, p. 53. Charles C. Thomas, Springfield, Illinois.
16. Todd. R. B. (1845): *Anatomy of the Brain, Spinal Cord and Ganglions*. p. 269. Sherwood, Gilbert & Piper, London.
17. Hutchinson, E. C., and Yates, P. O. (1956): The cervical portion of the vertebral artery—a clinico-pathological study. *Brain*, 79:319.
18. Liddell, E. G. T. (1960): *The Discovery of Reflexes*, p. 75. Clarendon Press, Oxford.
19. Todd, R. B. (1845): *Anatomy of the Brain, Spinal Cord and Ganglions*. p. x. Sherwood, Gilbert & Piper, London.
20. Gowers, W. R. (1892): *A Manual of Diseases of the Nervous System*, 2nd ed., Vol. 1, p. 398. Churchill, London.
21. Todd, R. B. (1845): *Anatomy of the Brain, Spinal Cord and Ganglions*. p. x. Sherwood, Gilbert & Piper, London.
22. Purser, J. M. (1863): *On disease of the spinal cord and medulla oblongata*. Ms of unpublished prize-winning essay in Library of Royal College of Physicians of Ireland.
23. Todd, R. B. (1847): *Cyclopaedia of Anatomy and Physiology*, Vol. 3, p. 721R. Longmans & Roberts, Longman, Brown, Green, London.
24. Romberg, M. H. (1853): *A Manual of the Nervous Diseases of Man*, Vol. 2, p. 395. Sydenham Society, London.
25. Todd, R. B. (1849): *London Med. Gaz.*, 8:668.
26. Meyer, J. S., and Portnoy, H. D. (1959): Post-epileptic paralysis. *Brain*, 82:162.
27. Todd, R. B. (1849): On the pathology and treatment of convulsive diseases. *London Med. Gaz.*, 8:663.
28. Jefferson, G. (1953): The prodromes to cortical localisation. *J. Neurol. Psychiatr.*, 16:59.
29. Todd, R. B. (1849): On the pathology and treatment of convulsive diseases. *London Med. Gaz.*, 8:668.
30. Todd, R. B. (1849): On the pathology and treatment of convulsive diseases. *London Med. Gaz.*, 8:726.
31. Todd, R. B. (1849): On the pathology and treatment of convulsive diseases. *London Med. Gaz.*, 8:767.
32. Todd, R. B. (1849): On the pathology and treatment of convulsive diseases. *London Med. Gaz.*, 8:772.
33. Todd, R. B. (1849): On the pathology and treatment of convulsive diseases. *London Med. Gaz.*, 8:815.
34. Todd, R. B. (1849): On the pathology and treatment of convulsive diseases. *London Med. Gaz.*, 8:820.
35. Todd, R. B. (1849): On the pathology and treatment of convulsive diseases. *London Med. Gaz.*, 8:821.
36. Jefferson, G. (1953): The prodromes to cortical localisation. J. Neurol. Psychiatr., 16:59.
37. Todd, R. B. (1849): On the pathology and treatment of convulsive diseases. *London Med. Gaz.*, 8:841.
38. Todd, R. B. (1853): Farewell address at King's College. p.6. W. Tyler, London.

Historical Aspects of the Neurosciences,
edited by F. Clifford Rose and W. F. Bynum.
Raven Press, New York ©

History of Narcolepsy

David Parkes

University Department of Neurology, King's College Hospital and Institute of Psychiatry, London, U.K.

For only Og King of Bashan remained of the remnant of giants; behold his bedstead was a bedstead of iron: is it not in Rabbath of the children of Ammon?

Deuteronomy 3:11

Sleepy giants were recognized in Biblical times, but symptoms of narcolepsy were not defined until the last century, when at least three famous novelists described characters with narcoleptic symptoms (1). Poe, who may have suffered from sleep paralysis, described in "The Premature Burial," a character with "a species of exaggerated lethargy . . . without ability to stir." Melville in *Moby Dick* drew a picture of narcolepsy, while George Eliot described the paralysis with surprise of Silas Marner. The Victorian hero and missionary explorer David Livingstone had a similar experience when frightened by a lion. As well as the men of action and of letters, the physicians, and in particular the neuropsychiatrists, of the 19th century recorded their curious cases of sleep disorders. The problem was Linnean, one of classification.

AFRICAN SLEEPING SICKNESS

The endemic disease known as sleeping sickness, hypnosia (2), and various other names seems to have been first observed by Winterbottom in 1819 as being very common among the slaves in the Bay of Benin on the West Coast of Africa. Clark in 1840 found it common in Sierra Leone among the Free Africans, and by other observers it was found in the Niger, in the Antilles, with an endemic area from Senegal to the Congo, and in the Sierra Leone district. According to various medical observers, only Negroes were affected, with more cases inland than on the coast, with pathological sleep usually manifest after prolonged and fatiguing work had exhausted the victim's strength. The result was death. De Manacéine (3) describes the condition being first shown by enlarged lymph nodes and drooping of the eyelids. "Initially the subjects can be roused but periods of sleep become longer and more frequent, until at last sleep is almost continuous, food is refused, and death ensues in the course of weeks or months." The brain was described as "anaemic and unusually firm, with inflammation of the membranes" (2), although we now know the disease is due to nests of trypanosomes which colonize the choroid plexus and the surrounding brain. Semelaigne, in comment of a case of Caffé (4), rejecting a diagnosis of the "sleep sickness" in a French patient plagued by hallucinations and an overpowering need to sleep, concludes his argument by saying, "I'm sure that you would be inclined to agree with me, my dear colleague, that we would be better off leaving sleep disease to the blacks, at least temporarily anyway, since whites have plenty of problems to contend with without that one too."

However, the problem could not be left to the blacks. At least a century previously, Oliver (5), in the *Philosophical Transactions* of 1704 and 1705, had related the history of "an extraordinary Sleepy Person at Timsburg, near Bath," and many similar and singular cases were observed. These fell into two groups: patients with remarkably prolonged and profound sleep likened to hibernation (6), such as in the dormeuse d'Okno (7), or alternatively, patients with short sleep episodes, from which they were easily aroused.

TRANCE

On January 31, 1897, the gates of Rochefort Hospital admitted a sleeper by the name of Victorine Doirat. She was carefully watched, and shamming was put out of question. During a month, she was plunged more or less in sleep, remaining in a cataleptic condition for five consecutive days without eating or drinking or satisfying any of the wants of nature. The day on which she was taken to the hospital, she had an attack of somnambulism, and she frightened her neighbors by going to them moving like an automaton with shut eyes. The morning after her admission, the *chef de service* going on his rounds found her asleep. By means of stimulants and suggestions, she was awakened and induced to take some soup and drink some milk. An hour afterwards, she fell into a cataleptic sleep. The condition continued, interrupted by intervals of waking, which were very variable. Sometimes they occurred several times a day, at others after two or three days of sleep. She opened her eyes and asked for food; if not immediately satisfied, she fell asleep. In order to oblige her to take nourishment, she was awakened by stimulating the median and ulnar nerves, but her eyes closed again almost as soon as they opened. At 20 years of age, her excited condition obliged her family to put her in an asylum. At 28, she married a deaf and dumb man. Her appearance was healthy. The eyelids constantly trembled, the body was rigid, and the limbs remained for several hours in the position in which they were placed (*Lancet*, May 8, 1897).

NARCOLEPSY

In contrast to such cases of prolonged sleep, Graves (8) described a Dublin gentleman with the habit of falling asleep in his soup, and Lasègue (3) described a young waiter who suddenly fell asleep while serving and stood sleeping with the glass in his hand, after which he awoke and continued serving. De Manacéine (3) also records two patients, both illiterate and of slow intellect. One of them, a housemaid of 19 years of age, was a very sound sleeper at night, and in the daytime one could never be sure of her remaining awake. "I have seen her going to sleep in the very act of announcing a visitor and in bringing in a tray with cups full of coffee. The other was a woman of 50, who was a nurse until in one of her sleeping paroxysms she dropped an infant on the floor and nearly killed him. In both, the pulse was remarkably slow: in the girl, it varied between 50 and 70 beats when awake; in the woman of 50, between 40 and 60. Every excitement caused, instead of an acceleration, a retardation of the heartbeats, the pulse falling to 35 in the woman and to 40 in the girl."

CATALEPSY

In addition to these cases of trance or prolonged pathological sleep and briefer attacks of paroxysmal sleep often considered to be of an epileptic or neurotic character, other less definable disturbances in consciousness, sometimes accompanied by changes in muscular tone, were documented. To this group belongs catalepsy, of which an outbreak raged endemically for several years at Billinghausen, near Würzburg, and was described by Vogt. Half the inhabitants suffered from catalepsy, often lasting for a few minutes, during which the face became intensely pale, the limbs motionless, speech embarrassed and consciousness, if not altogether abolished, much obscured. The attacks were liable to occur at any moment and fixed the patient in the position in which they caught him. All those who were attacked showed a very feeble physical and intellectual development. The disease was transmitted by heredity, not immediately by parents to children, but atavistically, by skipping a generation, from grandparents to grandchildren. Those attacked by this cataleptic disorder were commonly called *die Starren* (the rigid ones). Gélineau must have known of this endemic disease when he described as cataplexy (not catalepsy) the similar behavior of an agoraphobic patient, white with anxiety and paralyzed by the fear of mutilation or death due to a possible carriage accident on traversing the streets and squares of Paris.

GÉLINEAU AND THE NARCOLEPTIC SYNDROME

The principle event in this period was the introduction of the name "narcolepsy" by the French neuropsychiatrist Gélineau in 1880 (9,10) who regarded it as a separate disease entity. The term was derived from ναρχωσιζ, meaning "somnolence," and λαμβανειν, meaning "to seize." The patient described by Gélineau in two reports to the *Gazette des Hôpitaux* was a Parisian retailer of casks or hogsheads who attended his clinic on February 15, 1879. The history commenced with an unhappy *affaire*, after which frequent and disabling narcolepsy set in, attacks usually lasting for a few minute, sometimes half an hour or more. There were as many as 200 attacks a day, all exhibiting the characteristics of normal sleep in an intense degree. Attacks could be brought on in a number of ways—by walking or other muscular exertion, by emotion, by sexual excitement—and they were particularly common during thunderstorms. The patient also had a lively sense of humor, and the sight of a grotesque person or a visit to the theater made him weak with laughter. Unlike the patient with agoraphobia, surprise or emotion provoked loss of muscle tone with falls rather than rigidity and fixed posture. These falls were named "astasia" by Gélineau and only later as "cataplexy" by Henneberg in 1916 (11). Gélineau considered that emotions influence the onset of sleep attacks and the nature of falls, or astasias. "The fall associated with a sleep attack is similar to that of a drunk or of a child who falls asleep. It is a collapse preceded and induced by sleep, whereas in the epileptic seizure, sleep follows the fall." To alter the activity of the intracerebral circulation, Gélineau investigated the action of amyl nitrate in narcolepsy and also that of a number of unrelated drugs including apomorphine, picrotoxin, and strychnine. However, it seems probable that only his treatment with caffeine had much success.

NARCOLEPSY AND STRUCTURAL LESIONS

During the first decades of this century, many structural lesions of the nervous system associated with disordered sleep were described. These included neoplasms, and in particular, those around the aqueduct and periventricular areas, pineal tumors, and other tumors affecting the hypothalamus, brain stem, and third ventricle as well as those causing increased intracranial pressure; many vascular disorders, including vascular lesions of the brain stem and diffuse cerebrovascular disease; a host of parainfective disorders such as brain abscess, syphilis, and Sydenham's chorea; and a number of diverse degenerative conditions, including senile dementia, Alzheimer's disease, as well as *chorée fibrillaire de Morvan*, myriachit of the Orient, and jumping Frenchmen of Maine. More recently a case of mixed salivary tumor in the right tonsillar fossa near the carotid sheath has been described, removal of which abolished narcolepsy and cataplexy. A Balinese method of inducing sleep is for specialized masseurs to put bilateral pressure on the carotid triangles (15). Narcolepsy has also been described in patients with disseminated sclerosis and cerebellar tumors, although in the last condition, an operation may not alter narcolepsy (16). In individual subjects with narcolepsy, congenital ocular paresis, temporal lobe epilepsy, familial tremor, and peptic ulcer have occurred (17,18). Passouant (13) describes how Mauthner, studying cases of possible encephalitis with sleep disturbance in 1890, assumed that drowsiness was due to involvement of the mesencephalon and diencephalon, and it became customary to refer to these regions as Mauthner's area. Previously, Gayet (19) had identified lesions in the mesencephalic and hypothalamic areas of the brain in a patient with encephalitis, but not until the work of von Economo and Grippe (20) was the importance of lesions in the caudal part of the third ventricle and the upper brain stem recognized. Using only cases with well-localized anatomical lesions, Lhermitte and Tournay (21) described cases of excessive hypersomnia from a lesion within the pons.

ENCEPHALITIS LETHARGICA

The acute phase of encephalitis lethargica was often associated with reversal of the sleep-walking rhythm. Symonds (22) and Adie (23) both described patients who developed fairly typical narcolepsy following undoubted encephalitis lethargica. Symonds' patient was a native of Iceland, who presented the characteristic parkinsonian facies, and his posture and gait, though less severely affected, were typical of the same condition. With this were associated bilateral ptosis and a blinking tic. His chief complaint was of insomnia. He said that on getting up at about 9:00 a.m., he became so sleepy that he had to go to bed again; he was at his best in the evening, seldom getting off to sleep until well on in the early hours of the morning. This illness followed a mild attack of influenza in December 1918. Not until the summer of 1919 did the patient complain of excessive sleepiness, followed by a period of delirium and visual hallucinosis. After this, he noticed that whenever he laughed or was excited he fell down, and subsequently he developed signs of parkinsonism. He began to improve in 1922 but remained liable to falling attacks. Symonds described what he took to be an attack of petit mal: "A little twitching of the facial muscles, short interval of silence, then talked vaguely in Icelandic; then said, 'I can't move my arm'." In this case, there seems no doubt of the association of both narcolepsy and cataplexy with encephalitis lethargica, despite the tendency for the condition to improve. However, with other structural lesions of the nervous system, sleep reversal was more common than daytime narcolepsy, and cataplexy very uncommon.

NARCOLEPSY WITHOUT ENCEPHALITIS

Despite the description by Gélineau (9,10), Caffé (4), Graves (8), Westphal (12), and many others, narcolepsy was little known and rarely recognized until the second decade of the 20th century (13). Gowers (14) thought that most attacks of narcolepsy occurred in hysterical subjects, and that for every 15 cases of narcolepsy, 30,000 cases of epilepsy would come under observation. He described the case of a 22-year-old girl "without neurotic heredity," who had brief attacks of rapidly deepening sleepiness without sufficient reason, apart from the scarcely sufficient cause of early rising. These attacks commenced with sudden yawning and heaviness of the eyes, so that she found it impossible to keep them open: In a minute or two she was asleep and dreaming vividly. Attacks occurred in clusters every one or two months, and the victim was possibly the first recorded example of the occasional association between narcolepsy and menstruation. Gowers, like Gélineau, found an effective treatment in citrate of caffeine, and he also stressed the beneficial effect of mountain and sea air on sleep.

Published cases of narcolepsy without any structural lesion became more and more numerous following the 1917–1926 encephalitis epidemic: 43 by Wilson in 1928 (24), 45 at the Mayo Clinic (25), then about 100 (26), and then more than 200 (27). Adie's paper in *Brain* (23) began with this dramatic sentence: "The disease I am about to describe is characterised by the occurrence of attacks of irresistible sleep without apparent cause, and curious attacks on emotion in which the muscles relax suddenly so that the victim sinks to the ground, fully conscious, but unable to move." In this paper, the whole description of the malady was crystallized, and Adie rightly contended that the term "narcolepsy" was best confined to the condition, with its peculiar and unmistakable features, that he had observed in eight cases, supplemented by some 15 published reports. Adie considered that the feeling of powerlessness was merely an exaggeration of that helplessness or inability for action that may overcome normal people or animals under strong emotion, or with laughter, fear, or horror.

Patients were found to be mentally and physically normal, although Redlich (28) drew attention to possible signs of ductless gland disorder in some of the cases: a small pituitary fossa, slight acromegalic signs, obesity, delayed sexual development, and periods of amenorrhea. These examples surely include patients with sleep apnea, acromegaly, and hyperprolactinemia, which accounted for infertility.

CATAPLEXY

When Adie's paper was published (September 1926), it was specifically remarked that no patient had been examined by a competent neurologist while in the cataplectic state. However, in the same year, Mankowski reported absent reflexes including an extensor plantar response during cataplexy, and Mussio Fournier described total electrical inexcitability of the facial muscles. It remained for Wilson to give the classic account of cataplexy (24):

> The clinical value of this striking case of combined narcoleptic and emotional attacks is enhanced by the fact that I was able to observe one of the latter from beginning to end and to examine the patient's neurological condition during it. Dr. MacDonald Critchley, the present registrar at the National Hospital, was with me at the time and helped materially in the examination which was of necessity hurried.
> *Description of attack of "powerlessness"*—while I was occupied with another patient, E.C. was sitting behind me and as afterwards appeared was endeavouring to keep himself from falling asleep. Suddenly I heard a slight groaning noise coming from him and at once looking around I saw his head nodding gently on his chest as he sank forward into a bend position and a moment or two later slid or "slithered" off the chair to the floor. The arms were by the side and the fingers semiflexed; the eyes were closed. Lifting the arms I found them absolutely atonic and flaccid. When let go they fell like lumps of lead by his side. The legs similarly were absolutely atonic sprawling out on the floor. Lifting the eyelids I observed that the pupils reacted to light slightly but definitely, while the eyelid muscles were so toneless that little or no reflex contraction took place on my touching the cornea. Testing the knee jerks I found them completely abolished on both sides. In the meantime, Dr.

> Critchley had hurriedly taken off the patient's shoe and sock on the left side and testing the plantar reflex obtained a slight but definite left extensor response which he demonstrated to me and which I corroborated.
> Just as we were finishing this rapid examination the patient suddenly said "I am alright sir" in his ordinary voice and with a faint smile. Muscular power came back; he moved his limbs, got onto the chair and told us that he had been conscious the whole time.

SLEEP PARALYSIS

It would be wrong to object that this was an attack of sleep paralysis rather than cataplexy, and Wilson was aware of the closest resemblance between these phenomena. With the exception of Westphal (12), previous writers on narcolepsy had not referred to the much discussed question of nocturnal paresis or paralysis, which formed the subject of an interesting study by Weir Mitchell (29), and was considered a transient physiological rather than pathological event, the spell to be instantly broken by an acute mental effort to move. Lhermitte (30) described sleep paralysis as "waking cataplexy" and Daniels (31) described it as "hypnagogic cataplexy." The close similarity between cataplexy and sleep paralysis was maintained, but sleep paralysis was considered to be a borderline normal phenomenon.

CATAPLEXY OR CATALEPSY?

Loss of muscle tone and reflexes during certain sleep phases were described by Lombard in 1887 (32), who also made the repeated observation that a dream of active movement was associated with a very violent knee kick. About the same time, Rosenbach (33) systematically observed the reflexes excited in children by tickling the palm of the hand, the sole of the foot, the tendon reflexes, and the pupil reaction during different sleep and waking phases. The connection between loss in muscle tone and reflexes during sleep and cataplexy was, however, obscure during this period. Since head movement (28) and trembling, grimaces, and tongue protrusion (12) were occasionally found during cataplexy or sleep paralysis, a possible relationship between cataplexy and epilepsy or chorea was considered. However, during this period, a clear distinction emerged between cataplexy with loss of muscle tone, and catalepsy with increase in tone resulting in fixed postures, which could be maintained without fatigue for long periods, although both were accompanied by paralysis of movement. Catalepsy was frequently associated with epilepsy and hysteria; the rigid and waxy state disappeared with the onset of sleep. Attempts were made to localize the lesion responsible for catalepsy when due to organic cause; this appeared to be anywhere between and including the mammillary bodies and the corpus striatum. The ability to retain certain postures for longer than normal suggested that a special type of plastic tonus not usually shown by skeletal muscles rather than a contractile tonus leading to fatigue was present.

DREAMS

The absence of dreams during narcoleptic sleep or prolonged trance was noted by de Manacéine (3), who remarked that the subjects almost never dream and, on awakening, cannot recall any sensations experienced during sleep. However, this proved incorrect, and hypnagogic hallucinations were added to the recognized manifestations of narcolepsy (34–36). The occurrence of hallucinations had been described during the encephalitis epidemic by Levy (34), and false sensory perceptions occurring unexpectedly before or without sleep attacks were described by Alajouanine and Baruk (37). Hypnagogic hallucinations had been considered a normal event by Maury (38), who remarked that the best moment to observe the influences of the visual apparatus in producing dreams was the moment before going to sleep. At this time, a whole variety of imagery would pass before the eyes—luminous phenomena in some people, human forms in others, while still others most often saw flowers or landscapes or the capricious play of arabesques or geometrical figures. To concentrate was to cause the vision to vanish. Weir Mitchell (39) remarked that from childhood he had been able to summon visions before falling asleep, but that once present they could not be controlled and would change and disappear of themselves. During the half-awake stage, subjects could cease to feel the bed and would experience the illusion of being unsupported, leading to dreams of falling or flying, especially common in children. In contrast to these not unpleasant dreams, hallucinosis in narcoleptics sometimes had a horrific quality, as in a patient who witnessed "flames licking the wall, skeletons, heads of dead bodies" (30).

AUTOMATIC BEHAVIOR

Another manifestation of narcolepsy recognized during this period was automatic behavior, likened in many ways to somnambulism or half-awakening. Maury (38) thought that this intermediate state between sleeping and waking, when consciousness itself was inert, was mainly due to too short a natural sleep or one interrupted by force and that it could be diminished by intellectual pursuits. As such, it was a normal state when the time for rest was insufficient. Half-awakening was particularly common in children belonging to the working class. De Manacéine (3) observed that 27 of 84 persons she saw with this condition came from Finland, which she explained by the fact that among the natives of Finland, it was nearly impossible to find a person of sanguine temperament.

Periods of automatic behavior are common in people with narcolepsy. This half-awake syndrome can cause great anxiety and even jeopardize life. Patients are unable to perceive the alteration in consciousness, and complete amnesia associated with automatic activity results in medical diagnoses ranging from temporal lobe epilepsy to hysteria. A common feature is a sudden burst of words sometimes without meaning and always without any relationship to what the patient might have just been saying. Loss of all sense of passage of time occurs, a feature also of sleep paralysis. Guilleminault et al. (40) gave the case history of a patient who left Reno alone at 10:00 a.m. en route to Tahoe, a 70-mile drive: "I remember perfectly what happened to Carson City (30 miles away). After that I had a complete blackout. I found myself at the reception desk of the hotel at Tahoe knocking on the desk and the receptionist asked me what he could do to help. I suddenly 'came back.' I could not remember why I was in that hotel, where I had parked my car and what had happened in the past 90 minutes." Such memory lapses occur in about half of all narcoleptic patients and may sometimes be responsible for the not infrequent automobile accidents that occur.

NATURE OF NARCOLEPSY

The auxiliary signs of narcolepsy were all recognized as occasionally occurring in normal subjects. The only distinction was one of frequency. Adie (23) considered that "patients so far overstep the arbitrary limits of the normal that we are justified in saying that they suffer from disease." However, by the time Adie and Kinear Wilson's papers appeared, it was apparent that most people with narcolepsy had no history or sign of endemic encephalitis or other brain disorder despite the later demonstration by Daniels (31) that many people with narcolepsy and also cataplexy attending the Mayo Clinic did have a history of encephalitis. Was narcolepsy a common symptom of many disorders and due to inhibition spreading throughout the cerebral hemispheres and to the subcortical centers? Against this view and despite occasional confusion with petit mal or chorea, narcolepsy was different from epilepsy, pyknolepsy, and hysteria and also certain conditions such as pituitary or other cerebral tumors. The main diagnostic difference from epilepsy was that the cataplectic attacks were brought on immediately by a recognizable exciting cause, namely, emotion, whereas attacks of epilepsy came on without any exciting cause. In ruling out hysteria, reliance was placed on the absence of undoubted hysterical manifestations and on the failure of every kind of suggestion to banish the attacks. The leader writer in the *Lancet* (Nov. 13, 1926) concluded that narcolepsy was a specific physiological disturbance arising from a disorder of the pituitary or related structures.

DIAGNOSTIC CRITERIA

The establishment of strict diagnostic criteria for narcolepsy was the achievement of Yoss and Daly (41). They demonstrated that the diagnosis of narcolepsy with the associated symptoms of cataplexy, sleep paralysis, and hypnagogic hallucinations was based on sound clinical criteria. At the Mayo Clinic between 1950 and 1954, 241 cases were seen. Of all the patients with narcolepsy, 68% had cataplexy, 24% had sleep paralysis, and 30% had hypnagogic hallucinations. These symptoms were combined in different ways, and only 11% of patients had the complete picture. Symptoms could develop at any age, although usually in the second and third decades. The onset of cataplexy could be delayed by many years and was not considered essential for the diagnosis of the narcoleptic syndrome. Other studies have shown a greater frequency of accessory symptoms, probably dependent on the perseverance with which they were sought. Once present, the condition persisted for life. The tendency to excessive sleep during the day was manifested in one of two ways. Most patients gave the classic story of almost irresistible episodes of actual sleep occurring from a few to many times each day. Others were drowsy much of the time and yet did not actually fall asleep. In contrast to the convulsive disorders, attacks of sleep were never paroxysmal.

Following Yoss and Daly and in the era up to 1960, the diagnosis of narcolepsy rested entirely on the history, although some aspects remained controversial, and separation of normal from abnormal behavior was not always easy. The achievement of the last quarter of a century has been to resolve a wealth of clinical detail. Largely in America and France, and assisted by physiological as well as clinical criteria, the nature of narcolepsy has been clarified and its genetic basis and frequency determined.

GENETIC BASIS

Impressive data have been collected showing that narcolepsy has a genetic basis. Westphal (12) described a man with narcolepsy and sleep paralysis whose mother had similar attacks. "A brick is said to have fallen on her head some time ago. Attacks occur when she is sitting quietly, when sewing, eating, when drinking coffee from her saucer, etc." Krabbe and Magnussen (42) described a family in which four of 12 sibs had a sleep disorder, and reviewing other reports, they found 54 narcoleptics belonging to 19 families with a single dominant mode of inheritance. However, the diagnosis of the narcoleptic syndrome was uncertain in some patients. Yoss and Daly (41), using more exact diagnostic criteria, found 30% of subjects with narcoleptic syndrome had an affected relative, Sours (43) 12%, Bruhova (44) 32%, and Kessler et al. (45) 52%.

Several interesting case reports have described families with only one symptom of the narcoleptic syndrome. Gelardi and Brown (46) described a family in which 15 members had cataplexy, three members sleep paralysis, and three members possible narcolepsy; Rushton (47) described a family with isolated sleep paralysis. Daly and Yoss (48) described a family in which 12 members with narcolepsy occurred in four generations, but only three of the subjects had cataplexy. Too few twins with narcolepsy have been reported to give a reliable estimate in monozygotic and dizygotic pairs; Imlah (49) described identical twins who both developed narcolepsy and cataplexy at the age of 13, but one pair of discordant monozygotic twins has also been reported (50). Although Yoss and Daly (51) suggested that narcolepsy was at one extreme of the normal distribution of vigilance and was polygenically determined, the pattern of inheritance suggests a single dominant gene in some families (52). There remains no certain method of identifying which, if any, of the children of parents with narcolepsy will develop the condition.

FREQUENCY

The frequency of narcolepsy in the general population is not known with certainty, and recent estimates of 100,000 narcoleptics in the United States and perhaps 20,000 in the United Kingdom are based on small samples. However, in view of the large case series described (41,53,54), there seems little doubt that narcolepsy is common and may occur at a rate of four cases per 10,000 with no gender dominance. Relatives of narcolepsy index cases have a 60-fold greater risk of having the disease than individuals in the general population (55).

REM NARCOLEPSY

Narcolepsy is a disease of REM sleep. REM sleep was discovered in 1953 by Aserinsky and Kleitman (56), and Vogel in 1960 showed that the night sleep of people with narcolepsy began with a period of REM sleep, unlike normal subjects (57). This finding of Vogel was confirmed by Rechtschaffen et al. (58) and by Takahashi and Jimbo (59). Many factors, including change in posture, change in setting, stimulant drug, or drug withdrawal, may alter the timing or occurrence of REM sleep, and initially the significance of this finding was controversial, although it proved of practical diagnostic significance. Over 90% of people with narcolepsy and cataplexy have sleep-onset REM periods on a single-nap recording (60), and if multiple or 24-hour recordings are done, this abnormality is present in practically all subjects. The appearance of REM sleep within 10 minutes of sleep onset can be considered as evidence for narcolepsy.

The discovery that people with narcolepsy and cataplexy have REM sleep at the onset of an attack and at the start of night sleep explained many features of the disease. Vivid dreams with loss of muscle tone and paralysis of movement are features of REM sleep as well as of narcolepsy and cataplexy. Since patients are not usually asleep during cataplectic attacks, the normal association between awareness and motor control is lost during cataplexy and also during sleep paralysis.

TWO KINDS OF NARCOLEPSY

Narcolepsy can occur with or without auxiliary symptoms. Some patients with narcolepsy alone have a typical history and often affected relatives; they usually have sleep-onset REM periods and may eventually develop cataplexy. In these subjects, narcolepsy is the single manifestation of the narcoleptic syndrome.

Other patients with essential hypersomnolence have recurrent daytime sleepiness but often do not have sleep attacks; these subjects may have frequent automatic behavior, prolonged and "sound" nocturnal sleep, often with difficulty in arousal or "sleep drunkenness," but they do not have sleep-onset REM periods (61). There is often a family history of hypersomnolence. This condition may not respond to CNS stimulants, which can aggravate associated symptoms of migraine, headache, nausea, and syncope, but may improve with methysergide, which is of no value in narcolepsy (55). The two kinds of narcolepsy, REM narcolepsy (the narcoleptic syndrome) and non-REM narcolepsy (essential hypersomnolence) appear to be separate disorders with different clinical as well as polygraphic features, a different biochemical basis, and different treatments.

SLEEP APNEA

The introduction of polygraphic studies allowed the identification of another disorder associated with daytime somnolence and previously often confused with narcolepsy. Hypersomnolence occurs in a high proportion of subjects with respiratory disorders due to either upper airway obstruction or a central cause. The classic example was described by Dickens in the *Posthumous Papers of the Pickwick Club*. Joe was a grotesquely fat boy who kept falling asleep. The Pickwickian syndrome is one of gross obesity with an enormous appetite, impaired respiration, perhaps owing to fat deposition, periodic respiration, cyanosis, secondary polycythemia, right ventricular hypertrophy, and sometimes right heart failure. Sleep is associated with a rise in threshold of response to carbon dioxide by the respiratory center, and these patients fall asleep for 10 to 12 second periods throughout the day. The EEG is usually normal, that of light sleep.

In patients with sleep apnea, respiration is highly irregular during sleep, with multiple and frequent pauses, and many hundred brief periods of apnea may occur each night with restlessness and loud snoring. This is accompanied by somnambulism, nocturnal enuresis, and difficulty in arousal, as well as by profound daytime sleepiness and frequent automatic behavior. The diagnosis is based on the history, but many EEG, cardiac, respiratory, and hemodynamic abnormalities occur during sleep. The condition must be distinguished from narcolepsy. It is apparently common, and with the help of polygraphic studies, Guilleminault et al. (60) found 44 patients with upper airway obstruction, apnea, and hypersomnolence in 235 patients with excessive daytime sleepiness. Many different obstructive and central disorders have been associated with sleep apnea, including acromegaly, myotonic dystrophy, and cerebral tumors. In some cases, no cause is apparent. Occasionally, sleep apnea may be accompanied by cardiac arrhythmias; hypertension is present in approximately 40% of the cases, and heart failure may be severe. The condition can be lethal (55).

The separation of REM narcolepsy from non-REM narcolepsy, the identification of sleep apnea, and the distinction among the different causes of daytime sleepiness have been major achievements of sleep laboratory studies. These achievements have been a powerful stimulus for the development of these studies with a recent dramatic increase in knowledge of different sleep disorders, particularly in the United States. However, there may recently have been an overemphasis on the need for patients to be evaluated in such clinics, which are expensive and time consuming and often contribute only minimally to patient management (62).

BIOCHEMISTRY OF NARCOLEPSY

It seems probable that the narcoleptic syndrome is due to an inborn error of metabolism, but the nature of this has not been demonstrated. There is no consistent abnormality in urinary catecholamine content, urinary estrogens, blood sugar levels, and cerebrospinal fluid concentration of the dopamine metabolite homovanilic acid, the serotonin metabolite 5-hydroxy indole acetic acid, and various amino acids (63). Blood gas alterations with mild hypoxia and hypercapnia (64) may at least partly result from sleep apnea.

TREATMENT OF NARCOLEPSY

The amphetamines belong to the general group of sympathomimetic drugs. Evidence for the use of these drugs can be found as early as 5,000 years ago, when in China the herb ma huang (*Ephedra vulgaris*) was used as a stimulant and for the treatment of respiratory diseases. Approximately 75 years ago, ephedrine was isolated from ma huang but was considered too toxic for clinical use. In attempting to make a synthetic substitute for ephedrine, Gordon Alles synthesized amphetamine in 1927 (65). The drug's stimulant action was first described by Alles, and Prinzmetal and Bloomberg (66) first used the drug to treat narcolepsy. Despite the widespread epidemic of amphetamine misuse in many countries, this drug and related compounds remain the most effective treatment for narcolepsy yet discovered. Methyl amphetamine, the *n*-methyl analogue of dextrorotary amphetamine, was synthesized long before amphetamine and is the most potent central stimulant drug known.

Many other drugs have been tried in narcolepsy although with limited success. Willis in 1685 used caffeine to increase alertness. The drugs *l*-amphetamine, methylphenidate, the monoamine oxidase inhibitor phenelzine, *l*-dopa, amantadine, carbamazepine, 5-hydroxy tryptophan, clonidine, ascorbic acid, thiamine, aspartic acid, and glutamate, the appetite suppressant drug Mazindol, and naturally occurring hypnotic gamma hydroxy butyrate have all been given in attempts to improve narcolepsy (67–69). However, amphetamines remain the treatment of choice for most narcoleptics, although they do not abolish cataplexy. The use of tricyclic drugs and, in particular, clomipramine has proved very effective in the treatment of both cataplexy and sleep paralysis. The antiepileptic drug clonazepam will also sometimes abolish cataplexy (70,71).

Descartes, Leibnitz, and Kant taught that we think and dream continually during sleep, although we frequently forget we have done so. "In sleep the mind is not engaged with thoughts but with molecular processes, and these processes are the great factor in the etiology of dreams" (72). Despite the philosophical speculation, the function of sleep and dreams remains unknown. There is still too little recognition that narcolepsy is a crippling disease, which may cause patients to sleep their lives away.

ACKNOWLEDGMENTS

I am indebted to the King's College Hospital and Medical School Research Committee for support of investigation of narcolepsy, to Dr. M. Schachter for helpful suggestions, and foremost, to Dr. P. Passouant, whose classic history of narcolepsy (13) is unrivaled.

REFERENCES

1. Zarcone, V. (1973): *N. Engl. J. Med.*, 288:1136.
2. Forbes, C. (1894): *Lancet*, 1:1185.
3. De Manacéine, M., (1894): *Sleep: Its Physiology, Pathology, Hygiene and Psychology*, p. 96. Walter Scott, London.
4. Caffé (1862): *J. Connaiss. Méd. Pharmaceut.*, 29:323.
5. Oliver, W. (1704): *Phil. Trans., London*, 24(304):2177.
6. Gimson, W. G. (1863): *Br. Med. J.*, 1:616.
7. Fröderström, M. (1912): *Nouv. Icon. de la Salpêtr.*, 25:267.
8. Graves, R. J. (1851): *Dubl. J. Med. Sci.*, 11:1.
9. Gélineau, J. (1880): *Gaz. Hôpitaux*, 53:626.
10. Gélineau, J. (1880): *Gaz. Hôpitaux*, 54:635.
11. Henneberg, R. (1916): *Neurol. Zbl.*, 30:282.
12. Westphal, C. (1877): *Arch. Psychiat. Nervenkr.*, 7:631.
13. Passouant, P. (1976): In: *Narcolepsy*, edited by C. Guilleminault, W. C. Dement, and P. Passouant, p. 3. Spectrum Publications, New York.
14. Gowers, W. (1907): *The Borderland of Epilepsy*, p. 93. Churchill, London.
15. Schlager, E., and Meier, T. (1947): *Acta Trop. (Basel)*, 4:127.
16. Tridon, P., Montaut, J., and Picard, L. (1969): *Rev. Neurol.*, 121:186.
17. Lössner, J., and Zeit, W. (1967): *Psychiat. Neurol. Med. Psychol. (Lpz.)*, 19:381.
18. Berg, O., and Hanley, J. (1963): *Acta. Neurol. Scand.*, 39:252.
19. Gayet, M. (1875): *Arch Physiol.*, 7:341.
20. Von Economo, C., and Grippe, C. (1919): *Wien. Klin. Wochenschr. (suppl.)*, 32:393.
21. Lhermitte, J., and Tournay, A. (1927): *Rev. Neurol.*, 1:751.
22. Symonds, C. P. (1926): *Lancet*, ii:1214.
23. Adie, W. J. (1926): *Brain*, 49:257.
24. Wilson, S. A. K. (1928): *Brain*, 51:63.
25. Cave, M. (1931): *Arch. Neurol. Psychiat.*, 26:50.
26. Redlich, E. (1931): *Z. ges. Neurol. Psychiat.*, 136:129.
27. Levin, M. (1933): *J. Neurol. Psychopathol.*, 14:1.
28. Redlich, E. (1915): *Monatschr. Psychiat. Neurol.*, 37:85.
29. Weir Mitchell, S. (1897): *Clinical Lessons on Nervous Diseases*, p. 58, Lea Brothers, Philadelphia.
30. Lhermitte, J. (1930): *Progrès. Med.*, 962.
31. Daniels, L. (1934): *Medicine*, 13:1.
32. Lombard, W. P. (1887): *Am. J. Psychol.*, 1:1.
33. Rosenbach, O. (1881): *Z. Klin. Med.*, 2:17.
34. Levy, G. (1922): Contributions à l'etude des manifestations tardives de l'encéphalite épidémique. Thèse, Vigot Freres, Paris.
35. Leroy, E. (1933): *Les Visions du Demi-sommeil*. Alcan, Paris.
36. Lhermitte, J. (1922): *Rev. Neurol.*, 1:1369.
37. Alajouanine, T., and Baruk, H. (1926): *Progrès. Med.*, 639.
38. Maury, (1848): *Ann. Médico-psychol.*, 11:27.
39. Weir Mitchell, S. (1896): *Br. Med. J.*, 2:1625.
40. Guilleminault, C., Billiard, M., Montplaisir, J., and Dement, W. C. (1975): *J. Neurol. Sci.*, 26:377.
41. Yoss, R. E., Daly, D. D. (1957): *Proc. Mayo Clin.*, 32:320.
42. Krabbe, F., and Magnussen, G. (1942): *Acta Psychiat. Neurol.*, 17:149.
43. Sours, J. (1963): *J. Nerv. Ment. Dis.*, 137:525.
44. Bruhova, S. (1973): *Acta Univ. Carol. Med. (Praha)*, 18:109.
45. Kessler, S., Guilleminault, C., and Dement, W. C. (1974): *Acta Neurol. Scand.*, 50:503.
46. Gelardi, J. A. M., and Brown, J. W. (1967): *J. Neurol. Neurosurg. Psychiat.*, 30:455.
47. Rushton, J. G. (1944): *Med. Clin. N. Am.*, 28:945.
48. Daly, D. D., and Yoss, R. E. (1959): *Proc. Mayo Clin.*, 34:313.
49. Imlah, N. W. (1961): *J. Neurol. Neurosurg, Psychiat.*, 24:158.
50. Mitchell, S., and Cummins, L. (1965): See ref. 52.
51. Yoss, R. E., Daly, D. D. (1960): *Trans. Am. Neurol. Assoc.*, 85:239.
52. Baraitser, M., and Parkes, J. D. (1978): *J. Med. Genet.*, 15:254.
53. Guilleminault, C., Carskadon, M., and Dement, W. C. (1974): *Arch. Neurol.*, 30:90.
54. Parkes, J. D., Baraitser, M., Marsden, C. D., and Asselman, P. (1975): *Acta Neurol. Scand.*, 52:337.
55. (1979): *Sleep, Vol. 2*. Association of Sleep Disorders Centers. Diagnostic Classification of Sleep and Arousal Disorders, 1st ed., pp. 1–137.
56. Aserinski, E., and Kleitman, N. (1953): *Science*, 118:273.
57. Vogel, G. (1960): *Arch. Gen. Psychiat.*, 3:421.

58. Rechtschaffen, A., Wolpert, W., Dement, W., Mitchell, S., and Fischer, C. (1963): *Electroenceph. Clin. Neurophysiol.*, 15:599.
59. Takahashi, Y., and Jimbo, M. (1963): *Folia Psychiat. Neurol. Jpn. (suppl.)*, 7:343.
60. Guilleminault, C., and Dement, W. C. (1977): *J. Neurol. Sci.*, 31:13.
61. Passouant, P., Popovichiu, L., Velok, G., and Baldy-Moulinier, M. (1968): *Rev. Neurol.*, 113:43.
62. Soldatos, C. R., Kales, A., and Kales, J. D. (1979): In: *Annual Review of Medicine*, edited by W. P. Creger, C. H. Coggins and E. W. Hancock, Vol. 30, p. 301. Annual Reviews, Palo Alto, Calif.
63. Parkes, J. D., Fenton, G., Struthers, G., Curzon, G., Kantamaneni, B. D., Buxton, B. H., and Record, C. (1974): *Quart. J. Med.*, 43:525.
64. Birchfield, R. L., Sieker, H. O., Heyman, A. (1958): *Neurology (Minneapolis)*, 8:107.
65. Kornetsky, C. (1969): *Sem. Psychiat.*, 1:227.
66. Prinzmetal, M., and Bloomberg, W. (1935): *J. Am. Med. Assoc.*, 105:2051.
67. Parkes, J. D. In: *Narcolepsy*, edited by C. Guilleminault, W. C. Dement. and P. Passouant, p. 643. Spectrum Publications, New York.
68. Parkes, J. D., and Schachter, M. (1979): *Acta Neurol. Scand.*, 60:250.
69. Broughton, R., and Mamelak, M. (1979): *Canad. J. Neurol. Sci.*, 6:1.
70. Hishikawa, Y. Ida, H., Nakai, K., and Kaneko, Z. (1966): *J. Neurol. Sci.*, 3:453.
71. Parkes, J. D., and Schachter, M. (1979): *Lancet* ii:1085.
72. Cane, F. E. (1889): *Lancet* ii:1331.

Historical Aspects of the Neurosciences,
edited by F. Clifford Rose and W. F. Bynum.
Raven Press, New York ©

Elizabeth Garrett Anderson and Migraine

Marcia Wilkinson

Regional Neurological Unit, Eastern Hospital (St. Bartholomew's Teaching Group), The City and East London Area Health Authority, London E9 6BY, U.K.

Elizabeth, the second daughter of Newsom and Louisa Garrett, was born in London in 1836. When she was 4 years old, her parents moved to Aldeburgh in Suffolk, a place with which she was closely associated for the rest of her life. Louisa and her sister Elizabeth were first taught by a governess but were later sent to a boarding school at Blackheath run by the Misses Browning, aunts of the celebrated poet Robert Browning. At fifteen Elizabeth's education was supposed to be over, but that year she worked at home on Latin and mathematics with the tutors who came to coach her brothers. She decided to become a doctor after hearing a lecture by Dr. Elizabeth Blackwell, who had taken her degree in America. She was encouraged in this decision by Emily Davies, the daughter of the Rector of Gateshead, who was afterwards the Principal of Girton College, Cambridge. Elizabeth found endless difficulties put in her way. She went to the Middlesex Hospital, where she stayed for about a year, acting partly as a nurse but spending the greater part of her time in medical studies. At the end of the year, she applied for admission into the school of the Middlesex Hospital after having tried the Westminster, London, St. Mary's, etc., all of which had refused her. She also applied to the College of Physicians, the College of Surgeons, and to the Society of Apothecaries, but again she was refused. She was advised that the Society of Apothecaries could not legally refuse, so she applied again, saying that she would ask for a "mandamus." The Society consulted their counsel Sir James Hannen who confirmed this, and she was told that the Apothecaries Society would make no objection to her receiving private tuition from the recognized teachers in the school provided that she did not attend the classes with the other students.

She followed this plan and found some lecturers willing to teach her. She went to Scotland and asked the College of Physicians and the Medical Schools for admission as a student and the right to graduate, but again she was disappointed and later she tried at St. Andrew's with the same result. She continued to work on her own for another six months and later managed to spend four months in the Maternity Hospital in Edinburgh. On her return to London, she went to the London Hospital in Whitechapel, where she studied anatomy, although nominally attending as a nurse.

By these various means, she completed the course and made up the regular number of lectures, and in October 1865, she received the L.S.A. diploma and began to practice in Upper Berkeley Street. From the outset Elizabeth Garrett Anderson's aim was to provide a hospital for women staffed by women. In July 1866, she opened St. Mary's Dispensary in Seymour Place, Marylebone; from the first it was a great success and within a few weeks, approximately 60 to 90 women and children were attending each session. As well as running the dispensary, she also visited patients in their own homes and took charge of midwifery cases in the district. As the work increased, the need for in-patient treatment became overwhelming, and in 1872 a ward of 10 beds was opened by Lord Shaftesbury and St. Mary's Dispensary became the New Hospital for Women. These premises were rapidly outgrown, and three houses in the Marylebone Road were bought, which when converted provided 26 beds. The hospital remained there until 1899, when it moved to its present site in Euston Road.

Elizabeth Garrett Anderson was at first the only one able to undertake any major operations. The position of women in medicine had become even more difficult when in 1866 the Society of Apothecaries amended its regulations to prevent the admission of women. It was not until 1878 that they were admitted by the University of London and 1882 that the first two women graduated.

Because of the regulations in England at this time, Elizabeth Garrett Anderson also had difficulty in getting her Doctor's degree. She was determined to have one, as she wished to be as well qualified as any of her male colleagues. She found that the only way she could get a degree was by taking it in France at the Sorbonne, and thus she submitted her thesis on "Migraine" on June 15, 1870 and later defended it satisfactorily.

Elizabeth Garrett Anderson considered that "migraine was essentially a disturbance of the central nervous system and that there was an associated weakness or disorder in some part of the neurovisceral system, most frequently that of the gastro-intestinal tract. The two lesions the one cerebral the other peripheral reacted one upon the other, neither of the two being invariably the main cause of the attack."

Elizabeth Garrett Anderson was a very good clinical observer and obviously had treated successfully a large number of patients with migraine and other types of headache. She says that migraine is a malady that can be defined as "an acute pain in the head which makes itself felt from time to time, which lasts from 3/4-hour to twelve hours, and sometimes, though more rarely, from 24 to 36 or even 72 hours. There is no fever but it is nearly always accompanied by dizziness, nausea, and vomiting. The pain is usually unilateral with frontal intensity in the region of the eye and temple on the affected side. The intellectual faculties remained perfectly normal during the attack." She was obviously intrigued by the dual nature of the symptoms and goes on to say that neither simple neuralgia nor ordinary gastric disorder, but a combination of both, occurs in migraine, and she wonders why two groups of symptoms, one springing from the brain and one from the stomach should occur in the same disorder. She goes on to speculate on their relationship: "which is the cause and which the effect? Are they rather the result of a more obscure cause? Formerly one would have said the stomach produces the illness, the digestion is upset and the brain suffers in sympathy. But it is necessary to determine first the true sense of the words. What does one mean by the brain suffering in sympathy? What is meant by sympathy in pathological terms and why should it be the brain and not the stomach which is attacked by sympathy? It is essential in order to understand the points raised by these questions to examine more closely the symptoms and history of the attack which we are proposing to analyse."

She then goes on to describe some of the clinical features and epidemiology and says that, in the first place, migraine is nearly always hereditary, and she notes that "the first attacks are usually felt before the age of twenty years, sometimes even before seven or eight, but more often between thirteen and eighteen. The attacks become more and more frequent, increasing in intensity up to fifty or fifty-five years of age, then decreasing, and after the seventieth year becoming quite rare. The gastric symptoms are most marked at the height of the attack, but they occur rarely and with less severity at the beginning and the end of an attack. The attacks vary in the same individual but usually, except in those caused by exceptional excitement, the patient enjoys a fairly constant period of immunity." She goes on to quote examples where there has been a remarkably regular occurrence, and one of the cases she sites is that of Tissot, who had a patient who was a monk who for three years and seven months had a migraine attack each Monday. It was thought that these attacks were probably caused by an excess of fatigue, Sunday being a day of painful and spiritual toil for the patient in question. When this fatigue ended, the periodicity also disappeared.

Her remarks on the association of migraine with the menstrual period are also interesting. She says that "Amongst women migraines often recur during the menstrual period but this periodicity probably also depends on the regular return of the same causes of excitement. True periodicity seems to be very rare since in the majority of cases there is not an absolute respite." She then goes on to consider the early symptoms and says that "these symptoms vary considerably from case to case. They are an abnormal appetite, pyrosis or vomiting of an acid liquid, sensory deafness or a buzzing in the ears, a pronounced aversion both for certain foods and for tobacco, extreme depression, lowering of mental faculties, disturbed sleep, troubled dreams, irritability, poor vision and numbness of the hand, arm or leg usually on the affected side. Of these warning symptoms many recur in the majority of chronic migraine sufferers. The prodromes are rarely felt more than 24 hours before an attack, usually considerably less. Several patients have told me that they have experienced a sudden awakening and extreme lassitude, and it seems possible to assert that this, as well as a marked change in the appetite, are the most frequent warning symptoms. The headache usually begins during sleep, but this rule has numerous exceptions.

"The pain is almost always felt on one side only, more often on the left than the right; it changes places, but sometimes it is localised. At other times it is more general and it does not reach its maximum intensity all of a sudden, but during an hour or more it will get worse and will reach the climax over a period of several hours. When the attack begins the patient becomes chilly, pale, and the pulse rate slows and often he will experience slight shivering. In certain cases the temperature rises. When the pain reaches its climax there is an almost feverish reaction; the face flushes, the conjunctiva become congested, the carotid pulse faint, but in most cases the temperature falls before vomiting begins. During the attack all effort is intolerable, the patient, who dreads noise, light or the slightest movement, is tormented by the vibration of a pendulum. During this crisis flashing lights are seen and there is humming in the ears. The muscles of the affected side contract spasmodically. The patient cannot open his mouth or speak without pain and all attempts to take nourishment or medicine aggravate his sufferings. In this state violent nausea is experienced followed by vomiting. When the attack comes after several hours of sleep the stomach is empty and the vomit contains only gastric mucus which mixes with bile introduced into the stomach after the diaphragmatic contractions. In the majority of cases vomiting is followed by some easing of the headache. This will occur even though the vomited material contains nothing but mucus, so that the act of vomiting must be considered as important as the evacuation of the stomach. After several hours of suffering the pain gradually subsides and during this time the patient often drops off to sleep and after several hours wakes up perfectly recovered."

The emphasis Elizabeth Garrett Anderson puts on the value of sleep is interesting because it is only relatively recently that sleep has become a well-recognized part of the treatment of a migraine attack. In fact, the use of caffeine in so many of the preparations of ergotamine now on the market have on the whole militated against sleep.

TREATMENT

Elizabeth Garrett Anderson also had very definite ideas on the way a migraine attack should be treated. She starts by saying that the curing of migraine is seldom more than partial and that in her experience, where there is a family history, the attacks will tend to occur. "The external influences (including medical treatment) being incapable of altering to any great degree the visible resemblance of children to their parents or altering, for example, the shape of the hands, the development of bony tissue, the colour of the hair. It is not going to be easy to alter the visible origin of the attack. That is not to say that recourse cannot be had to medical science in the presence of inherited nervous tendencies. Faced with nervous temperaments science has a double duty—to maintain the original nervous nutrition and to remove, as far as possible, any condition or inference tending to provoke a weakness of this function.

"In the treatment of migraine one should have recourse to remedies directed more against the alterations in the nervous system rather than those of the digestive system. Unhappily it is very difficult to find remedies which can act directly and in a constant manner on the morbid condition of the action or the nervous nutrition. It is a fact that patients are in the habit of turning all their attention to the upsets of the digestive system which so often gives them their migraine.

"It is nevertheless very important in theory and in practice, not to lose sight of a nervous element even when the initial remedies employed aim at the secondary or exciting causes. It is necessary to prevent the attacks or at least to dispel the previous predisposition and for this one should not neglect the warning signs. Habit probably has a powerful influence in maintaining a state of sickness rather than of health. Each nervous attack increases the predisposition to future attacks and creates a new difficulty in changing the abnormal molecular conditions of the nervous system. It is necessary to remove all the causes which experience has shown to be likely to bring on an attack. In cases where the attacks appear to depend on abnormal condition of the digestive system, these conditions should immediately be dispersed.

"The upset of the digestive system which so often accompanies migraine and even seems to produce it, can be combated in several different ways. The following treatment is that which I have followed with great success. As a general rule alcoholic stimulants of all kinds should be forbidden, the patient taking nothing but a half-glass of cold water with each meal. An exception to this rule can be made if the patient loses his appetite, then a glass of red wine may be permitted twice a day. Food should be simple, nourishing and varied. Meat should be eaten twice during the twenty-four hours, but not in a large quantity and never reheated. The two main meals should each consist of only two courses, toast or biscuits being preferred to ordinary bread. There should not be a very long interval, say more than four hours, between breakfast, which should preferably be light, and lunch which should be a proper meal like supper, but neither one nor the other should completely satisfy the appetite. An interval of five hours or more should separate lunch and supper, and it is good to have a small cup of tea towards four or five o'clock in the afternoon. If the patient's work obliges him to lead a sedentary life, one would recommend ten minutes of lively exercise before lunch and supper . . ."

She goes on to say that in the majority of cases, if these prescriptions are followed, the attacks of migraine will be considerably diminished and then goes on to extol the virtues of fresh air and exercise. She considers that such agents are capable of combating the morbid conditions that predispose to migraine. She then goes on to expand this idea and says that "the tonic influence of fresh air on the nervous system is just as important as that of exercise. It is this influence to which poor agricultural workers probably owe their comparative immunity and strong nerves. Despite their often inadequate diet and hard life, and constant exposure to the vagaries of the weather, cases of epilepsy, hysteria, spasmodic asthma and migraine are very rare in the country, as compared with those met with among workers in the town. It is difficult to attribute to fresh air much effect as a cure against neuroses in a country such as England, where for nine or ten months the temperature is too low to be healthy or agreeable."

She then recommends "a prolonged stay in a climate warm enough to allow the patients to spend eight or ten hours a day in the open air. Failing this particular attention must be paid to ventilation. The amount of air ordinarily entering the best-aired houses (except in summer) is far from sufficient for general health, and above all for nervous or tuberculous people. Unhappily the low temperature of the English climate makes suitable ventilation almost impossible, at least without artificial methods. The discovery and popularisation of a procedure which would allow an abundant quantity of warm fresh air to enter bedrooms and other apartments when it was too cold outside for the windows to be widely opened, would be the best remedy for neuroses and the best preventative against nervous illnesses and tuberculosis."

After she has mentioned natural means, such as air and exercise, she discusses treatment with electric current, and the next part of her thesis is devoted to a description of such treatment. Her aims and treatment of migraine were largely preventative because she says "one should scarcely ever have recourse to treatment during the duration of an attack. The urging of friends to take nourishment, stimulants or remedies can only increase the suffering. Generally there is nothing for the patient but air, quiet, solitude, and a darkened room. All noises torture, even the noise of footsteps or the ticking of a watch." She does, however, suggest that static positive electricity might be used. For the vomiting, she recommends a large quantity of very hot tea, both as an emetic and purgative, and for the sedative action of the heat on the gastric and duodenal nerves. The only medicaments she mentioned are bicarbonate of soda or aromatic spirits of ammonia in half a glass of very hot tea.

The interest in migraine at the Elizabeth Garrett Anderson Hospital continues, and there has been a migraine clinic there since 1958; it was there that Edda Hanington did her original work on tyramine and the use of clonidine in migraine. I think that Elizabeth Garrett Anderson would be pleased to know that her interest in migraine continues at her hospital.

BIBLIOGRAPHY

1. Anderson, Elizabeth Garrett (1870): *Sur la Migraine*. Theses, École de Medecine de Paris.
2. Anderson, Louisa Garrett (1939): *Elizabeth Garrett Anderson, 1836–1917*. Faber, London.
3. Manton, J. (1965): *Elizabeth Garrett Anderson*. Methuen, London.

Historical Aspects of the Neurosciences,
edited by F. Clifford Rose and W. F. Bynum.
Raven Press, New York ©

The Development of Concepts Concerning Cerebral Circulation

Marek Gawel

Department of Neurology, Charing Cross Hospital, London W6, England

THE CIRCULATION OF THE BLOOD

Without an understanding of the development of ideas concerning the systemic circulation of the blood, it would be impossible to understand the significance of the anastomotic circle that supplies the brain. The fact that blood vessels are pulsatile has been known since antiquity (1), but it was Herophilus who first made use of a water clock to measure the pulse rate. He studied the rhythm for several minutes at a time and, if it was not regular, he tried to match it to the beat of the playing of a harp or flute provided by slave women. He also differentiated between arteries and veins (ca. 280 B.C.) and observed the heart and blood vessels leading from it.

The fact that the cardiac valves are unidirectional was known before Hippocrates, and these valves are further described by Erasistratus (ca. 260 B.C.),who dissected the blood vessels and followed their courses into various organs. Erastistratus believed that air reached the nervous system through the blood vessels of the brain, there to be transformed into a different kind of pneuma, which was called animal pneuma. He thought that three different kinds of substances made their way outward from the center: blood by way of the veins, life pneuma by way of the arteries, and soul pneuma by way of the nerves. He was faced with a conceptual problem, in that after death there was only a small amount of blood in the arteries besides air, while in a living person, blood gushes out in profusion. He explained this by deciding that the blood permeated the limbs and organs through the veins into the arteries at invisible small spots, and he said that the veins and arteries terminated in minute pores opening opposite each other, which were normally closed. Following fever, eating and drinking too much, or other activities leading to an excess of blood, these mouthlike endings, anastomoses, would open, and blood could flow from the veins into the empty arteries.

Galen (129–ca. 200 A.D.) severed an artery and found that blood poured from it, gushing out rhythmically with every pulse beat, and there was no time for the anastomoses postulated by Erasistratus to open. This suggested that the blood was already in the arteries. Ligaturing an artery in fact abolished the pulse beat, and loosening the ligature caused resumption of the pulse beats, and therefore these beats had to originate from the heart. He isolated an artery, tied it at two points, and found that blood in the arteries was present all the time and that it was pushed into them by the left ventricle. Unfortunately, he chose a very complex explanation, which necessitated a link between the right and the left ventricles, air via pores entering the left ventricle from the lungs, and blood flowing into it from the right ventricle. There the matter rested despite the work of Ibn au-Nafis, who decided after experimentation that the descriptions of Galen were made after faulty observation.

Leonardo da Vinci made many observations on blood vessels and noticed that in old age their straight course became increasingly twisted and bent and the arteries became thicker. The question arises, he said, why the vessels should become winding where they were straight before, and why their walls should thicken to such an extent as to hinder or prevent the flow of blood, and if, without any actual disease, this might itself be the cause of death of old people. He was also interested in the brain's structure and made a wax model of the ventricular cavities by filling them with molten wax and removing the brain itself after the wax had set. He made a model of the heart out of glass, thus making possible the direct observation of the flowing process starting out of the heart. He stuck small membranes in place of the valves in his model and was able to study the swirls produced within the aorta and the closing of the semilunar valves. He could not explain the seeming paradoxes of Galen's theories but commented that these things were very hard to explain.

In 1537, Andreas Vesalius passed his final examinations and the following day gave his first lecture as a professor. He rediscovered what had been described by Ibn au-Nafis, namely, that the small holes in the septa dividing the two ventricles could not be seen. Similar statements were made by Servetus, who went on to say that, in a pulmonary blood vessel, blood does not flow in every direction but in one only.

Like many discoveries in science, the concept of the circulation of the blood dawned on several of Harvey's contemporaries and predecessors, but he was the first to formulate it. Many of Harvey's ideas came from the original work by Fabricius, who studied the valves in the opened-up veins of the leg. At that time in Padua, there was much discussion about the movement of the blood and the role of the valves. Following Harvey's discovery that blood did in fact circulate, it becomes easy to see how functional significance could be ascribed to anatomical descriptions of such structures as the circle named after Willis.

THE ANATOMY OF THE CEREBRAL BLOOD SUPPLY

Wepfer

In 1658 Wepfer (4) published *De Apoplexia*. Wepfer had been appointed Physician to the city of Schafhausen and had conferred upon him the privilege of performing postmortem examinations. He was a dedicated scientist and, among other things, he studied the pathological results of toxic agents on animals and demonstrated that the heart devoid of blood could be kept in motion for some moments after death by the action of certain substances. Although *De Apoplexia* was published at Schafhausen in 1658, reprinted there in 1675, and in Amsterdam in 1681, 1710, and 1724, it is curious that the observations in this volume seem to have been little noticed in England. They are not mentioned in the controversies that arose concerning the stroke, which was the beginning of the fatal illness of Charles II, nor does Willis (23) allude to them in *De Cerebri Anatome* (1664).

Wepfer writes: "I shall give here the histories of four cases of apoplexy to which I have added a dissertation concerning the place affected in this disease. Incidentally, I set forth the proximate causes of the same, and to the best of my ability have accommodated all to the laws of the circular motion of the blood." The ages of his patients were 45, 70, 60, and

50 years, and in each of them a cerebral hemorrhage was found. A great part of Wepfer's dissertation is directed against John Riolan. Riolan taught, like Galen, that in man the internal carotid arteries, having entered the skull, immediately divided outside the dura into a number of small communicating branches and formed thereby the so-called rete mirabile. From these, the vital spirits instilled into the ventricles of the brain, where they were transformed into animal spirits, whence they were carried by the nerves to various parts of the body.

What Wepfer really says then is that if you look carefully and dissect out the branches of the carotid artery instead of the supposed rete, you find that each internal carotid artery proceeds intact and undivided along the sides of the sphenoid bone and pituitary gland and that it perforates the dura mater intact. It then divides into several branches that penetrate different parts of the brain; not a drop of blood from it reaches the dura mater. He investigated the course of the artery in two ways. First, having incised the dura and divided the artery, he introduced the stylus into it at a point where he perforated the dura mater and followed the artery from the pituitary gland to its canal in the bone. In other cases, he followed the carotid artery to the styloid process and observed that there it bent and, having entered the canal in the petrous bone, it proceeded obliquely forward. Having emerged from the canal, the artery ascended and turned a little posteriorly. Then, bending again, it descended by the pituitary gland, once more ascending and having been covered by, and held in, a deep and conspicuous sinus beneath the anterior apophysis of the hippocampus. It then turned upward and perforated the dura mater near the infundibulum. Throughout this whole course, it remained intact.

Thus, by careful observation, Wepfer flatly disproved Riolan's ideas, which were that from the rete mirabile innumerable branches were given off, coursing through the dura mater and serving as channels to convey the blood upward to the meningeal sinuses. Wepfer ends by stating: "Therefore, I, together with all those who favour the circulation of the blood even in the brain, declare to Riolan that the arteries of the dura mater everywhere poured their own blood into its venous sinuses, accordingly what will he have left over for the ventricles and how will he prove that they are the true store-houses of the animal spirits, for all the blood carried to this sinus naturally proceeds to the heart through the jugular veins and not a drop of blood distils from them from the brain or to the ventricles and moreover, if this should occur it would result in the gravest injury to the individual." Wepfer was constrained to postulate circulation of the blood in the brain as well as in other parts of the body.

Wepfer described the method of opening the cranium and removing the brain and its vessels; he also described the vessels of the dura mater of the vertebral arteries and of the internal carotid arteries with their branches, and in this connection he describes accurately the arterial circular anastomoses that afterward came to bear the name of Willis. However, he did not in fact recognize this as being a complete anastomosis in each case and to this point we shall return.

Wepfer also tried to explain the purpose of the ventricles, denying that they were the site of animal spirits but stating rather that they were receptacles of excrementous products from the brain, and from this he stated that, since the brain is of large size, it stands in need of much nourishment, and there will be a copious amount of excrement, which can be contained only in ventricles like those of the brain. Otherwise, a man would have to expectorate constantly.

Concerning apoplexy, Wepfer was more scientific; he stated that apoplexy was produced in the first place either because the influx of the blood through the arteries is denied to the brain or because the influx of animal spirits in the cerebrum and cerebellum to the nerves and spinal cord is hindered or in certain cases prevented completely. He said that the privation of blood must resolve in a loss of power of action. Not only is there loss of motion, but the mind is also disturbed, which occurs for the reason that some part of the brain is deprived of its blood. Anything, therefore, that prevented the influx of blood to the brain through the carotid or vertebral arteries and its return to the jugular veins was capable of producing apoplexy. This influx of blood may be hindered by obstruction of the internal carotid or vertebral arteries by compression of these arteries or by blood extravasated within the brain. He probably described atheroma, talking about certain small fibrous bodies found in the carotid and vertebral arteries as well as in the heart, and he noted that the people most liable to develop these are those who lead an idle life, those who are obese, and those whose hands and face are livid and whose pulse is constantly unequal. A second cause of obstruction could be found in the composition of the blood, stating that in certain circumstances, blood could be so mixed with viscid phlegm that its constant propulsion through the small arteries would produce obstruction and consequently apoplexy.

Apoplexy caused by intracerebral hemorrhage is another entity. Wepfer observed blood extravasated within the cranium and when it was copious in amount lying in the deeper parts above the base of the brain, he maintained that the hemorrhages deposited their blood not only in the substance of the brain, but also in the cavities of the ventricles, so that it was easy to understand how so great an outpouring of blood could cause apoplexy. He also thought that there was some link between apoplexy and circulation of CSF or serum, stating that if it was found in too great an amount, it would block off the pores that led through the animal spirits and hence destroy them. He suggested that several factors would predispose the brain to a sensitivity to this effect of the serum, and he mentioned narcotics, especially opium, cannabis, and wine. He observed that daily indiscretions in drinking predisposed to apoplexy. Thus, Wepfer made enormous advances in the understanding of cerebral circulation as well as in the causes of cerebrovascular disease, and indeed it may be said that very little real advance was made for many hundreds of years.

Willis

There is some controversy as to who in fact described the so-called circle of Willis. Thomas Willis, who illustrated the circle in his book *De Cerebri Anatome* in 1664, was not the first to describe it, and many continental authors hold that Wepfer was first. While Wepfer clearly knew in detail the anastomoses that made up the circle, he gave no illustration of the arterial circle but referred to an illustration in *Sintagma Anatomicum* of J. Vesling (22), saying that "He does not explain in full everything which has been said and still remains to be said in . . . dealing with these arteries. . . ." Vesling himself in 1647 published an illustration of the arterial circle, but a substantial union of the anterior branches of the carotid artery is missing, though small vessels seem to be running between the two arteries in the depth, nor in the explanatory text is there any mention of a junction of these arteries. The posterior communicating arteries appear as a direct continuation of the basal artery after its redivision without any indication of the existence of the posterior cerebral artery. Fallopius also described the union and the later division of the vertebral artery and the union of the anterior rami of the carotid arteries, corresponding to the anterior cerebral arteries. He described about two-thirds of the posterior communicating artery, stating that it only had an indirect connection with the external branch of the carotid (which corresponds to our middle cerebral artery).

Before this date, the concepts of the arteries and veins of the brain blur into an ill-defined mirage, the rete mirabile described as a strongly interwoven tissue with fine arteries miraculously duplicated, multiplicated, and alternatively interwoven with branches of the ascending arteria apoplectica. In this rete or its veins were contained the vital spirits which ascended from the heart to the brain in order to become animal spirits. For this reason, the rete was composed of the smallest and most subtle veins or arteries, so the spirit contained in them may be easily changed by the brain and be converted into the form of the animal spirit, although it would acquire greater perfection than the cerebral ventricles, like the blood in the ventricles of the heart. In this context, it must be said that Riolan, who in fact defended the existence of the rete mirabile in man, described four arteries ascending and entering the brain and said that the junctions of these four arteries form that plexus which is indeed mirabilus or reticularis.

On this basis, especially on the contributions of Fallopius, Thomas Willis, assisted by Richard Lower and Christopher Wren, gave the first indisputably complete illustration of the circle in both man and sheep in his *De Cerebri Anatome*. Posterior cerebral arteries in both figures are missing, but the total presentation of the vessels of the base of the brain and the relationship between blood vessels and cranial nerves is the most accurate that had ever been presented, and Willis' main contribution is the physiological significance of this. He said that "there is another reason far greater than this of these manifolding graftings of the vessels to which there may be a manifold way for the blood to go into diverse regions of the brain that if by chance one or two should be stopped there might easily be found another passage instead of them, as for example, the carotids of one side being obstructed, the vessels of the other side might provide for either province so that if both carotids should be stopped, the offices of each might be supplied through the vertebrals." He described later a patient who used to have frequent headaches on the left side and at postmortem an old thrombosis of the right carotid artery was found. Willis makes the point that it was remarkable that this man had not died of a stroke but had been protected from it by the action of the other arteries contributing blood to the brain. It is puzzling that Willis did not quote Wepfer, but it is equally interesting that Willis' immediate successors in the field did not quote him either nor indeed anybody else as the discoverer of the arterial circle, although most of them made some comment on *De Cerebri Anatome* (16).

In 1774, Bonheller speaks of the "circulum qui dictur Willise." Even in current research, a similar and simultaneous discovery is common. It is therefore not surprising that there have been many contenders for the title of discoverer of the anastomotic circles; however, like many of these things, the process was a gradual one of increase in awareness, but Willis should certainly have the credit of first recognizing the physiological significance of his circle.

AFTER WILLIS: PHYSIOLOGY AND ANATOMY

Following the discoveries of Willis, extensive anatomical work was done, but most of it served to define the smaller branches of both internal and external carotid arteries and the anastomoses between them. Similarly, much comparative anatomical work was done which showed that the extent to which animals are protected by the anastomotic circle and other anastomoses is very different between species. I shall not dwell on the nature of the so-called blood-brain barrier, e.g., Del rio Hortega describing oligodendrocytes alongside blood vessels. The other advance in the anatomy of the cerebral circulation is the relationship of the autonomic nervous system to the extra- and intracerebral arteries. McNaughton (18) in

1938 reviewed the origin of these nerves, and the diagram he used to summarize the known connections, together with the question marks which he employed, can be reproduced today without much modification. Huber in 1899 and again Clerk in 1929 stated that the source of sympathetic vasoconstrictive fibers is the plexus of nerves on the vertebral and carotid arteries. The role of this sympathetic innervation was unclear but, more recently, it has been shown that sympathetic stimulation increases the limits between which autoregulation to pressure is affected; it has also been shown that hypertensive patients autoregulate at higher mean arterial pressures than normotensive patients.

THE MONRO-KELLIE DOCTRINE AND AUTOREGULATION

The unyielding nature of the skull led Alexander Monro in 1783 (17) to suppose that expansion of the cranial contents was severely limited and that active changes in the caliber of cerebral vessels was unlikely. He said that as the substance of the brain, like that of other solids of our body, is nearly incompressible, the quantity of the blood within the head must be the same or very nearly the same at all times, whether in health or disease, in life or after death. The confirmation of Monro's concept by Kellie in 1824 (10) became known as the Monro-Kellie doctrine and indeed was misinterpreted by many people. Hill, for instance, in 1896 (8), concluded that the whole circulatory system of the brain will assimilate itself into a system of tubes, and he felt that the cerebral circulation passively followed the change in the general arterial and venous pressures. Despite this, some of his own experiments suggested that there might be independent vasomotor activity in cerebral vessels. However, Burrows pointed out that while the brain was incompressible, there were changes in brain volume possible at the expense of other fluids, and indeed this is exactly what happens when changes in posture occur. The recognition of the multifactorial control of cerebral blood flow led to a new understanding of its control, and the work of Kety and Schmidt with Shenking in 1948 (11-13) demonstrated that cerebral autoregulation did in fact occur. This autoregulation was essentially regulation in the face of differences in perfusion pressure.

The homeostatic function of CSF was first described by Merritt and Fremont Smith in 1937 (15) and Masserman in 1934 (14). Further control of cerebral blood flow and perfusion pressure was described by Cushing in 1901 (3) in a situation that raised intracranial pressure. Here ischemia of the vasomotor center resulted in an increase in perfusion pressure and led in fact to a systemic hypertension.

Recognition that the properties of the blood itself were important was present in Wepfer's work, though it was not until the 1940s and 50s that the effect of viscosity in cerebral blood flow was recognized. This relationship was not straightforward; hence the original observations of Fähraeus and Lindquist in 1931 (5), which have since been confirmed, showed that the apparent viscosity of blood diminished in proportion to the radius of the tube through which it was passing.

STUDIES IN FUNCTIONAL PHYSIOLOGY

Ridley in 1700 (20) was probably the first to undertake a systematic study of pulsations of the brain and concluded that they are arterial in origin. Haller (1755) was first to use trephine holes in the human skull (7) and Ravina (1811) (19) converted the trephine method into a skull window technique. These studies sparked interest in the direct observation in vasomotor reactions, so that the foundations were laid for the current interest in cerebral blood flow and its relationship to metabolism and mental activity.

Early clinical studies were made by Fulton (1928) (6), who gave an account of the responses of blood flowing through an angioma of the occipital cortex to an increase in illumination. The patient had noticed an increased noise in the head whenever he used his eyes, and Fulton was able to demonstrate an undoubted increase in the frequency in amplitude of vibrations from the tumor when the patient read newsprint after dark adaptation.

Cobb and Talbott (1927) (2) estimated the capillary density in the motor cortex, olfactory bulb, and visual area in animals, which immediately before death were subjected to olfactory stimulation. In stimulated animals, there was an increased number of capillaries, this increase being maximal when ammonia had been used. This suggested that mental stimulation increased the blood flow in some way. It is well known that mental activity causes changes in the EEG pattern and decreases synchronicity, but it was not until sensitive methods of cerebral blood flow estimation were developed by Ingvar and Risberg in 1967 (9,21) that regional cerebral blood flow differences could be observed. The link between neuronal activity and regional cerebral blood flow is as yet poorly understood, and many theories have been put forward, none wholly satisfactory. It is clear, however, that in certain circumstances, for example, schizophrenia, there seems to be a breakdown in this particular relationship, there being very little regional cerebral blood flow differences when various activities are undertaken. These findings agree with other studies of a synchrony of the EEG in schizophrenia.

It is uncertain at this point whether this failure of linkage between regional cerebral blood flow and neuronal activity is a primary result of the schizophrenia process or whether it may be a cause. Such studies have opened a new dimension in the relationship between the blood flow and neuronal metabolism as well as enabled the localization of functional areas within the brain, undertaken systematically by the Scandinavians with great success. More recent work involving the use of radioactive glucose and oxygen in the positron emission scanner enables areas of poor metabolism to be identified. These areas do not always correspond to either areas of infarction on the CT scan or areas of poor blood flow as such.

CONCLUSION

From this rather short summary of the history of the cerebral circulation, a number of points are apparent. First, before any idea of cerebral circulation had developed, it was necessary to have a concept that the blood circulated at all. Before this idea was current, the complicated network of veins and arteries in the brain was only perceived as a rete, a network containing some vital spirit. Once the concept of circulation of the blood had been accepted, people were forced to look at these arteries and veins more closely. The second point is that until Willis described the physiological function of the anastomotic circle that now bears his name, although it had been described more or less by other authors, nobody paid very much attention to its structure. This applies to many areas of science, and understanding functional significance throws a new light and expands interest in areas previously neglected. Finally, the intriguing questions raised by the finding of the close interrelationship between neuronal metabolism and cerebral regional circulation raises many fascinating questions. It may be that many disorders of function, both neurological and psychiatric, are in some way caused by breakdown in this link mechanism.

REFERENCES

1. Burrows, G. (1846): *On Disorders of the Cerebral Circulation and on the Connection Between Affections of the Brain and Diseases of the Heart.* Langman, London.

2. Cobb, S., and Talbott, J. H. (1927): Studies in cerebral circulation II. A quantitative study of human capillaries. *Trans. Assoc. Am. Physns.*, 42:255–262.
3. Cushing, H. (1901): Concerning a definite regulating mechanism of the vasomotor centre which controls blood pressure during cerebral compression. *John Hopkins Hosp. Bull.*, 12:290–292.
4. Dorley, J. E. (1909): John James Wepfer, a Renaissance student of apoplexy. *John Hopkins Hosp. Bull.*, 20 (214):1–9.
5. Fähraeus, R., and Lindquist, T. (1931): The viscosity of the blood in narrow capillary tubes. *Am. J. Physiol.*, 96:562–568.
6. Fulton, J. F. (1928): Observations on the vascularity of the human occipital lobe during visual activity. *Brain*, 51:310–320.
7. Haller, A. von (1755): *Dissertation on the Sensible and Irritable Parts of Animals*, pp. 20,21. Nourse, London.
8. Hill, L. (1896): *The Physiology and Pathology of the Cerebral Circulation. An Experimental Research*, p. 208, Churchill, London.
9. Ingvar, D. H., and Risberg, J. (1967): Increase in regional cerebral blood flow during mental effort in normals and in patients with focal brain disorders. *Exp. Brain Res.*, 3:195–211.
10. Kellie, G. (1824): Reflections of the pathology of the brain. *Trans. Edin. Med. Chir. Soc.*, 1:123–169.
11. Kety, S. S., and Schmidt, C. F. (1948): The effect of altered arterial tensions of carbon dioxide and oxygen on cerebral blood flow in man: theory, procedure and normal values. *J. Clin. Invest.*, 27:484–492.
12. Kety, S. S., Shenkin, H. A., and Schmidt, C. F. (1948): Blood flow, vascular resistance and oxygen consumption of the brain in essential hypertension. *J. Clin. Invest.*, 27:511–514.
13. Kety, S. S., Shenkin, H. A., and Schmidt, C. F. (1948): The effects of increased intracranial pressure on cerebral circulating effects in man. *J. Clin. Invest.*, 27:493–499.
14. Masserman, J. H. (1934): Cerebral spinal hydrodynamics IV. Clinical experimental studies. *Arch. Neurol. Psychiat., Chicago*, 32:523–553.
15. Merritt, H. H., and Fremont Smith, F. (1937): *The Cerebral Spinal Fluid.* Saunders, Philadelphia.
16. McNaughten, F. (1938): The innervation of the intraarterial blood vessels and dura mater. *Res. Publ. Assoc., Res. Nerv. Ment. Dis.*, 18:178–200.
17. Meyer, M., and Hierons, R. (1962): Observations on the history of the "Circle of Willis." *Med. Hist.*, 6:119–130.
18. Monro, A. (1783): *Observations on the Structure and Functions of the Nervous System.* W. Creech, Edinburgh.
19. Ravina, A. F. (1811): Specimen de moti cerebri. *Mermone. Accad. Sci. Torino, Memoires presentée*, 20:16–93.
20. Ridley, H. (1700): An experiment to discover the cause of the motion of the dura mater. *Phil. Trans. Roy. Soc.*, 5:199–202.
21. Risberg, J., and Ingvar, D. H. (1968): Regional changes in cerebral blood volume during mental activity. *Exp. Brain Res.*, 5:72–78.
22. Vesling, J. (1651): *Sintagma Anatomicum*, p. 195. Framissiti, Padua.
23. Willis, T. (1664): *De Cerebri Anatome.* Martin and Allestry, London.

Historical Aspects of the Neurosciences,
edited by F. Clifford Rose and W. F. Bynum.
Raven Press, New York ©

Congestion of the Brain

Simon Behrman

Department of Neurology, Guy's Hospital, London, England

> "And yet you incessantly stand on your head—
> Do you think at your age, it is right?"
> "In my youth," Father William replied to his son,
> "I feared it might injure the brain."
> *Alice's Adventures in Wonderland*
> Lewis Carroll

Pietro Fasolati, aged 62, an engraver in Padua, retired to bed after eating a hearty supper and, two hours later, was found by his wife to be dead. Giovanni Morgani (1682–1771) examined the body to discover the cause of death. He found such an unusual quantity of blood distending all the cerebral vessels that he did not remember ever having seen the like before; even the small vessels, usually imperceptible, were extremely large and turgid. Morgani, in his remarks upon this case, refers to the opinion of Galen and many other ancient physicians that apoplexy was induced by too great repletion of arteries, veins, and sinuses of the brain. This case was included by Morgani in his *De sedibus et causis morborum* (1), a collection of clinicopathological correlations published in 1761. The book made an immense impact on medical thought, and congestion of the brain came to be recognized as a condition in which an abnormal accumulation of blood in the vessels of the brain might cause apoplexy—a disorder of brain function—or death.

Included in *De sedibus et causis morborum* was also a case in which Morgani found "blood filled cavities in the brain." He claimed: "We must take it as strong evidence that here is the seat and cause of contralateral hemiplegia." The juxtaposition of these two cases led to a firmly held supposition that congestion of the brain, apoplexy, might eventually lead to brain hemorrhage manifesting as stroke with contralateral hemiplegia.

Some reassurance that the transition from congestion of the brain to brain hemorrhage was not inevitable was found in George Kellie's axiom: "to whatever extent the one set of vessels (in the head) is becoming overcharged, to the same extent, it seems probable, is the other set voided." No "greater quantity of blood can be forced within the vessels of the brain without an equivalent compression or displacement" (2). This axiom was the direct corollary of the doctrine that Monro, Kellie's teacher, had formulated some years earlier, as follows (3):

> For as the substance of the brain, like that of the other solids of the body, is nearly incompressible, the quantity of blood within the head must be the same, or very nearly the same, at all times, whether in health or disease, in life or after death . . . It does not, however, follow from this that every individual artery or vein within the head is constantly the same

> size . . . For whilst the heart is performing its systole, the arteries here as elsewhere may be dilating and in the meantime the quantity of blood, equal to that which is dilating them, is passing out of the head by the vein.

Morgani's other conclusion that "the seat and cause of hemiplegia" was a contralateral cerebral hemorrhage remained unshaken. As recently as 1843, that great clinician, Robert Graves, wrote as follows (4):

> To quote one of many examples I myself have seen: a man named Thomas Lynch was admitted into Sir Patrick Dun's Hospital afflicted with symptoms indicative of cerebral disease. During his residence in the hospital he suffered four or five attacks of hemiplegia, in every respect complete, and depriving him of the use of his speech. Some of these attacks lasted only fifteen minutes, while the longest continued about an hour and a half; they ceased as suddenly as they commenced, and left no trace of hemiplegia behind them. The circumstances of this case evidently prevents us from assigning each attack to a separate effusion of blood: for were it owing to this cause, it would be impossible to account at once for the sudden appearance and sudden cessation of so extensive and complete a paralysis. Let it not be imagined, however, that I wish to throw doubts upon the beneficial influence of morbid anatomy on the diagnosis and treatment of diseases of the brain—my object in making these observations is not to retard, but to advance the progress of morbid anatomy by pointing out errors of some generally received opinions.

Four years after Robert Graves voiced his bewilderment, Virchow put forward in a paper, published in the first volume of his newly founded *Archiv* (5), the concept of "ischaemic apoplexy," of which embolism was the most important cause.

The phenomenon of congestion of brain vessels was demonstrated in the rabbit in 1850 by Frans Cornelius Donders, with the aid of a cranial window. Having replaced part of the skull by a piece of transparent glass, he was able to view the cortical and pial vessels with a microscope in the intact and inexpansible skull. He noted that filling of these vessels became greatly increased by suffocation and by "hanging the animal with its head down" (6).

It may be noted that little interest in the effects of the head-down position had been taken by clinicians until recently. The single exception seems to have been M. Bricheteau, who described a student whose memory was treacherous, and who was in the habit of placing himself not merely in the horizontal position but with his lower extremities elevated and his head dependent, when he wished to study with most effect (7).

This head-down position, previously only assumed by children and acrobats, has now become of interest to students of the effect of exposure to varying levels of gravity. The effects of the head-down position, now known as the foot-to-head negative G, is experienced by a pilot when his aircraft is performing the loop. On the arterial side, negative G manifests as slowing of the heart; on the venous side, as nasal obstruction and appearance of petechiae (8). The reflex slowing of the heart under this condition has been found effective in the treatment of paroxysmal tachycardia that fails to respond to the standard forms of treatment (9).

John Abercrombie (1780–1844) described in his *Pathological and Practical Researches on Diseases of Brain and Spinal Cord* (1827) (10) several cases of "simple apoplexy," where he could not account for the coma and subsequent death. Case 100 is of particular interest. Upon the dissection of the head, the veins on the surface of the brain were found turgid, and its substance, when cut into, exhibited a remarkable degree of vascularity.

Sir George Burrows' *Disorders of Cerebral Circulation*, published in 1846, is almost entirely devoted to a discussion of brain congestion (11). He begins his book with a detailed criticism of George Kellie's reasonings that the absolute quantity of blood within the cranium is at all times nearly the same. Little is known of Kellie before 1802, when he began his surgical apprenticeship in Edinburgh. About this period in his life, he recorded (2): "One of my oldest physiological recollections is the second Monro exhibiting a hollow glass ball filled with water. Not a drop of water escaped when he inverted the sphere with the aperture pointing downwards." After graduation, he set up in practice in Leith, where he died suddenly in 1829. Burrows listed Kellie's three arguments that form the basis of the doctrine of the invariable quanity of blood in the cranium and then demolished them one by one.

1. A state of bloodlessness is not discovered in the brains of animals that have died by hemorrhage. In reply, Burrows cites Mr. Lawrence of Bedlam Hospital, that in 53 out of 72 cases examined, the vessels of the brain were found congested, sometimes they were turgid, at other times extremely so. Cerebral vessels were found exsanguined, i.e., "unusually empty," only once, and in this case death was caused by hemorrhage from bursting of a femoral aneurysm. "When we learn that in autopsies of seventy-two insane patients the cerebral vessels were found unusually empty only once, and that this patient bled to death, can we give credence to the statement that the quantity of blood in the cerebral vessels is always nearly the same or that artificial abstraction of blood does not diminish the actual quantity in the cerebral vessels?"

2. Congestion of the cerebral vessels is not found in those instances where it might be most expected, as in persons who die by hanging. The bodies of two pirates who were hanged at Leith were dissected by Monro and Kellie. The bodies were examined while still warm; the limbs were not rigid; the countenances were livid and eyeballs suffused. In each body, on the division of the scalp, blood flowed from the vessels in such quantity as to afford ample proof of congestion of the external parts of the head. The sinuses of the dura mater contained *no* extraordinary quantity of blood; the large vessels on the surface of the brain were but moderately filled; the pia mater was paler and less vascular than is found in ordinary cases. No sooner was the brain removed from the skull than blood, still warm, began to flow profusely from the divided sinuses and vessels at the base of the skull. Burrows claimed that "in opposition to such a conclusion it would not be difficult to cite numerous well-authenticated instances of death by hanging where the brain and its membranes have presented all the usual appearances of congestion and even apoplexy to a striking extent." This he proceeded to do.

3. Kelly's next statement was "that if there be repletion or depletion of one set of vessels (arteries or veins) in the cranium, there will be an opposite condition of the other set of vessels." Burrows argued that this concept of reciprocal equilibrium of the intracranial contents is based on the assumption that "the anatomical structure of the human cranium is a complete sphere capable of removing the contents from the influence of atmospheric pressure. The numerous fissures and foramina for the transmission of vessels and nerves appear to me to do away with the idea of the cranium being a perfect sphere like a glass globe . . . If the brain is defended from atmospheric pressure, should we not expect to find the functions of that organ disturbed in some way when part of the wall of the sphere is wanting? But in children with open fontanelles and in adults who have lost part of the cranium we observe no peculiar disturbance of functions of the brain from a gap in the walls of the imaginary sphere."

The peculiar opinions of Kellie, Abercrombie, and other British physicians upon the cerebral circulation have not escaped the attention of the industrious Germans. In one of the latest and best summaries of the present state of medical opinions in Germany, we find the following remarks written by Dr. Carl Canstadt (11):

> English physicians have come to the conclusion, that the quantity of blood in the vessels of the brain cannot alter, but remains always the same. In states of hyperaemia and apoplexy, they only admit a stagnation of circulation, but not an increase of the quantity of blood there, because, as they assert, there is no room for such an increase on account of the unyielding nature of the walls of the cranium."

Burrows summarized his views as follows:

> On the vast majority of cases of apoplexy, coma is attributable to pressure induced by brain congestion. But, if this derangement of circulation of the brain is alone capable of producing so serious a result as coma, it may be properly asked why is not apoplectic coma produced by those frequently recurring causes of determination of blood to the brain, such as violent exercises, strong mental emotions and intemperance.
>
> The explanation, according to Abercrombie, is that arteries of the brain pass through tortuous bony canals. Therefore a sudden momentum of blood flowing to the cranium may be diminished and sinuses of dura mater which channel blood from the brain are kept constantly pervious.
>
> I therefore infer that in the larger number of cases of apoplexy accompanied with extravasation of blood, the coma is to be attributed to antecedent or coexisting cerebral congestion, while the paralysis which is more durable is dependent upon the limited local mischief produced by extravasation.

Burrows considered that venesection was indicated as the first step in the treatment of brain congestion. He then proceeded to suggest two rather more fanciful courses of treatment, namely, ligature of the common carotid artery and the application of Erasmus Darwin's rotatory machine.

Treatment by ligature was based on Caleb Parry's success in employing digital compression of the carotid artery to "subdue mania, headaches and vertigo." Caleb Parry (1755—1822), described by his contemporaries as "vir probus, medicus sagax," recorded in 1792 how he came to discover the therapeutic value of carotid compression (12). Under the pretence of feeling the pulse of the neck he took the opportunity to press strongly with his thumb on the carotid artery, a little below the larynx. On this carotid compression, Caleb wrote the following (12):

> I do not remember having experienced a philosophical pleasure in any degree comparable to that which this experiment afforded to me. No sooner was the pressure made than the austerity of the countenance disappeared. At the same time headache and undue sensibility with regard to light and sound were altogether wanting. It nearly totally removes the hemicrania of the side on which the compression is made.

Burrows evidently preferred to ligature the common carotid, though this procedure is attended with risk to life in some cases (perhaps in the proportion of one death in four operations). "Still, experience proves that where proper precautions have been taken the operation is not so dangerous as many suppose. Therefore in violent hopeless cases which are characterized by extreme cerebral congestion, it appears to me that other remedies failing this operation may be fairly resorted to. I am aware of the responsibility of advocating a remedy attended with risk to life, but are not all our best remedies most violent poisons in the hands of the unskilled?"

Burrows' third remedial measure was to make use of a rotatory machine that he contended had been invented by Dr. Erasmus Darwin (1731–1802). Burrows then described the mode of application of this machine. "The patient is laid on his back with his head close to a column or pivot around which the bed is made to revolve with considerable velocity. A centrifugal force is thus generated which from the position of the patient drives the blood from the head toward the lower extremities. The centrifugal force thus suddenly created powerfully diminishes the momentum of the blood moving into the cranium. The diminished arterial pressure on the cerebral substance soon produces a sense of exhaustion or complete syncope." In a footnote, Burrows gives the page of *Zoonomia* (13) on which further details could be found. In fact, there is no such reference to this rotatory bed in *Zoonomia*. However, on page 237 in Volume 1 of Darwin's work can be found the germ of Burrows' fabrication. The passage reads as follows:

> Another way of procuring sleep mechanically was related to me by Mr. Brindley, the famous canal engineer, who was brought up to the business of a mill-wright. He told me that he had more than once seen the experiment of a man extending himself across the large stone of a corn-mill and that by gradually letting the stone whirl, the man fell asleep before the stone had gained its full velocity and he supposed would have died without pain by the continuance or increase of the motion. In this case the centrifugal motion of the head and feet must accumulate the blood in both those extremities of the body and thus compress the brain.

The most recent authoritative article on congestion of the brain (14) was written by Russell Reynolds (1828–1896) and Charlton Bastian (1837–1915), both physicians to the National Hospital for the Paralysed and Epileptics, and was published in 1868. Like Burrows, whom they cite extensively, they were critical of the Monro-Kellie doctrine. The perivascular spaces, which had recently been discovered by Robin and His, were put to use by them to explain how the varying amounts of blood in the cerebral vascular system could be accommodated within the cranium without increased pressure. "In order to make room for an increased amount of blood in the cerebral vascular system, a corresponding amount of fluid must be driven out of the enveloping lymphatic vessels." Of the conditions capable of bringing about a state of cerebral congestion, they said: "Some are strictly mechanical phenomena due to some impediment to the proper return of blood from the brain; in some the condition of hyperaemia seems a vital phenomenon as when it is the result of prolonged study and mental work." Bastian also included the following among likely causes: "alcoholic intoxication, exposure to the sun's rays in hot summer weather and the suppression of accustomed fluxes whether menstrual or others."

They considered that cerebral congestion is most intimately related to cerebral hemorrhage. They quoted with approval these statements made by Laborde in his book on congestion of the brain (published in 1866): "that the links which bind cerebral congestion and cerebral haemorrhage together are frequently the minute aneurysms described by Bouchard. Congestion may have something to do with their formation as it certainly has with their final rupture leading to effusion of blood." They concluded the article by an enjoinder to avoid "sudden change of posture or strain, and to prevent the head and shoulders from sinking down to the level of the bed" (14). Two foremost physicians in mid-19th century London, Burrows and Reynolds, were therefore greatly concerned in the detailed examination of the concept of congestion of the brain. At the time, it was regarded as a cornerstone in the pathology of vascular diseases of the brain.

George Burrows (1801–1887) and John Russell Reynolds (1837–1896) were both physicians to Queen Victoria, on each of whom she had conferred a baronetcy. They had both been Presidents of the Royal College of Physicians. Having amassed gold medals as a student at University College Hospital, Reynolds set up in practice in Leeds, but he was soon afterwards persuaded by Marshall Hall to take over the lease of 38, Grosvenor Street, London, W.1., on his retirement. Reynolds eventually died in this house, and the following appreciation appeared in the *Lancet*: "He appeared at a transition period when order in neurology was just discernible—forming itself out of chaos—and he was largely responsible for that order." Congestion of the brain as a nosological entity was still widely accepted as recently as 1891, as is testified by papers published in that year (15,16).

Erasmus Darwin's medical treatise, *Zoonomia*, was based on the analogy between genera of living things and diseases. It would appear that congestion of the brain, like the dodo, has become an extinct species. Reynolds and Bastian bemoaned that "we cannot see the brain while the symptoms of congestion of the brain last." This is no longer true since there are now available two methods capable of measuring intravascular blood volume of the brain without resorting to any invasive maneuvre. In the normal brain, this was found to be 3% of the brain volume (17,18). Any figure in excess must presumably be regarded as indicative of "brain congestion."

REFERENCES

1. Morgani, G. B. (1761): *De sedibus et causis morborum*. Venice.
2. Kellie, G. (1824): *Trans. Med.-Chir. Soc. Edinburgh*, 1:84–169.
3. Monro, A. (Secundus) (1783): *Observations on the Structure and Functions of the Nervous System*. Edinburgh.
4. Graves, R. J. (1884): *Clinical Lectures on the Practice of Medicine*. New Syndenham Society, London.
5. Virchow, R. (1847): *Archiv Pathol. Anat. Physiol. Klin. Med.*, 1:272.
6. Donders, F. C. (1850): *Ned. Lancet (The Hague)*, 5(2nd ser.):521.
7. Bricheteau, M., quoted by G. Burrows (1846): *On Disorders of Cerebral Circulation*. Longman, London.
8. Wilkins, R. W., Bradley, S. E., and Friedland, C. K. (1950): *J. Clin. Invest.*, 29:940.
9. Constantiniu, I. (1972): *Am. J. Cardiol.*, 30:310.
10. Abercrombie, J. (1827): *Pathological and Practical Researches on Diseases of Brain and Spinal Cord*. Edinburgh.
11. Burrows, G. (1846): *On Disorders of Cerebral Circulation*. Longman, London.
12. Parry, C. H. (1792): *Memoirs Med. Soc. London*, 3:77.
13. Darwin, E. (1794): *Zoonomia*, Vol. 1, p. 237.
14. Reynolds, J. R., and Bastian, H. C. (1868): *System of Medicine*, Vol. 2, p. 413. Macmillan, New York.
15. Whitley, G. W., (1891): *Lancet*, ii:1333.
16. Gay, J. (1891): *Lancet*, i:1148.
17. Grubb, R. L., Phelps, M. E., and Ter-Pogossian, M. M. (1973): *Arch. Neurol.*, 28:38.
18. Penn, R., and Kurtz, D. (1977): *J. Neurol.*, 46:282.

Historical Aspects of the Neurosciences,
edited by F. Clifford Rose and W. F. Bynum.
Raven Press, New York ©

Transient Cerebral Ischemia: A Historical Sketch

Vladimir Hachinski

Department of Clinical Neurological Sciences, University of Western Ontario, London, Ontario, Canada

> Everything has been discovered before. The difficulty is to discover it again.
>
> Goethe

FROM ANTIQUITY TO THE 19TH CENTURY

Although the term "transient ischemic attacks" has been coined recently (1), the syndrome has been recognized since antiquity. Hippocrates noted that "unaccustomed attacks of numbness and anesthesia are signs of impending apoplexy" (2). But description does not equal understanding. The term apoplexy was used to describe any sudden catastrophic event resulting in death, coma, or paralysis. It is likely, therefore, that "apoplexy" included, but was not limited to, cases of acute cerebral ischemia. In addition to this terminological imprecision, "the physician of the Hippocratic School paid less attention to precise and local diagnosis, despite his clinical acumen. He believed that disordered bodily function was a generalized process, and his approach was directed primarily toward prognostic rather than diagnostic considerations" (3). Nevertheless, apoplexy was considered a disease of the brain and a disorder of black bile. Greek and Roman medical writers added variety but not substance to the Hippocratic descriptions. Thus, Caelius Aurelianus, in paraphrasing the work of Soranus, describes apoplexy as "a sudden collapse, as if from a deadly blow. It is a sudden seizure, in general without fever, and it deprives the body of all sensation. . .In some cases there is no visible indication before the coming of the attack, but in others there are certain signs that point to this disease, e.g., a feeling of heaviness or pain in the head, dizziness, ringing in the ears, difficulty in making accustomed motions, sadness of facial expression, quivering of the parts, and of the lips more than of the other parts; trembling voice, words indistinctly pronounced, a breaking off without any reason in the midst of speaking, or forgetfulness of what has just been said; face full; evacuations painful" (4). This description mixed symptoms that may be interpreted as transient ischemic attacks ("difficulty in making accustomed motions, words indistinctly pronounced, breaking-off without any reason in the midst of speaking") with a number of nonspecific symptoms. The writer himself recognized the general nature of some of the symptoms, since he notes that "the same antecedent signs appear also in cases where the patient is found to be on the verge of epilepsy or mania."

Interestingly, while the classic medical writers were composing their learned tomes, Greek mountebanks were amusing audiences by tying up and relaxing the carotid arteries of goats. The animals would fall and rise with the occlusion and release of their brain feeding arteries. The term "carotid" comes from the Greek word "karos" meaning deep sleep, probably coined by someone watching goats rendered motionless by compression of their carotid arteries. Leonard Hill (5) observes that "It was a custom among the Assyrians to compress these arteries in their young men before circumcision so that they might feel less pain." However, it was not until the 19th century that there was enough knowledge and an appropriate intellectual framework to relate these examples of induced transient cerebral ischemia to spontaneous ischemic attacks.

McHenry (2) states that "Although a few additional clinical features had been presented during the Middle Ages and Renaissance, little was added to the ancient descriptions and concepts of apoplexy." The same holds true for transient cerebral ischemia, at least in Western medical literature. In 1658, Wepfer stated that he had seen patients who had recovered from hemiplegia in a day or less (6). These instances may well represent cases of transient ischemic attacks, although Wepfer most clearly relates apoplexy to cerebral hemorrhage. However, he does discuss a number of other causes of apoplexy, including certain small fibrous bodies in the carotid and vertebral arteries (corpora fibrosa), resulting in narrowing or occlusion that would interfere with the delivery of "animal spirits" to the brain. He noticed that "To this variety of apoplexy those are most liable who lead an idle life, those who are obese and those whose face and hands are livid and whose pulse is constantly unequal" (7). In the 18th century, Hermann Boerhaave also noted "stenochoria in chondrogonia arteriae, i.e., narrowing due to cartilaginous change of the artery" (8). But he regarded a change in the composition of the blood as the main cause of apoplexy.

The 18th century also provided the first self-reported case of transient ischemic attack. Jean Paul Grandjean de Fouchy, writing in 1783 at the age of 76 years, stated that "Toward the end of dinner, I felt a little increase of pain above the left eye, and in that very instant I became unable to pronounce the words that I wanted. I heard what was said, and I thought of what I ought to reply, but I spoke other words than those which would express my thoughts, or if I began them I did not complete them, and I substituted other words for them. I had nevertheless all movements as freely as usual . . . I saw all objects clearly, I heard distinctly what was being said; and the organs of thought were, it seemed to me, in a natural state. This sort of paroxysm lasted almost a minute" (9).

In the same year of 1783, Dr. Samuel Johnson, at the age of 73, wrote "Thus I went to bed, and in a short time waked and sat up as has long been my custom, when I felt a confusion and indistinctness in my head which lasted, I suppose about half a minute; I was alarmed and prayed God, that however he might afflict my body he would spare my understanding. This prayer, that I might try the integrity of my faculties I made in Latin verse. The lines were not very good, but I knew them not to be very good, I made them easily, and concluded myself to be unimpaired in my faculties" (10).

One week after this event, Dr. Johnson wrote: "My friends tell me that my power of utterance improves daily, and Dr. Heberden declares that he hopes to find me almost well tomorrow." A careful and masterful analysis by Macdonald Critchley (10) of the handwriting of these letters shows that Johnson repeated some words and showed other discrepancies, suggesting that he had sustained a cerebral infarction rather than merely experiencing transient ischemia. Although Dr. William Heberden looked after Johnson during the latter's illness, we have no record of this physician's thoughts on the matter. Nevertheless, Heberden did know about transient cerebral ischemia. He stated that a complete paralysis may be preceded by "A faltering and inarticulation of the voice, drowsiness, forgetfulness, a slight delirium, a dimness of sight, or objects appearing double, trembling, a numbness gradually propagated to the head, a frequent yawning, weakness, a distortion of the mouth, a palpitation, a disposition to faint; some, or most of these have preceeded a palsy for a few minutes, or for some hours, or even for a few days; in a weakness of the limb, or of one side, has been many months, or a few years, gradually increasing to a perfect loss of one side, or a hemiplegia. I have known a sleepiness and duplicity of objects with violent pains and tightness of the head for two days, then the senses and voice were lost on the third and the man expired. A numbness of the hand has come on the first day, and on the second a faltering of the voice, and a palsy on the third" (2). There is no evidence, however, that Heberden or any other 18th century physician had a clear idea of pathophysiology of the premonitory symptoms of stroke.

THE 19TH CENTURY TO THE PRESENT

During the 19th century, a number of reports established the association between apoplexy and disease of the brain arteries. The cervical portions of the carotid and vertebral arteries were seldom examined; perhaps this contributed to misunderstandings about the relationship of arteriosclerosis to transient or permanent cerebral ischemia. At other times, medical writers concentrated on a secondary aspect of the relationship, such as pain. Richard Bright (11), for example, states that "It very frequently happens, when listening to the detail of symptoms, in connection with deranged cerebral circulation and threatened apoplexy, that we find the patient laying considerable stress upon a constant or frequently recurring pain diffused over the occiput . . .". Furthermore, he thought that "this pain would, of itself, chiefly direct our suspicions to disease of the vertebral arteries."

Textbooks of medicine continued to confuse probable symptoms of transient cerebral ischemia with vague and nonspecific complaints. George McClellan (12) observed that "In some instances, a numbness is felt in the fingers or in one side of the body shortly before the attack supervenes." But he goes on to say that "In general, the symptoms which announce the approach of an apoplectic attack, indicate an unusual determination of blood to the head. Of these symptoms, however, vertigo, ringing in the ears, dimness of sight, and pain and heaviness in the head, are by far the most common precursors of an attack of this disease." These and failures of attention, inability to do accustomed work, and insomnia were often attributed to a generalized softening of the brain. Hughlings Jackson (13) protested: "I know nothing of general or universal softening of the brain," and he argued that the diagnosis of softening of the brain could not be made "unless the patient has certain local paralytic symptoms, as hemiplegia, or some other symptoms implying a local cerebral lesion, such as affection of speech. . . ." Jackson, while discussing "hemiplegia from clot," stated that "this form of palsy arises in the vast majority of instances from bad cerebral arteries; they break or get blocked up. Hemiplegia is the common arteriocerebral symptom partly because an embolus can more easily get into the middle cerebral artery for anatomical causes, and partly because this vessel lies more directly in the way of strain from the heart, and thus is the most diseased and most easily ruptured. . . ." He goes on to quote Prevost and Cotard, who found that "tobacco-seeds injected into a dog's carotid most often lodged in the animal's middle cerebral artery." He thought that "Suddenly occurring and transitory slight symptoms, such as affections of speech, unilateral numbness, may be owing to little foci of softening (or rather to thrombosis of small arteries, which in due time lead to local softening), just as much as permanent paralysis may be owing to extensive softening." He adds that "At the same time it is only an inference that such slight and transitory paralytic symptoms depend on small foci of softening; for there is no, or practically no, morbid anatomy of such slight symptoms." The search for the morbid anatomy of transient ischemic attacks would generate three main pathophysiologic theories: vasospasm, hemodynamic, and thromboembolic.

THE VASOSPASM THEORY

Raynaud (14) in 1862 postulated that intermittent cerebral arterial spasms caused transient loss of vision. This mechanism was invoked to account for transient neurological symptoms in a paper on "Relations between arterial diseases and visceral changes" by Peabody in 1891 (15). The thinking behind the vasospasm theory was exemplified in an article on "Intermittent closing of cerebral arteries: Its relation to temporary and permanent paralysis" by William Russell in 1909 (16). He described a 50-year-old farmer who suffered "three attacks, characterised by tingling in the right arm and hand, a stiff and numb feeling in the right side of the face, and difficulty in articulating." The patient had other transient focal neurological symptoms and eventually experienced a right homonymous hemianopia. "The pulse was 84, regular, and of moderate force, brachial pressure was 210. . . ." Russell went on to discuss the differential diagnosis. He dismissed the possibility of cardiac embolism because of the lack of coexisting mitral or aortic disease. He discounted hemorrhage as a cause because the paralysis occurred without loss of consciousness. The possibility of thrombosis was considered but dismissed: "thrombus, once formed, does not break up and disappear in some mysterious way; it is a difficult thing to get rid of, and we cannot appeal to recurring formation and disappearance of thrombi to explain our clinical phenomena." By contrast, modern neurologists explain most transient ischemic attacks as the result of recurrent formation and breakup of thrombi. Russell concluded that the likeliest cause was local closing of arterial channels. This phenomena could be seen in "the local syncope of 'dead fingers,' in the 'local syncope' of Raynaud's disease, in some cases of migraine . . . and in temporary partial blindness seen to be due to closing of a branch of the retinal artery." Russell believed that "There must be some vessel constriction, local in site, varying in degree and in extent, coming and going, intermittent."

William Osler doubted initially that arterial spasm could occur in sclerotic vessels, but by the time that he published his article on "Transient attacks of aphasia and paralysis in states of high blood pressure and arterio-sclerosis" in 1911 (17), he did not think that ". . . any other explanation was more plausible than that these attacks represent vascular crises. We have plenty of evidence that arteries may pass into a state of spasm with obliteration of the lumen and loss of function in the parts supplied."

Although the vasospastic theory had its detractors, it remained the predominant explanation for transient ischemic attacks in the first half of the 20th century. The vasospastic theory also provided the rationale for the use of cervical sympathetic block and vasodilators in an attempt to overcome the alleged transient vasoconstriction. But Pickering in 1948 (18) argued that arterial spasm was an unlikely explanation for transient ischemic attacks. He pointed out that the cerebral vessels were among the least reactive in the body and that when they did react, they did so in response to a local stimulus. No such stimulus could be identified. The introduction of cerebral arteriography (19) and the development of the hemodynamic and the thromboembolic theories (see below) made vasospasm a plausible mechanism only in subarachnoid hemorrhage and in classic migraine. In subarachnoid hemorrhage, vasospasm usually lasts hours or days, rather than minutes, as is usual in transient ischemic attacks. In migraine, although cerebral blood flow may significantly decrease, it is unclear whether this decreased perfusion is due to vasospasm or to metabolic depression with subsequent diminished blood flow (20).

HEMODYNAMIC THEORY

William Stokes in 1846 (21) reported the case of a 68-year-old man with "Repeated pseudo-apoplectic attacks, not followed by paralysis: slow pulse, with valvular murmur." The patient was prone to episodes wherein he "was suddenly seized with a fainting fit, in which he would have fallen if he had not been supported." Attacks came on several times a day and lasted "seldom more than four or five minutes, and sometimes less." To avert an attack, "he directly turns on his hands and knees, keeping his head low, and by this means, he says, he often averts what otherwise would end in an attack." Stokes noted "that on listening attentively to the heart's action, we perceived that there were occasional semibeats between the regular contractions, very weak, unattended with impulse, and corresponding to a similar state of the pulse, which thus probably amounts to about 36 in the minute, the evident beats being only 28." This report remains one of the most lucid accounts relating cardiac disturbances to transient cerebral ischemia.

Although Carl Rokitansky emphasized the importance of cardiac dysfunction in the production of apoplexy, it is uncertain whether or not he had any clear pathophysiological ideas about the production of transient ischemic attacks. He thought, for example, that congestion of the brain would "give rise to the transient or protracted attacks, which simulate apoplexy, and are so frequent in old age" (22). Nevertheless, Rokitansky made major contributions to the understanding of the role of arterial disease in the production of stroke.

Ramsay Hunt in 1914 (23) suggested that transient cerebral ischemic attacks were a form of cerebral intermittent claudication by analogy with symptoms produced by exercise in patients with severe femoral arterial disease. This view did not gain wide currency, and it was only with increasing use of cerebral arteriography in the 1940s that interest in the pathophysiology of transient cerebral ischemia was revived.

Denny-Brown in 1951 wrote a paper on "The treatment of recurrent cerebrovascular symptoms and the question of 'vasospasm'" (24). Therein he attacked the concept of "vasospasm" and suggested that "circulatory insufficiency due to carotid or basilar stenosis, are related to anatomical defects in collateral circulation'." In 1953, Corday et al. introduced the concept of "Cerebral vascular insufficiency" (25) by analogy with cardiac insufficiency and based on experimental work. They ligated the carotid vessels of monkeys either partially or completely. The blood pressure was lowered, and electroencephalographic changes occurred in the site of ligation, with restoration of the tracing to normal when the blood pressure was normalized. Later in the decade, Meyer et al. in 1956 (26) showed by a tilt-table technique that while the majority of patients with symptomatic carotid and basilar disease developed electroencephalographic changes with decreased blood pressure, only two out of 23 patients developed symptoms. The likely explanation for this is that cerebral perfusion is independent of systemic blood pressure above a mean blood pressure of 55 mm Hg (28), and the lumen of the internal carotid artery has to be decreased below 5 mm or more before there is any decrease in blood flow (29). It is now recognized that hemodynamic factors are probably important only in cases of severe cardiac arrhythmias, orthostatic hypotension, carotid sinus hypersensitivity, tight aortic stenosis with falling left ventricular function, and in cases of multiple cervical artery occlusions (30).

THROMBOEMBOLIC THEORY

Virchow and his pupils laid down the foundations of our understanding of thrombosis and embolism during the third quarter of the 19th century (8). Virchow (31) debunked the belief that thrombosis is an inflammatory process, and his pupil Julius Cohnheim (32) demonstrated elegantly the effects of embolization by injecting wax globules into a frog's tongue arteries. This produced lesions that we would now call "ischemic necrosis" and "hemorrhagic infarct," respectively. Later in the century, others were to apply Virchow's and Cohnheim's concepts to specific clinical situations.

Cervical Arteries

Penzoldt (33) in 1881 was the first to diagnose carotid occlusion "in vivo." Chiari, in a classic but neglected article, pointed out "the relative frequency of thrombosis resulting from 'endarteritis chronica deformans,' occurring at the bifurcation of the carotis communis and the origin of the internal carotid, whence embolism of the cerebral arteries often occurs, and on the other hand, the not infrequently early and also isolated occurrence of 'endarteritis chronica deformans' at the bifurcation of carotis communis and the origin of carotis interna" (34). Ramsay Hunt in 1914 (23) also drew attention to the carotid arteries by describing two patients with neck wounds that resulted in carotid thrombosis with a contralateral hemiplegia and ipsilateral pallor of the optic disc. Although other reports appeared in the literature, e.g., Moniz et al. in 1937 (19), Kubik and Adams in 1946 (35), and Denny-Brown and Meyer in 1951 (41), it was not until the publications of Miller Fisher (1,36,37), that the importance of carotid disease was appreciated. In his 1954 paper (37), Miller Fisher described patients with prodromal symptoms, but he was uncertain about the precise etiology. A year later, Millikan et al. (38) in 1955 reported seven patients with transient ischemic attacks that stopped after treatment with anticoagulant therapy. The authors suggested that "the newly formed clot becomes dislodged before symptoms occur, travels to a place where the vessels branch, lodges for a few minutes (symptoms produced), and then fragments and is carried away." In 1959, Miller Fisher (39) observed a white body passing slowly through the retinal arteries during attacks of transient blindness, which supported the idea that transient ischemic attacks were indeed caused by emboli. The whitish appearance and apparent friability of the embolus suggested that it was largely made up of platelets.

Florey in 1925 (40) showed that platelet emboli could be produced experimentally by injury to the rabbit's cortical and mesenteric vessels. Denny-Brown and Meyer in 1951 (41) reported platelet emboli moving across the pial circulation after injury to the middle cerebral artery in the monkey. In 1960 Denny-Brown (42) suggested that these platelet emboli were responsible for transient ischemic attacks. Ross Russell in 1961 (43) described further cases of transient white emboli in the retinal circulation during attacks of amaurosis fugax. Gunning and coworkers in 1946 published a well-documented paper on "Mural thrombosis of the internal carotid artery and subsequent embolism" (44). The understanding of this important pathophysiological mechanism in the production of transient ischemic attacks led to attempts to prevent cerebral infarction by the use of anticoagulants and of platelet suppressant agents. The latter has resulted in some success (45) and continues to be a fruitful field for investigation. A more direct attack on the problem was first attempted in 1954 by Eastcott and coworkers (46), who operated on a patient with transient ischemic attacks and with an internal carotid artery stenosis. Carotid endarterectomy has become a widespread but as yet unproven procedure. A surgical operation for transient ischemic attacks and other manifestations of cervical and cerebral arterial disease that is being evaluated consists of anastomosing the temporal artery with a branch of the middle cerebral artery (47).

An atheromatous plaque can be a site for thrombus and a source of emboli. W. W. Meyer in 1947 (48) and Winter in 1957 (49) were the first to describe atheromatous emboli in the cerebral circulation. This material was identified in the retinal arteries by Witmer and Schmid in 1958 (50) and labeled "bright plaques" by Hollenhorst in 1961 (51). David and coworkers (52) recognized in 1963 that these bodies contained cholesterol esters. Embolization can also occur from the site of an occluded subclavian (53) or internal carotid artery (54). These transient ischemic attacks may be due to embolization from the white tail of a thrombus (55) or due to hemodynamic factors (56).

Cardiac

Gowers in 1875 (57) described a case with embolism to the left middle cerebral artery and a small embolus to the central retinal artery. The source of the embolus was the auricular appendage in a case with mitral stenosis. Subsequently, it became well established that cardiac valvular lesions could result in cerebral embolism, leading to transient or permanent cerebral symptoms. Decline in the incidence of rheumatic valvular disease has decreased awareness of the heart as a potential source of emboli in transient ischemic attacks. Recent work has emphasized the importance of atrial myxoma and myxomatous degeneration of the mitral valve as possible causes of transient ischemic attacks. Atrial myxoma is uncommon but often presents with transient ischemic attacks. The evidence that a prolapsing mitral valve can lead to transient cerebral ischemia is strong (58). What remains to be determined is how the few cases at risk of developing cerebral symptoms are to be differentiated from the many who are not.

Aorta

Although the aorta is one of the earliest sites for formation of atherosclerosis, we know little about the role of the aortic arch in the production of transient ischemic attacks. This disparity between hypothetic possibility and empiric difficulty in supporting or dismissing this viewpoint exemplifies a problem faced by physicians over the centuries—intelligent supposition lacking the means of proof.

SUMMARY

Symptoms of transient cerebral ischemia have been recognized since antiquity, but no cohesive etiological explanation was offered until the 19th century. Since that time, the vasospastic, hemodynamic and thromboembolic theories have held sway in turn.

ACKNOWLEDGMENT

I thank Professor H. J. M. Barnett for helpful comments during the preparation of this manuscript.

REFERENCES

1. Fisher, C. M. (1958): In: *Cerebral Vascular Diseases*, edited by I. Wright and C. H. Millikan. Grune & Stratton, New York.

2. Coan Prenotions 466 (1950): *The Medical Works of Hippocrates*, edited by J. Chadwick and W. N. Mann, p. 260. Oxford Univ. Press. Oxford, England.
3. Clarke, E. (1963): *Bull. Hist. Med.*, 37:301–314.
4. Caelius Aurelianus (1950): *On Acute Diseases and on Chronic Diseases*, edited and translated by E. I. Drabkin, Acute Diseases e. 48f, p. 239. University of Chicago Press, Chicago.
5. Hill, L. (1896): In: *The Physiology and Pathology of the Cerebral Circulation: An Experimental Research*, edited by J & A Churchill, London.
6. Gurdjian, E. S., and Gurdjian, E. S. (1979): *Arch. Neurol.*, 36:340.
7. Donley, J. E. (1909): *Bull. Johns Hopkins Hosp.*, 20:1–8.
8. Schiller, F. (1970): *Med. Hist.*, 14:115–131.
9. Benton, A. L., and Joynt, R. J. (1960): *Arch. Neurol.*, 3:109–126.
10. Critchley, M. (1962): *Med. Hist.*, 6:27.
11. Bright, R. (1836): *Guy's Hosp. Rep.*, 1:9.
12. McClellan, G. (1849): In: *A Treatise on the Practice of Medicine*, by John Eberle, edited with notes and additions, by George McClellan. Grigg, Elliot & Co., Philadelphia.
13. Jackson, J. H. (1875): *Lancet* (Sept.):335–339.
14. Raynaud, A. (1862): as quoted by Loeb, C. (1980), *Eur. Neurol.*, 19:1.
15. Peabody, G. L. (1891): *Trans. Assoc. Am. Physns.* 6:154–195.
16. Russell, W. (1909): *Br. Med. J.*,(Oct.):2546–2547.
17. Osler, W. (1911): *Canad. Med. Assoc. J.*, 1:919–926.
18. Pickering, G. W. (1940): *J. Am. Med. Assoc.*, 137–423.
19. Moniz, E., Lima, A., de l'Acerda, R., (1937): *Nouv. Presse Med.*, 45:977.
20. Hachinski, V. C., and Norris, J. W., (1980): In: *Clinical Applications of Non-Invasive Xenon Studies in Cerebral Blood Flow*, edited by R. H. Ackerman and W. D. Obrist, William & Wilkins, Baltimore (*in press*).
21. Stokes, W. (1846): *Dublin Quart. J. Med. Sci.*, 2:73.
22. Rokitansky, C. (1856): *A Manual of Pathological Anatomy*, 1842–44. Published for the Sydenham Society, London.
23. Hunt, J. R. (1914): *Am. J. Med. Sci.*, 147:704.
24. Denny-Brown, D. (1951): *Med. Clin. N. Am.*, 35:1457–1474.
25. Corday, E., Rothenberg, S. F., and Putnam, T. J. (1953): *Am. Med. Assoc. Arch. Neurol. Psych.*, 69(5):551–570.
26. Meyer, J. S., Leiderman, H., and Denny-Brown, D., (1956): *Neurology*, 6.
27. Kendell, R. E., and Marshall, U. (1963): *Br. Med. J.*, 2:344–348.
28. Lassen, N. A. (1959): *Phys. Rev.*, 39:183–238.
29. Brice, J. G., Dowsett, D. M., Lowe, R. D. (1964): *Br. Med. J.*, 2:1363.
30. Barnett, H. J. M. (1979): *Med. Clin. N. Am.*, 63(4):649.
31. Virchow, R. (1856): In: *Gesammelte Abhandlungen zur wissenschaflichen Medizin*, edited by A. M. Meidlinger, p. 478. Frankfurt.
32. Cohnheim, J. (1872): In: *Untersuchungen uber die embolischen process*, edited by Hirschwald, Berlin.
33. Penzoldt, F. (1881): *Dtscht. Arch. Klin. Med.*, 28:80–93.
34. Chiari, H. (1905): *Verh. Dtsch. Pathol. Ges.*, 9:326.
35. Kubik, C. S., and Adams, R. D. (1946): *Brain*, 69:73.
36. Fisher, C. M. (1951): *Arch. Neurol. Psych.*, 65:346–377.
37. Fisher, C. M. (1954): *Arch. Neurol. Psych.*, 72:187–204.
38. Millikan, C. H., Siekert, R. G., and Shick, R. M. (1955): *Proc. Mayo Clinic*, 30:578.
39. Fisher, C. M. (1959): *Neurology*, 9:333–347.
40. Florey, H. (1925): *Brain*, 48:43.
41. Denny-Brown, D., and Meyer, J. S. (1951): *Neurology*, 7:567.
42. Denny-Brown, D., (1960): *Arch. Neurol.*, 2:194.
43. Ross Russell, R. W. (1961): *Lancet*, 2:1422.
44. Gunning, A. J., Pickering, G. W., Robb-Smith, A. H. T., Ross Russell, R. W. (1946): *Quart. J. Med.*, 33:155–195.
45. Canadian Cooperative Study Group (1978): *N. Engl. J. Med.*, 299:35.
46. Eastcott, H. H. G., Pickering, G. W., Rob, C. C. (1954): *N. Engl. J. Med.*, 2:994.
47. Barnett, H. J. M. et al. (1980): *12th Princeton Conference*, edited by J. Moosey (*in press*).
48. Meyer, W. W. (1947): *Arch. Pathol. Anat.*, 314:616.
49. Winter, W. J. Jr., (1957): *Arch. Pathol.*, 64:137–142.
50. Witmer, R., and Schmid, A. (1958): *Arterieller Embolus Ophthal.*, 135:432.
51. Hollenhorst, R. W. (1961): *J. Am. Med. Assoc.*, 178:23–29.
52. David, N. J., Klintworth, G. K., Friedberg, S. J., and Dillon, M. (1963): *Neurology (Minneapolis)*, 13:708–713.
53. (1927): *Proc. Roy. Soc. Med.*, 20:1244.
54. Barnett, H. J. M., Peerless, S. J., and Kaufmann, J. C. E. (1978): *Stroke*, 9:448–456.
55. Finklestein, S., Kleinman, G. M., Cuneo, R., and Baringer, J. R. (1980): *Neurology*, 30:84–88.

56. Sundt, T. M. Jr., Siekert, R. G., Piepgras, D. G., Sharbough, F. W., and Houser, O. W. (1976): *Mayo Clin. Proc.*, 51:677.
57. Gowers, W. R. (1875): *Lancet*, 2:794.
58. Barnett, H. J. M., et al. (1976): *Arch. Neurol.*, 33:777–782.

Historical Aspects of the Neurosciences,
edited by F. Clifford Rose and W. F. Bynum.
Raven Press, New York ©

Spinal Cord Arteries Described by Willis

J. Trevor Hughes

Department of Neuropathology, Radcliffe Infirmary, Oxford OX2 6HE, England

Thomas Willis is well known for his descriptions of the anatomy of the brain based on dissections and detailed examinations of most of the components of the brain with an important description of the cranial and spinal nerves. What is less recognized is that his publications include the first accurate descriptions of the vascular supply of the spinal cord. The present chapter singles out this part of his work from the better known account of the anatomy of the brain in his book *Cerebri Anatome: cui accessit Nervorum Descriptio et Usus*, published in 1664.

THOMAS WILLIS AND HIS COLLEAGUES

During his active research period in Oxford, Willis had as associates or pupils a remarkable group of scientific workers. Among these were Robert Hooke, John Locke, Edmund King, William Petty, Richard Lower, Thomas Millington, and Christopher Wren. In that part of Willis' work that concerns the anatomy of the blood vessels of the spinal cord, Richard Lower took a prominent part, and Thomas Millington and Christopher Wren were involved to a lesser degree.

Thomas Willis was born in 1621 in Great Bedwyn in Wiltshire but moved as a boy to North Hinksey very near Oxford. He came as a pupil to Christchurch, Oxford, in 1636, graduated B.A. in 1639 and M.A. in 1642. After the disturbances of the civil war, he returned to Oxford, where he set up medical practice and was appointed Sedleian Professor of Natural Philosophy in 1660. His researches on neurological anatomy date from this period, and his famous book *Cerebri Anatome* was published in 1664. He moved to London in 1667 where he died in 1675 of pneumonia.

Richard Lower was born in 1631 and, like Willis, was educated at Christchurch, Oxford, proceeding to M.A. in 1655 and M.D. in 1665. It is clear from Willis' writings and also from letters of Richard Lower that a great part of the anatomical dissection and some of the drawings in *Cerebri Anatome* were done by Lower. Willis himself in the preface to his book gives fulsome acknowledgment: "And here I made use of the Labours of the most Learned Physician and highly skilled Anatomist, Dr. Richard Lower, for my help and Companion; the edge of whose Knife and Wit I willingly acknowledge to have been a help to me for the better searching out both the frame and offices of before hidden Bodies."

Sir Christopher Wren (1632–1723), originally a pupil of Willis, made many of the drawings in Willis' book. He probably did not draw those that illustrated the vascular supply of the spinal cord, which probably were drawn by Lower. At the time of this collaboration, Wren

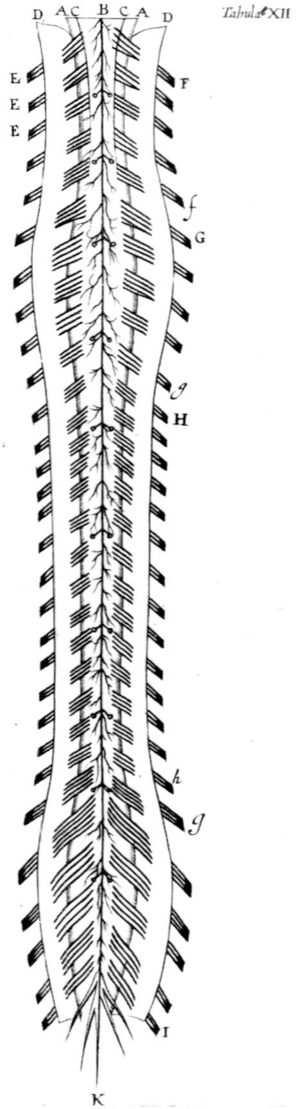

FIG. 1. Table XII from Willis' *Cerebri Anatome* (1664). The figure shows the anterior aspect of the spinal cord. The translated legend reads "Shows the Spinal Marrow whole taken out of its bony Den, and half taken from the Membrane cloathing it." The letter *B* signifies "The Spinal Artery seen to descend through the whole marrow which however is made up of Arteries, brought into it from between several joyntings of the Vertebrae."

was Savilian Professor of Astronomy at Oxford and, from mathematics, astronomy, and science, he was now turning to architecture, being busy with the designs of the new Sheldonian Theatre. One further contribution of Wren should be noted. Wren devised various techniques for carrying out intravenous injections in animals, and these methods were used in the first successful blood transfusion in man by Richard Lower and Edmund King. Injections of india ink and other fluids were used with considerable advantage by both Willis and Lower to show up the blood vessels to the brain and spinal cord. Wren contributed by advice and assistance in these injection studies.

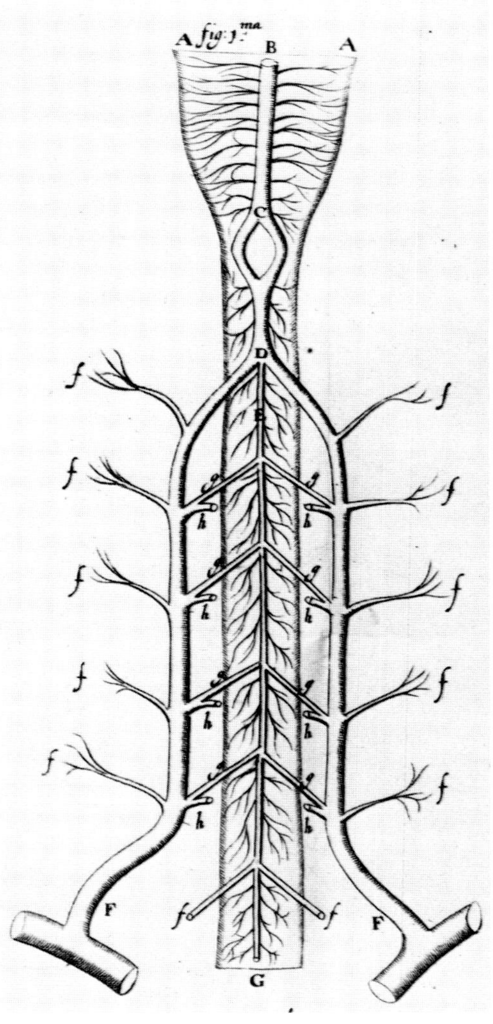

FIG. 2. Table XIII, figure 1, from Willis' *Cerebri Anatome* (1664). The figure shows the vertebral arteries and their branches forming the anterior spinal artery. The translated legend reads "Shows the branchings forth of the Vertebral Artery reaching out on both sides into the superior parts of the Spinal Marrow." The letter *D* signifies "The first joyning together of the Vertebral Artery above the spinal Marrow, from which place the spinal Artery descends." The letter *g* represents "Shoots sent in the Spinal Marrow which joyn together from either side in the Spinal Marrow nigh the several joynings of the Vertebrae." The letters *f* are given as "Two Arteries sent down from the Aorta into the Spine."

Thomas Millington (1628–1704) graduated at Trinity College, Cambridge, and moved to Oxford in 1657 when he took his M.D. He was elected a Fellow of All Souls in 1659. In the preface to his book, Willis describes the contribution of Millington and Wren in terms that suggest that their contribution was equal. He said "it becomes me not to hide how much besides I did receive from these most famous Men, Dr. Thomas Millington, Doctor in Physick and Dr. Chr Wren, Doctor of Laws and Savill Professor of Astronomy; both which were wont frequently to be present at our Dissections and to confer and reason about the uses of the Parts. Besides the former most Learned Man, to whom I from day to day proposed privately my Conjectures and Observations, often confirmed me by his Suffrage, being uncertain in my mind, and not trusting to my own opinion. But the other most renowned Man, Dr. Wren, was pleased out of his singular humanity, wherewith he abounds, to delineate with his own most skillful hands many Figures of the Brain and Skull, whereby the work might be more exact."

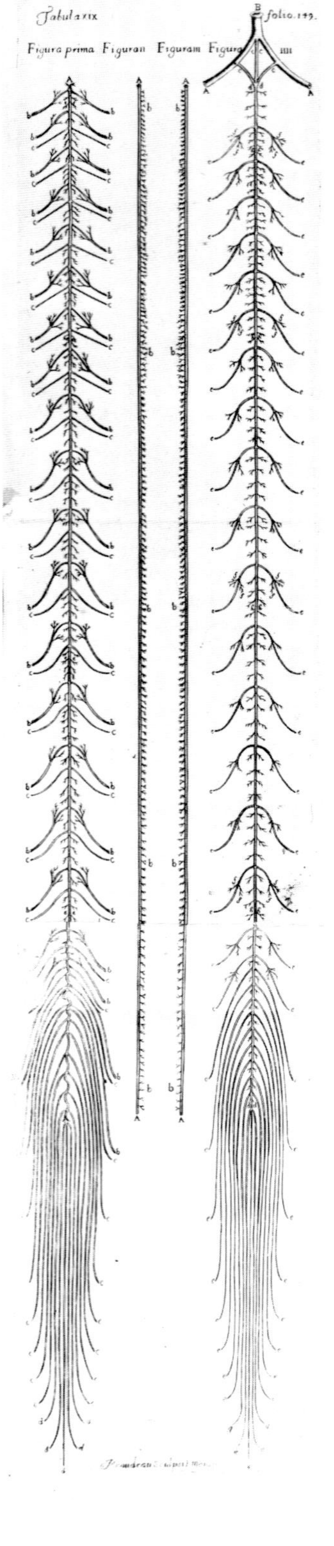

FIG. 3. Tabula XIX, folio 149, from Vieussens' *Neurographia Universolis* (1684), Lugdum, Joannen Certe. The figures show the anterior (right) and posterior (left) spinal arteries.

To summarize the distribution of work, Willis appears to have been the originator and driving force behind the anatomical work, Richard Lower was the skillful prosector, preparing and injecting specimens and possibly drawing some of them, and Christopher Wren made a major contribution by his technique of injecting, and also in the drawings, some of which have a distinctive style attributed to him. Millington was an anatomist of profound knowledge and was of considerable help in discussion on the structure and function of the brain.

THE ANATOMICAL WORK

The work of anatomical dissection was based on necropsies of patients, and these frequently had been in the practice of the group of doctors concerned. In some accounts, symptoms and signs of a terminal illness are given, and in one famous example, the necropsy revealed a cerebral hemorrhage. Doubtless these necropsies were used as opportunities for anatomical dissection. Preservation of the tissue was probably obtained by the use of spirits of wine, which was pioneered by Robert Boyle in Oxford. Willis and Lower probably injected the preservative into the vessels as well as using it for immersion, a considerable advance in preserving the brain, which consequently was spared the distortion evident in earlier work.

The examination of the spinal arteries was far from easy. Willis writes "But by what means these Vessels proceed on both sides from the Trunk of the Vertebral artery, and also the blood-carrying Veins, which are destinated to the whole spinal Marrow, and the inferior portion of its arterious passages, doth not so plainly appear; because the boney Cloisters of the Vertebra are not broken through without much labour, especially in grown up living Creatures; and in that work the beginnings and branchings out of very many Vessels are want to be blotted out." Willis resorted, as many have since, to fetal material: "But that we might more accurately search in these hid things, we made the Dissections of several Embryons, in which we are able to dissect the Vertebrae as yet soft, and to take out of them the Marrow whole, and look more narrowly into all the recesses of the bones." Willis and Lower indicate clearly the success of their injection experiments by this passage: "further, that all the tracts and branchings out of them might be the better perceived in all the Vessels, we did cast in divers coloured Liquors. And we had our desired wish: for presently we found with much admiration, that those kind of vessels, viz. arteries, Bosoms, and veins which respect the head, belong also the spinal marrow with no less a noted disposition of provision." Willis is clear that the vertebral arteries not only supply the hinder part of the brain but also the upper part of the spinal cord. "But the Vertebral Artery pays to the superior part of the Spine as great Tributes of Blood as to the Head itself." Willis also understood that while the vertebral arteries supplied the upper part of the spinal cord, the supply below came directly from the aorta. The following passage is crucial: "The Arteries which carry the Blood toward the Spine, are disposed after one manner above the Heart, and after another below it. As to the first, whereas the Trunk of the Aorta being there cleft presently to many branches, departs from the Region of the Spine, therefore the Vertebral Artery is produced on both sides from its axillary branches, which ascending straight into the hinder part of the Head sends forth a branch into the meeting together of every Vertebra. But below the Heart, forasmuch as the Aorta, in its whole descent, lyeth on the Spine, two arteries are received into the Spine from its bottom nigh its Internodia or spaces between the knots of the Vertebrae; so that if the trunk of the Aorta be cut open long-ways, there will appear a series of double holes through its whole tract."

THE ANATOMICAL ILLUSTRATIONS

The pictures of the spinal cord vascular supply appear in tables 12 and 13. Table 12 is an anterior aspect of the spinal cord seen after the dura has been opened in the midline and

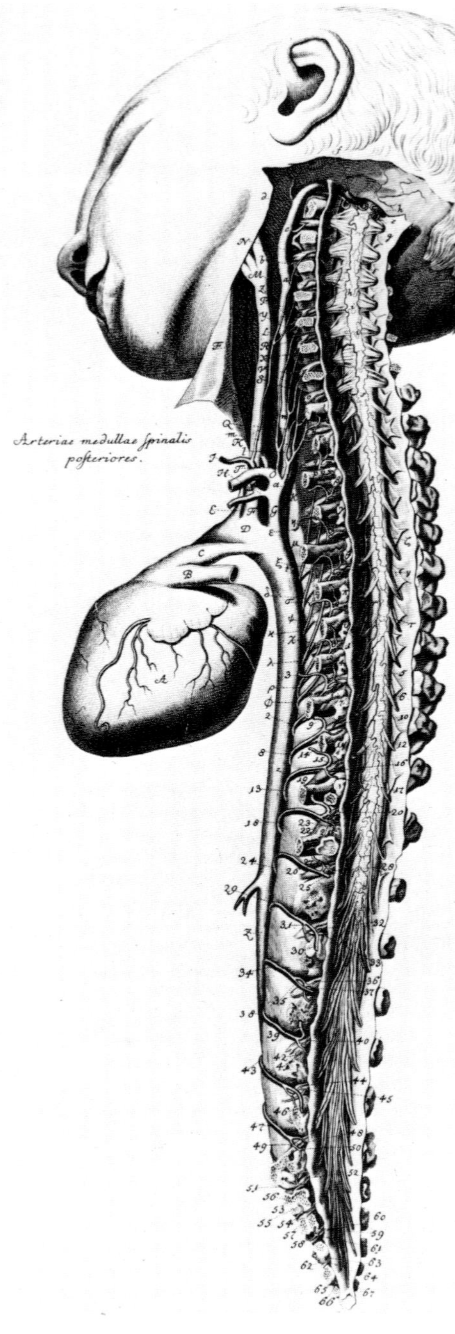

FIG. 4. Tabula IV from Haller's *Iconum Anatomicarum Corporis Humani* (1754), Göttingen. The figure shows a drawing of a dissected and injected specimen displaying the anterior spinal arteries.

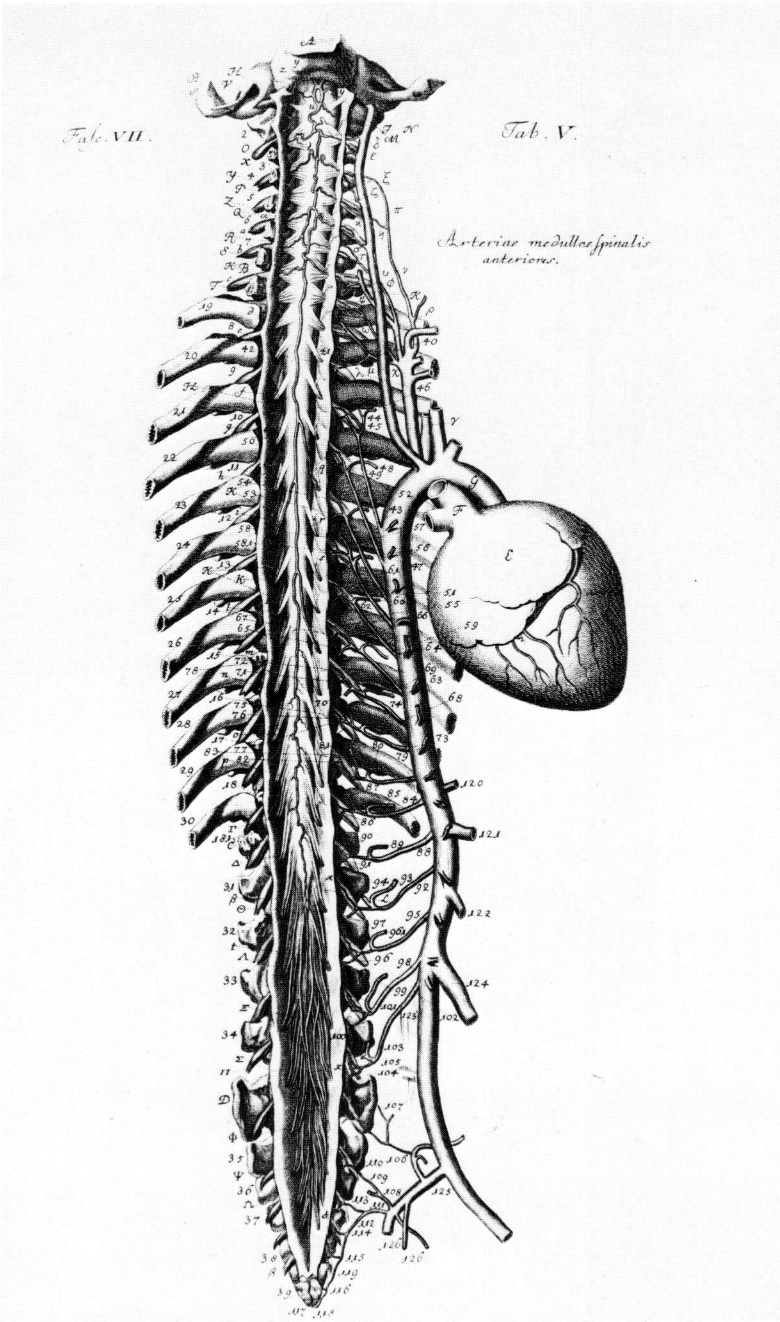

FIG. 5. Tabula V from Haller's *Iconum Anatomicarum Corporis Humani* (1754), Göttingen. The figure shows a drawing of a dissected and injected specimen displaying the posterior spinal arteries.

reflected. The appearances are those of the spinal cord of a human or animal fetus, the nerve roots of which enter and exit almost transversely through the dural sleeves. The 13a table contains five important parts. Figure 1 of table 13 is the famous illustration showing the origin of the anterior spinal artery from tributaries of both vertebral arteries. This figure shows a considerable understanding of the anatomical complexity of the spinal cord vasculature. A modern criticism would be that the anterior spinal cord artery and its tributaries are shown as regular structures with equal tributaries, whereas they are irregular with grossly differing size of the arterial tributary vessels. Figure 2 also shows the spinal veins, the upper part of which are shown to drain into the jugular veins. Figure 3 shows the posterior aspect of spinal arteries throughout the whole extent of the cord, and the plexus of arterial tributaries are indicated. Again the error is in portraying them as regular mathematically arranged structures. Figure 4 shows the plexus of veins throughout the spinal canal. Figure 5 is a detail of a venous sinus in a dog.

THE BOOK

The work referred to above was published in a book that has attained great fame, and some words about its production are of interest. The text was written by Willis and the drawings are by Richard Lower and Christopher Wren, possibly with additions by Willis and others. Probably completed in 1663, the work was first published in 1664. The first edition was in quarto, was published by John Martyn and James Allestry, who used the printer James Fletcher of London for the quarto edition, and Thomas Roycroft for a cheaper octavo edition, also produced in 1664. Fifteen plates were included in the first edition, and the engraver was probably David Loggan, who lived near Oxford at that time and subsequently became engraver to Oxford University. Plates 12 and 13 are those with the illustrations of the blood supply of the spinal cord, but these are the last two plates, as two unnumbered plates were inserted following plates 6 and 8.

Following the first two London editions, there were several Amsterdam editions, beginning with one also issued in 1664. The contemporary importance of the work is emphasized by the number of editions that followed, and these have been analyzed by H. R. Denham of the Wellcome Historical Medical Library. The only English translation is Samuel Pordage's, first published in London in 1681 in a collected work entitled "The Remaining Medical Works of Dr. Thomas Willis." This is now accessible in a facsimilie edition published by the McGill University Press in 1965 and edited by William Feindel. This modern work is in two volumes, and the first volume contains valuable notes by Feindel on Willis, his work, and his medical and scientific colleagues.

THOMAS WILLIS' SUCCESSORS

The publication of the work described above, on the anatomy of the spinal cord vessels, was followed by several similar accounts. Most of these accounts, until that of von Haller, were derived from Willis.

Gerard Blasius (1626–1692) knew the works of Thomas Willis well and reedited them for publication in Amsterdam. His own book *Anatome Medullae Spinalis, et nervorum* was published in 1666 and contains the same plate that appeared in Willis' book. Although he made his own observations on the spinal cord vessels, he is chiefly known for his distinction of the anterior and posterior nerve roots and the gray matter from the white matter of the spinal cord. Molinetti, in his work *Dissertationes anatomico-pathologicae* in 1675, described the union of two spinal branches of the vertebral arteries into one "rete mirabile," which he called the spinal artery. He showed how several small branches of the vertebral artery and the descending aorta contribute to the spinal artery.

Vieussens (1684) studied the vascular supply of the spinal cord. He produced many drawings of his findings, and these showed the anterior spinal artery beginning as a union of three tributaries, one from each vertebral artery and one from the basilar artery. He drew the anterior spinal artery as a regular longitudinal structure with regular tributaries accompanying each spinal nerve root and in this way perpetuated the error of Willis. He also studied the vessels of the posterior aspect of the spinal cord and showed how the cephalic origin of these was from a vessel on each side arising from a cerebellar artery. He drew the posterior spinal arteries as a single vessel throughout most of their course with regular tributaries accompanying each posterior nerve root. In this regular reinforcement of the spinal cord blood supply of the posterior spinal artery, Vieussens made errors similar to those of Willis.

I shall close this chapter with a note on the work of Albrecht von Haller (1708–1777). Albrecht von Haller was an admirer of Willis and first used the phrase "circle of Willis." He studied with great care the spinal cord vascular supply, making drawings remarkable in quality and accuracy (see Figs. 4,5). Although he undoubtedly knew of the works of Thomas Willis, his studies show no evidence of following earlier errors, and with his diagrams we arrive at the understanding of the spinal cord blood supply that we have today.

ACKNOWLEDGMENT

I wish to acknowledge the administrators of the Bodleian Library, Oxford, England, for the use of the reproductions of the illustrations that appear in this chapter.

Historical Aspects of the Neurosciences,
edited by F. Clifford Rose and W. F. Bynum.
Raven Press, New York ©

History of Syringomyelia

J. B. Foster

Department of Neurology, Newcastle University, Newcastle General Hospital, Newcastle, England

It is generally accepted that Estienne (1) in *La Dissection des Parties du Corps Humain* (1546) first described cavitation of the spinal cord. Many years later, Portal (2) recognized the clinical phenomena associated with cavitation but the pathology of the cavitation had been described by Brunner (3) in 1688 and Morgagni (4) in 1761, respectively, in a child and an adult. Schliep (5) would have us believe that the first clinical description of syringomyelia concerned the Roman, Mucius Scaevola, who apparently demonstrated his fearlessness to the King of the Etruscans, Porsenna, when he put his hand into a blaze. The term "syringomyelia" is credited to Charles P. Ollivier d'Angers (6), when in a monograph entitled *La Moelle Épinière et ses Maladies*, published in 1824, he described the pathological dilatation of the central canal of the cord in continuity with the cavity of the fourth ventricle. Syringomyelia denotes cavity formation in the cord. In a later two-volume work, *Traité de la Moelle Épinière et de ses Maladies*, he described cord cavitation, "Syringomyelie ou cavite centrale dans la moelle," and this is cited as the first published use of the term "syringomyelia" by Ballantine et al. (7).

Ollivier used the term to describe pathological dilatation of the central canal as a developmental anomaly. After Stilling (8) had demonstrated in 1859 that the central canal could persist in childhood and into the adult life of all vertebrates, conditions of pathological dilatation came to be referred to as hydromyelia and the term "syringomyelia" was less commonly used [Gull (9), Schüppel (10), Virchow (11)]. Central cord cavities seen in pathological specimens unconnected with the central canal and associated with myelitis were described by Hallopeau (12) in 1870 and telangietatic tumors and gliosis were recognized, with Simon (13), suggesting in 1875 that the term "syringomyelia" be reserved for such cavities and that hydromyelia be restricted to dilatation of the central canal. Leyden (14) offered the suggestion that the two conditions were identical, and this view was supported by Virchow (15) in 1863 and Kahler and Pick (16) in 1879. Schultze (17) gave an account of the clinical syndrome in 1882, outlining the clinicopathological correlation between cysts of the cord and the clinical symptomatology and, in particular, stressing the reduced sensibility to pain and temperature, i.e., dissociated sensory loss. Although earlier descriptions of the features of the condition had been offered by Gull (9), Clarke (18), and Clarke and Johnson (19), the clinical presentation of syringomyelia was well recognized and fully described by Gowers (20) in his *Manual of Diseases of the Nervous System* (1886). Many other clinical descriptions followed, notably those of Bäumler (21), Hoffmann (22), and Schlesinger (23). Today's clinician believes that the symptom complex of syringomyelia follows a characteristic pattern and a similar course and prognosis [Schaltenbrand (24), Andre (25), Alsen (26), Wells et al. (27), Erbslöh (28), and McIlroy and Richardson (29)].

The unitary hypothesis of the pathogenesis of syringomyelia was supported by Chiari (30) in 1888. He confirmed that in most cases the syrinx connects with the central canal of the cord. The description by Langhans (31) in 1881 of a case associated with cerebellar deformity was followed by Chiari's description in 1891 of the anomolies associated with congenital hydrocephalus, "concerning changes in the cerebellum due to hydrocephalus of the cerebrum." Chiari divided the eponymous malformations into three anatomical categories of increasing severity. In the first group (type I), he described an extension of the cerebellar tonsils into the spinal canal. He later (32) described 14 further cases, some with an associated hydromyelia. It was many years before Russell and Donald (33) in 1935 noted the association between hydromyelia and the Chiari malformation. Gardner and Goodall (34) found hydromyelia in 13 out of 17 adult cases of Chiari malformation in 1950.

In a series of papers from Cleveland (35–39), W. J. Gardner and his colleagues suggested what has come to be known as the hydrodynamic theory of the development of syringomyelia. Cystic dilatation of the cord originates in embryonal life and results from overdistention of the central cavity in the neural tube because of a partial or complete obstruction at the foramen of Magendie. Resulting dilatation of the central canal (hydromyelia) or a ramifying diverticulum (10) was the product. In Gardner's 74 cases of syringomyelia, obstruction at the foramen of Magendie was due to a Chiari malformation in 68, Dandy-Walker malformation in three, and a cyst in a further three.

Gardner's theory has been reviewed by Newton (40, 41) and others, notably Bernard Williams (42) and the Newcastle Group (43). In 1973, we were able to record our clinical experience with a consecutive 100 cases of syringomyelia with pathological material available and the results of surgical management of those associated with Chiari malformation.

It is now generally accepted that syringomyelia may be broadly classified into groups. First, there is the so-called communicating syringomyelia, where there are associated developmental anomalies of the foramen magnum or in the posterior fossa, and those associated with acquired abnormalities at the base of the skull, i.e., arachnoiditis, posterior fossa tumors, and cysts. Noncommunicating syringomyelia is a late sequel to trauma of the spinal cord, and there is a form of syringomyelia associated with tumors of the cord, either intramedullary or extramedullary. There is a final variety, making up 8% of cases, where none of the above named abnormalities can be demonstrated, where myelography is normal. These constitute an uncertain group of idiopathic cases of syringomyelia.

With a prevalence of 8.4 per 100,000, the disease is rare, but recent investigation and surgical treatment has led to the belief that early recognition will allow arrest of the progressive dissection of the cord following upon breeching of the dilated central canal. Most authorities now agree that syringomyelia is a complication of hydromyelia secondary to an anomaly at the foramen magnum, i.e., the Chiari malformation or hindbrain hernia, and the argument of the true pathogenesis is frequently enjoined. We have, to date, in Newcastle, had the opportunity to study 180 cases. Many of these have been subjected to operative decompression at the foramen magnum and the results were subsequently reported. Recent concern involves the role of birth trauma in the genesis of syringomyelia; again our findings are to be reported separately.

The pathological and clinical descriptions of this rare but classical neurological disease have not been bettered in recent reviews, but due to Gardner's interest in the condition and subsequent interest expressed by Conway (44), Appleby et al. (45), and colleagues in the United Kingdom, we have come to understand much more about the pathogenesis of the communicating variety of syringomyelia. Recent advances in radiology, in particular the use of metrizamide myelography, and the combined use of metrizamide myelography and

CAT scanning has allowed not only the demonstration of the filling defect at the foramen magnum, but the visualization of the tonsillar tissue itself, the cavitated and dilated spinal cord and, in some cases, on CAT scanning, contrast medium in the syrinx.

REFERENCES

1. Estienne, C. (1546): *La Dissection des Parties du Corps Humain*, Chap. 3. Simon de Colines, Paris.
2. Portal, A. (1804): *Cours d'Anatomie Médicale*, Vol. 4, pp. 111–120, Baudouin, Paris.
3. Brunner, J. C. (1688): In: Boneti, T. (1700), *Sepulchretum Book*, 2nd ed. Vol. 1, p. 396, Cramer & Perachon, Geneva.
4. Morgagni, G. B. (1761): *De sedibus et causis morborum* (The Seats and Causes of Disease) translated by B. Alexander. Millar and Cadel, London (1769).
5. Schliep, G., and Ritter, J. (1971): *Fortschr. Neurol. Psychiat.*, 39:53–82.
6. Ollivier d'Angers, C. P. (1824): *De le Moelle Épinière et de ses Maladies*, p. 116. Paris: Chez Crevot, Paris.
7. Ballantine, H. T., Jr., Ojemann, R. G., and Drew, J. H. (1971): *Progr. Neurol. Surg.* 4:227–245.
8. Stilling, B. (1859): *Neue Untersuchungen über den Bau des Ruckenmarks*, pp. 13–19. Hotop, Kassel.
9. Gull, W. W. (1862): *Guys Hosp. Rep.*, 3rd ser., 8:244.
10. Schüppel, O. (1865): *Arch. Heilk.*, 6:289–315.
11. Virchow, R. (1863): *Arch. Pathol. Anat. Physiol.*, 27:575.
12. Hallopeau, F. H. (1870): *Gaz. Méd. Paris*, 25:183.
13. Simon, T. (1875): *Arch. Psychiat. Nervenkr.*, 5:120.
14. Leyden, E. (1876): *Arch. Pathol. Anat. Physiol.*, 68:1.
15. Virchow, R. (1863): *Arch. Pathol. Anat. Physiol.*, 27:575.
16. Kahler, O., and Pick, A. (1879): *Vjschr. prakt. Heilk*, 142:20–41.
17. Schultze, F. (1882): *Virchows Arch. Pathol. Anat.*, 87:510–540.
18. Clarke, J. L. (1865): *Med.-Chir. Trans.*, 48:255.
19. Clarke, J. L., and Johnson, Z. (1869): *Med.-Chir. Trans.*, 51:249.
20. Gowers, W. J. (1886): *A Manual of Diseases of the Nervous System*, Vol. 1, p. 433. Churchill, London.
21. Bäumler, A. (1887): *Deutsche Arch. Klin. Med.*, 40:443.
22. Hoffman, J. (1893): *Deutsche Z. Nervenheil.*, 3:427.
23. Schlesinger, H. (1902): *Die Syringomyelie*. Deuticke, Leipzig and Vienna.
24. Schaltenbrand, G. (1951): Syringomyelie. In: *Lehrbuch der Neurolgie*, p. 147. Georg Thieme, Stuttgart.
25. André, M. J. (1951): *Acta Neurol. Psychiat. Belg.*, 51:665.
26. Alsen, V. (1957): *Deutsche Z. Nervenheil.*, 177:156.
27. Wells, C. E. C., Spillane, J. D., and Bligh, A. S. (1959): *Brain*, 82:23.
28. Erbslöh, F. (1963): In: *Differential diagnose neurologische Krankheit*, edited by G. Bodechtal, p. 710. Georg Thieme, Stuttgart.
29. McIlroy, W. C., and Richardson, J. C. (1965): *Canad. Med. Assoc. J.*, 93:731.
30. Chiari, H. (1888): *Deutsche Med. Wocherschr.*, 17:1172.
31. Langhans, T. (1881): *Arch. Pathol. Anat. Physiol.*, 85:1.
32. Chiari, H. (1896): *Denkschr. Acad. Wiss. Wien*, 63:71.
33. Russell, D. S., and Donald, C. (1935): *Brain*, 58:203.
34. Gardner, W. J., and Goodall, R. J. (1950): *J. Neurosurg.*, 7:199.
35. Gardner, W. J., Abdullah, A. F., and McCormack, L. J. (1957): *J. Neurosurg.*, 14:591.
36. Gardner, W. J., Karnosh, L. J., and Angel, J. (1957): *Trans. Am. Neurol. Assoc.*, 82:144.
37. Gardner, W. J., and Angel, J. (1958): *Clin. Neurosurg.*, 6:131.
38. Gardner, W. J. (1965): *J. Neurol. Neurosurg. Psychiat.*, 28:247.
39. Gardner, W. J. (1967): *Clin. Neurosurg.*, 15:57.
40. Newton, E. J. (1962): *J. Neurol. Neurosurg. Psychiat.*, 25:185.
41. Newton, E. J. (1969): *Ann. Roy. Coll. Surgeons of England*, 44:194.
42. Williams, B. (1970): *Lancet*, ii:41.
43. Barnett, H. J. M., Foster, J. B., and Hudgson, P. H. (1973): *Syringomyelia*, W. B. Saunders, Philadelphia.
44. Conway, L. W. (1961): *Trans. Am. Neurol. Assoc.*, 86:206.
45. Appleby, A. et al. (1968): *Brain*, 91:131.

Historical Aspects of the Neurosciences,
edited by F. Clifford Rose and W. F. Bynum.
Raven Press, New York ©

Historical Concepts of Spinal Cord Pathways Subserving Pain

Robin Illingworth

Charing Cross Hospital, London, and The Regional Department of Neurosurgery, Central Middlesex Hospital, London, United Kingdom

The recognition of the spinal cord as a large nerve has been ascribed to Galen, who believed that it functioned in two separate halves related to the same sides of the body. Little further advance in understanding its functions occurred until the early 19th century, when Sir Charles Bell, François Magendie, and others elucidated the function of the spinal nerve roots and suggested corresponding division of functions of the anterior and posterior spinal columns.

Paul Broca, writing on the animal experiments of Brown-Séquard in 1855 (1), had a more modern concept of the intricacies of spinal cord function when he described it as "a nervous centre with its own action, and a pathway designed to put the organs in communication with the brain." He recognized that reflex actions occurred in the central gray matter and that the posterior white matter columns were concerned with sensory conduction, and the anterior and lateral columns with motor functions. These concepts of unilateral functions and broad anatomical divisions for motor and sensory functions were overturned by the animal experiments of Brown-Séquard, performed originally on rabbits, and later repeated before a committee of scientific observers, including Paul Broca and Claude Bernard, on a variety of animals, including horses, sheep, and pigs (1). Various spinal cord sections were performed on unanesthetised animals, and the general conclusions were that division of the posterior columns produced increased sensitivity of the body below the level of section and that division of all the spinal cord except the posterior columns resulted in loss of sensation.

Within a few years, clinical verification of these observations was made by Dr. John Ogle, Physician to St. George's Hospital, who in 1859 described seven patients with partial spinal cord lesions (2). Ogle recognized that the posterior columns were not the sole route for sensation and that at least some sensory fibers decussated at every level immediately after entry into the spinal cord. It is clear from reading these accounts that Ogle was aware of dissociated sensory loss and that some touch sensation could be retained despite loss of pain sensation. This new concept, that as a result of spinal cord injury, a part of the body could lose appreciation of one modality of sensation while retaining others, took some years to be appreciated, and even Brown-Séquard, writing nearly 10 years later and describing cases of spinal hemiplegia, appears to have been unaware of the concept of dissociated sensory loss (3). Brown-Séquard described cases of hemiplegia with contralateral sensory loss, but he made no distinction between pain and light touch sensations. He still felt that while sensation was lost on the opposite side to the cord injury, it was actually increased on the same side as the lesion.

During the next 40 years, as a result of clinical observations often confirmed by autopsy studies and increasingly by degeneration studies following selective spinal cord and nerve root sections in animals, these simple concepts of anatomical pathways in the spinal cord were refined and corrected. William Gowers, writing in his monograph *Diseases of the Spinal Cord* in 1881 (4), suggested that all sensations passed through the posterior columns, but that there was some evidence to suggest that pain passed via the lateral columns in animals; however, there was no evidence to suggest that this occurred in man. On the other hand, he demonstrated sections of the spinal cord showing the pattern of degeneration after a cord crushing injury, noting symmetrical degeneration in the anterolateral quadrant above the level of the crush, though he clearly did not recognize the significance of this. Writing later in 1886 (5), he again referred to the anterolateral ascending tract and stated that the fibers may come from the posterior roots of the opposite side, crossing in the posterior commissure of the cord. He described a unilateral lesion of the cord produced by a bullet wound at C3, causing compression of the cord by a spicule of bone, where he detected complete contralateral loss of pain, with intact sensation to light touch on both sides. He referred to a complementary case described by Kobner in 1885 (6), in which a stab wound of the spinal cord had divided both posterior columns and one-half of the spinal cord, producing bilateral loss of light touch and contralateral loss of pain sensation. Gowers also referred in his textbook to spinal tumors producing contralateral loss of pain sensation and suggested that one day such lesions might be removed surgically.

In 1895, Frederick Mott, Lecturer in Physiology and Physician at Charing Cross Hospital, described the results of degeneration studies on the spinal cord following unilateral sections of lumbosacral roots in seven monkeys and one cat (7). He was able to demonstrate degeneration in the ipsilateral posterior column and also occasionally in the contralateral anterolateral quadrant. He was uncertain of the significance of this latter observation, but he suggested that the pathway for pain and temperature might be separate from light touch and could be through the cord gray matter via the anterior commissure to the anterolateral quadrant of the cord and hence to the lateral lemniscus. The anatomical evidence for this pathway had previously been reviewed by Edinger in 1890 (8), and a large collected clinical series of 93 partial spinal cord injuries was reviewed by Petren in 1910 (9). Head and Thompson in 1906 (10) published meticulous records of sensory loss in patients with spinal cord lesions, and proposed their concept of protopathic and epicritic sensory pathways.

Interesting as these observations were in relation to spinal cord function, the therapeutic possibilities for the relief of pain appear to have been first recognized by Spiller, Professor of Neuropathology and Assistant Professor of Neurology at the University of Pennsylvania, in a case report of a patient with bilateral tuberculomas of the spinal cord (11). The opening sentence in this paper, published in 1905, 50 years after the report of Brown-Séquard's animal experiments, reads as follows: "Many believe the tracts of Gowers may contain the fibres for the sensations of pain and temperature, but evidence supporting this opinion has been sadly deficient." Spiller described a patient with spinal tuberculosis with normal light touch sensation in the lower limbs but bilateral absence of pain and temperature sensations, and he was able to show at autopsy bilateral tuberculomas involving only the anterolateral quadrants of the spinal cord. This was for him conclusive proof, and six years later he persuaded Dr. E. Martin to operate on a 47-year-old man with a spinal cord tumor producing flaccid paralysis of the legs and also severe pain. Initial exploration in November 1909 showed the tumor to be inoperable, and on January 19, 1911, bilateral anterolateral cordotomies were performed in the middorsal region with relief of pain in the legs for two months (12). Spiller and Martin described the cut as being 2 × 2 mm, 3 mm anterior to the entry of the posterior roots, and they suggested that unilateral cordotomy might be suitable for unilateral pain and that cordotomy should be made sufficiently high to allow for decussation of the fibers within the spinal cord. They asked whether sensibility to heat and cold may be lost independently, and also asked: "Are fibres of pain confined to one system within the spinal cord, and if so can pain sensation be conveyed by other systems when the fibres usually employed for the purpose are destroyed?" We are still asking this question today.

Although the account Spiller and Martin gave in their paper does not read very convincingly, it clearly initiated anterolateral cordotomy as a surgical procedure for the relief of pain, and Frazier, writing in 1920 (13), described six more cases with successful relief of pain for up to three years. He described the surgical technique in detail and gave an illustration of the extent of the cordotomy, which I am sure must be erroneous. Clearly, if he were to have made the section illustrated, this would be likely to produce paralysis of the ipsilateral leg with little prospect of contralateral pain relief.

Despite the opportunities for clinical observation in patients with therapeutic spinal cord lesions, progress in recognition of the anatomy of the spinal cord was slow. Foerster and Gagel (14), writing in 1932, illustrated the spinal cord with all sensations including light touch in the anterolateral quadrant, and the fibers arranged segmentally from the outside inward. This was also the view of Walker (15), who in 1940 produced what is probably the most generally accepted scheme of the anatomical arrangement of the fibers, but again he separated pain from temperature. At about the same time, Le Gros Clark (16) performed degeneration studies in the spinal cord and brain stem of the Macaque monkey and traced the ascending anterolateral tract through the lateral lemniscus as high as the thalamus.

The results of anterolateral cordotomy in man allowed other spinal cord functions to be identified. Peat (17) in 1933 was able to show that bilateral cervical cordotomy interfered with the descending respiratory pathways and could be associated with sudden death due to cessation of respiration. More recently, Nathan and Smith have studied patients after cordotomy to identify the pathways for bladder (18) and bowel (19) control and sensation and the descending respiratory pathways. White and Sweet (20) documented the results of cordotomy in terms of pain relief and such undesirable effects as limb weakness and sensory disturbance. They pointed out the tendency for pain and sensation to return in patients with pain due to nonfatal conditions, suggesting that alternative routes might be found within the spinal cord, the same question raised by Spiller and Martin in 1912. Anterolateral cordotomy for unilateral pain in the lower limbs remains a most satisfying and worthwhile procedure and has been modified by the introduction of a percutaneous method, initially proposed by Mullan et al. (21), using a radioactive source, and later modified by Rosomoff et al. (22) by the use of radiofrequency to make the lesion.

Looking back through the publications of 125 years, I have been impressed by two things. First, one notes the eminence of many of the authors who have contributed to this subject. Gowers, Mott, and Head were all Fellows of the Royal Society, and also holders of the Fothergillian Gold Medal, awarded triannually by the ancient Medical Society of London. I was also impressed by how slowly our understanding has evolved during this time and how little we still know about the anatomical pathways and physiological mechanisms concerned with pain perception. In conclusion, I would like to quote again from William Gowers: "Our knowledge of the sensory path in the cord is far less definite than that of the motor path." These words that were written nearly 100 years ago still appear to be relevant today.

REFERENCES

1. Broca, P. (1855): *Proprietés et Fonctions de la Moelle Epinière. Rapport sur quelques experiences de M. Brown-Séquard.* Bonaventure et Ducessais, Paris.
2. Ogle, J. W. (1859): *Br. For. Med.-Chir. Rev.*, 24:500.
3. Brown-Séquard, C. E. (1868): *Lancet*, 2:593, 659, 755, 821.
4. Gowers, W. R. (1881): *The diagnosis of Diseases of the Spinal Cord.* J. & A. Churchill, London.
5. Gowers, W. R. (1886): *A Manual of Diseases of the Nervous System, Vol. 1. Diseases of the Spinal Cord and Nerves.* J. & A. Churchill, London.
6. Kobner, H. (1885): *Deutsche Arch. Klin. Med.*, 19:169.
7. Mott, F. W. (1895): *Brain*, 18:1.
8. Edinger, L. (1890): *Deutsche Med. Wochenschrift.*, 16:421.
9. Petren, K. (1910): *Arch. Psychiat. Nervenkrankh.*, 47:495.
10. Head, H., and Thompson, T. (1906): *Brain*, 29:537.
11. Spiller, W. G. (1905): *J. Nerv. Ment. Dis.*, 32:318.
12. Spiller, W. G., and Martin, E. (1912): *J. Am. Med. Assoc.*, 58:1489.
13. Frazier, C. H. (1920): *Arch. Neurol. Psychiat.*, 4:137.
14. Foerster, O., and Gagel, O. (1932): *Z. gesamte Neurol. Psychiat.*, 138:1.
15. Walker, A. E. (1940): *Arch. Neurol. Psychiat.*, 43:284.
16. Clark, W. E. Le Gros (1936): *J. Anat.*, 71:7.
17. Peat, M. M., Kahn, E. A., and Allen, S. S. (1933): *J. Am. Med. Assoc.*, 100:448.
18. Nathan, P. W., and Smith, M. C. (1951): *J. Neurol. Neurosurg. Psychiat.*, 14:262.
19. Nathan, P. W., and Smith, M. C. (1953): *J. Neurol. Neurosurg. Psychiat.*, 16:245.
20. White, J. C., and Sweet, W. H. (1955): *Pain.* Charles C. Thomas, Springfield, Illinois.
21. Mullan, S., Harper, P. V., Hekmatpanah, J., Torres, H., and Dobbin, G. (1963): *J. Neurosurg.*, 20:931.
22. Rosomoff, H. L., Carroll, F., Brown, J., and Sheptak, P. (1965): *J. Neurosurg.*, 23:639.

Historical Aspects of the Neurosciences,
edited by F. Clifford Rose and W. F. Bynum.
Raven Press, New York ©

History of Muscle Disease

Victor Dubowitz

Department of Paediatrics and Neonatal Medicine, and Jerry Lewis Muscle Research Centre, Hammersmith Hospital, London, W.12, England

The name of Duchenne has become so intimately associated with the childhood form of muscular dystrophy that he has almost assumed the position of patron saint of muscle disease in childhood (Fig. 1). He described his first case in 1861, in the second edition of his famous book, *De l'électrisation localisée et de son application à la pathologie et à la thérapeutique*, under the title "Paraplégie hypertrophique de l'enfance de cause cerébrale" (1) (Fig. 2). Because of associated intellectual impairment in that child, Duchenne thought that the condition might have a cerebral origin. The following year, Duchenne (2) published a remarkable series of clinical photographs, in his *Album de Photographies Pathologiques*, perhaps all the more remarkable in that he personally was the photographer. The illustration of a child with "congenital muscle hypertrophy" is probably of his first case of muscular dystrophy (Fig. 3). Duchenne subsequently gave a comprehensive account of the disease, based on a study of 13 cases, in a series of papers in the *Archives Générales de Médecine*

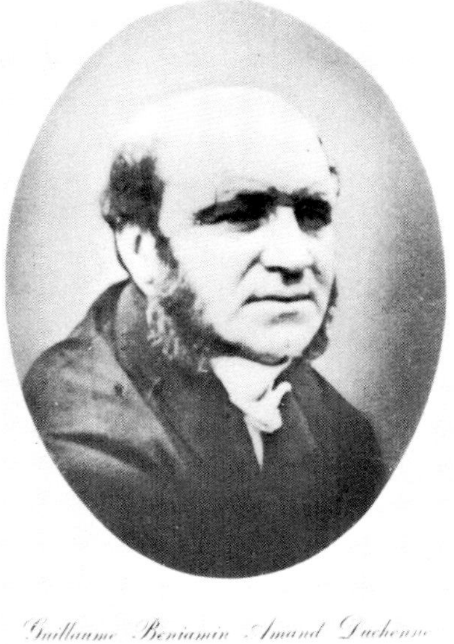

FIG. 1. Duchenne (de Boulogne).

in 1868 (3). He suggested the name "paralysie musculaire pseudohypertrophique" to draw attention to the unusual muscle enlargement in association with the muscle weakness and the term "paralysie myosclerosique" to highlight the extreme fibrosis in the muscle. In the third edition of *L'électrisation localisée*, published in 1872 (4), he included a comprehensive section on pseudohypertrophic muscular paralysis, together with some excellent illustrations.

Duchenne was looked upon as a somewhat eccentric physician, who came from a seafaring family in Boulogne. He studied medicine in Paris but in 1831 returned to practice in Boulogne until moving back to Paris in 1842. He had no formal appointment to any of the Parisian hospitals, but he was allowed to visit the outpatient clinics in order to apply his diagnostic procedures to a wide range of patients with chronic neurological disorders.

Duchenne made two other major contributions to medicine. He was the first to apply electricity to the study of disease, both from a diagnostic point of view and also from a therapeutic aspect, and he became a well-known figure around the clinics of the Paris hospitals carrying his little box of faradic stimulation equipment (Fig. 4). He was also the first to introduce biopsy as a technique into clinical medicine, and he designed his ingenious muscle biopsy needle (Fig. 5), which was the forerunner of all subsequent biopsy needles and which also bears a very close resemblance to the currently used Bergstrom type muscle biopsy needle (Fig. 6).

It seems to be axiomatic in medicine that if someone's name becomes attached to a particular disease, he inevitably turns out to be the second person to have described it. Muscular dystrophy is no exception. Pride of place for the first accurate and detailed description should probably go to a London physician, Meryon, who in 1852, some 10 years ahead of Duchenne, described in lucid detail a family in which four boys were affected with the condition (5). Meryon had a flair for clinical description, and one can practically visualize

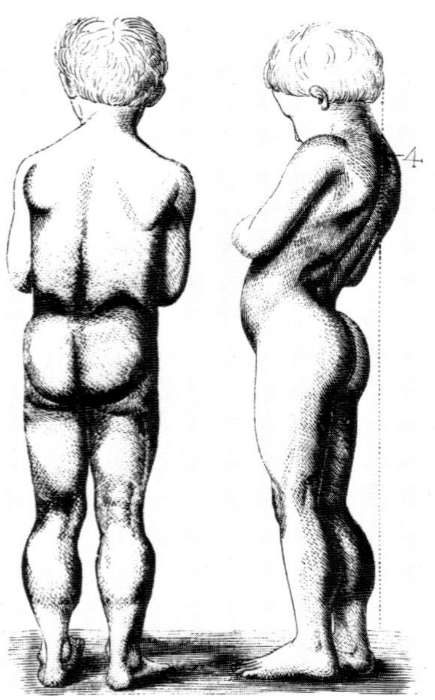

FIG. 2. Illustration of child in the second edition of Duchenne's *De l'électrisation localisée* (1). Note that the figure on the left is identical to that in Fig. 3.

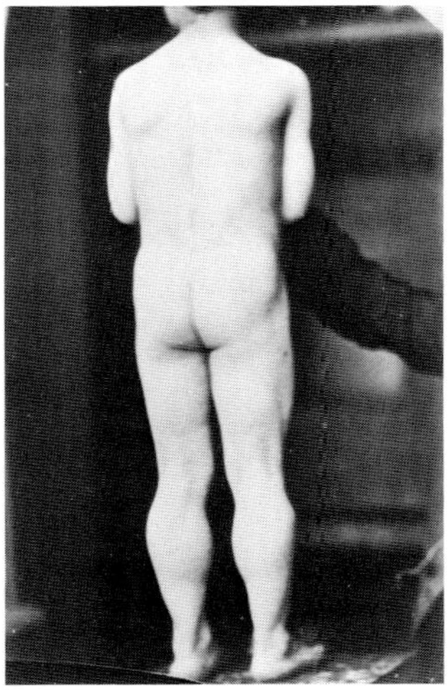

FIG. 3. Photograph taken by Duchenne of child with "congenital muscle hypertrophy." This is probably the first case of muscular dystrophy referred to by Duchenne (1).

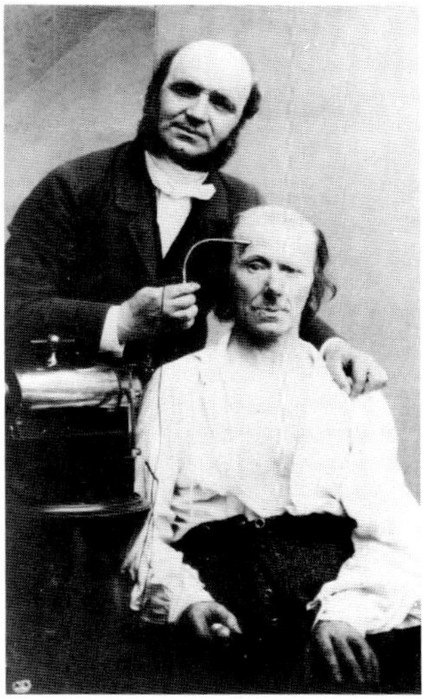

FIG. 4. Duchenne applies faradism to a patient (model ?).

the progression of the disease in his record of one of his patients: "In May 1847, when nearly nine years of age, he walked from Bruton Street to Westminster Bridge, but in November 1848, he could neither walk nor stand, and in 1850 his arms were fast losing power." In addition to the superb clinical documentation, Meryon also pointed out the striking pathological changes within the muscle, on which his title, "On fatty and granular degeneration of the voluntary muscles," was based. He also did a necropsy on one of the cases and noted the apparent normality of the central nervous system.

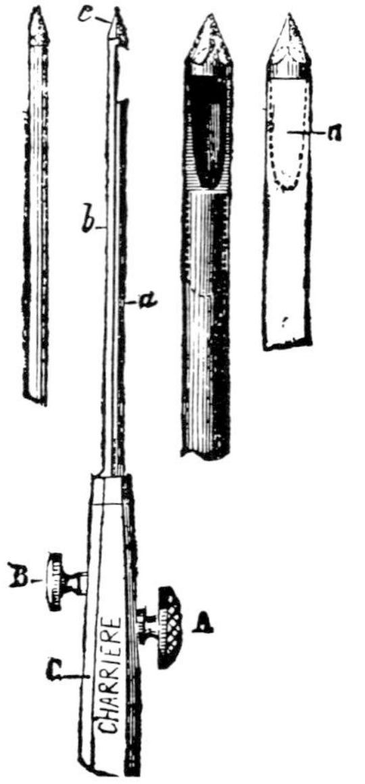

FIG. 5. Duchenne's biopsy needle.

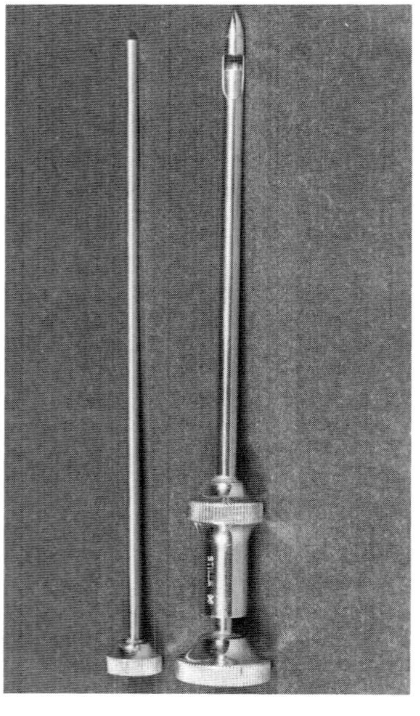

FIG. 6. Bergstrom's modern biopsy needle.

It is very difficult to find much detail on the life of Meryon, but judging from his obituary in the *Lancet* in 1880, he was obviously a well-known, well-liked, and respected physician. He trained at University College Hospital and in Paris, and he was Lecturer in Comparative Anatomy at St. Thomas's Hospital. He later was also appointed Physician to the Hospital for Epilepsy and Paralysis at Portland Terrace. In tracking his progress through sequential years of the Medical Register, one notes that in the year 1880 his address changes from "14

Clarges Street, W." to "14 Clarges Street, Mayfair, W. and Atheneum Club, Pall Mall." He had obviously made the grade!

Meryon was quite a prolific writer, and in 1864 he put together an interesting volume on various forms of paralysis (6). He also wrote an early book on the history of medicine but did not get further than the first volume (7). In addition to his medical career, he was also a Fellow of the Geological Society.

There may possibly be an even earlier description of muscular dystrophy. In the 1839 issue of *Schmidt's Jahrbücher der In-und Aüslandischen gesamenten Medicin* (8), Schmidt refers under the title "Krankhafte Hypertrophie des Muskelsystems" to the record by Coste and Gioja in the 1838 volume of the Italian journal *Annali Clinici dell'Ospedale degl'Incurabili Napoli* of two brothers with progressive weakness of the lower limbs starting at the age of 10 years and later becoming generalized and associated with striking enlargement of several muscles. I spent a very interesting day in the leather-bound isolation of the reading room of the British Museum but unfortunately failed to discover the paper by these authors in all five volumes of the journal published prior to 1839. In any event, the clinical description suggests that these two affected brothers may well have had a milder type of dystrophy, more closely resembling the Becker than the Duchenne type.

The next giant in the field of muscular dystrophy is undoubtedly Gowers, who gave us so much in clinical neurology. In 1879, he gave a series of five clinical lectures, delivered at the National Hospital for the Paralysed and Epileptic, to the students of University College, on "Pseudo-hypertrophic muscular paralysis," and he described with masterly clarity and color the features of 21 personal cases, and he reviewed a further 139 published cases of previous authors (9,10). His poetic and almost photographic word pictures of the disease have never been equaled (9):

> The disease is one of the most interesting,
> and at the same time most sad,
> of all those with which we have to deal;
> interesting on account of its peculiar features and mysterious nature;
> sad on account of our powerlessness to influence its course,
> except in a very slight degree,
> and on account of the conditions in which it occurs.
> It is a disease of early life and of early growth.
> Manifesting itself commonly at the transition from infancy to childhood,
> it develops with the child's development,
> grows with his growth—
> so that every increase in stature
> means an increase in weakness,
> and each year takes him a step further
> on the road to a helpless infirmity,
> and in most cases to an early and inevitable death.

Gowers also included some excellent illustrations of his patients (Figs. 7 and 8), and among these was the method by which children with Duchenne dystrophy get up from the floor (Fig. 9), now well known as the Gowers maneuver.

Gowers popularized the term "pseudo-hypertrophic," coined by Duchenne, and this remained in use until comparatively recently. It has now been dropped as a descriptive title, since it is not specific to the Duchenne type dystrophy but also occurs in many other forms of dystrophy, and indeed prominence of muscles may also be seen in some of the neurogenic atrophies such as spinal muscular atrophy (Kugelberg-Welander disease).

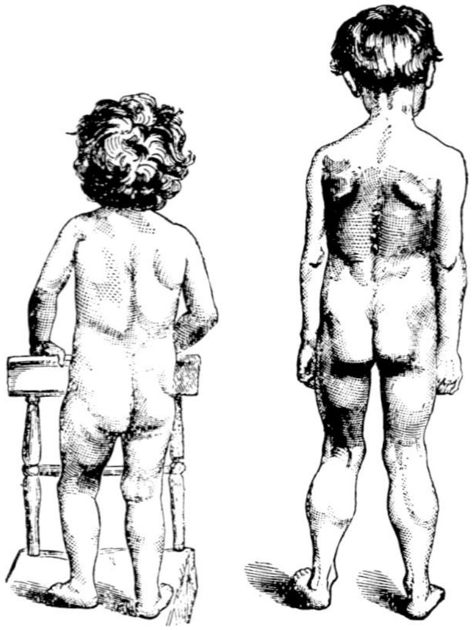

FIG. 7. Patient with "pseudo-hypertrophic paralysis." (From Gowers, ref. 10.)

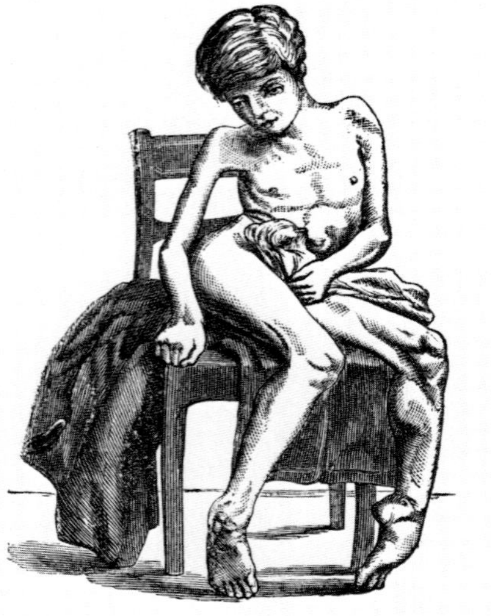

FIG. 8. Patient with "pseudo-hypertrophic paralysis." (From Gowers, ref. 10.)

There are a number of other names that have become associated with different forms of muscular dystrophy. In 1877, Leyden (11) drew attention to an atrophic pelvifemoral form of muscle weakness, and Möbius (12) subsequently commented on the similarity of this condition to the pseudohypertrophic muscular paralysis of Duchenne. These early descriptions formed the basis of the Leyden-Möbius, or limb girdle, form of muscular dystrophy.

Around that time, Erb in Heidelberg was also writing very prolifically about muscle disorders and in 1891 produced two articles on "dystrophia muscularum progressiva" in the first volume of *Deutsche Zeitschrift für Nervenheilkunde* (13), which ran to almost 200 pages. As Erb was also the editor of the journal, one presumes he may not have been subject

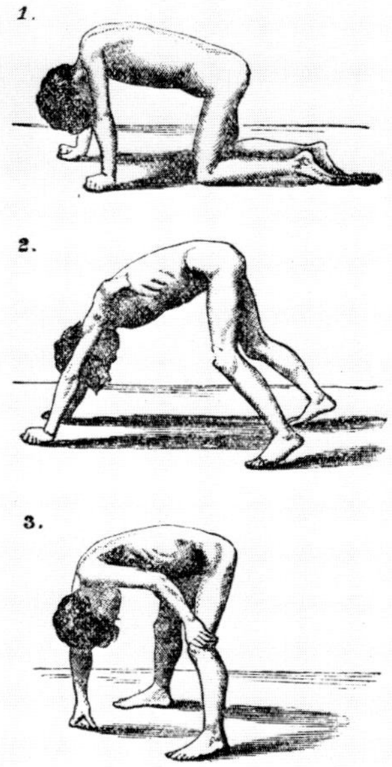

FIG. 9. Gowers' sign. (From Gowers, ref. 10.)

to the same constraints on space that contemporary authors would be. He was the first person to try to bring together all the different clinical forms of muscular dystrophy under one pathological blanket, and he gave an excellent description of the pathological changes. His name is usually associated with the so-called "juvenile form" of muscular dystrophy, which he considered distinct from those described before and affecting more the scapulohumeral than the pelvic girdle.

The names of Landouzy and Déjerine (14) are usually linked with the facioscapulohumeral type of myopathy, of which they gave an excellent description. They were in fact beaten to the post by Duchenne himself who, in the third edition of his book (4), had already described nine cases of this form of muscular paralysis and had pointed out the early involvement of the facial muscles, often before any limb girdle involvement. One of the cases in Duchenne's atlas (2) also looks like a facioscapulohumeral myopathy (Fig. 10).

There are a number of other eponymous diseases that I think are of interest and worthy of some comment. In a magnificently detailed and well-documented series of papers, Werdnig (15,16), of the Institute of Pathology of the University of Graz in Austria, and Hoffmann (17–20), attached to Erb's clinic in Heidelberg, described the infantile form of spinal muscular atrophy that bears their name. By striking contrast, in a rather poorly documented, brief and anecdotal paper, Oppenheim in Berlin (21) claimed to have seen a number of floppy infants who had a better prognosis than those with Werdnig-Hoffmann's disease. He suggested the term "myatonia congenita" for this condition, and this subsequently wreaked absolute havoc in the confusion and chaos in terminology that surrounded the floppy infant syndrome. Initially, Oppenheim's "myatonia congenita" became confused with myotonia congenita (Thomsen's disease), and Collier and Wilson (22) came to the rescue with the suggestion of an alternative title "amyotonia congenita." This remained firmly entrenched, particularly in the pediatric literature, until some 10 to 15 years ago but caused endless

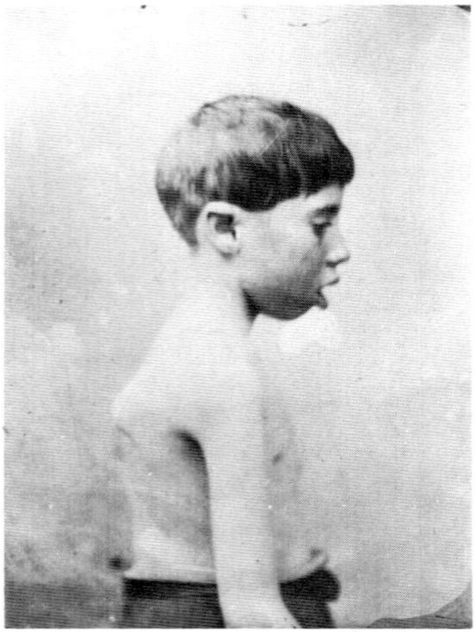

FIG. 10. Illustration from Duchenne's pathological photographs (2), showing child with facioscapulohumeral dystrophy.

confusion as many pediatricians used it synonymously with Werdnig-Hoffmann's disease, as did many of the early pathologists (23). Fortunately, with the more rigid and well-defined delineation of various neuromuscular disorders following the application of histochemistry and later electron microscopy to the analysis of muscle biopsies, nonspecific descriptive terms such as "amyotonia congenita," "Oppenheim's disease," and "universal muscular hypoplasia" have been appropriately relegated to oblivion (24).

The latter part of the 19th century and the turn of the century also saw the recognition of a number of additional muscle disorders. In 1876, Thomsen described "his" disorder, myotonia congenita (25). It was literally his disorder, as he had personally been affected, and it had been well recognized through five generations of his family. What in fact prompted Thomsen to document the disease, at the age of 61 years, was apparently the refusal of the Prussian army medical officers to accept Thomsen's medical certificate that his affected son, who had been conscripted into the Prussian army, was unfit for military service. Thomsen described the disease as "tonic cramps," and he also highlighted the "psychotic disposition," which ran concurrently in his family and which he considered an integral part of the condition. We now know that this was probably purely a coincidental feature.

In 1886, Wilhelm Erb wrote an exhaustive monograph on *Die Thomsen'sche Krankheit (myotonia congenita)* (26) to commemorate the 500th anniversary of Heidelberg University. He described for the first time the production of myotonia by electrical stimulus and also gave a description of the histological features of the disease. Around the same time, Eulenburg (27,28) drew attention to "paramyotonia congenita" in a study of 26 members from six generations of a family in East Germany, in whom the myotonia was characteristically brought on or aggravated by cold. Subsequent to these reports, a number of case histories appeared with associated weakness and other features, which we now know to be associated with dystrophia myotonica, but it was not until the description of Steinert in Germany in 1909 (29), which was concurrent with that of Batten and Gibb (30), that dystrophia myotonica became clearly delineated as a distinct clinical syndrome.

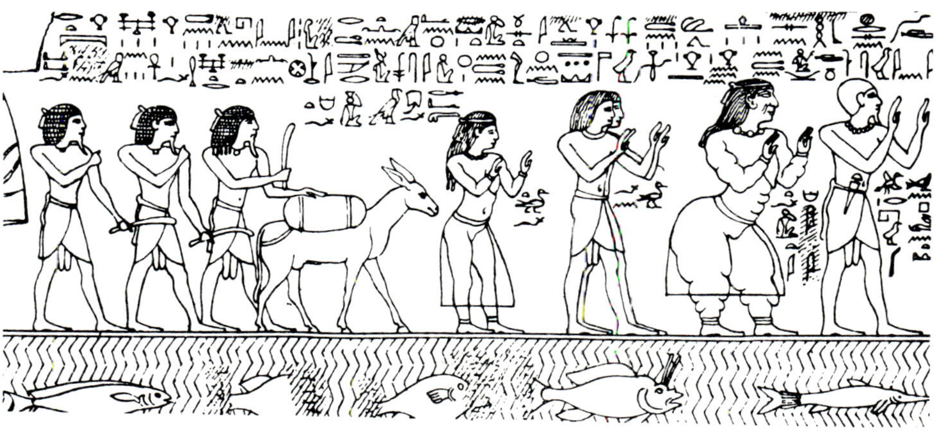

QUEEN OF PUNT. TEMPLE OF HATSCHEPSUT

FIG. 11. The Queen of Punt (second from right) and her family and entourage receiving the royal visitors from Egypt (1500 B.C.). (From Poch and Becker, ref. 31.)

There was a fair hiatus subsequent to this time, and it was not until the 1940s that a new impetus came into the whole field again, and in recent years, there has been considerable expansion and recognition of many new syndromes and variations on the theme of muscle disorders, as a result of the introduction in the early 1960s of histochemistry as a standard technique for the investigation of muscle biopsies and subsequently the additional use of electron microscopy. However, it might be of interest perhaps to delve back again for a moment into the past and look at a possible very early description of muscle disease in ancient Egypt (31).

In Egypt, on the Temple of the Queen Hatshepsut, who reigned between 1500 and 1480 B.C., there is a relief showing the expedition to Punt, which the Egyptians had undertaken during her reign (Fig. 11). On this particular relief one sees the Queen of Punt (the lady to the right in the picture), together with various members of her family and her entourage, welcoming the visitors from Egypt. The striking appearance of this lady is immediately apparent and though the superficial appearances are of obesity rather than muscle pseudohypertrophy, she does also have a rather lordotic posture. It is perhaps of interest as well that the artist has chosen to depict nasolabial folds on her face, which are not present on any of the other individuals, suggesting perhaps that there was some abnormality of her facial appearance as well. The other thing of interest is her family. Her two sons behind her look quite normal in their posture, whereas the daughter also shows a somewhat lordotic posture. It thus appears that the Queen of Punt, back in the 15th century before Christ, may have been a case of muscular dystrophy, possibly of the facioscapulohumeral variety with a dominant inheritance. Perhaps this needs a bit of a stretch of the imagination as the visual pictorial description could go equally well for some other disorders but, if nothing else, at least this type of documentation stresses the importance of good pictorial records of disease for retrospective diagnosis later.

REFERENCES

1. Duchenne, G.-B. (1861): *De l'électrisation localisée et son application à la pathologie et à la thérapeutique*, 2nd ed. Bailliere et Fils, Paris.

2. Duchenne, G.-B. (1862): *Album de photographies pathologiques*. Bailliere et Fils, Paris.
3. Duchenne, G.-B. (1868): *Arch. Gen. Med.*, 6 ser., 11:5,179,305,421,552.
4. Duchenne, G.-B. (1872): *De l'électrisation localisée et son application à la pathologie et à la thérapeutique*, 3rd ed. Bailliere et Fils, Paris.
5. Meryon, E. (1852): *Med.-Chir. Trans.*, 35:73.
6. Meryon, E. (1864): *Practical and Pathological Researches on the Various Forms of Paralysis*. Churchill, London.
7. Meryon, E. (1861): *The History of Medicine*, Vol. 1, Longman, London.
8. Schmidt, C. C. (1839): *Schmidts Jahrbücher der in- und aüslandischen gesamenten Medicin*, 24:176.
9. Gowers, W. R. (1879): *Lancet*, ii:1,37,73,113.
10. Gowers, W. R. (1879): *Pseudohypertrophic Muscular Dystrophy: A Clinical Lecture*. Churchill, London.
11. Leyden, E. (1876): *Klinik der Ruchenmarks-Krankheiten*, Vol. 2, p. 447, Hirschwald, Berlin.
12. Möbius, P. J. (1879): *Sammlung klin. Vortrage*, 171:1505.
13. Erb, W. H. (1891): *Dtsch. Ztschr. Nervenh.*, 1:13,173.
14. Landouzy, L., and Déjerine, J. (1884): *Comp. Rend. Acad. Sci., Paris*, 98:53.
15. Werdnig, G. (1891): *Arch. Psychiat. Nervenh.*, 22:437.
16. Werdnig, G. (1894): *Arch. Psychiat. Nervenh.*, 26:706.
17. Hoffmann, J. (1893): *Dtsch. Ztschr. Nervenh.*, 3:427.
18. Hoffmann, J. (1897): *Dtsch. Ztschr. Nervenh.*, 10:292.
19. Hoffmann, J. (1900): *Munch. Med. Wschr.*, 47:1649.
20. Hoffmann, J. (1900): *Dtsch. Ztschr. Nervenh* , 18:217.
21. Oppenheim, H. (1900): *Mschr. Psychiat. Neurol.*, 8:232.
22. Collier, J., and Wilson, S.A.K. (1908): *Brain*, 31:1.
23. Greenfield, J. G., and Stern, R. O. (1927): *Brain*, 50:652.
24. Dubowitz, V. (1980): *The Floppy Infant*, 2nd ed. SIMP/Heinemann, London.
25. Thomsen, J. (1876): *Arch. Psychiat. Nervenh.*, 6:702.
26. Erb, W. (1886): *Die Thomsen'sche Krankheit (myotonia congenita)*. Leipzig.
27. Eulenburg, A. von (1886): *Neurol. Zentralbl.*, 5:265.
28. Eulenburg, A. von (1916): *Med. klin.*, 12:505
29. Steinert, H. (1909): *Dtsch. Ztschr. Nervenh.*, 37:58.
30. Batten, F. E., and Gibb, H. P. (1909): *Brain*, 32:187.
31. Poch, H., and Becker, P. E. (1955): *Nervenarzt*, 26: 528.

Historical Aspects of the Neurosciences,
edited by F. Clifford Rose and W. F. Bynum.
Raven Press, New York ©

History of Myasthenia Gravis

Johan A. Aarli

Department of Neurology, University of Bergen, Bergen, Norway

Our concept of the clinical manifestations of myasthenia gravis was formed mainly by German neurologists in the last two decades of the 19th century. There are reports containing case histories of patients with undoubted myasthenia gravis before this time, but they have not contributed to the development of neurologic nosography. These studies may, however, throw some light upon the diagnostic capabilities of skilled physicians at a time when a systematic description of diseases was almost nonexistent.

THE FORERUNNERS

Thomas Willis (1621–1675) was a professor in Oxford and later a successful and respected practioner in London. Although an anatomist whose name is associated with the anastomotic arterial circle at the base of the brain, his reputation is mainly based upon his endeavors in clinical medicine. In his treatise on physiological and pathological aspects of disease, *De anima brutorum* (1), translated into English in 1685 (2), he wrote:

> Nevertheless, those labouring with a want of Spirits, who will exercise local motions, as well as they can, in the morning are able to walk firmly, to fling about their Arms hither and thither, or to take up any heavy thing; before noon the stock of the Spirits being spent, which had flowed into the Muscles, they are scarce able to move Hand or Foot. At this time I have under my charge a prudent and an honest Woman, who for many years hath been obnoxious to this sort of spurious *Palsie*, not only in her Members, but also in her tongue; she for some time can speak freely and readily enough, but after she has spoke long, or hastily, or eagerly, she is not able to speak a word, but becomes as mute as a Fish, nor can she recover the use of her voice under an hour or two.

The description, emphasizing many of the essential features of myasthenia gravis, such as dysarthria, increased fatiguability with physical exercise and recovery at rest, shows that Thomas Willis had recognized the disease 200 years before Erb. It made, however, apparently no impact upon the contemporary medical world and was probably never intended to represent a description of a definite clinical entity. The report was forgotten and then recalled by Guthrie in 1903 as a case of myasthenia gravis in the 17th century (3).

Two hundred years later, Samuel Wilks published an article entitled "On cerebritis, hysteria and bulbar paralysis, as illustrative of arrest of function of the cerebro-spinal centres" in *Guy's Hospital Reports* (4). Here he described cases of evidently widely varying etiologies as being due to general cerebral involvement, in contrast to symptoms resulting from focal brain lesions. One of his patients was a young girl with strabismus and difficulties in speech and movement, who then developed dysarthria and dysphagia and died of acute respiratory paralysis. The description is incomplete, but the patient may well have suffered from myasthenia gravis. The report contains an account of the autopsy, and the medulla oblongata "appeared quite healthy to the naked eye and the microscope discovered no manifest changes in the tissue."

Both Willis' and Wilks' reports were rediscovered at a time when the principal symptoms of myasthenia gravis were recognized and defined due to detailed and systematic case histories published by German neurologists.

Motor neuron disease in its various disguises was identified as a clinical entity mainly by the work of French neurologists around 1850. The first descriptions of cases of myasthenia gravis came 30 years later. They all have as their point of origin comparisons with progressive bulbar paralysis, which was well known around 1880. It is not surprising that cases of myasthenia gravis at this time were first diagnosed as bulbar paralysis. The heedful observers would, however, soon recognize clinical aspects that were incompatible with this diagnosis, and the reports show how the concept of the new disease gradually emerges with clinical features distinctly different from those of motor neuron disease.

THE GERMAN SCHOOL

Neurologists and psychiatrists from the southwestern part of Germany attended their annual meeting, the III Wanderversammlung, in Wildbad, May 18 and 19, 1878. At the first day of this meeting, Wilhelm Erb, a 38-year-old physician working at Friedreich's clinic in Heidelberg, reported on a condition he had encountered in three patients, all with symptoms of bulbar paralysis but with clinical features indicating a new syndrome. He gave a full account of this syndrome, based upon observations of two men of 55 and 47, and a woman of 30 years, all of them with similar symptoms and signs. There can be no doubt that they all had myasthenia gravis. Like other patients with bulbar paralysis, they had difficulties in chewing and swallowing. But what was unique with this syndrome were several symptoms and signs not commonly encountered in bulbar paralysis. They all had ptosis, and a prominent finding was the weakness of the neck muscles. Erb also noted the paresis of the extremities and that the symptoms were fluctuating and not slowly progressive as in bulbar paralysis. Two of the patients, followed only for a short period of time, made an apparent recovery. Erb, a pioneer of electrotherapy and not fully aware of the natural history of the disease, attributed the recovery to the electric treatment given. His third patient, a 30-year-old woman, died suddenly at night after 1½ years of the disease, which included a period of recovery. According to Erb, the cardinal symptoms were ptosis, weakness in chewing, and weakness of the neck. He also reported some symptoms that later were regarded as less relevant than the neuromuscular weakness, such as headache, vertigo, and hyperacusis.

Erb was convinced that the cause of the disorder was to be found within the central nervous system. On the basis of anatomical considerations, he tried to localize the lesion within the brain stem but gave it up and concluded that a topographic diagnosis could first be given when there was an autopsy finding. When he presented his paper, he stressed that it was incomplete and in many ways premature, but he wished to bring it to the attention of his colleagues (5).

The prognosis of the disorder described by Erb was in many cases very serious, and the next cases reported supplemented Erb's paper by containing autopsy details. Hermann Oppenheim, a 27-year-old neurologist working in the nerve clinic at the Charité in Berlin under Professor Westphal, gave a lecture to the Society for Psychiatry and Neurology in Berlin in 1887 on "a case of chronic progressive bulbar paralysis without anatomical findings," printed in *Virchow's Archiv* the same year (6). He had had for 1½ years under his care at the nerve clinic a 29-year-old woman, who first developed weakness of arms and legs, followed by difficulties in speech and swallowing, and weakness of the facial muscles. She had, however, no ocular symptoms but showed a marked fluctuation in the severity of the muscular weakness and died of respiratory insufficiency. For some reason, Oppenheim did not mention and may not have been aware of the three cases described by Erb nine years earlier. On the other hand, he reprinted word for word Wilks' case of possible myasthenia gravis (4). Clinically, the condition described by Oppenheim was characterized by a glosso-pharyngo-labial paralysis. Oppenheim, just as convinced as Erb that this was "eine Erkrankung des Nervensystems," was clearly surprised that the central nervous system was normal at autopsy.

Although Erb's description is detailed, it was quite natural that he should miss some important clinical features, which were added by his colleagues in the following years. Oppenheim gave his paper in March 1887. In August, the same year, Carl Eisenlohr, one of Erb's pupils, now working in Hamburg, reported in *Neurologisches Centralblatt* the case of an 18-year-old girl with ptosis and diplopia (7). Eisenlohr observed that the ocular symptoms varied both during the day and from time to time, and he was the first to emphasize the variation in muscular strength as a part of the clinical picture. His patient developed weakness in the hands and difficulties in swallowing and died after two years from respiratory insufficiency. At autopsy, the central nervous system was found to be normal. Eisenlohr referred to his case as a parallel to that which Oppenheim had described only a few months earlier. Both Eisenlohr and Oppenheim regarded their cases as due to a "neurosis," which at that time only meant that the symptoms were typical of an organic lesion in the central nervous system but lacked the anatomical correlate. Like Oppenheim, Eisenlohr was also surprised and apparently disappointed at the negative autopsy findings. Neither of them mentioned Erb's description of the same disorder nine years earlier.

In England, Shaw reported in *Brain* another case of "bulbar paralysis without structural changes in the medulla" (8). His patient has been regarded as a case of myasthenia gravis. Shaw observed that at the symptoms of his patient "became more evident as the day advanced," but his description is not typical for myasthenia gravis. The patient had a bulbar paresis, and no ocular symptoms; the tendon reflexes were exaggerated with ankle clonus on the right side, so that it might be, as supposed by Shaw, a case of bulbar paresis. Shaw's patient died with paralysis of the respiratory muscles and his report is remembered because it includes the first report of artificial respiration, which was tried without effect.

An American from Cincinnati, Ohio, Hermann Hoppe, had for some time worked with Oppenheim in Berlin. He was apparently the first to realize that Eisenlohr's and Oppenheim's papers should be seen together with that of Erb because of the autopsy reports. Hoppe cited Eisenlohr, Oppenheim, and Wilks' cases and added a similar case of his own, a 40-year-old man with symptoms typical of a generalized myasthenia gravis. He drew attention to the differences from chronic progressive bulbar paralysis:

1. The lack of muscular atrophy and the difference in response to electrical stimulation.
2. The affection of upper facial and the oculomotor nerves.
3. The infrequent affection of the hypoglossal nerve.
4. The distinct remissions and the variation in the intensity of symptoms even in the course of the day.
5. The lack of anatomical findings.

Hoppe was the first to discuss the pathogenesis of the disease. He dwelt briefly with the possibility that the weakness was due to a chronic intoxication with some internally produced toxin specific for the motor centers, but he found no evidence for this and concluded, like his predecessors, that the symptoms were neurogenic in origin (9).

A few more cases were reported in the following years, adding little to what was already known about the condition. The best comprehensive clinical delineation was given by Samuel Goldflam from Warsaw, who had worked in Lambl's clinic for internal medicine. Being especially interested in neurology, he had for some time studied with Westphal in Berlin and with Charcot in Paris. Back in Warsaw, he established out of his own earnings a polyclinic for poor patients with neurological disorders. In 1891 and 1892, he saw three patients in his polyclinic, which he reported in *Deutsche Zeitschrift für Nervenheilkunde* in 1893 (10). He discussed the cases reported by Wilks, Erb, Oppenheim, Hoppe, and Eisenlohr, and he found that the disorder was a separate clinical entity, different from bulbar paralysis as described by Duchenne. He reemphasized all the clinical features that we know today, including the increased fatiguability and the undulating course of the disease. Thus, Goldflam realized that the recovery in some patients was not due to a therapeutic effect of galvanic stimulation but to a remission of the disease. He stressed that the diagnosis of this special and in many cases benign disorder can be made on the basis of certain clinical symptoms. According to Goldflam, when bulbar symptoms occur and progress rapidly in a young individual, and the trunk and the extremities are less affected, when the bulbar paralysis differs in many ways from the type described by Duchenne, when the chewing muscles are affected to a high degree and early in the course of the disease without weakness of the facial muscles, when there is ptosis or paresis of the external ocular muscles, but not atrophy, fibrillations and changes in the electrical irritability, when difficulties in respiration and attacks of dyspnea constitute an important part of the clinical picture and the pareses show an increased fatiguability, when the symptoms change not only from day to day, but also during the day, when there are considerable remissions and exacerbations and deep reflexes are normal, then we have a case of this special disease (10).

Goldflam pointed out that it had for some time been fashionable among neurologists to diagnose hysteria in cases offering diagnostic difficulties. To prove this diagnosis, a prerequisite is that the subject "has to be a hysteric." He was the first among many neurologists to warn against the diagnosis of hysteria in patients with neuromuscular weakness and increased fatiguability. After Goldflam, little has been added to the clinical description of the disease, and his paper still stands out as one of the best descriptions of the symptoms and signs in myasthenia gravis. Among the pioneer reports, Erb's is the first and Goldflam's the most comprehensive, and the eponym Erb-Goldflam symptom complex is therefore appropriate. Goldflam was just as convinced as his predecessors that the condition was due to a nondetectable disturbance of the central nervous system, possibly to an effect of toxins.

In Berlin, Oppenheim had been in charge of the clinic at the Charité during Westphal's protracted illness. After Westphal's death, Oppenheim was nominated as his successor, but due to internal political circumstances at that time, he was not appointed and had to leave the Charité to open his own private clinic. Friedrich Jolly became Westphal's successor. At a meeting of the Berliner medicinische Gesellschaft in 1894, Jolly demonstrated a 14-year-old boy who developed bilateral ptosis when he was tired with difficulties in swallowing, and general muscular fatiguability and weakness, features typical of the disorder, and he suggested the name "pseudoparalysis myasthenica" (11). In a subsequent paper from 1895, he changed this name to "myasthenia gravis pseudoparalytica" (12). Jolly examined the reaction of the muscles to electric stimulation and demonstrated the decremental response by tetanic indirect stimulation. He even concluded that the muscles were in a pathological condition, which was opposite to that of myotonia. However, he believed that the disorder was primarily cerebral and that the symptoms could be caused by substances which were released from the brain during metabolism and acted as toxins upon the muscles. Concerning the treatment, he suggested that alkaloids like physostigmine could be used, but he did apparently not apply them himself. Now we have the disease and its name, but its pathology remained unknown.

THE PATHOLOGY OF MYASTHENIA GRAVIS

The main changes in myasthenia gravis are confined to the neuromuscular junction and the thymus. The endplate changes, although crucial for pathogenesis, are only seen at the electron microscopical level with refined immunological techniques (13). A thymoma is found in approximately 10 to 15% of cases while 85% of the remaining cases have a follicular hyperplasia (14), knowledge that has accumulated only gradually from the turn of the century.

Because of similarities with progressive bulbar paralysis, myasthenia gravis was first regarded as a disease of the central nervous system. Although no lesions of the nervous system had been reported in autopsies performed before 1900, all investigators who described new cases of myasthenia gravis concluded that the condition was due to a disturbance of the brain function. At the end of the century, Campbell and Bramwell (15) summed up what was known about the clinical features of the disease. They reviewed the whole literature to 1900, including clinical details of 60 published cases. They were aware of the negative findings at autopsy, and they regarded the etiology as probably connected with a "toxin probably of microbic origin, circulating in the blood" and acting "selectively upon the lower motor neuron, so as to modify its functional activity." Later studies on the central nervous system in myasthenia gravis have not given any clues as to the cause of the disease. It is true that Mott and Barrada in 1923 described minor changes in the brain from a patient who died from definite myasthenia gravis in 1919 (16). The findings they described were neuronal degeneration, especially in the thalamus, but also in the third nerve nucleus. There were no lymphorrhages in the brain. Similar changes had not been observed by other investigators and were rejected as irrelevant for the pathogenesis, as the link with thymus was at that time already firmly established (17,18). In 1899, Oppenheim had reported on a patient with myasthenia gravis and a mediastinal tumor (19). The neoplasm, which was found at autopsy and was diagnosed as a lymphosarcoma, was apparently regarded as irrelevant for the myasthenic condition and did not lead to any etiological considerations.

Very little was therefore known about the pathology of myasthenia gravis when neurologists and psychiatrists from southwest Germany again came together at the Wanderversammlung, this time in Baden-Baden in June 1901. Leopold Laquer from Frankfurt reminded the audience that 21 years now had passed since Erb at a similar meeting had described the clinical features of the disease. At 21, myasthenia gravis had now reached adult status, and contributions leading to an increased understanding of myasthenia gravis should therefore be expected. Laquer reported another case of myasthenia gravis, a 30-year-old man who developed classical symptoms of the disease and died within one year after the appearance of the muscular weakness (20). Geheimrat (privy councillor) Carl Weigert, Ehrlich's cousin, then 55 years of age and one of the leading pathologists of his time, especially known for his staining techniques, gave the results of autopsy findings (21). The central nervous system was normal, as were most organs, except for an aspiration pneumonia. In the anterior mediastinum was a tumor 5 × 5 × 3 cm in size and adherent to the pericardium and the left pleura. The tumor consisted of lymphoid and a few epitheloid cells, and was of thymic origin. Biopsies of the deltoid and the diaphragm muscles showed lymphoid cells infiltrating the muscle fibers. There were similar, but not so prominent, changes in the heart, especially near the pericardium. Weigert regarded these lymphocyte infiltrations as metastases from the malignant thymus tumor. He considered the histological changes in the muscles so conspicuous that he excluded the possibility that similar changes could have been overlooked by previous investigators. Accordingly, he believed that the changes he had described were present only in some patients with myasthenia gravis.

That myasthenia gravis was connected not only with thymoma, but also, and presumably more often, with other types of thymus pathology, was demonstrated by Buzzard in 1905 (22). He examined muscles from myasthenic patients and found small lymphocyte accumulations (lymphorrhages) distributed in between the muscle fibers. He also observed an inconstant increase of lymphoid cells in the thymus from the patients he had studied. Like several of his predecessors, he believed that the findings were caused by a toxic, "possibly autotoxic" agent, and he considered it most fruitful now to direct attention to the lymphatic system. Norris later found such lymphorrhages in nearly two-thirds of the cases and only in the muscles of patients with myasthenia gravis (23); he therefore regarded them as pathognomonic for this disease.

In 1917, Herzog had, on the basis of results of electric stimulation of muscle in myasthenic patients, suggested that the cause of the muscular weakness was in the muscles and not in the nervous system (24). This view was further substantiated by Marburg, showing myositic changes in biopsies of patients with this disorder (25). Around 1920, myasthenia gravis was therefore mainly regarded as a primary disease of the striated musculature of the body.

The association between myasthenia gravis and thymus pathology was supported by many reports of both thymoma and thymic hyperplasia in myasthenia gravis patients. In the 1920s, several investigators had been convinced of an important link between the thymus and myasthenia gravis. Thus, at a meeting at the Royal Society of Medicine in 1923, Gordon Holmes (17) stated that there were either tumors or enlargements of the thymus in six of the eight cases of myasthenia gravis that he had examined at autopsy. It seemed to him that it was only from further studies of the physiology of the thymus that one could expect more light on the pathology of this disease. At the same meeting, Greenfield (18) reported that the thymus was persistent in three cases in which he had recently performed autopsies.

In 1917, Bell presented a systematic treatise on the thymic tumors in myasthenia gravis (26). He stated that the thymic tumors occurring in myasthenia gravis formed a distinct group. He concluded that some form of thymic involvement seems to occur in nearly half the cases of myasthenia gravis. Very few studies on the correlation between thymus and myasthenia gravis then appeared until the pathologist Norris published a broad review on thymus pathology in myasthenia gravis in 1936 (23). He regarded the pathologic findings in the thymus as conditions of greater or lesser degrees of epithelial hyperplasia. Norris was of the opinion that "pathologic changes may be found in the thymus in cases of myasthenia gravis in direct ratio to the care with which they are sought."

A possible link between striated muscle and the thymus had been presented by the Swedish pathologist Hammar in 1905, when he described myoid cells in the central medulla of thymus, especially from reptiles and birds. These cells, with round heads and fusiform tails, had striations identical to those of skeletal muscle in the tails and radial striations in the cytoplasm surrounding the nucleus in the rounded head (27). His observation was overlooked until van der Geld et al., almost 50 years later, showed that sera from some patients with myasthenia gravis contained antibodies that reacted both with skeletal muscle and with the myoid cells of the thymus (28,29). The linkage between thymus and myasthenia gravis was then established. In the meantime, more support had been dramatically gained by the results of thymectomy.

REMOVAL OF THE THYMUS

The first thymectomy in a patient with myasthenia gravis was performed in 1911 in Zürich by Professor Ferdinand Sauerbruch (30). The patient was a 20-year-old woman who within one year had developed severe hyperthyroidism and generalized myasthenia gravis; conservative treatment available at that time had no influence upon her condition, nor was there any improvement after ligation of the right superior thyroid artery and vein. The same year, Capelle and Bayer (31) had reported that thymus extirpation could induce a remission of a thyrotoxicosis (31). Aware of this and of the linkage between myasthenia gravis and thymus hyperplasia, Sauerbruch believed that a thymectomy was indicated, and he succeeded in removing an enlarged thymus. Histological examination showed no neoplastic elements but hyperplasia with a cellular distribution corresponding to that of the fetal thymus. There was an improvement both of the myasthenic symptoms and of the hyperthyroidism. The thyroid symptoms recurred, and it became necessary to perform a subtotal thyroidectomy with subsequent improvement of both diseases.

A few years later, Haberer reported the results of combined partial thyroid and thymectomies in 40 patients with hyperthyroidism. The thymectomy was apparently always partial (thymus reduction) and was performed under local anesthesia. In one patient, a 27-year-old man with myasthenia gravis, only a partial thymectomy was performed; the thymus was described as involuted. Neurological examination three years after the operation revealed that the condition had clearly improved (32). In the 1930s, Sauerbruch, now at the Charité in Berlin, performed a thymectomy in two patients with both thymoma and myasthenia gravis; both had tumors the size of a man's fist. The tumors, classified as lymphoepithelioma, were encapsulated, and a radical extirpation was possible in both cases. They died, however, five and eight days postoperatively from mediastinitis (33,34).

The first successful removal of a thymic tumor in a patient with myasthenia gravis was reported by Blalock and his coworkers in 1939 (35). The patient was a 20-year-old woman who had suffered from a severe and generalized myasthenia gravis for five years, and the effect of prostigmin treatment was unsatisfactory. X-ray examination revealed a mass in the anterior mediastinum. At operation, an encapsulated 6 × 5 × 3 cm cystic tumor was found and removed. Due to X-ray irradiation given preoperatively, the central parts of the tumor were necrotic, and there was no microscopic evidence of thymic tissue left. The patient recovered rapidly after the operation and became apparently symptom free. This paper introduced the era of thymectomy for myasthenia gravis, not only for thymoma, but also in myasthenia gravis with thymus hyperplasia (36).

THE NEUROMUSCULAR TRANSMISSION IN MYASTHENIA GRAVIS

Myasthenia gravis was first believed to be a disease of the central nervous system, was then regarded as an entity whose picture was produced by metastases from a malignant thymoma, and then as a primary disease of the striated musculature of the body (23). Around 1935, several events drew attention to the neuromuscular transmission as the site of the basic defect. Back in the 1850s, Claude Bernard had examined the paralytic effect of curare and found that one site of action was the neuromuscular junction. Eighty years later, Mary

Walker was struck by the similarities between the symptoms of myasthenia gravis and those of curare poisoning and gave physostigmine (eserine), a drug known to antagonize curare. The dramatic effect upon the motor weakness led her to suppose that the fatiguability was due to a poisoning of the motor endplates rather than to an affection of the muscle itself (37).

The results of neurophysiological examinations led Lindsley to a similar conclusion. He observed that both the rate and rhythm of the motor unit potentials remained unaltered during voluntary muscle contraction while the amplitudes varied considerably. He concluded that the function of the motor nerves was normal but that there was a block of the transmission of nerve impulses at the motor endplate (38).

A few years later, Harvey and Masland described the decremental response of muscle action potentials to repetitive nerve stimulation (39). Thus, both pharmacological and neurophysiological evidence now pointed toward a defect of the neuromuscular transmission. A discussion whether this defect was pre- or postsynaptic followed. Electromyographic data were interpreted as evidence of a presynaptic defect, and this was supported by the demonstration of neurogenic muscle atrophy in cases of long-standing myasthenia gravis. On the other hand, the structural changes found in the muscle tissue were more in favor of a postsynaptic cause of the disease. Then, unexpectedly, this question was elucidated from a new point of view, that of immunology.

THE IMPACT OF IMMUNOLOGY

In 1960, at a time when the idea of autoimmunity had inspired thinking in clinical medicine, John Simpson postulated that myasthenia gravis was due to an autoimmune attack upon a protein of the motor endplate (40). Almost simultaneously, a young American medical student, Arthur Strauss, showed that sera from some patients with myasthenia gravis contained antibodies that reacted with the cross-striations of skeletal muscle (41). It soon became clear that these antibodies were not ubiquitous in myasthenia gravis, but were mainly found in sera from patients with myasthenia gravis and thymoma. As they do not react at the neuromuscular junction, they could not explain the basic defect in myasthenia gravis.

In 1973, it was demonstrated that antibodies against the acetylcholine receptor protein could interfere directly with the neuromuscular transmission. That year, Patrick and Lindstrom reported in *Science* that they had produced a disease in rabbits by immunization with purified acetylcholine receptor protein (42). The disease had so many clinical features in common with myasthenia gravis that it was termed "experimental autoimmune myasthenia gravis."

It was later shown that similar antibodies are also present in sera from patients with myasthenia gravis. It is today reasonable to assume that the basic defect in myasthenia gravis is caused by a loss of acetylcholine receptor protein from the postsynaptic membrane. This loss is partly caused by the effect of complement-mediated antibody-dependent membrane destruction and partly by the effect of sensitized lymphocytes (43). The reason why this immune attack is initiated remains unknown.

NONSURGICAL TREATMENT

Wilhelm Erb was one of the pioneers of electrotherapy, being only 27 when he published his first study on the effect of electricity upon brain and spinal cord. He pursued the idea that electric stimulation could give strength to paretic muscles, and he tried to give a scientific basis to electrotherapy in his classical work *Handbuch der Elektrotherapie und Elektrodiagnostik* (1882). Although critical by nature, Erb's attitude toward electrotherapy was enthusiastic and optimistic, an attitude not always shared by his colleagues. In myasthenia gravis, he attributed any improvement in the condition to the therapeutic effect of the galvanism. His pupils carried on his ideas for some time, but it was soon realized that electrotherapy had little to offer. This treatment was therefore supplemented with various drugs in common use at that time, in the hope of inducing a remission of the disease.

In addition to electrical treatment, Eisenlohr had treated his patient with myasthenia gravis with subcutaneous injections of strychnine (7). The doses were not given in the report, and the injections had apparently no effect upon the patient's condition. Strychnine had at that time a reputation as a useful therapeutic agent, having gained wide usage as a "tonic" for various chronic diseases. Therapeutic doses of strychnine have, however, no detectable effect on skeletal muscle. Only high doses have an effect upon the neuromuscular junction as a part of the combined effects upon the synaptic transmission. The dosage employed for the treatment of myasthenia gravis was for several years up to 0.25 g daily in subcutaneous injections (44). This treatment was in use until the introduction of physostigmine in the 1930s.

Hoppe used iodine in addition to electrotherapy (9). At this time, iodine compounds were also used for a series of different disorders. The drug, most commonly administered as a compound solution with 5% elemental iodine and 10% potassium iodide in aqueous solution, seems to have been without clinical effect.

Arsenic also had an undeserved reputation of being an effective stimulating drug, but all attempts to demonstrate such a tonic action in animals have consistently met with failure. Inorganic arsenic, when added to the diet of experimental animals, will not improve their nutritive state. Nevertheless, a combination of presumed tonic agents were in use for the treatment of myasthenia and of various other diseases as late as the 1920s, as recommended in a standard textbook of neurology from 1925 (44):

> The treatment consists in complete rest, careful attention to feeding, and the use of iron, arsenic, strychnia, the calcium salts and intestinal disinfectants. In some cases excellent results are obtained by injections of massive doses of strychnia, up to gr 1/4 *ter die* hypodermically. By one or other of these measures, all patients if seen reasonably early can be relieved or cured.

Harriet Edgeworth, a physician who had suffered from myasthenia gravis for many years, in 1929 took ephedrine for menstrual cramps and noted a degree of muscular improvement much greater than had occurred for many months. She found that she increased in strength on a daily dose of 48 mg and reported this observation in a letter to *JAMA* in 1930 (45). The letter introduced ephedrine in the treatment of myasthenia gravis and it soon became the most effective drug available at that time.

The trials of so many drugs, all of them now obsolete, clearly showed the desperate need for an effective agent. They also illustrate the neurologist's dilemma, being able to diagnose a serious disease but unable to help. In 1894, Friedrich Jolly had discussed on a purely theoretical basis the possible use of physostigmine in the treatment of myasthenia gravis. Apparently afraid of its side effects, he did not try it on his patients. One year later, Morri had recorded alleviation of myasthenic symptoms after the administration of physostigmine (46), but for some reason, this observation was not followed up.

Prostigmine, a synthetic analogue of physostigmine, was first synthesized around 1930 and was employed for the treatment of myasthenia gravis by Laser Remen in Münster (47), who published his report in 1932. Only one of his three patients had definite myasthenia gravis while the two others had central nervous system diseases with myasthenic features. The myasthenic patient was a 49-year-old man, who for three years had experienced periods with diplopia and then developed ptosis, dysphagia, and weakness in arms and legs. He was given prostigmine injections (dose not reported). The author described that the patient one hour after the injection could open his eyes better than before the injection and was able to swallow and to stretch out his hands. The effect lasted only for one hour. Remen's report was, however, mainly a study on the effect of glycine upon the creatine/creatinine metabolism. The prostigmine effect, his most important observation, was played down and not mentioned at all in the discussion.

It was therefore up to Mary Walker, then a resident physician at St. Alfege's Hospital in London, to report to the world that dramatic effect of cholinesterase inhibitors upon myasthenia gravis, in what has later become known as "the miracle at St. Alfege's." A 56-year-old woman with myasthenia gravis was given a hypodermic injection of 1/60 g physostigmine salicylate (37):

> In from half an hour to an hour after the injection the left eyelid "goes up," arm movements are much stronger, and jaw drops rather less, swallowing is improved, and the patient feels "less heavy." The effect wears off gradually in from 2-3 hours.

Mary Walker's report introduced the first really effective drug in the treatment of myasthenia gravis. Besides, it focused the attention upon the motor endplate as the site of the basic defect in myasthenia gravis. Physostigmine was, because of side effects, soon replaced by prostigmine, the main drug in the treatment of myasthenia gravis until the introduction of pyridostigmine in the 1950s.

Both steroids and corticotrophin were tried in severe cases in the late 1940s. The effect could be dramatic but was incalculable, and the drugs fell soon into disrepute. It was von Reis and his colleagues who reintroduced corticotrophin as the short-term ACTH course with a paper at the myasthenia gravis conference in New York in 1965 (48), a paper which also opens another aspect of the disease, that of the patient. The early reports on cases of myasthenia gravis show, with their detailed reports on the development of death by suffocation and respiratory paralysis, how the neurologists at that time were touched by the sufferings of their patients. There was something more dramatic about the myasthenia gravis patient because of the rapid and often unexpected appearance of the exacerbations. Most reports are seen from the clinician's point of view. There is one example of a poet's description of his life and sufferings with myasthenia gravis.

THE POET AND HIS DISEASE

Case 1 in von Reis' paper, H. G., was Hjalmar Gullberg, an outstanding poet and a member of the Swedish Academy, "the eighteen." At the age of 59, he developed classical myasthenia gravis with general muscular weakness and his condition deteriorated rapidly. Prostigmine treatment restored his strength only temporarily and gave the well-known side effects, which he described in private letters, telling about his inability to swallow, his hanging lower jaw and the constant stream of saliva dripping from his mouth except for a couple of hours after he was given atropine. The disease had become manifest while he was completing a collection of Dante-inspired *terza rima*, giving the latter part of his book a premonition of imminent death.

After a brief remission, a dramatic exacerbation followed. The Swedish poet became bedridden, tracheostomy was performed, and he was given artificial ventilation (49). He was, however, able to continue his writing, and he wrote his last volume of poetry, *Eyes, lips*, partly when being on a respirator. There are few poems taken from the hospital situation, but in a few lines he admits to "an amateur poet, sending his verses and confiding his mental distress," that "a diseased body/ is a reality in a way which differs/ from that of a soul in distress."

He was then given a corticotrophin course, which resulted in a dramatic change of his condition. His friends had regarded a remission as nothing less than miraculous, as he was apparently brought back to life. But during the treatment which saved his life, he had been through three tracheostomies, once as an emergency operation, being hypoxic and more or less unconscious (50). The corticotrophin courses had added days and months of grace to his life, but when he felt that the myasthenic symptoms were returning and he became unable to talk or swallow, he wrote to his friends that he would not go through a fourth tracheostomy and the sufferings of another stay in a respirator, but preferred to die. This was repeated in a poem "just one wish." On his last evening, he listened once more to Brahms' *Ein deutsches Requiem*. The next morning, he walked down to a lake near his home, perhaps the same lake he had written about in his youth, which he described in these lines:

> there is a lake
> thereafter—nothing more.

REFERENCES

1. Willis, T. (1672): *De anima brutorum*. Theatro Sheldoniano, Oxford, England.
2. Willis, T. (1685): *The London Practice of Physick, or the whole practical part of physick contained in the works of Dr. Willis*. London.
3. Guthrie, L. G. (1903): *Lancet*, I:330.
4. Wilks, S. (1877): *Guy's Hosp. Rep.*, 22:7.
5. Erb, W. (1879): *Arch. Psychiat. Nervenkr.*, 9:336.
6. Oppenheim, H. (1887): *Virchow's Archiv*, 108:522.
7. Eisenlohr, C. (1887): *Neurol. Centralbl.*, 6:337,361,389.
8. Shaw, L. E. (1890): *Brain*, 13:96.
9. Hoppe, H. H. (1892): *Berl. klin. Wschr.*, 29:332.
10. Goldflam, S. (1893): *Dtsch. Z. Nervenheilk.*, 2:312.
11. Jolly, F. (1895): *Neurol. Centralbl.*, 14:34.
12. Jolly, F. (1895): *Berl. klin. Wschr.*, 32:1.
13. Engel, A. G., Lambert, E. H., and Howard, F. M. (1977): *Mayo Clin. Proc.*, 52:267.
14. Castleman, B. (1966): *Ann. N.Y. Acad. Sci.*, 135:496.
15. Campbell, H., and Bramwell, E. (1900): *Brain*, 23:277.
16. Mott, F. W., and Barrada, Y. A. (1923): *Brain*, 46:237.
17. Holmes, G. (1923): *Brain*, 46:239.
18. Greenfield, J. G. (1923): *Brain*, 46:240.
19. Oppenheim, H. (1899): *Dtsch. Z. Nervenheilk.*, 15:1.
20. Laquer, L. (1901): *Neurol. Zbl.*, 20:594.
21. Weigert, C. (1901): *Neurol. Zbl.*, 20:597.
22. Buzzard, E. F. (1905): *Brain*, 28:438.
23. Norris, E. H. (1936): *Am. J. Cancer*, 27:421.
24. Herzog, F. (1917): *Dtsch. Arch. klin. Med.*, 123:76.
25. Marburg, O. (1931): *Wien. klin. Wschr.*, 44:413.
26. Bell, E. T. (1917): *J. Nerv. Ment. Dis.*, 45:130.
27. Hammar, J. A. (1905): *Anat. Anz. (Jena)*, 27:23.
28. Geld, H. W. R. van der, and Strauss, A. J. L. (1966): *Lancet*, I:57.
29. Geld, H. W. R. van der, Feltkamp, T. E. W., Logheim, J. J. van, Oosterhuis, H. J. G. H., and Biemond, A. (1963): *Lancet*, II:373.
30. Schumacher, E. D., and Roth, M. (1913): *Mitt. Grenzgeb. Med. Chir.*, 25:746.
31. Capelle, W., and Bayer, R. (1911): *Beitr, klin. Chir.*, 72:214.
32. Haberer, H. von (1917): *Arch. klin. Chir.*, 109:193.
33. Adler, H. (1937): *Arch. klin. Chir.*, 189:529.

34. Obiditsch, R. A. (1937): *Virchow's Arch. Pathol. Anat.*, 300:319.
35. Blalock, A., Mason, M. F., Morgan, H. J., and Riven, S. S. (1939): *Ann. Surg.*, 110:544.
36. Keynes, G. (1949): *Br. Med. J.*, 2:611.
37. Walker, M. (1934); *Lancet*, I:1200.
38. Lindsley, D. B. (1935): *Brain*, 58:470.
39. Harvey, A. M., and Masland, R. L. (1941): *Bull. Johns Hopkins Hosp.*, 69:1.
40. Simpson, J. A. (1960): *Scot. Med. J.*, 15:8.
41. Strauss, A. J. L., Seegal, B. C., Hsu, J. C., Burkholder, P. M., Nastuk, W. L., and Osserman, K. E. (1960): *Proc. Soc. Exp. Biol.*, (New York), 105:184.
42. Patrick, J., and Lindstrom, J. (1973): *Science*, 180:871.
43. Lennon, V. A. (1976): *Immunol. Commun.*, 5:323.
44. Dana, C. L. (1925): *Text-book of Nervous Diseases*, 10th ed. William Wood, New York.
45. Edgeworth, H. (1930): *J. Am. Med. Assoc.*, 46:1136.
46. Rowland, L. P., Hoefer, P. F. A., and Aranow, H. (1960): In: *Neuromuscular Disorder*, edited by R. D. Adams, L. M. Eaton, and G. M. Shy, p. 548–600. Williams & Wilkins, Baltimore.
47. Remen, L. (1932): *Dtsch. Z. Nervenheilk.*, 128:66.
48. Reis, G. von, Liljestrand, Å., and Matell, G. (1966): *Ann. N.Y. Acad. Sci.*, 135:409.
49. Fehrman, C. (1967): *Hjalmar Gullberg*. PAN/Norstedt, Stockholm.
50. Holmberg, O. (1969): *Hjalmar Gullberg—en vänbok*. Bonnier, Stockholm.

Historical Aspects of the Neurosciences,
edited by F. Clifford Rose and W. F. Bynum.
Raven Press, New York ©

Sir Victor Horsley: Father of Modern Neurological Surgery

Irving S. Cooper

Department of Neurosurgery, New York Medical College, New York, New York 10029

I am grateful for the opportunity of contributing to this volume, which pays tribute to Dr. Macdonald Critchley on the magnificent occasion of the eightieth anniversary of his birth. The subject of this occasion, The History of Neurology, is particularly fitting since Dr. Critchley's career has indelibly engraved his name in the history of neurology in this century.

Macdonald Critchley's manifold contributions in clinical research; his unsurpassed art and science as practicing physician; his erudite, literate, and creative publications; his unequaled mastery as lecturer and teacher to his students and his peers; and his long period as statesman and spokesman for neurologists throughout the world are already legendary.

It has been one of the great privileges of my own life and career to know Macdonald Critchley in all of these roles. I have been fortunate even beyond that, for during the past two decades, I have known Macdonald Critchley as a charming and brilliant companion and a respected friend, upon whom I look with great esteem and affection.

The first time I ever saw our honored guest in person, he was presenting the opening address to a combined meeting of the British Neurosurgical Society and the Neurosurgical Society of America in the renowned lecture hall of the National Hospital at Queen Square. He spoke on that occasion of Sir Victor Horsley, saying: "Horsley was a man who could have been great in any calling. He chose the virgin field of surgical neurology, but there is no field in the arts, in science, or in politics in which his greatness would not have flourished. Had he turned to religion as his calling one can well visualize him as an Archbishop, or as a Cardinal." These words spoken by Dr. Critchley of Sir Victor Horsley can, in turn, be said of Dr. Critchley himself. I can imagine no field in which he would not have distinguished himself. It is our good fortune that he elected the Divine Banquet of the Brain (1) as his discipline and as his art.

Any contribution which I might hope to add to our comprehension and appreciation of the historical role of Sir Victor Horsley must necessarily be a modest one, since his life and contributions to surgical neurology have been the subject of many published studies. Moreover, as will become evident, my essay will reflect my own parochial interests within the field of neurological surgery, which deal with the role of clinical neurophysiology.

Horsley has been the subject of two thorough biographical studies (2,3). The obituaries written by his own friends and peers immediately following his untimely death give evidence that his greatness and pioneering role was apparent to the most knowledgeable neuroscientists and physicians of his own time.

His rightful place as the father of neurosurgery was proclaimed by Gilbert Horrax, longtime first assistant to Harvey Cushing. Dr. Horrax stated: "It seems to me that there can be no possible dispute to the right of Sir Victor Horsley to be called the father of neurosurgery. It was he above all who pointed the path to the advancement of this newest branch of surgery by his physiological experiments in addition to his clinical and pathological contribution. Furthermore he was the first surgeon ever to devote the bulk of his time to neurological surgery." This judgment withstands any challenge.

No neurosurgeon, living or dead, has been more frequently imitated, followed, enlarged upon, taught by—knowingly or unknowingly—than Victor Horsley. Although he died almost half a century before I entered neurosurgery, I have long regarded him as a true hero and one of my greatest teachers.

Horsley was born in 1857, the son of an artist, whose own father was a composer. This heritage was combined with several generations of physicians on his mother's side. His character, personality, and genius encompassed the artistic, creative, scientific, and humanistic elements of his parents and their antecedents.

He entered medical school at the age of 20 at University College, London, where he trained extensively in experimental physiology. While still a student, he assisted two of his illustrious teachers, Bastian and Gowers, in the publication of neurological reports. Also, while still a student, he was awarded a prize for his independent study of the structure of the intervertebral disks.

By 1886, aged 29, he became an assistant professor at University College and superintendent of the Brown Institution. In the latter position, he carried out basic neurophysiological research of far-reaching importance. The same year he was elected as neurosurgeon to the staff of the National Hospital at Queen Square.

During the next decade, his laboratory research and innovative clinical studies in the operating theater were prodigious. Surgical treatment of brain tumors had already been carried out by Macewen in Glasgow and Godlee in London. Horsley extended this aspect of brain surgery and then introduced virtually every procedure that would eventuate in the emergence of the variegated surgical approaches to the entire nervous system, thereby creating the specialty of neurosurgery.

In collaboration with Hughlings Jackson, he performed ablative operations upon the brain for epilepsy. Six years later, like most innovators, he complained that little notice had been given to his results. He concluded that patients with Jacksonian epilepsy should receive surgical treatment, since no other satisfactory therapy was available to them.

In 1887, the year after introducing surgery for epilepsy, he collaborated with another giant of medical neurology, William Gowers. Horsley performed his famous laminectomy and successful removal of a spinal cord tumor, which was paralyzing Gower's patient Captain Golby, the diagnosis having been made by Gowers (4).

In 1891, having introduced the semicircular scalp incision, the use of bone wax to control bleeding from the skull, and having developed a technique to expose the pituitary gland, he also performed the first operation to relieve craniostenosis, and he developed the operation of section of the posterior root of the trigeminal nerve to alleviate the unbearable pain of tic douloureux. In the same year, Horsley delivered the Croonian Lecture on The Function of the Cerebral Cortex.

Were there no other creative contributions after 1891, Horsley would have earned his place in neurological history many times over. However, what may be his most illustrious and compelling contributions are found in the further application of his profound understanding of neurophysiological principles which he, and generations following, could apply to surgical therapy and to an increased understanding of disabling neurological diseases due to aberrations of brain mechanisms.

In the laboratory, Horsley carried out experiments to study the effects of extirpation of the pituitary gland (5). An extension of this investigation by Bernardo Houssay of Argentina led to a Nobel Prize for the Argentinian researcher. Today neuroendocrinology is still an embryonic burgeoning therapeutic and investigative field, fulfilling the promise of Horsley's pituitary investigation, in itself a monumental work.

Complementing his classical studies of the functional localization within the cerebral cortex, Horsley turned his attention to the cerebellum. In 1897, in collaboration with Lowenthal, he reported the fact that electrical stimulation of the cortex of paleocerebellum relieved experimental decerebrate rigidity in animals (6). This exciting revelation was reported independently by Sherrington the same year. Risien Russell, working in Horsley's laboratory, demonstrated an important physiological relationship of cerebellar malfunction to epileptic seizures. The importance of these cerebellar investigations in human clinical neurophysiology is presently emerging (7).

In order to investigate deeper structures within the brain, Horsley collaborated with the anatomist R. H. Clarke to develop an instrument that could accurately guide electrodes and other delicate surgical instruments into these profound structures with insignificant trauma to the brain (8). The Horsley-Clarke stereotactic instrument revolutionized neurophysiological laboratory investigations throughout the world. A modification of this unique concept was introduced into human neurosurgery by Spiegel and Wycis (9). The horizons of the usefulness of Horsley and Clarke's stereotaxis are constantly expanding.

Horsley's genius and intuitive grasp of the physiology of the human brain are summarized in the brilliant Linacre Lecture of 1909, entitled "The Function of the 'So Called' Motor Area of the Brain." Paying tribute to the preceding studies of Hitzig and Frisch, which were extended by Ferrier, as well as to the hypothesis of Hughlings Jackson, Horsley summarized much of his life's work in this master lecture given only seven years before his death.

He demonstrated that the concept of isolated motor and sensory centers within the cerebral cortex was incorrect. He destroyed the dogma of motor centers, which had held back progress in understanding of brain function, by describing a quarter of a century of laboratory and clinical investigations, which he had begun with Beevor in 1885.

Citing the first electrical excitation of cerebral cortex by Beevor and himself, Horsley elaborated the thesis, later extended by Sherrington, that stimulation of the postcentral gyrus was capable of facilitating a motor response elicited from the precentral gyrus. While pointing out that "physiologically considered, an electrical stimulus is a crude method of exciting a nerve centre," Horsley presented evidence that the precentral gyrus was a seat of highly important sensory as well as motor functions. Horsley inevitably reminded his audience that it was Hughlings Jackson who first enunciated the principle that every center in the nervous system must be sensorimotor, which Horsley's laboratory and clinical experience substantiated.

It was not until 1908 that Horsley was able to prove conclusively this thesis by surgically ablating the precentral gyrus in a young boy of 14, which was done in an attempt to relieve intractable involuntary movements of the left upper limb. Following extensive electrical stimulation of the precentral gyrus, the entire portion of the gyrus representing the arm was excised. Following surgery, the involuntary movements disappeared and were still absent 13 months later at the time of this memorable Linacre Lecture. Moreover, Horsley reported the remarkable fact that within a month after the operation, voluntary movements of the hand returned, in spite of the fact that the Betz cell area for the upper limit had been removed. Further, Horsley observed a degree of astereognosis and tactile anesthesia in the left hand, providing proof in this daring operation "that in the same region of the cortex cerebri sensory and motor representation exist together."

Horsley expounded upon this finding by pointing out that this sensorimotor cortex is the principal funnellike outlet for afferent impressions coming from many parts, including the thalamus. In this particular, he anticipated the role that thalamic surgery—employing the Horsley-Clarke instrument—would play in relieving the same type of involuntary movements half a century later (10).

In his Linacre Lecture of 1909, Horsley crowned a quarter of a century of innovative neurosurgery that encompassed the perfecting of intracranial surgery for brain tumors; initiation of laminectomy for spinal cord tumor; trigeminal root section for relief of the pain of tic douloureux; investigation of the intervertebral disk; surgery for craniostenosis; cortical ablation for epilepsy; experimental physiological studies of the cerebellum; experimental ablation of the pituitary gland and a detailed study of its effects; development of stereotactic surgery of the brain; and the first major step in the alleviation of involuntary movement disorders. Horsley's greatness and genius is self evident in the remarkable, continuing, original, and profound accomplishments of his relatively brief career.

Victor Horsley was a man of deep personal attributes, which paralleled his scientific stature. He generously and intelligently championed the investigations of Pasteur and of Lister at a time when many of his colleagues ridiculed them. Although well born and named for Queen Victoria, he was a staunch individualist and often took positions that were in conflict with the establishment. He openly renounced his religious affiliation, declaring himself to be agnostic. Yet, his devotion to his family, his patients, his students, and his country reveal him to have harbored deep religious feelings.

Although he was knighted in 1902, he continued to speak openly on subjects that brought him into open conflict with the General Medical Council. When he urged consideration of health legislation that would benefit the poorer classes he was disgracefully hooted from the podium at a meeting of the British Medical Association.

At the age of 57, he volunteered for military service in World War I. The world's greatest neurosurgeon, unpopular among the political medical establishment, was given a military rank beneath that of his former house officer Dr. Francis Walshe. Horsley, the father of neurosurgery and the champion of antiseptic surgery, was sent, as though in exile, to Mesopotamia, where his principal duty was to institute hygienic conditions in a desert outpost. There, he had an appointment in Amara where, on July 15, 1916, he contracted a severe tropical fever which took his life the following day.

Neurologists, neurophysiologists, endocrinologists, neurosurgeons, and, above all, humanity, stand in immeasurable debt to the heritage which Sir Victor Horsley, scientific genius and profound humanist, has left us.

REFERENCES

1. Critchley, M. (1979): *The Divine Banquet of the Brain*. Raven Press, New York.
2. Paget, S. (1919): *Sir Victor Horsley. A Study of His Life and His Work*. Constable and Co., London.
3. Lyons, J. B. (1966): *The Citizen Surgeon: A Biography of Sir Victor Horsley*. Dawnay, London.
4. Gowers, W., and Horsley, V. (1888): *Trans. Roy. Med.-chir. Soc.*, 1:XXI.
5. Lyons, J. B. (1967): Sir Victor Horsley. *Med. Hist.*, XI:4.
6. Lowenthal, M., and Horsley, V. (1897): *Proc. Roy. Soc. London*, 61.
7. Cooper, I. S. (1978): *Cerebellar Stimulation in Man*. Raven Press, New York.
8. Horsley, V., and Clarke, R. H. (1908): *Brain*, 31.
9. Spiegel, E., and Wycis, H. (1962): *Stereoencephalotomy*. Grune & Stratton, New York.
10. Cooper, I. S. (1969): *Involuntary Movement Disorders*. Hoeber, New York.

Historical Aspects of the Neurosciences,
edited by F. Clifford Rose and W. F. Bynum.
Raven Press, New York ©

The First Attempts at Removal of Brain Tumors

J. M. S. Pearce

Department of Neurology, Hull Royal Infirmary, Hull, United Kingdom

THE GLASGOW EXPERIENCE

On July 27, 1879, Dr. William Macewen performed a remarkable operation. Macewen was a surgeon and lecturer in surgery to the Royal Infirmary Glasgow and surgeon to the Hospital for Sick Children in Glasgow. He admitted to Ward 22 a patient, aged 14, with swelling over the left eye. This little girl had been admitted one year previously with a supraorbital periosteal tumor which had been removed, following which she had been well for three months. She then developed headaches, and after six months the swelling over the eye recurred. It increased in size and she was readmitted.

"On the 27th of July a series of convulsions occurred the initial stages of which were carefully recorded by a nurse without which the key to the brain lesion as indicated by the convulsions would have been lost, as when seen by me they had become generalised and threatened speedy dissolution. The convulsions were at the outset strictly limited to the right side, commencing in the face and arm and confined to these two parts during the initial attacks. The leg on the same side was affected during the third seizure and ultimately the convulsions became general with complete loss of consciousness. These phenomena were construed as indicating extension of the irritation to the lower middle portions of the ascending convolutions; and when this was considered along with the former evidence it was concluded that an irritative lesion existed in the left frontal lobe. On these grounds it was resolved to trephine midway between the centre of the ascending convolution and the anterior part of the cranium. At this point a minute nodule the size of a barley grain was detected on the outside of the skull. A large trephine was applied a disc of bone removed and a tumour of the dura mater which was exercising pressure on the brain was exposed. It was half an inch in thickness at this point gradually becoming much thinner and spreading all over the anterior two-thirds of the frontal lobe. The tumour was, after a prolonged operation, carefully dissected out along with the brain membranes where they were involved in the neoplasm. The patient rapidly recovered, was restored to perfect health, and subsequently was able to gain her own livelihood. She lived for eight years afterwards ultimately becoming affected with chronic Bright's disease from which she died. The skull and brain were examined and there was no trace of further tumour growth."

This case was published by Macewen in 1879 in the *Glasgow Medical Journal* (1). By 1888, Macewen published in the *British Medical Journal* the initial history of cerebral surgery and recounted in detail the following cases (2):

1. Case in which symptoms of focal cerebral disease led to diagnosis of lesions in Broca's lobe, 1876, brain abscess. Operation performed post-mortem, refused in life.
2. Case in which motor phenomena were the sole guides to cerebral lesion, 1879, subdural haematoma, cure.
3. Case in which the symptoms exhibited pointed to lesion in frontal lobe, 1879, described above, meningioma, cure.
4. Cerebral abscess in temporo-sphenoidal lobe involvement of motor area, 1881, abscess size of tennis ball, patient greatly relieved, died from exhaustion.
5. Intracranial effusion of blood diagnosed from motor symptoms alone, 1883, traumatic cerebral haematoma and cure.
6. Syphilitic tumour in paracentral lobule diagnosed from motor symptoms alone, 1883, lesion removed, patient recovered with slight hemiplegic gait.
7. Focal lesion in ascending convolution recognised by motor symptoms alone, 1883, intracerebral haematoma, cure.
8. Jacksonian epilepsy due to post-traumatic cyst, removal, improvement.
9. Protospasm of the hallux preceded by sensory impressions and followed by paralysis, removal of tuberculoma, and cure of fits.
10. Brachiocrural monoplegia, removal of post-traumatic cyst.
11. Psychical blindness, homicidal impulses and deep melancholy, removal of depressed fracture from angular gyrus.
12. Removal of temporosphenoidal abscess, 3 ozs. of pus, cure.

When Macewen published his collected experiences in 1888, he had operated on 21 cerebral cases exclusive of fracture of the skull in which operations had been performed. There were then three deaths and 18 recoveries. Macewen's main concern in the absence of any ancillary investigations was the correct localization of the lesion prior to surgery. His second major concern was the strict application of the aseptic techniques still relatively new from Lister's controversial teachings.

THE LONDON EXPERIENCE

The most celebrated removal of a brain tumor was that by Rickman J. Godlee in 1884. Godlee performed his operation at the Hospital for Epilepsy and Paralysis, now known as the Maida Vale Hospital. Godlee was the nephew of Lord Lister, whose recent discovery of antisepsis had no doubt sustained the young surgeon in his endeavors. He had been on the staff of University College Hospital for seven years and was by training an anatomist of unusual skill as well as an accomplished surgeon and an assiduous teacher. Among his contemporaries at U.C.H. were Arthur Barker, who drained one of the earliest otogenic brain abscesses, and Victor Horsley, who was among the pioneers of removal of spinal tumors.

But what of the man himself? Those who were apprenticed to him described him as precise, patient, and an extraordinarily lucid teacher. As a surgeon he can be given no higher praise than the words of Wilfred Trotter: "He was a true and single-minded clinician, for whom the task of a surgeon was to teach and practise the established doctrines and rules of the art. His attitude to surgery was therefore in the best sense academic and authoritarian, and his work, well controlled by caution and scepticism, had the distinction conferred by a capacious and instructed mind."

It is to Trotter (3) and his contemporary, D'Arcy Power, that we are indebted for the description of the operation. The patient was a 25-year-old man called Henderson, from Dumfries. For three years, he had a succession of focal motor fits, which would now be called Jacksonian epilepsy. The limited attacks were first in the left side of the face and tongue and then in the left hand and arm. There had been occasional attacks with unconsciousness. For six months, weakness of the left arm had been noted, and for three months prior to hospital admission on November 3, he had to give up work because the left arm was useless.

"From the time of admission there had been slight weakness of the left leg and severe pressure symptoms had set in, namely, paroxysmal headache and vomiting and well marked papilloedema with haemorrhages. The diagnosis was made of a tumour 'probably of limited size involving the cortex of the brain and situated at the middle part of the fissure of Rolando'."

"On November the 25th, the tumour was found and removed by operation through an opening immediately over and but little larger than the tumour itself. Only one cerebral convolution was exposed—the ascending parietal as was afterwards proved—it was slightly yellow and avascular. When it was incised a tumour was disclosed at the depth of ⅛ inch. This showed an apparent encapsulation but was enucleated piecemeal and subsequently described as a glioma."

The postoperative course initially was excellent. The patient's weakness increased a little, but his other symptoms were relieved and his mental faculties were unimpaired. Sadly, this triumph of diagnostic precision and technical virtuosity was not to remain unmarred. Wound infection developed and was complicated by meningitis, from which Henderson died four weeks later.

The potential importance of this operation was clearly recognized at the time, for there were present a number of distinguished onlookers. Among these was Hughes Bennett, a physician whose father had commended the use of cod liver oil for rickets, 80 years before the discovery of vitamin D. The famous Hughlings Jackson and David Ferrier were also present, and it was doubtless the efforts of these two great pioneers that made possible Godlee's task. The localization of cerebral lesions was then, as it is today, an essential prerequisite to intracranial surgery. The attribution of certain symptoms and signs to dysfunction arising at an identifiable focal point in the brain was the basis for clinicopathological correlation and hence for rational treatment. This art was not new. Heberden (1816), Dax of Montpelier (1836), and Auburtin had related speech disturbance and hemiplegia to lesions of the dominant hemisphere. John Hughlings Jackson, of Green Hammerton near York, had left the now extinct medical school at York and in 1862 joined the staff of the National Hospital, Queen Square, as it is now known. He, above all the distinguished doctors of his generation, combined the arts of minute clinical observation and recording with a remarkably perceptive and speculative intelligence, which permitted him visions of neurological physiology that have only of recent years been accredited and validated by scientific proof. These qualities allowed him to propose the clinical significance of epileptic attacks of diverse patterns, to regard epilepsy as a symptom and not a disease, and to speculate about the disturbed neuronal physiology underlying the epileptic events. His deduction of a hierarchy of neural functions, and the concepts of evolution and dissolution of the nervous system in development and disease, have been handed down and, more remarkably, almost invariably proved to be accurate by succeeding generations. His work on cerebral localization was thus to be an invaluable ingredient in the treatment of Rickman Godlee's patient.

The other distinguished spectator was Ferrier, one of the originators of neurophysiological experiments in animals. Fritsch and Hitzig had shown in 1870 that electrical stimulation of the anterior half of the brain could induce neuronal excitation. Ferrier, in a classic paper in the Medical Report of the West Riding Lunatic Asylum (1873) described his own work on experimental excitation of the brain, and his results were the first objective confirmation of some of Jackson's concepts. At this time, Jackson's work was in large part speculative and, until Ferrier's brilliant experiments, was incapable of proof or rejection.

The presence of Jackson, the observer, scientist and philosopher, and of Ferrier, the clinician and pioneer neurophysiologist, was thus in every way appropriate to the momentous operation, executed on that memorable day by Rickman Godlee. The unfortunate patient should not be neglected. He was to add his name to the exiguous list of those by whose misfortune or endurance the world has directly gained. As a footnote, one may add that Hughlings Jackson, though not renowned for his sense of humor, remarked to Godlee at the end of the operation: "You've missed a great opportunity. You have opened a Scotsman's head and neglected to put a joke in."

REFERENCES

1. Macewen, W. (1879): Tumour of the dura mater—convulsions—removal of tumor by trephining—recovery. *Hospital Practice, Glasgow Med. J.*, 210–213.
2. Macewen, W. (1888): An address on the surgery of the brain and spinal cord (delivered at the annual meeting of the British Medical Association, held in Glasgow, August 9th, 1888). *Br. Med. J.*, 302–309.
3. Trotter, W. (1941): A landmark in modern neurology. In: *Collected Papers*, pp. 33–46. Oxford Medical Publications, Oxford, England.

Historical Aspects of the Neurosciences,
edited by F. Clifford Rose and W. F. Bynum.
Raven Press, New York ©

The Decline of Osteology and the Rise of Surgical Neurology in the Management of Head Injuries

Eugene S. Flamm

Department of Neurosurgery, New York University School of Medicine, New York, New York 10016

Let me have a surgeon;
I am cut to th' brains.
King Lear, IV, vi.

Long before Shakespeare, traumatic lesions of the head were regarded as surgical problems. Management of patients with head injuries is discussed in the earliest examples of medical literature. Thirteen of the 48 cases described in the Edwin Smith Papyrus deal with skull fractures and other severe head injuries (1). Such neurological sequelae as aphasia, meningitis, and hemiparesis are described. The concept of prognosis and outcome, so much a part of current work on head injury, was also considered (2), and the surgeon advised to avoid cases with predictably poor outcome.

The Hippocratic writing, *De Vulneribus Capitis*, is the first work that can truly be said to be a systematic approach to head injuries (3–6). There is a void of almost 1,500 years between the writing of these two works, so we do not know how the early Greek physicians arrived at their methods. Unfortunately for those interested in medical and surgical neurology, this cornerstone of the history of head injuries might better be regarded as a tract on cranial osteology. The bulk of the work concerns itself with distinguishing the characteristics of various types of skull bruises and fractures. Five categories are described: linear fracture, contusion, depressed fracture, hedra (or dent) occurring both with and without fracture, and contrecoup fracture.

In addition to describing these lesions, the writer does mention certain features of the skull, such as the sutures, and proposes indications for trephination based on the type of fracture discovered. The technical aspects of ascertaining that a fracture is present are stressed, since this, more than any other aspect of the patient's condition, determined the need for trephination. Basically, those wounds that produced bruises of the skull, but no fracture, required trephination, while surgical intervention could be omitted if a fracture was present since the fracture would provide room for egress of any collection formed beneath the bone. The greater the injury to the skull, the less the need for trephination. This can be transformed into an aphorism that if no hole is present in the skull, one should be created.

From a surgical standpoint, the work is a curious mixture of sound advice, which is applicable today, and incomprehensible admonitions. The advice to cool the trephine with water is still practiced today, although the reasons for doing this may yet be unclear. The surgeon is advised to trephine if the wound crosses a suture but is warned not to apply the trephine to the suture itself or in the temporal area. The danger of injuring the underlying dura mater was appreciated. In fact, the surgeon was advised to leave a thin shell of the bone in place and allow it to exfoliate. Perhaps because of this practice, no mention of the purpose of the trephination to evacuate a collection in the epidural or subdural space is to be found. It is hard to believe that these hematomas were not encountered, but no mention of them appears in the work.

Although the major emphasis of *De Vulneribus Capitis*, as indicated in the title, is on wounds of the head, in contradistinction to wounds of the brain, several glimpses of knowledge of the organization of the nervous system are found. The occurrence of seizures involving the side of the body opposite the head injury can be singled out as the earliest sign of decussation of neural control. The major emphasis of these surgical interventions was to prevent the complications of inflammation, not to treat the results of cerebral trauma.

As one traces the history of writings on head injuries, two separate pathways can be followed. For 2,000 years after the Hippocratic writings, most authors repeated the same classification of *De Vulneribus Capitis* and added their own commentaries. These dealt with injuries of the scalp and skull that were regarded ends in themselves. Surgery that was advised was prophylactic, in theory to prevent the formation of epidural collections but, in fact, often to become the cause of an infected collection. Little regard was given to the effects of head injuries on the brain. Thus, there is a vast literature that can be regarded as the orthopedic approach to head injuries or cranial osteology.

What is of greater interest to those of us interested in the neurosciences is the development of concepts about the effects of trauma on the function of the nervous system. Although scattered examples appear in the 16th century, it is not until the 18th century that we find the beginning of a literature devoted to the effects of trauma on brain function. It is for this reason that I have chosen to address myself to these origins of surgical neurology and the treatment of head trauma in the 18th century.

From the early 16th century onward, many individual works devoted to the anatomy and surgery of the head appeared, as did sections within general surgical texts. Some of these were simply reworkings of *De Vulneribus Capitis*, while others represented small advances based on the commentaries by surgeons with first-hand experience. Thus, we find Lanfrancius, as early as the end of the 13th century, introducing the concept of concussion, an injury to the brain without any fracture (7). This was dealt with in greater detail by Berengario da Carpi in the first separate work on head injuries to appear after the Hippocratic tract. Once again, the title indicates the primary concern with skull fracture, i.e., *Tractatus de Fractura Calve Sive Cranei*, which appeared in two 16th-century editions and was reprinted in the 17th century (8,9). There was no advancement of diagnostic acumen beyond the ability to detect fractures. That surgeons had to deal often with these lesions is attested to by the extensive repetitious discussions that appear in works by Paré, Fallopius, Fabricius ab Aquapendente, and Croce (10–13).

A most celebrated case of the head injury sustained by Henri II of France was related by Paré, who attended the King and was present at his autopsy. A large subdural hematoma was found and Paré proposed the tearing of bridging cortical veins as the cause of the accumulation. His clinical observations of the dying King included many of the signs of increased intracranial pressure: headache, blurred vision, emesis, decreased level of consciousness, and ultimately decreased respiration.

Paré attributed these signs and symptoms to the injury itself when they appeared within the first few days. When they developed many days after the wound, they were due to inflammation of the brain and "putrefaction of the blood poured forth upon it" (10). This inability to distinguish between a collection, resulting from the head injury, and one developing because of infection secondary to the injury or surgical intervention was to remain a major obstacle to accurate diagnosis of cerebral compression and the timing of surgical intervention until well into the 19th century. It is this very point, the ability of the surgeon to diagnose cerebral compression and utilize this symptom as an indication for surgical intervention, that represents a turning point in the establishment of surgical neurology as a discipline. I shall return to this point when I discuss the contributions of several 18th-century surgeons.

The importance of trephination and treatment of head injuries during the 16th and 17th centuries can be judged from the number of publications dealing with them and the amount of space in general surgical works devoted to head injuries. The management of head injuries occupied one-third of a late 16th-century work by Andrea dalla Croce (13). Also included in this book were three large woodcuts depicting a trephination in progress (Fig. 1). Except for the decor and domestic touches, the procedure does not appear to have changed very much. It was the surgical judgment, the indications for performing such a procedure, that constituted the advances of the next two centuries.

Except for such insights as shown by Paré in explaining a mechanism for the formation of a subdural hematoma, there was a surprising lack of innovative ideas in this whole area. The overwhelming burden of the Hippocratic emphasis on the fracture as the focal point in head injuries and the inability to distinguish between traumatic clots and secondary collections appears to have been sufficient to distract many observers from the underlying implications of alterations in neurologic findings and the time course of their development (4,5).

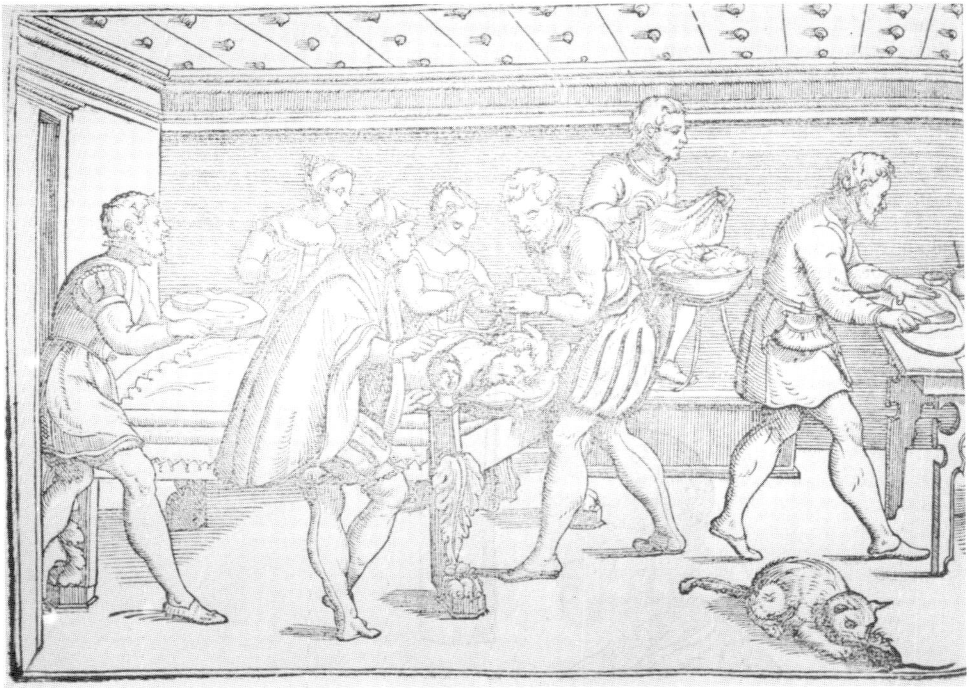

FIG. 1. Sixteenth-century trephination. (From Croce, ref. 13.)

Although it is difficult to find any sophistication in neurological evaluation of patients in works of the 16th and 17th centuries, I have elsewhere noted a curious neurological finding that appeared in an illustration in a surgical work of this period (14). The development of a third nerve palsy and contralateral facial palsy ought not to be an unusual finding in patients sustaining severe cerebral trauma. Nevertheless, it did not appear in the writings on trauma to the head until the 18th century.

The importance of including the illustrations that appear in medical books as part of the history of medicine of a period has been stressed by Herrlinger (15). Gersdorff's *Feldbuch der Wundartzney* has been regarded as the first printed book to illustrate actual surgical procedures (16). It went through many editions and must have been frequently consulted, since the illustrations were used by other writers for their own texts. On folio XXII, recto and verso, two woodcuts showing the method of elevating depressed skull fractures appear. I have suggested that the first illustration shows anisocoria (Fig. 2) and that the second one shows a more nearly complete third nerve palsy and contralateral facial weakness (Fig. 3). Since there is no comment in the text about these findings, I can only conclude that this was a direct observation of the artist and did not attract the attention of Gersdorff or any of the later surgeons who borrowed freely from this work and actually repeated these same illustrations. A version appears in Croce, as well as in works by Paaw and Pott in the 17th and 18th centuries (13,17,18). One of these drawings is actually embossed on the cover of a recent work on the history of medical illustrations (19).

It is difficult to notice a clear progression from surgery based on osteology to one determined by neurologic signs and symptoms. This is further obscured by the inability of the proponents and critics of trephination during the 17th and 18th centuries to separate the results of surgery from the results of infection, both primary and resulting from surgical intervention. In pre-Listerian times, the perfect operation performed for all the correct indications was often doomed to failure.

In France, at the turn of the 18th century, surgery emerged once again as an independent discipline under the patronage of Louis XIV and Louis XV. The story has been told many times (20–22). Surgery was separated from the Faculty of Medicine in 1724, the Royal Academy of Surgery was chartered in 1731, and in 1743, by royal decree, surgery could only be performed by those trained in the discipline.

Among the group of French surgeons of this period, several can be singled out as having special interest in the problem of head injuries and their management. One surgeon is cited by all of his contemporaries for introducing the concept that the time course of the appearance of alteration in the level of consciousness following a head injury might serve as an indication for trephination. This is Jean-Louis Petit. Clearly the leading surgeon of Paris during the first half of the 18th century, Petit drew a clear-cut distinction between the loss of consciousness accompanying a blow to the head and the drowsiness *(assoupissement)* that appeared later. The first he attributed to concussion, the latter to the formation of a collection or effusion (*épanchement)* producing compression of the brain.

Petit's accomplishments in general surgery are noted in many of the standard works on the history of medicine (20–22). He introduced an improved screw tourniquet and was the first to open the mastoid for the treatment of mastoiditis. A work on diseases of the bones, published in 1705, presented good descriptions of osteomalacia and the management of fractures with splinting and traction, as well as a description of a fracture that has since been known as Pott's fracture (23). An indication of Petit's position in French surgery was his appointment as the first Director of the Royal Academy of Surgery from its inception in 1731 until 1738.

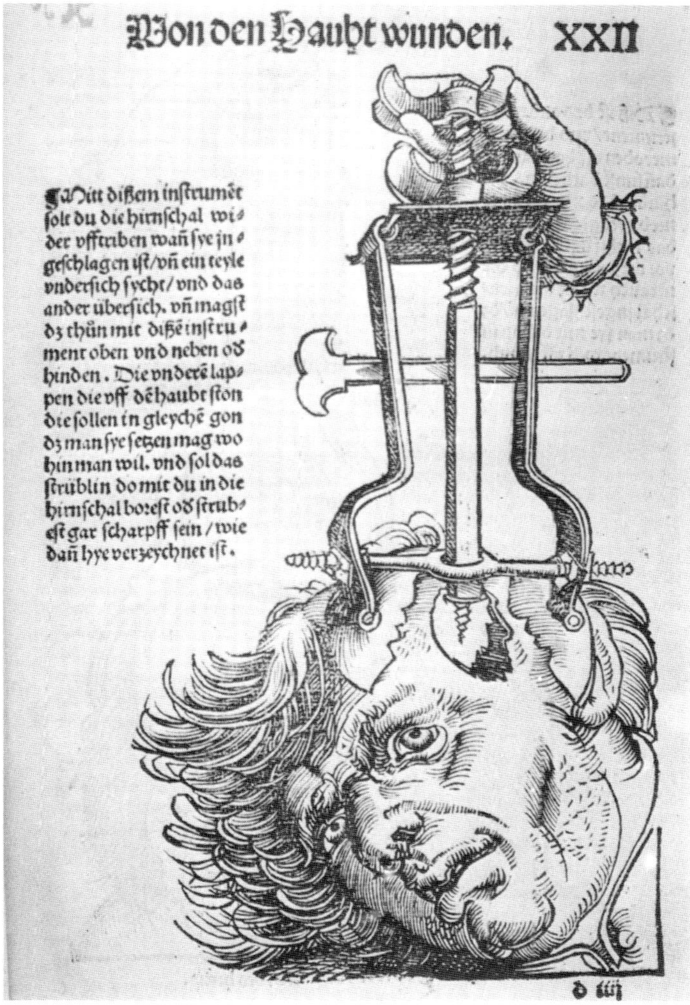

FIG. 2. Elevation of degressed skull fracture. Note the suggestion of anisocoria. (From Gersdorff, ref. 16.)

To regard Petit as an early neurosurgeon, we must remember that he, too, like his contemporaries, still labored under the impression that the diagnosis and disclosure of skull fractures themselves played an important role in the management of this group of patients. Furthermore, the inability to separate traumatic lesions from those resulting from infection, either because of or in spite of the surgical intervention, made it very difficult to evaluate the results of these surgical interventions.

To determine Petit's priority for the observation that a lucid interval between head injury and decrease in level of consciousness often bespoke a collection of blood that required trephination, we must rely on a number of secondary sources. Petit's own surgical works were not published until 1774, 24 years after his death (24). His only paper on a neurosurgical topic was published in 1743 in the *Mémoires de l'Académie Royale de Chirurgie* (25). This introduced the design of a new elevator for dealing with depressed skull fractures. The

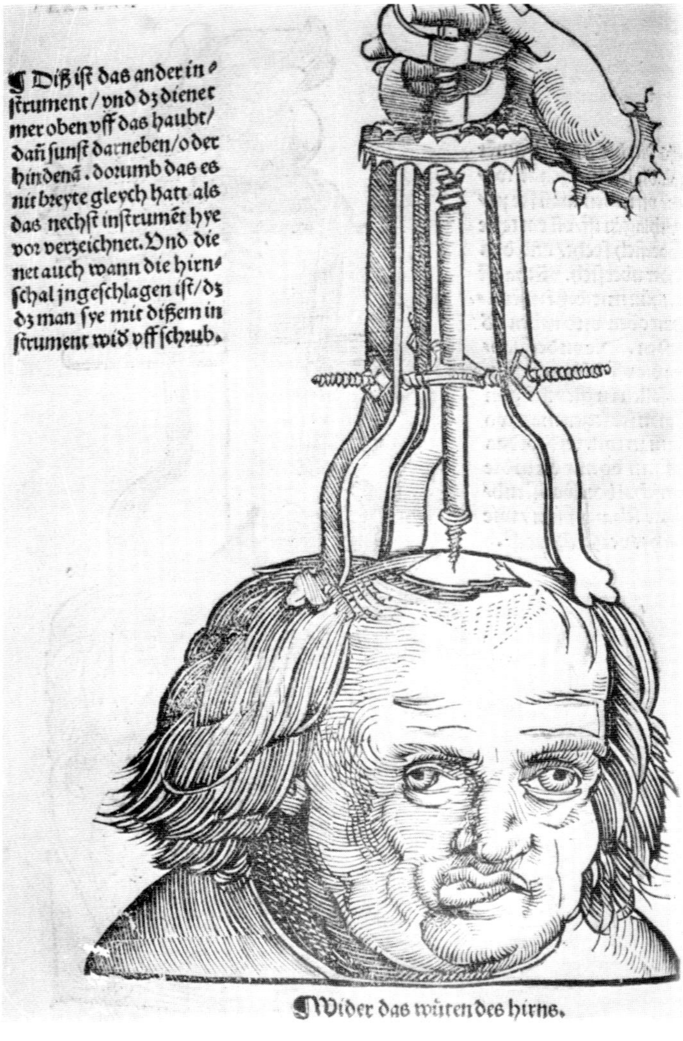

FIG. 3. Elevation of depressed skull fracture. Note the presence of a right third nerve palsy and a left seventh nerve palsy. (From Gersdorff, ref. 16.)

principle was that, unlike earlier examples of elevators, the pressure was applied to the stable portion of the skull and not to the free fragment. This eliminated the risk of further compression of the brain during the course of the operation.

The earliest reference to Petit as the originator of the idea that concussion and compression of the brain could be separated by their clinical presentations was in a work by Louis François Manne, a surgeon in Avignon (26). In the foreword, Manne suggested that the danger to the patient with a head injury comes not from the fracture, but from concussion and compression due to an effusion. On page 100, he attributed this observation to Petit. Later, he summarized his position that fractures of the skull are no different from fractures of bones elsewhere; the true danger to the patient results from an effusion of blood between the skull and dura, which must be removed by trephination.

> After all that we have said, it seems that there must be an indisputable surgical principle, that fractures of the skull are no different from fractures of other bones, that the lacerations of the brain and its coverings are wounds in themselves neither dangerous or mortal if they are free of concussion and effusion.[1]

Appended to this work are letters to the author from several surgeons to whom he had submitted his manuscript. These are La Peyronie, Morand, and Petit, all leaders in the foundation of the Royal Academy of Surgery in Paris.

Petit commented that the principle that wounds of the head are dangerous only because of effusion *(épanchement)* and concussion *(commotion)* had always served as a rule for him in arriving at a prognosis. This letter was dated February 12, 1729. It marks a turning point in the surgical approach to head injuries since it establishes the importance of injury to the brain either primarily from the impact or secondarily from compression rather than relying on the type of fracture, which had guided prognosis and therapy for 2,000 years.

Several other sources support the priority of Petit in establishing this important neurosurgical principle. A contemporary manuscript in my collection consists of the lecture notes of Jean Monpillier from Anjou, entitled "Principes de Chirurgie démontrés dans l'amphithéâtre de St. Côme par M. Petit—maitre chirurgien juré, membre de l'Académie royale des Sciences et démonstrateur royal à Paris" (Fig. 4). It is dated 1730. In the section on wounds of the head, he divides the signs into those related to injury of the skull, the dura, and the brain. A separate section lists the signs of compression of the brain due to a collection of blood. The one most clearly stressed is drowsiness *(assoupissement).*

Among the papers dealing with head injury that appeared in the *Mémoires de l'Académie Royale de Chirurgie* was a report by Quesnay in 1743 on the use of the trepan (27). This was translated into English and published by the Sydenham Society in 1858 (28). Referring to Petit, Quesnay wrote:

> This observation brings to our remembrance a very appropriate work of M. Petit's respecting insensibility and stupor, which deserves great attention. That able practitioner thinks that these affections are due only to concussion of the brain, when they occur immediately after the blow; and that, on the contrary, when they come on at a later period they are due to an effusion which has taken place under the skull in consequence of the blow.

Quesnay added that Petit was preparing a "Treatise on Operations," which would appear shortly and contain more details of Petit's ideas. This did not appear until 31 years later.

Petit was not alone among the surgeons of 18th-century France in recognizing that signs of cerebral compression, rather than bony lesions, should serve as the indication for trephination. Henri François Le Dran, another founding member of the Royal Academy of Surgery, published his surgical observations in 1731 (29). He pointed out that drowsiness must not be attributed to the fracture of the skull but to injury of the brain and that the delayed appearance of drowsiness was a sign of compression due to a collection of blood beneath the skull. In describing a case requiring trephination, Le Dran cited his determination to attempt an operation, not in itself dangerous, rather than to miss the opportunity of a cure (Obs. XVIII).

Thus, by 1731, two of the leading surgeons on the continent were aware of a very important principle in surgical neurology, one that had escaped many experienced surgeons for hundreds of years. It is hard to establish how this principle became obvious to Petit and Le Dran, unless it was an original insightful observation.

---

[1]Author's translation of p. 234, ref. 26.

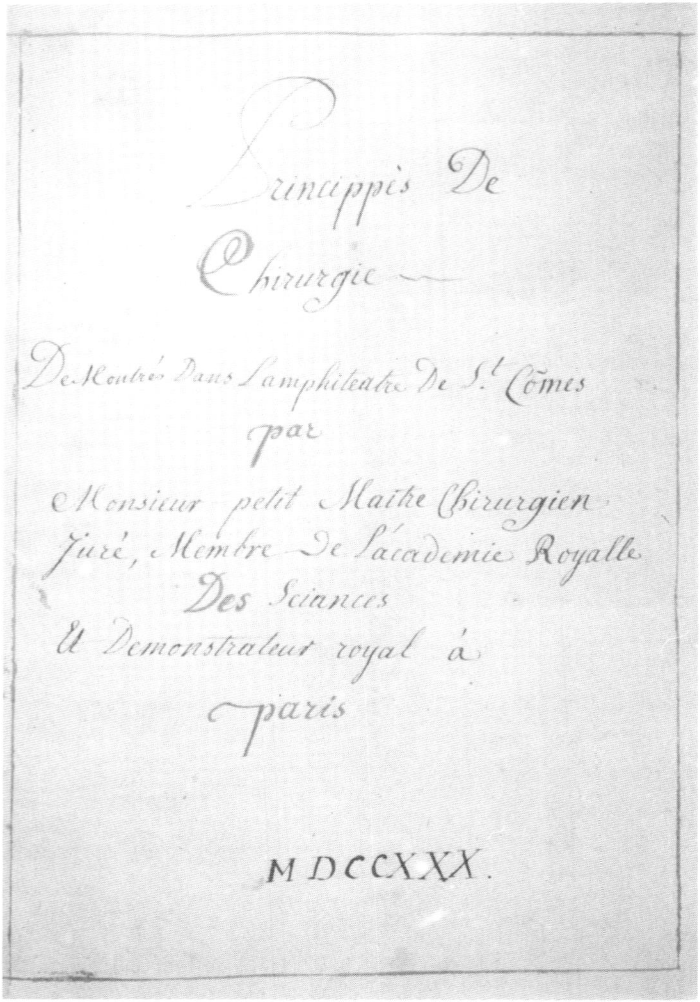

Princippes De Chirurgie

Demontrés Dans l'amphiteatre De St Cômes

par

Monsieur petit Maitre Chirurgien Juré, Membre De l'academie Royalle Des Sciences

Et Demonstrateur royal à paris

MDCCXXX.

FIG. 4. Title page of manuscript of lectures delivered by J.-L. Petit in 1730.

Nothing appears in the 17th- and early 18th-century works by Hildanus, Scultetus, Wiseman, Dionis, or Heister that gives any suggestion of an understanding of the temporal events associated with head injury (30–34). These authors' works are in the osteologic tradition and describe a variety of fractures that should or should not be trephined. To be sure, many surgeons utilized trephination as a last resort when the patient was moribund, but none before Petit and Le Dran attempted to establish clinical criteria. It is for this reason that I have focused on this period in the history of French surgery as a possible start of the specialty of surgical neurology.

How was this concept taken up by colleagues and by the next generation of these surgeons? Since factors other than timing of surgical intervention alone determined the outcome of trephination, it is not surprising that this principle soon became elaborate and confusing to many of the surgeons of this period. The inability to separate the ravages of infections as a consequence of surgery performed for proper indications became a major stumbling block for the ready acceptance of this clear surgical indication.

The major supporter of an aggressive approach to head injuries was Percival Pott (18). He credited Le Dran for calling attention to the lucid interval that occurs prior to the onset of coma due to cerebral compression from an epidural collection.

It was apparent to Le Dran and also to Pott that the depression of consciousness following a concussion could merge with that of a collection causing cerebral compression. Thus, it became difficult at times to separate these two causes of what might present as a prolonged period of unconsciousness. A further source of confusion lay in the inability of surgeons of this period to separate the depression of consciousness due to a blood clot from those due to the formation of an epidural abscess or subdural empyema. Pott tried to distinguish between epidural clot and infection by noting that the latter was more often associated with a febrile course and localized pain. In addition, he noted that symptoms due to an infected collection developed later than those due to extravasated blood.

The lack of any understanding of the nature of infectious processes continued to confound this group of surgeons. Since the 17th century, most writers believed that any extravasation of blood would suppurate (4). Pott denied this and advanced the hypothesis that damage to vessels bridging between the skull and dura or dura and brain was the cause of inflammation and suppuration. Based on this hypothesis, he advocated early trephination for most head injuries even if this meant an unnecessary operation for some. Although Pott was aware of the significance of the delayed appearance of drowsiness following a head injury, he was unable to discard all of the old osteologic indications for neurosurgical intervention. Pott felt there was still a role for prophylactic trephination. Speaking of undepressed fractures of the skull, he wrote (18):

> The reasons for trepanning in these cases are first, the immediate relief of present symptoms arising from pressure of extravasated fluid; or second, the discharge of matter formed between the skull and dura mater in consequence of inflammation; or third, the prevention of such mischief as experience has shewn, most probably, be expected from such kind of violence offered to the last-mentioned membrane.

Other surgeons of the latter part of the 18th century had difficulty in reconciling the importance of the clinical signs of cerebral compression and the results of surgical intervention. In England and Ireland, Dease and O'Halloran, while recognizing the importance of distinguishing between concussion and compression, concluded that the results of trephination were worse than when expectant treatment, which utilized bleeding and purging, was used (35,36). In France, a similar backlash occurred, and Desault, the successor to Petit as the leader of French surgery, went so far as to forbid the use of the trephine at the Hôtel-Dieu (20). This reactionary position was forced upon these surgeons not because of an error in understanding the significance of cerebral compression, but because of the limitations of surgery due to infection in the pre-Listerian era.

The final chapter in the development of an awareness of neurological signs in head injury as a surgical indication was written by Benjamin Bell. If we contrast the title of Pott's work, "Observations on the Nature and Consequences of those Injuries to which the Head is liable from External Violence" (18), with Bell's "On affections of the Brain from External Violence" (37), we see that the emphasis has finally been directed to the proper seat of the disorder. Bell stressed the importance of relieving compression of the brain, be it caused by bone, blood, or pus. Of even greater importance is the emphasis he placed on the use of the trephine when symptoms of compression are present, even if no sign of injury to the head is evident (38). This is a bold surgical principle based on an understanding of neurological symptoms. Finally, brain surgery began to emerge from the 2,000-year history of skull surgery. Bell writes:

> But although it is proper to enquire into the nature of the cause by which a fracture is produced, yet we are not to imagine that any material advantage is to be derived from it . . . As it is impossible to ascertain the extent of any injury done to the brain by this circumstance alone, little or no dependence should be placed upon it . . .

For Bell, surgery was to relieve compression of the brain, which could be diagnosed by the neurological signs and symptoms of the patient, and which he most carefully observed and recorded:

> . . . the most frequent, as well as the most remarkable are the following: giddiness, dimness of sight, stupefaction, loss of voluntary motion, vomiting, an apopletic stertor in breathing, convulsive tremors in different muscles, a dilated state of the pupils, even when the eyes are exposed to a clear light, paralysis of different parts, especially the side of the body opposite to the injured part of the head, . . . an oppressed, and in many cases an irregular pulse. . . .

Finally, a surgeon was aware of a fixed, dilated pupil in association with trauma and cerebral compression almost 300 years after a 16th-century artist had noted a third nerve palsy. Bell was no less precise in dispelling the age old concept of prophylactic trephination:

> For although I am clearly of opinion, that the trepan should be applied with freedom wherever it is indicated by symptoms of a compressed brain, and where these symptoms must in all probability prove fatal if the cause which produced them is not soon removed; yet I am equally satisfied, that it is the presence of such symptoms only which can warrant this operation; and that it should never be employed, as it too frequently has been, merely with a view to prevent them.

Although the ability of surgeons to diagnose and treat head injuries at the end of the 18th century was still primitive, the foundation of our current methods of utilizing neurological symptoms and signs to arrive at a proper course of action began to be utilized by a number of these early surgical neurologists. Their opinions were not accepted by all of their contemporaries, but they began to introduce the principles of neurosurgery upon which we rely today.

REFERENCES

1. Breasted, J. H. (1930): *The Edwin Smith Surgical Papyrus*, 2 vols. University of Chicago Press, Chicago.
2. Ciba Foundation Symposium (1975): *Outcome of Severe Damage to the Central Nervous System*, 354 pp. Elsevier, Amsterdam.
3. Hippocrates (1923–1931): In *Works*, English translation by W. H. S. Jones and E. T. Withington, Vols. 1–4. Loeb Classical Library, Heinemann, London.
4. Mettler, F. A., and Mettler, C. C. (1945): *Proc. ARNMD*, 24:1.
5. Courville, C. B. (1946): *L.A. Neurol. Sci.*, 11:1.
6. Ballance, C. (1922): *Lancet*, I:111,165.
7. Lanfrancius (1565): *A moste excellent and learned woorke of chirurgery called chirurgia porva Lanfranci*. T. Marshe, London.
8. Berengario da Carpi, J. (1518): *Tractatus de fractura calve sive cranei*. H. de Benedictis, Bologna.
9. Berengario da Carpi, J. (1535): *Tractatus perntilis et completus de fractura cranei*. J. A. de Nicolinis de Sabio for J. B. Pederzanus, Venice.
10. Paré, A. (1634): *The Workes*, translated by T. Johnson. T. Cotes and R. Young, London.
11. Fallopius, G. (1584): *Opera quae adhuc extant omnia*. A. M. Haer and A. Wecheli, Frankfurt.

12. Fabricius ab Aquapendente, H. (1619): *Opera chirurgica*. P. Megliettum, Venice.
13. Croce, G. A. dalla (1573): *Chirurgiae libri septem*. G. Ziletti, Venice.
14. Flamm, E. S. (1972): *Med. Hist.*, 16:194.
15. Herrlinger, R. (1970): *History of Medical Illustration*. Editions Medicina Rara, New York.
16. Gersdorff, H. (1517): *Feldbuch der Wundartzney*. J. Schott, Strassburg.
17. Paaw, P. (1616): *Succenturiatus Anatomicus*. J. à Colster, Leyden.
18. Pott, P. (1773): *Observations on the Nature and Consequences of those Injuries to which the Head is Liable from External Violence*, 3rd ed. L. Hawes, W. Clarke and R. Collins, London.
19. Hahn, A., and Dumaitre, P. (1962): *Histoire de la Médecine et du Livre Médical*. Olivier Perrin, Paris.
20. Zimmerman, T. M., and Veith, I. (1967): *Great Ideas in the History of Surgery*. Dover Publications, New York.
21. Garrison, F. H. (1929): *An Introduction to the History of Medicine*, 4th ed. W. B. Saunders and Co., Philadelphia.
22. Mettler, C. C. (1947): *History of Medicine*. Blakiston, Philadelphia.
23. Petit, J.-L. (1705): *L'art de guérir les maladies des os, où l'ontraite des luxations et des fractures avec les instruments nécessaires et une machine de nouvelle invention pour les réduire, ensemble des exostoses et des caries, des ankyloses, des maladies des dents, et de la charte au rachites, maladie ordinaire aux enfans*. L. d'Houry, Paris.
24. Petit, J. -L. (1774): *Traité des maladies chirurgicales et des opérations qui leur conviennent*, 3 vols. P. F. Didot le jeune, Paris.
25. Petit, J.-L. (1743): *Mem. Acad. roy. Chirurg.*, 1:302.
26. Manne, L. F. (1729): *Observation de Chirurgie au Sujet d'une Playe à la Tête avec Fracas, et une pièce d'os implantée dans le cerveau pendant un mois sans aucun simptome, accompagnée d'une dissertation au sujet des playes de tête avec fracture et du plusiers autres observations dans ce genre, suive des lettres des sçavans, qui ont été consultez à ce sujet par l'auteur*. F. Girard, Avignon.
27. Quesnay, F. (1743): *Mem. Acad. roy. Chirurg.*, 1:188
28. Ottley, D. (1858): *Observations on Surgical Diseases of the Head and Neck*. Sydenham Society, London.
29. Le Dran, H.-F. (1731): *Observations de chirurgie*, 2 vols. C. Osmout, Paris.
30. Fabricius Hildanus, W. (1646): *Opera quae extant omnia*. A. M. J. Beyer, Frankfurt.
31. Scultetus, J. (1655): Χειροπλουηχη *seu armamentarium chirurgicum*. B. Kühnen, Ulm.
32. Wiseman, R. (1676): *Severall chirurgicall treatises*. R. Royston, London.
33. Dionis, P. (1707):*Cours d'opérations de chirurgie, demonstrée au Jardin Royal*. L. d'Houry, Paris.
34. Heister, L. (1743): *A General System of Surgery*. J. Whiston, L. Dawes and C. Reymers, London.
35. Dease, W. (1776): *Observations on wounds of the Head with a particular enquiry into the parts principally affected in those who die in consequence of such injuries*. G. Robinson, London.
36. O'Halloran, S. (1793): *A new treatise on the different disorders arising from external injuries of the head*. G. C. and J. Robinson, London.
37. Bell, B. (1785): In: *A System of Surgery*, vol. 3, p. 1. C. Elliott, Edinburgh.
38. Forster, F. M. (1944): *Bull. Hist. Med.*, 15:298.

Historical Aspects of the Neurosciences,
edited by F. Clifford Rose and W. F. Bynum.
Raven Press, New York ©

The History of Neuroradiology

J. W. D. Bull

Department of Neuroradiology, National Hospital for Nervous Diseases, London WC1, England

In the decade before Röntgen's discovery, Sir William Gowers (1) wrote in his famous textbook:

> The nervous system is almost entirely inaccessible to direct examination. The exceptions to this are trifling. The termination of one nerve, the optic, can be seen within the eye. Some of the nerve trunks in the limbs can be felt; a few, as the ulnar, in the normal state; others only when enlarged by disease.

Radiology came very slowly on the scene of neurology, particularly in England, and it was not until 1924 [29 years after Röntgen's (2) discovery] that any serious neuroradiological discussion took place in England. I will refer to this in more detail shortly. The long-established English clinical school of medicine, which was perhaps second to none in the world, has always accepted new paraclinical methods of investigation very slowly.

Before summarizing the evolution of neuroradiology, I would like to draw attention to the fact that man is very lucky to be able to apply Röntgen's discovery to his own ends. It so happens that the largest members of our species approach the critical level of x-ray photography. It is well known how difficult it is to obtain a satisfactory radiograph of the abdomen of a very large obese human subject. To put it another way, one cannot x-ray the abdomen of a pig or a horse; it is too thick. With regard to the brain, again man is fortunate phylogenetically that his face has shrunk relative to the remainder of his skull and his frontal bone has ascended well above his paranasal sinuses. This is a great advantage in taking a frontal radiograph of the brain.

The father of neuroradiology was undoubtedly Arthur Schüller. He was born in Brunn, Bohemia, then part of the Austro-Hungarian Empire. His father was a doctor, an ear, nose, and throat specialist, and a friend of Politzer. Young Schüller was a brilliant student, graduating in Vienna with the highest honors and receiving a prize presented at a special audience with the Emperor Franz Joseph for outstanding merit. It was given only twice during his 60-year reign.

Schüller qualified soon after the discovery of x-rays by Röntgen at Würzburg in November 1895. He was attracted to the study of this revolutionary development in medicine and was introduced to its practice by Holzknecht, the founder of the Viennese School of Radiology. In 1905 he published *Die Schädelbasis in Röntgenbilde* (3) and in 1912 *Röntgendiagnostik der Erkrankungen des Kopfes* (4), concerning radiological diagnosis of diseases of the head. These classic works still form the basis of x-ray examination of the skull. This latter book was translated into English in 1918 by Dr. Fred Stocking (5) and published by Mosby of St. Louis, but it received little attention in England.

It should be made clear that Schüller was trained in neurophysiology. In 1910, in the *Wiener Medizinische Wochenschrift*, he published a paper entitled "Durchtrennung der Rückenmarksstränge" (6), about the section of the spinal tracts, or what we would call cordotomy. Schüller practiced surgery only on dogs, but this was the forerunner of Sjöquist's (7) tractotomy. In association with Erdheim, he studied pituitary tumors. Not being a surgeon, he persuaded his friend to operate by the transnasal approach. Schüller devised three operations, cordotomy, transnasal pituitary ablation, and posterior cisternal drainage of the hydrocephalic third ventricle, and his name is attached to three diseases of bone, Schüller-Christian disease, osteoporosis circumscripta, and cephalhematoma deformans.

He possessed independent means and did not bother much about private practice until after World War I when he had lost everything. Then he earned most of his living teaching foreign postgraduates who flocked to Vienna at that time. Though a Catholic, having some Jewish blood, he decided to leave Vienna in 1938, spent a few months in Oxford, and then went to Melbourne, where he lived until his death in 1957. Schüller never interested himself much in contrast methods, but there was no one like him for analyzing the skull.

Radiology developed slowly as an adjunct to neurology. But as early as 1907, Fedor Krause, a German surgeon, published a three-volume textbook entitled *Surgery of the Brain and Spinal Cord* (8) (translated in the U.S.A. in 1910), which said of x-rays: "Above all other means of diagnosis it furnishes the most useful in tumors with calcareous or bony deposits, as for instance in exostosis and any injury to the skull may bring on epileptic seizures . . . whenever possible x-ray examination should be made; it is frequently a great aid in clearing up the diagnosis. Even in other forms of epilepsy röntgenography is of urgent need." This view of Krause was very advanced then. In my early days at the National Hospital after World War II, it was by no means routine to x-ray a patient's head for epilepsy.

In 1912, a young Swedish pathologist, Folke Henschen, soon to become a professor and later one of the world's leading neuropathologists, added an important contribution. He was already well known as an authority on acoustic tumors, the surgery of which was subsequently mastered by Cushing (9). In his communication, Henschen (10) gave an excellent up-to-date account (1912) of the value and limitations of radiology in the diagnosis of brain tumors and went on to describe how he had found at autopsy that acoustic neuromas always widened the internal auditory meatus. He felt convinced that this feature should be demonstrable radiographically in life, and he sought the aid of his radiological colleague, Dr. Forssell, who was later to become a professor. In passing, it could be added that in the opinion of many, Forssell was the greatest personality that the world of radiology has yet seen, and he did more for its progress and status than anyone before or since.

In February 1910, Henschen had a case of suspected acoustic tumor that he submitted to radiography. Unfortunately, only one side of the head was x-rayed, and the patient was allowed to depart. Henschen had to wait just over a year for another case (March 1911). On this occasion he obtained two radiographs, one of the normal and the other of the abnormal meatus. The patient died in April, and Henschen confirmed the radiographical findings at autopsy.

In the following year, 1912, on November 24th, a middle-aged man was admitted with a head injury to a New York hospital under the care of Dr. W. H. Luckett (11). He was x-rayed by Dr. W. H. Stewart, who detected a fracture in the posterior wall of the frontal sinus. The patient was treated conservatively and discharged from hospital, but he returned some three weeks later having suffered a relapse. On December 14th a further radiographical examination of the skull was undertaken by Dr. Stewart. He reported that these x-rays showed the ventricles enormously dilated by what was probably air or gas. As a result of these findings, Dr. Luckett operated and during the course of operation tapped one of the ventricles and noticed that air or gas was released. The patient died three days later, and at autopsy the fracture in the posterior wall of the frontal sinus was confirmed and part of the bone was found to be depressed about 1 cm.

The brain was removed in toto and placed under water. Bubbles emerged through a laceration in the base of the frontal lobe and this laceration was shown to communicate with the anterior horn of the ventricle. The fluid in the ventricle at the time of the operation was examined bacteriologically and found to be sterile. It was therefore assumed that air, not gas, was present. On his second admission to the hospital, the patient said that just previously he had sneezed, that this was followed by a terrific pain in his head, and immediately afterwards about a cupful of clear fluid came away from his nose. We know nowadays that this can be the classic story associated with so-called spontaneous pneumoencephalography.

In 1917, one year before Dandy's discovery, Dr. Gilbert Scott (12), radiologist to the London Hospital, reported a remarkable case in the *Archives of Radiology and Electrotherapy*. This case merits reporting at some length because it is important historically and has not received its due publicity.

The patient, a female aged 38, was referred to Dr. Scott. She complained of very severe headaches and said that her brain was splashing. "At first I ignored this symptom of brain splashing as a subjective sensation," wrote Dr. Scott, but after going on to take a more detailed history, he recorded, "my curiosity by this time being thoroughly roused, I took hold of her head in both hands and shook it vigorously. The sensation imparted to my hands, together with the sound produced by this procedure, was most extraordinary, not to say alarming, and I instinctively let go her head. Free fluid in considerable quantity could be felt moving about in the cranium, coming up with a resounding 'smack' against the frontal bone . . . as these signs indicated the presence of air and fluid in the cranium, I expected to find interesting radiographic appearances. In this I was not disappointed. The history was that nine years ago a bony tumor appeared in the inner and upper part of the orbit. An ophthalmic surgeon refused to touch it. She was then sent to a general surgeon who removed it with apparent success and she remained well until eight months ago when she developed unbearable headaches. The splashing was first noticed five months ago." Her mental state had remained quite normal and was so when Scott saw her in June 1915. The frontal bone was subsequently trephined, but this did not throw much light upon the condition. Scott lost touch with her after she left hospital. He postulated, probably correctly, that a small opening was made into the cranium through the orbit when the tumor was removed. Cushing (13) subsequently described the condition of pneumatocele associated with orbitoethmoidal osteoma.

In spite of Stewart's and Scott's findings of spontaneous pneumoencephalography, it is surprising that no one before Dandy used the procedure for diagnostic purposes. He was inspired by Dr. Halstead, a general surgeon and a senior colleague at his own hospital, Johns Hopkins, Baltimore. In his original paper (1918), Dandy (14) stated: "It is largely due to frequent comment by Dr. Halstead on the remarkable power of the intestinal gases to perforate bone on an X-ray that my attention was drawn to its practical possibilities in the brain." He went on to say that the chief value of ventriculography was in the diagnosis of internal hydrocephalus in infants and that he had not yet applied the method to adults, but he expected to do so in all cases where the diagnosis was obscure. In the light of our experience of the value of pneumography since 1918, this is a good example of the well-known reluctance by medical men to accept new methods wholeheartedly.

Within a year, Dandy had followed up his great discovery by another equally as great, that of encephalography (1919) (15). He described how by introducing air via the lumbar theca (lumbar puncture) after the removal of an equivalent amount of cerebrospinal fluid and by maintaining the patient in a sitting position, it was possible to outline the ventricles with air. At the same time, he predicted the procedure of air myelography for the localization of spinal tumors.

Meanwhile, we must go back in time to 1909 or 1910. In a paper published by Jacobaeus (16) in 1921 on myelography, he stated that in 1909 or 1910 he had replaced 100 ml of cerebrospinal fluid with air in cases of tuberculous meningitis. As there was no therapeutic effect apart from "whimsical improvement," as he put it, he gave it up and never published the method. Remembering this technique, in July 1919, three months before Dandy's second paper, he performed the first air myelogram, and in 1921 he published the results obtained in three cases in which spinal tumors were localized by air myelography, in the last two cases quite accurately. In the first case, the tumor was found to be two vertebrae higher than the top of the column of air, but the plain x-ray had revealed gross changes that enabled him to localize the lesion precisely. Then in the same year, Sicard (17), a Parisian neurologist, published his well-known paper using Lipiodol for myelography. His main interest was in the treatment of pain, for which he developed a great reputation and was the leading physician in France in this field. One of the substances he used for the treatment of sciatica and other neuralgias was Lipiodol. He noticed that it was an excellent x-ray contrast substance and was well tolerated without producing side effects when injected into the lumbar muscles. He then had the idea of using it diagnostically and started injecting it into the bronchi. In 1918, an American, Chevalier Jackson (18), a famous bronchoscopist, had tried using powdered bismuth, but this produced broncholiths.

When Sicard used Lipiodol for the treatment of sciatica, he observed radiologically that it tracked down the nerve sheath. It is said that one day, one of his pupils injected Lipiodol into the lumbar muscles and when he drew back the plunger of the syringe he noticed, to his horror,that he was withdrawing cerebral spinal fluid. He rushed off to Sicard to tell him what had happened, and Sicard merely asked him one question: "How is the patient?" He replied, "very well." "All right," said Sicard, "go and look at it on the fluorescent screen." Sicard screened the patient standing up and observed that the Lipiodol had dropped to the bottom of the spinal subarachnoidal space, and thus he had the brilliant idea of tilting the patient head down and observing the movement of the Lipiodol. There were no tilting x-ray tables in those days, so it must have been quite an exercise screening the patient partly upside down. Sicard and Forestier then stated that Lipiodol was apparently innocuous if introduced intrathecally.

It might be fair to describe Sicard as the father of positive contrast radiography. It should be remembered that up to the early 1920s, the only contrast method available was the bismuth, later barium meal. Barium meals are in a different category, as barium sulphate is inert and what is introduced by mouth all comes out unchanged and unabsorbed, so that it doesn't really enter the body. Lipiodol, on the other hand, soon came to be used for fistulas, sinuses, urethral and bladder injection, salpingography, the paranasal sinus replacement technique, and above all in the most sensitive of structures, the nervous system. Nowadays hardly any organ or tube is immune from radiological attack, so it is perhaps fair to say that it all stems back to Sicard.

Back in the early 1920s, when Dr. Critchley began practicing neurology, radiology provided scant aid to the neurologist. Neurosurgery was developing fast, and most surgeons were in the hands of the neurologist as to be told where the tumor lay. I referred at the beginning to the fact that no serious neuroradiological discussion took place in England until 1924, and there had been no significant papers published. In 1924, at the Royal Society of

Medicine, the Section of Neurology, under the presidency of Dr. James Collier, with Dr. Critchley in the audience, a discussion took place on Dandy's technique of ventriculography. It was noted that in some places in the United States the mortality was about 30%. The discussion was reported in *Brain* (19). A professor of medicine in Lisbon, Egaz Moniz (20), read the report. Clearly, he wrote later, the English were not altogether satisfied with ventriculography. This apparently spurred him on to seek help in another method of investigation and led to his great discovery of cerebral arteriography.

Moniz argued that it should be possible to outline the brain radiologically with some positive contrast substance, just as his Parisian friend Sicard had done with the spinal theca. As Moniz put it: "The brain was normally mute to x-rays"—the dark continent as he called it. He was also rather illogically stimulated by the recent work of Graham and Cole (21) of the Mallinkrodt Institute at St. Louis, whereby they succeeded in outlining the gall bladder following intravenous injection of a contrast substance. This of course depended upon a physiological concentration of the contrast substance in the bile in the gall bladder, and no parallel existed in the brain. Moniz had two methods in mind: (a) the opacification of the brain itself by intravenous or parenteral administration of a substance opaque to x-rays; and (b) the intraarterial injection of some opaque substance. He failed in the first but succeeded in the second. In order to opacify the brain, he attempted to flood it by the injection of a radiopaque substance. He injected large quantities of lithium bromide intravenously and also gave it by mouth in large doses. This failed and he then tried strontium bromide. Both substances were well tolerated by his patients but as no positive results ensued, this failure led him on to his second method, arteriography. In choosing a suitable substance, he considered Lipiodol, which Sicard had used for both myelography and ventriculography, but since it was oily Moniz realized that it might produce emboli.

Moniz therefore decided on an aqueous solution, an iodine or bromine salt, and favored iodine on account of its higher atomic weight and thus greater radiographic density. Having made a number of experiments on dogs and rabbits to assess the toxicity of various substances such as bromide and iodide of lithium, sodium, potassium, ammonium, and rubidium, he finally chose 25% sodium iodide. Fortunately, it was well tolerated by man when given intravenously, apart from producing some pain in the axilla when injected into an arm vein. He then pointed out that there was a precedent for intraarterial injection since Von Knauer (22) had injected neosalvarsan into the carotid artery percutaneously in 1919 for the treatment of general paralysis of the insane (GPI) without harm. This encouraged him to experiment on dogs, using strontium bromide and lithium bromide. At first, no contrast was seen on the radiographs, but he obtained a better x-ray machine and with shorter exposures achieved a satisfactory result. Then he passed on to the human cadaver in order to learn the normal radiographic anatomy. Having injected a number of corpses, he selected his first patient, a man suffering from GPI. Moniz himself suffered from gout in the hands and was unable to undertake arteriography, so this was performed by his pupil and successor Almeida Lima. It is interesting to recall that the injection was made percutaneously, just as Von Knauer had injected neosalvarsan into the carotid artery of a patient suffering from the same disease. Seven ml of 70% strontium bromide was injected without upsetting the patient, but the radiography showed nothing. They tried the percutaneous method of injection in three more cases but again without success, and in the last, Moniz thought that the contrast substance had been injected outside the artery. So thereafter it was decided to cut down on the artery. They were finally successful with the ninth case, a young man of 20 with a pituitary tumor, when 5 ml of 25% sodium iodide was injected and good pictures were obtained. Moniz then said: "Nous avons realisé notre desideratum."

This story has been recounted in some detail as it illustrates the tremendous determination of the man. Most people, had they had a similar experience, would have been deterred and abandoned the procedure long before they achieved success. This was in 1927, and he immediately went to Paris to read the paper to describe his success before his master and teacher, the great Babinski. Four years later, in 1931, he published a book (23) describing his first 90 cases. There were two deaths, both in arteriosclerotic patients. Babinski wrote the preface of the book and pointed out that Moniz made up his mind to put this project into execution and set forth courageously in his enterprise, as his compatriots Dias and Vasco de Gama had set forth across the ocean in their search for a route to the Indies. Surely no higher praise could be given to anyone, and perhaps only a Frenchman could express it so beautifully. Moniz had brought a new dimension to neuroradiology and helped very much to chart the dark continent.

Like Dandy's method of ventriculography, arteriography was accepted very slowly, particularly in the Anglo-Saxon countries. This may have been partly due to the fact that the investigation involved making two permanent scars, one on each side of the neck, unpleasant stigmata, particularly for an attractive woman to carry for the rest of her life, especially if the investigation proved negative. Moniz always insisted on undertaking bilateral arteriography and after his first three cases, he abandoned the percutaneous method for good. It was not until 1944 that the Norwegians Engeset and Christianson revived and firmly reestablished the method.

The history of the development of the technique of encephalography is of interest. For many years, huge amounts of air were introduced blind into the subarachnoid space by a doctor on the ward. There was often no idea of the size of the ventricles. Frequently, far too much air was introduced, making it extremely unpleasant for the patient.

In 1932, Leo Davidoff, the neurosurgeon, and C. G. Dyke, the radiologist, both of the Presbyterian Hospital in New York, published a paper entitled "An Improved Method of Encephalography" (24). The particular striking advance they made in technique was to carry out the whole examination in the x-ray department. The patient was set up and the head placed in the semiflexed position. Having introduced not more than 20 ml of air, they took a radiograph to see how much air was necessary in any particular case for a proper examination.

In 1941, Graeme Robertson of Melbourne further improved the method, which came to be known as controlled fractional air encephalography. Meanwhile, going back in time to the late 1920s, the technique of radiographing ventriculograms according to the method of Dandy had improved very little. Advances came from Stockholm, where Lysholm worked with Olivacrona. Lysholm's dictum in ventriculography was that the air should be placed up against the lesion in order to demonstrate the deformity of the ventricular system.

By placing the head in various positions and thus moving the air around the ventricular system, Lysholm was then able to make a synthetic drawing of the whole and, after studying hundreds of cases confirmed by operation or autopsy, he demonstrated that tumors produced characteristic deformities of the ventricular system according to their site. Night after night and year after year, he studied the ventriculograms with his assistants until, in 1935, he published the first part of his famous monograph, *Das Ventrikulogramm* (25). The first part was concerned with the normal ventricular system and the second, to be published, dealt with tumors involving the third ventricule, aqueduct, and fourth ventricle, of which he had 131 verified cases. In 1937 (26), he completed the work by publishing the findings of 398 verified supratentorial space-occupying masses. This classic work has stood the test of time and has not yet been and is unlikely to be superseded.

It all sounds simple, but filling the temporal horns, and particularly the aqueduct and fourth ventricle, could be difficult and one only has to glance at the literature to see how often it was not accomplished by radiologists not trained by Lysholm. He and his pupil Lindgren should be remembered for many advances. The Lysholm Skull Table is now known worldwide. Its proper use enabled one to take accurate projections and to repeat them exactly on a later occasion. It was he and Lindgren who also achieved the major advances in the technique of cerebral angiography, both carotid and vertebral. It should be remembered that Moniz only took lateral projections, while the Stockholm school developed accurate antero-posterior projections and also rapid serial angiography, thus deriving much information from the phlebograms in addition to the arterial phase.

By the late 1950s, the combination of plain x-rays, tomography, air studies, and angiography as undertaken at the major centers of the world enabled neurologists and neurosurgeons to have a fairly accurate picture of the size, shape, position, and often pathology of the lesion they were dealing with. These techniques had reached a point that made it difficult to imagine that radiology could help the neurologists and neurosurgeons any further. But it was not the end of the story. An entirely new dimension has since been developed. In February 1896, three months after Röntgen's discovery, Becquerel, (27,28) a Parisian physicist, discovered natural radioactivity. It was soon learnt that the naturally emitted rays from radioactive sources, so-called gamma rays, were of the same nature as x-rays. A few years after Becquerel's discovery, his rays were being used for medical treatment, radium being the source, but another half century was to pass before spontaneously emitted rays were used for diagnostic purposes. This is in large measure due to Rutherford's fundamental work, which ultimately led to the production of artificial radioactive isotopes.

World War II acted as a great spur to the development of nuclear physics, and by the mid-1940s, many artificial radioactive substances had been prepared. Their application to the diagnosis of disease began with the thyroid for two good reasons: (a) It was well known that iodine was taken up by the thyroid, and radioactive iodine isotopes were some of the first to be prepared; (b) The thyroid is a very superficial structure covered only by soft tissues, and thus the detection of any radioactivity within the gland was relatively simple. The brain was quite another problem in that it was not known to take up selectively any chemical compound or element, and even if a suitable isotope could be found, its rays would have to pass out through the skull bones. Not only would the skull grossly impede the radiation being emitted, but it would scatter it and thus add to the difficulties of precise localization.

It was George Moore (29), a young surgeon in Minneapolis, who solved the problem, and the story is fascinating. Having known previously that fluorescein was taken up selectively by certain tumors of the eye, Moore postulated that the same might apply to brain tumors. In cases of suspected glioma, immediately prior to operation, he injected a small quantity of fluorescein intravenously. It was found that it could be detected in tissues by ultraviolet light, using a Wood's lamp. When the brain was exposed at surgery, the ultraviolet light was shone on the cortex. Normal brain was given a grayish hue while a glioma appeared yellow in color and its edges could be clearly defined. Besides being successful in this project, Moore was able to delineate gliomas more clearly for neurosurgeons, since it is well known that the edge of a glioma is very difficult to determine macroscopically in that it often merges imperceptibly into normal brain.

Moore's next problem was to tag a radioactive substance to fluorescein. He prepared diiodofluorescein, the iodine being radioactive: ^{131}I. Having injected this substance intravenously, he attempted to detect the radioactive emissions from the tumor by means of a

Geiger counter, this being the tool used for the detection of radioactive emissions at that time. He was immediately successful and localized 12 out of 15 brain tumors. Thus it was that brain scanning, or isotope encephalography, came to be born in 1948. However, many years passed before the method became fully established. Other workers did not have the same success rate in detecting tumors, and over the next decade many apparatuses of gradually increasing sophistication were built in the United States. By 1960, a few American commercial firms had perfected scanning devices.

Until then, diagnostic radiology could be described as the study of shadows recorded on film after the passage of appropriate rays through the body. The value of the shadowgraph depended upon graduation of blackness, which was related to the different atomic numbers of elements contained in animal tissues. With the application of Becquerel's discovery, one could place the ray source within the body tissues and photograph the rays as they were emitted from the body. The great advantage of the isotope scan, as it came to be called, was its almost complete lack of morbidity and discomfort. The worst that could happen to a patient might be the inadvertant extravenous injection of a small quantity of the isotope. This could lead to local sloughing.

In the more recent history of neuroradiological advances, some mention should be made of catheter angiography with both diagnostic and therapeutic applications. The technique stems from cardiac radiology originally developed some 30 years ago. The applications began by injecting a contrast substance into the larger arteries. As techniques improved, smaller and smaller vessels were selectively catherized to both provide a better contrast effect and avoid the injection of unnecessary arteries. The new techniques also allowed the use of a smaller dose of contrast substance, as toxic effects to the delicate nervous system had always to be borne in mind. This can be illustrated by what one might call myeloangiography, or the outlining of vessels of the spinal cord. In earlier days, a bolus injection was made in the aorta in the hope that the spinal arteries would be opacified. If the main concentration of the contrast substance entered the spinal arteries, paraplegia sometimes ensued. The work of the Polish anatomist Adamkiewitz (30) was again remembered, and the artery that bears his name was the chief vessel supplying the lower part of the spinal cord. Its derivation from an intercostal artery was now shown to vary in level. This led to the selective catheterization and small volume (dose) injection of each of the 24 intercostal arteries in order to find Adamkiewitz's artery. The development of this work will always be associated with the name of Djindjian (31), a Parisian neuroradiologist. It was of course Thomas Willis (32) who first showed these vessels in stillborn infants some 300 years ago by using india ink as the outlining substance. Djindjian, and now many others, also applied this selective angiographic method to the branches of the carotid arteries, especially those of the external. This in turn led to the therapeutic application by embolizing the appropriate artery supplying the lesion. Various embolic substances have been used with differing degrees of success. The most popular at the moment is the balloon method developed by the Moscovite Serbinenko (33).

Lastly, we come to Godfrey Hounsfield's (34) great invention of computerized tomography. Without doubt it is the greatest advance in radiology since Röntgen's discovery in 1895. Above all other systems in the body, the central nervous system has benefited most. Up until 1971, it was impossible to explore this dark continent radiologically without causing real discomfort to a patient. By contrast, diseases of the chest and abdomen could be investigated by relatively benign means on outpatients. The benefits provided nowadays to explorers of the central nervous system by Hounsfield's methods are so well known that amplification is unnecessary. However, the work leading up to the present position should be recounted.

In 1967, Hounsfield had been working for some years in the Central Research Laboratories of EMI Limited at Hayes, Middlesex. He was very interested in pattern recognition and he sought to investigate how it could be acquired and then reproduced in a different form. He had previously worked on facial recognition and submitted a system to the police that he thought was as specific as fingerprints, but they were not interested. He then had the idea of considering a closed box containing a number of objects and finding a method of defining their size, shape, position and density, and relations to one another. Thus, he turned his attention to gamma rays or x-rays. It occurred to him that theoretically if readings were taken at all angles through the box, this would produce a large quantity of measurements that, when processed, would reveal the contents of the box. He decided that the most convenient way to examine the box would be to divide it into slices as in tomography. These, collectively, would give a three-dimensional representation of the tissue structure. It also meant that the transmission readings could be taken through a single plane.

One of Hounsfield's great breakthroughs in thinking was to dismiss the use of photographic film for producing an x-ray image. For nearly 80 years, one had always linked x-rays to photographic plates or films. Hounsfield knew that here the spectrum from black to white was very narrow. If he were to use simple crystals such as sodium iodide, which scintillated when exposed to x-rays, he could stretch the spectrum of density about 100 times, and thus soft tissues of varying densities could be differentiated. Interestingly enough, this quality of crystals had been known almost as long as x-rays themselves. The science of x-ray crystallography had been fully worked out very early in this century. The crystals would scintillate quantitatively relative to the attenuation of the emerging gamma ray or x-ray. Then, with the aid of photomultipliers and computers, he would obtain a digital printout, and with the use of a cathode ray oscilloscope and polaroid camera, he would obtain the first image.

Hounsfield's first experiment took nine days to complete. He then reduced it to nine hours, and with his prototype machine down to five minutes. Wondering what application it might have in human radiology, he consulted three radiologists, one interested in bones, the second in the chest and abdomen, and the third in the brain. It was ultimately decided that bone work would be limited, and chest and abdominal work would produce blurred pictures as no patient would be able to hold his breath for five minutes. Hounsfield therefore concentrated on the brain, which does not move with respiration. In October 1971, he and Ambrose obtained their first clinical picture, which was positive; this caused them to jump for joy like football players scoring a winning goal.

This new method swept the world in a manner almost unique in medicine. As is well known, improvements in manufacturing recurred rapidly, and the time required for producing a picture was later reduced to seconds, and thus a whole body machine was born. Finally, it is interesting to speculate as to whether or not Hounsfield's method would ever have reached maturity if it was not for the fact that the brain does not move.

REFERENCES

1. Gowers, W. R. (1886–1888): *Diseases of the Nervous System*, Vol. 1, p. 3. J. & A. Churchill, London.
2. Röntgen, W. C. (1895): *S.-B. phys.-med. Ges. Würzt.*, 132.
3. Schüller, A. (1905): *Die Schädelbasis in Röntgenbilde*,
4. Schüller, A. (1912): *Röntgendiagnostik der Erkrankungen des Kopfes*, Vienna & Liepzig.
5. Schüller, A. (1918): *Roentgen Diagnosis of Diseases of the Head*; translated by F. Stocking. C. V. Mosby, St. Louis.
6. Schüller, A. (1910): *Wien. Med. Wochenschr.*, 60:2291.
7. Sjöquist, O. (1938): Studies on pain conduction in the trigeminal nerve. *Acta Psych. Neurolog.*, Suppl. 17.

8. Krause, F. (1910–1912): *Surgery of the Brain and Spinal Cord.* 3 vols., translated by H. A. Haubold and M. Thorek. H. K. Lewis, London.
9. Cushing, H. (1917): *Tumors of the Nervus Acusticus.* W. B. Saunders, Philadelphia.
10. Henschen, F. (1912): *Fortsch, Röntgenstr.*, 18:207.
11. Luckett, W. H. (1913): *Surg. Gynec. Obst.*, 17:237.
12. Scott, G. (1917): *Arch. Radiol. Electrother.*, 21:237.
13. Cushing, H. (1927): *Surg. Gynec. Obst.*, 44:721.
14. Dandy, W. E. (1918): *Ann. Surg.*, 68:5.
15. Dandy, W. E. (1919): *Ann. Surg.*, 70:397.
16. Jacobaeus, H. C. (1921): *Acta Med. Scand.*, 55:555.
17. Sicard, J. A., and Forestier, J. (1921): *Rev. Neurol.*, 28:1264.
18. Jackson, C. (1918): *Ann. Otol. Rhinol. Laryngol.*, St. Louis, 27:1140.
19. (1924): *Brain*, 47:377.
20. Moniz, E. (1927): *Rev. Neurol.*, 34:ii, 72.
21. Graham, E. A., and Cole, W. H. (1924): *J. Am. Med. Assoc.*, 82:613.
22. Von Knauer, A. (1919): *München med. Wochenschr.*, 66:609.
23. Moniz, E. (1931): *Diagnostic des tumeurs cérebrales et épreuve l'encephalographie artérielles.* Masson, Paris.
24. Davidoff, L. M., and Dyke, C. G. (1932): *Bull. Neurol. Inst. N.Y.*, 2:75.
25. Lysholm, E. et al. (1935): *Das Ventrikulogramm II Teil.* Norstedt, Stockholm.
26. Lysholm, E. et al. (1937): *Das Ventrikulogramm III Teil.* Norstedt, Stockholm.
27. Becquerel, A. H. (1896): *C. R. Acad. Sci. (Paris)*, 122:420.
28. Becquerel, A. H. (1896): *C. R. Acad. Sci. (Paris)*, 122:501.
29. Moore, G. E. (1948): *Science*, 107:569.
30. Adamkiewitz, A. (1882–1885): *Sitzung d.k. Acad. d. Wissensch.* in WienMathNatKlasse, Vienna.
31. Djindjian, R. (1970): *L'Aagiographie de la Moelle Épinière.* Masson, Paris.
32. Willis, T. (1664): *Cerebri Anatome.* London.
33. Serbinenko, F. A. (1974): *J. Neurosurg.*, 41:125.
34. Hounsfield, G. N. (1973): *Br. J. Radiol.*, 46:1016.

Historical Aspects of the Neurosciences,
edited by F. Clifford Rose and W. F. Bynum.
Raven Press, New York ©

The Role of Neuropathology in the Neurosciences

Franz Seitelberger

The Neurological Institute, University of Vienna, Vienna, Austria

From the title of this chapter, it will be gathered that I look at neuropathology not only as at a medical discipline but, above all, as an essential area in the neurosciences. The nature of pathological changes of living matter is a fundamental part of biology, an integral and a constituent field of life itself. This is especially true for the pathology of the nervous system.

Several years ago, I put a question to a famous neurophysiologist: "What do you really understand by neuropathology?" He answered: "When at the end of a needle electrode a stereotactic coagulation has been made, then the consequent topographical localization and histological description of this lesion is neuropathology." This neurophysiologist looked at the nervous system according to the concept of a biological apparatus with numerous minute structural elements in a complicated wiring diagram, which could be explained by brain research. In this concept, neuropathology has the task of describing lesions and/or disorders understood as defects in the machinery and to localize them inside the neural apparatus. (Which elements are affected, where, and to what extent?) This idea of the nature of neuropathology, by reason of its simplicity, has many supporters and has contributed much to the devaluation of neuropathology in the Western world when compared with neurophysiology and neurochemistry. This interpretation of neuropathology is obviously wrong and insufficient in two aspects:

1. Pathology in general and neuropathology *eo ipso* does not deal only with lesions of normal organic structures. It is concerned principally with the regular protective processes against noxae of all kind, especially those originating environmentally, without which individual life could not exist.
2. In particular, the concept is insufficient in the case of the functional plurality of the nervous system, especially of the brain. The notion is related only to the level at which the nervous system is looked at as machinery and does not consider either the level of the living organ nor the level of specific functions. To characterize and to better define the propositions of neuropathology, we must consider the peculiarities of the structure-function relationship in the nervous system. I shall therefore make some general remarks on the set of models that constitute my concept of neuropathology.

The term "neuropathology" is understood to be the pathomorphology of the nervous system, i.e., the science of the morbid changes of the neural structures, tissues, and cells. Here belongs not only the quality of those changes and their course but also the conditions of their genesis and the causal connections of events, the so-called etiopathogenesis. Neuropathological findings and results are expressed in descriptions that are not only formal phenomena but also the causal and temporal reconstruction of the given process as comprised by synthetic interpretation. This morphological method of description must deal with the complexity of living structures and indicates the rational scientific method of research into biological entities of higher complexity; for the reestablishment of totality, it reconstructs its objects of research. Its range extends from the obvious area of living matter into its molecular dimension. Molecular biology itself, insofar as it has to do with structure-dependent qualities of organic molecules, can be looked upon as functional morphology at the molecular dimension.

Now let us turn to the object of neuropathology: Neuromorphology, including neuropathology, deals with the biological structures of the highest differentiation and complexity, the spectrum of functions seen nowhere else in the organic field. Were we to analyze the central nervous system, and consider the peripheral nervous apparatus, including the sense organs functioning as feeders of information or as effectors with limited competence, we would be able to distinguish it on three different levels of organization:

1. The nervous system is an organ of the body. A basic similarity exists with other organs as to the composition of cells, the metabolic requirements met by means of circulation, capacity of regeneration, and the factor of age dependent changes, growth, maturation, and ageing. The nervous system, however, corresponding to the differentiation and the peculiarities of its structure, shows its own pattern of these common qualities and its own dynamic reactions against noxae. This field of the behavior of the nervous system as a tissue under pathological conditions is the central core of neuropathology.

2. The nervous system at the same time is a biological system in the narrower technical sense of the term, i.e., the multiplicity of its nerve cells interconnected by dense intricate wiring to make a functional unity comparable to a technical device for data processing. The overall function of the nervous system can be characterized as central information processing for control of behavior. The system is constituted by an organ whose totality includes its functional elements, the nerve cells, which are interconnected according to a genetically defined wiring design. To the material substrate of the system must be added the contact adjustments (synapses) with the conductors of energy and substances effecting the transmission of excitation—the so-called transmitters. All this can be denoted by comparison with technical computer systems as "hardware." This aspect of the comparability of the nervous system with machinery was alone considered by the quoted neurophysiologist when he defined the neuropathologist as a fault-finding mechanic.

This is the level of the specific functions of the nervous system. In the technical comparison of data processing equipment, this is "software," i.e., the process whereby the form of information programs is projected to the nervous system. It is at this level where the particular position of the nervous system and the extraordinary range of the capacity and achievements of man are based. The possibilities of the program realizations, their complexity, and contents in meaning are related to those of the system, the number of its elements, the organization of partial systems, and the geometry of their connections. Structural parameters are essential conditions of function, not only on the organic level of causal physicochemical processes of life, but as limiting conditions in the meta-organic level of information as a functional reality.

In the functional spectrum of the nervous system, two provinces can be distinguished, which have their correspondence in the structure of the organ, namely, the modal and intermodal range, which comprises the primary processing of sensory input and the performance of movements, including speech. This could be denoted as the neurological domain. Further, there is the supramodal range comprising the higher levels of information processing together with the functions of conscious perception, speech, volitional movement, perhaps with use of tools, thinking, and finally, self-awareness. This range can be considered the neuropsychological domain.

3. Finally the specific human brain-dependent *meta-modal level* of the *products of the supramodal function of the brain* must be mentioned, namely, that of the abstractions of the real phenomena and of the realities modeled by the brain in language, techniques, science, art, sociology, law, and religion. These abstractions are available in symbolic form and represent the world of culture as created by the human brain.

These levels or organization of the nervous system represent models of interpretation as well as levels of scientific research with which different disciplines are associated. To derive from the above three levels the competence of the single neuroscientific disciplines, we can first confirm our statement that neuropathology as a morphological science has its primary tasks of research in the organic level of the nervous system. The accomplishment of the pathological anatomy of the nervous system will be reached in close interdisciplinary cooperation with the other sciences that analyze organic phenomena, especially neuroanatomy, neurophysiology, neurobiology, neurochemistry, neuroimmunology, etc. To this task pertain all problems of so-called general neuropathology, i.e., forms and conditions of the reactions of the single nervous elements, the types of tissue reaction such as edema, atrophy, demyelination, decay, regeneration, and so on, as well as all phenomena of special neuropathology, which concerns the complex picture of the diverse tissue changes underlying diseases of the nervous system. The task of integrative morphological description, in the sense stressed at the beginning of this chapter, is supported by the models of lesions and diseases as produced and causally studied in experimental neuropathology. The field of propositions is continuously spreading through alterations in the phenomenology of diseases as caused by the influence of environment and by the factor of civilization, e.g., neurotoxicological conditions, including iatrogenic ones.

How does neuropathology present itself on the level of the nervous system, if neuropathology is fault finding in the machinery of that nervous system? At the modal level, research into chemical transmission, electrophysiology, and functional neuroanatomy constitute the main field of the neurosciences. The structure-function analyses of the cerebral cortex done by interdisciplinary teams in recent years has achieved remarkable results, especially the demonstration of intrinsic modular organization within the cortex. Neuropathological research at this level must elucidate not only the quality and the course of the alteration but, above all, must localize and identify the affected part of the system. Neuropathology here investigates the functional pathology of the nervous system, the medical application of which is neurological localization. The task of neuropathology is not exhausted with the microscopic and submicroscopic dimension, e.g., in epilepsy research, the goal is not only the identification of morphological correlates of the propensity to epileptic fits, but the understanding of how the pathofunctional dimension of certain structural changes produces neural deafferentation or reduction in synaptic contacts. Remarkable experimental results in this area have already been achieved. Functional neuropathological statements are usually limited to the macroscopic level of larger conduction systems and areas of the brain. This may be because the most interesting pathological changes are not approachable by direct structure-function analysis. Above all, there is the fundamental problem of correlating a disorder of the "hardware" with sequelae in "software," a critical problem in an organ as complex as the brain. Consequently, accomplished exact descriptions of neuronal organizations, e.g., those of the cerebellar cortex, scarcely explain its function. We still need methods of structural description to grasp the causal connections of network systems with such complexity. Thus, the claim for pathofunctional statements based on the principle of complementing structure and function can be fulfilled only partially by neuropathology and therefore remains a permanent challenge.

The supramodal level of functions of the nervous system is beyond doubt the most suggestive to man searching beyond himself, so that neuropathological research at this level already has a long history. The term "Hirnpathologie" (brain pathology), still used at times, refers to the disorders of the higher supramodal cerebral activity. The morphological task here consisted in verifying localization, lateralization, and extension of the responsible lesions within the cerebrum. In functional neuropathology, progress announces itself because knowledge has followed not only neuropsychological research into the functions and their disturbances, e.g., perception, but also the analysis of the functional anatomy of the cerebral cortex, and in basic neurobiological research, especially in psychophysics. Morphological competence at this level is related to grasping the structural complexity of brain parts as the bearer of functions and distinct morphological types of disorders with a defined quality of disorder, e.g., different types of aphasia. In such cases, there is as yet no functional pathology of the cerebral cortex and, with regard to the elementary cortical functional unit of the so-called module, there is as yet no modular neuropathology.

It must not be thought that the functional level of information programs of the nervous system and the symbolic products of these functions decisive for behavior lie outside the direct competence of morphology. Since the neuropathology of psychiatric disorders is based on program faults and not on defects in the "hardware" of organic structure or transmission chemistry, there is not as yet a neuropathology of cultural behavior, although the possibilities and limits of the brain for the functions at each of these levels form the background and define the horizon of these phenomena.

Concluding this part of my remarks, I would like to state that the quality of structural changes of the nervous system in itself represents the object of research of morphopathology of the nervous system, which functionally corresponds to the vegetative behavior of the organ. In functional neuropathology and in neuropathopsychology, the so-called brain pathology, it is a case of constructive-structural, rather than the qualitative, definition of changes of the neural systems of information and of their functional correlates. In medicine, the results are applied by neurology and clinical neuropsychology. Finally, the neuropathological aspect of psychiatry in the narrower sense and of the pathology of behavior is related only to the structure-dependent proportions of capacity and complexity in the organic bearers of functions and to the material qualities of the organic apparatus but not to the functional processes themselves.

Having outlined the research field of neuropathology and the extent of its competence, we can now put the question regarding the relevance of its special contribution to the neurosciences. To do that I propose first to distinguish the historical relevance from the theoretical relevance for neuroscience:

1. The historical importance of neuropathology for the neurosciences is well known and cannot be overestimated. Medical observations of pathological disorders following lesions of the nervous system, especially of the brain, directed attention to this organ, long known

as the seat of the mental activities, but placed under taboo with considerable awe. Neuropathology, as the first medical neuroscientific discipline, created essential data and stimulated research into the differentiated fields of neuroscience today. For example, the neuropathological preoccupation with genetically determined diseases of lipid metabolism led to the development of successful sphingolipid research, and the functional neuropathological problems of Parkinson's disease developed research into biogenic amines, with their still unpredictable consequences. Other examples could be mentioned. Nor should it be forgotten that the relation between studies of the demyelinating diseases and immunology, as well as between neuropathology of the dementias and neurovirology, respectively, introduced the new scientific field of noninflammatory transmittable diseases.

2. Above all, I would like to stress the importance of neuropathology for scientific theory in general. Pathological phenomena in themselves represent an integral part of biology; they belong to the repertoire of behavior, while their structural correlates belong to the patterns of ordinary structural modification of living beings.

Concerning the peculiarities of the composition of the nervous system, e.g., the lack of mesenchymal stroma, the form and device of nerve cells and their processes, the behavior of glial cells, the peculiarity of the vessels and the blood-brain barrier, etc., all these are the conditions for the independent nature of its cellular and tissue reactions, which have no counterpart elsewhere in the body. Systemic degeneration, demyelination, and brain edema are incomparably specific complexes of events and therefore highly remarkable and unique conditions. This is even more true for the complex patterns of reactions and their temporal course in the diseases of the nervous system, e.g., demyelinating diseases. Because they are such a good example, I would like to consider them further.

In the case of multiple sclerosis, neuropathology defined precisely a peculiar tissue syndrome consisting in focal elective loss of myelin sheaths; the foci in the brain are irregularly distributed with a predilection for the surfaces and around venules of the white matter, connected with a subacute plasmolymphocytic inflammation, the organization of the foci leading to glial fibrillary scars: the plaque. Foci of different ages are met corresponding with the clinical course of the disease. The hypothesis derived from comparative studies of an autoimmunological process directed against a constituent of the myelin sheaths could be experimentally supported, although the exact pathogenesis and above all the etiology are still unclear. Recently, evidence of the following peculiar structure of a disease process is emerging: First, a viral infection in infancy leads to a change of immunological reactions (qualitative? quantitative? disorder of regulation?). Supported by other conditions in the second step, sensitization against certain antigens incorporated in the myelin sheaths and one's own myelin sheaths develops. In the third step, if antibodies of this kind or cells bearing antibodies invade the nervous system, which is normally protected by a barrier, then in the fourth step, an antigen-antibody reaction will result in destruction of the antigen-bearing structure of the myelin sheaths. With continuity of the antigen drift and production of antibodies, this event may occur repeatedly.

Thus, it is not the case of a uniform pattern of reactions but of a cascade which, by fitting constellations of conditions, more and more new levels of reactions and partial regulatory systems are incorporated. It cannot be spoken of as one cause or causes in the sense of a multifactorial genesis. It concerns a hierarchy of constellations of conditions of a different nature, the connection between which is established by specific, as yet unknown, factors; in addition to exogenous factors, there are also constitutional genetical prerequisites. The achievement of such a new concept of pathogenesis is an essential step in knowledge, which doubtless will attain therapeutic relevance.

Further examples are the so-called slow virus infections. Neuropathologically, among the progressive dementing processes of the adult, one type can be identified that is quite different from the degenerative type, where the primary attack on the neuronal element is missed, so that there is no parenchymal atrophy with loss of partial systems. Nor does it show the signs of a disorder of structural metabolism as found in, say, senile dementia. There are, however, prominent focal lesions of tissue with affection of several structural elements (nerve cells, glia, myelin sheaths) but without inflammatory reaction. The challenge offered by this syndrome to etiological research was accepted, and the consequent study and investigation of an hypothesis that appeared improbable at first sight has been rewarded by new knowledge of nonhereditary transmittable degenerative diseases of the nervous system. Here too is a case of a new principle of disease which, however, is not as yet sufficiently elaborated to be defined. The quality of transmittability alone is insufficient for such a definition.

As a further example of a neuropathologically based expansion of neurobiology, I can instance the ageing processes found in the nervous system. For long only a simple parenchymal atrophy had been known as a feature of ageing, i.e., the decrease in nerve cells and enlargement of the fluid tissue compartment. In the meantime, systematic studies demonstrated that the ageing process of the central nervous system comprises a cluster of different structural changes, with several processes leading to a final loss of neurons in a fashion different from that of simple atrophy. We now speak of neuronal dystrophies. Among them the so-called neuroaxonal dystrophies show remarkable features such as constant linear, age-dependent, changes of the distal parts of the axon of certain nerve cells. The special conditions of these complex structural dystrophies are not yet known, but their constancy indicates that they are based on an obligatory genetic program of resulting changes in the organ. These ageing dystrophies habitually provide a challenge for functional analysis, namely, what symptomatic expression has neuroaxonal dystrophy of the nuclei of the posterior funiculi in the medulla oblongata and of the substatia nigra-red nucleus in the ageing man? In this context, I would like to stress that all these single changes that regularly appear with ageing are borderline physiologically and may, under certain circumstances, constitute the substrates of defined diseases, e.g., neuroaxonal dystrophy. In the form of so-called infantile neuroaxonal dystrophy, these may appear in early age throughout the whole nervous system and produce a severe disorder with progressive loss of function, culminating in death.

The same holds true for other ageing dystrophies. Those individual changes in the ageing complex, when increased in intensity and occurring early, can become the substrates of disease in their own right. The condition for this shift from physiology to pathology are doubtless of genetic nature but are obscure. With that virtually pathogenetic quality of physiological phase-dependent changes, a third type of disease is outlined, only occurring in the nervous system, which, however, demonstrates general relations that possess relevance to neuroscience, medicine, and biology.

From these and other neuropathological experience, we can examine the concept of disease in the neurosciences and in medicine. Every scientific generation tries to elaborate a concept of disease based on the known facts, and I shall make a few remarks on this very difficult theme. Regarding a general definition of the medical concept of disease, we may say that it is a process connected with diminution of the active adaptability of man to the total circumstances of life and, in most cases, with the subjective awareness of illness and reduction of self-availability. Disease appears therefore as an organized and unity imposing process or complex of events:

1. Such a regulated pattern of reactions can occur as response to noxae (trauma, infections, stress, etc.) whereby the reaction brings in physiologically available programs of defense.

2. Diseases can be based on disorders of the course of reactions. Thus, the responses to different influences can be dynamically and quantitatively changed, so that inappropriate complex consequences of actions on the organism result. We speak of exogenous or endogenous disorders of regulation.

3. Finally, programs of higher order processes, as for metabolism, for the maintenance of structure or of the patterns of behavior, may be disturbed qualitatively by noxae at the molecular level. Such forms of programs may be of primarily genetic origin, i.e., conditioned by heredity, or more rarely, secondary or exogenous.

The example of multiple sclerosis shows that these factors may overlap or combine. In this disease, we must suppose a combination of genetic deviation, disorder of regulation, and of grouped physiologic reactions, at the end of which the morphologically very simple seeming event of selective disintegration of the myelin sheath occurs, a phenomenon which, when studied alone, gives no answer as to its pathogenesis.

These few examples demonstrate that diseases may be looked at as open systems of regulation, which in contrast to the open system of living beings, possess defined conditions of onset, namely causes, causal constellations, and so on. Thus, diseases are complicated regulating processes structured by the affected organism in interaction between disturbing factors and the programs of reactions. Step like development of disease, therefore, corresponds not to the realization of a program inherent in the disease itself, nor in its cause, but to the successive incorporation of a relatively self-governed partial program of reaction of a differentiated organism. One can also speak of organic learning processes in diseases, which apparently marshal the further course. The teleology of disease is therefore directed to a changed reorientated type of life of the organism. The identity of a disease derives from the affected organism, because it is structured by its pattern of reactions. Disease is partially reordered or reorganized life.

These examples demonstrate that this behavior of disease is true not only for organisms but also for certain organs, especially for the nervous system, whose complex structure-function relationship is reflected in its organ-specific disease states. Likewise, disease reveals the complexity and certain defined characters of the organ. Thus, multiple sclerosis teaches us about the quality of the self in the neural structure. The ageing changes prove that ageing is not a degenerative but a productive phase-specific process, and so on.

These examples selected from the nervous system show a spectacular complexity of form and progression. At the system level, disease usually causes a multiplicity of local disturbances in system-elements, conducting lines, and areas of integration. We can speak of system-related or system-specific disorders in the case of systemic faults, e.g., in the transmission of excitation caused by generalized changes of synapses or biochemical faults in transmission due to absent or false transmitters; probably also, if caused by a metabolic disorder, the basic metabolism of the nerve cells is generally changed (amaurotic idiocy, infantile neuroaxonal dystrophy). In all these types of disorder, not only is the vegetative function of the nervous system impaired, but also its function at the level of information. Connections between the substrates of disorder and the resulting disorders of function indicate a field for important future research. As to disorders on the supramodal level, it is especially true that the relation between the substrate and the quality of the disorder is still equivocal. The effect of a generalized nerve cell disorder on a modal function, e.g., a certain sensory integration, is defined precisely by physiology; the sequelae on the supramodal level, e.g., in the function of speech, however, are only capable of description. Here the nonreduceable categorical differences between bearers of information, programs of information, and meaning of information find their expression and indicate the limits of scientific analysis.

I hope that, despite the narrowness and incompleteness of my exposition, I have succeeded in giving a concept of the research field and the levels of competence of neuropathology. Pathology is a constituent and indispensible part of biological science, and neuropathology makes a claim for particular interest because it can substantiate and formulate statements about the nature of an organ with the highest degree of complexity, enclosing the whole range of functions from the physical up to the metaorganic level of mental activities. Neuropathology is therefore already, and increasingly so, relevant to man's self-knowledge, especially regarding the understanding of the higher conscious functions of the human brain. An increased and systematic incorporation of neuropathology into neuroscientific research therefore appears to me an urgent necessity.

Historical Aspects of the Neurosciences,
edited by F. Clifford Rose and W.F. Bynum.
Raven Press, New York ©

Sir Robert Carswell: Scotland's Pioneer Pathologist

*Peter O. Behan and **Wilhelmina M. H. Behan

**Department of Neurology, Glasgow University, Glasgow G12, Scotland; and **Department of Pathology, Glasgow University, Glasgow G12, Scotland*

What is fame? And how is it won? There are no simple answers to these questions. The contributions of some individuals are so fundamental that their names are indelibly written for posterity, but others with less achievements seem often to have the same good fortune. And there are also those whose works have great influence on thought and practice in their lifetime, and who are justly acclaimed by their peers and their monarch, but whose name fades into obscurity at death. We owe all the advantages of the present to the past and we have a duty to our forebears to celebrate their work. This may be a very difficult task because, with the passage of time, facts and fiction merge imperceptibly, and the truth may be difficult to extract. Thus, he who was once great and whose achievements were multiple may be concealed from us. Such a man is the subject of this essay, namely, Paisley's premier physician, Sir Robert Carswell, to whom posterity has been unkind. In his lifetime, his works were much admired and studied and his influence on pathology and neuropathology was profound. A brief record is given here as a humble tribute to his greatness.

Robert Carswell was born on February 3, 1793, in Thornliebank, just outside Glasgow. We know little of his family except that they moved early in his life to Paisley where his father, Allan Carswell, managed a store for Messrs. Crum. He had a good general education, representative of the high general level of education in Scotland at that time. The country had been well endowed with parish schools since the Act of 1696, which ordered a school to be set up in each parish in the land. Other schools in large towns were run by the Society for Propagating Christian Knowledge, and there were several excellent private academies. In Paisley, moreover, the famous Grammar School had been established since 1575, when it was granted a Royal Charter from James IV. All children in such schools received a grounding in English, writing, and arithmetic, and Latin and Greek were also taught. Education also depended on the locality and, living in Paisley, it is likely that Carswell had his unique artistic ability encouraged and nurtured by the school. Drawing was certainly one of the subjects taught at the time because, for instance, an advertisement for students to attend Jedburgh Academy stated that the school had "a rector, an assistant, a French master and a drawing master" (2).

It was possible to proceed directly from a parish school to a university, but Carswell finished school and, at a very early age, devoted himself to drawing and etching, and it is a measure of his exceptional ability that as a young man he was commissioned to sketch some of the plates for Robertson's book on Renfrewshire. His artistic ability was to stand

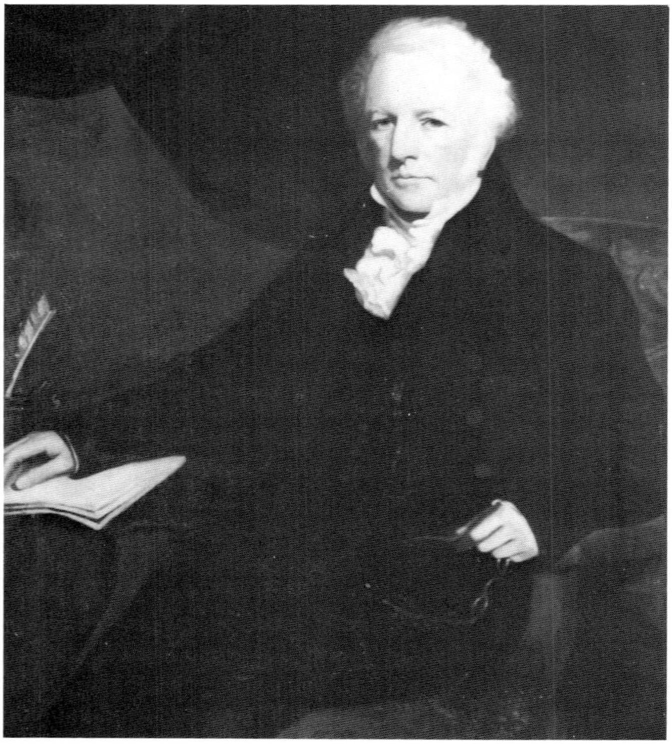

FIG. 1. Professor James Jeffray. (By kind permission of his surviving relative, Mrs. Johnstone of Dumfries.)

him in good stead and indeed, were it not for this gift, he would not have entered medicine nor made the contributions that he did to pathology.

Among his commissions at this time was one given him by Professor James Jeffray, Professor of Anatomy and Physiology at Glasgow University (Fig. 1), who asked the young man to make drawings for one of his inventions. Professor Jeffray was experimenting on a machine to propel boats up the Clyde, and Carswell, who was well known locally in Glasgow, was suggested to him. This meeting entirely changed the direction of the young man's life, and he bore Jeffray a debt of gratitude which he later made known publicly (Fig. 2). The invention was actually not a success; the boat sank and the project was abandoned, but the character, talent, and craftsmanship of the artist made an impression and he was commissioned further to make drawings of the professor's anatomical models. Jeffray was so pleased with the results that he encouraged Carswell to take up medicine, which he did at the age of 25.

A word here is appropriate about Professor Jeffray: He was the son of a Kilsyth merchant and came from a similar social background to Carswell. He had a thorough education at a parish school, and from there won a position as tutor to the family of Sir John Maxwell of Pollock. He entered medicine and made such a success of his career that at the age of 31, in 1790, he was appointed to the Chair of Anatomy and Physiology at Glasgow University. He was described as being a tall, handsome man whose nature alternated between aggressive vindictiveness and that of a gracious, dignified, and generous individual. Although severely

TO

JAMES JEFFRAY, M.D.

PROFESSOR OF ANATOMY AND PHYSIOLOGY IN THE UNIVERSITY OF GLASGOW, ETC. ETC.

My dear Sir,

The approbation with which you received my first attempts to represent, by coloured delineations, the healthy and diseased appearances of the human body, while attending your Lectures, and the encouragement and assistance which you afterwards afforded me in the prosecution of the subject, lead me to consider the publication of this work a befitting occasion on which to express my gratitude, and to acknowledge the influence you thus exercised in directing my attention in a special manner to the study of Pathological Anatomy. That this work, which embraces but a part of the subjects which derive illustration from a department of medicine to the cultivation of which I have devoted much time and labour, may also meet with your approbation, and be the means of extending our knowledge of diseases, is the desire,

My dear Sir,

Of your sincere and grateful servant,

ROBERT CARSWELL.

Berners-Street,
Oxford-Street, London,
15th December, 1837.

FIG. 2. From the frontispiece of Carswell's atlas.

criticized for some of his actions, he was acknowledged to be an original thinker, and he was almost certainly the most successful professor of the university, with no less than 352 students enrolled in his classes in the year 1813.

His scientific fame was attended also by notoriety: He had some involvement in body-snatching and was the last person to anatomize and dissect, in public, the body of a murderer, Matthew Clydesdale, who had been hanged. This he did in 1818. For this demonstration, he was garbed in a white gown and in front of the silent audience he first stimulated the corpse electrically, whereupon it sat up erect. Consternation reigned and several members of the audience fainted. Then Jeffray cut the neck with a knife and the unfortunate corpse fell to the ground. The Scottish Law Lords must have frowned on this performance because no more bodies were ever sent for public dissection.

Jeffray had in fact studied drama, and it was said that he lectured rather in the style of Garrick. He was not at all afraid of a fight; he opposed the Reform Act of 1832 and helped in the formulation of the Anatomy Act of the same year. In 1821, he had converted part of his official residence into a shop, about which this jingle was later written:

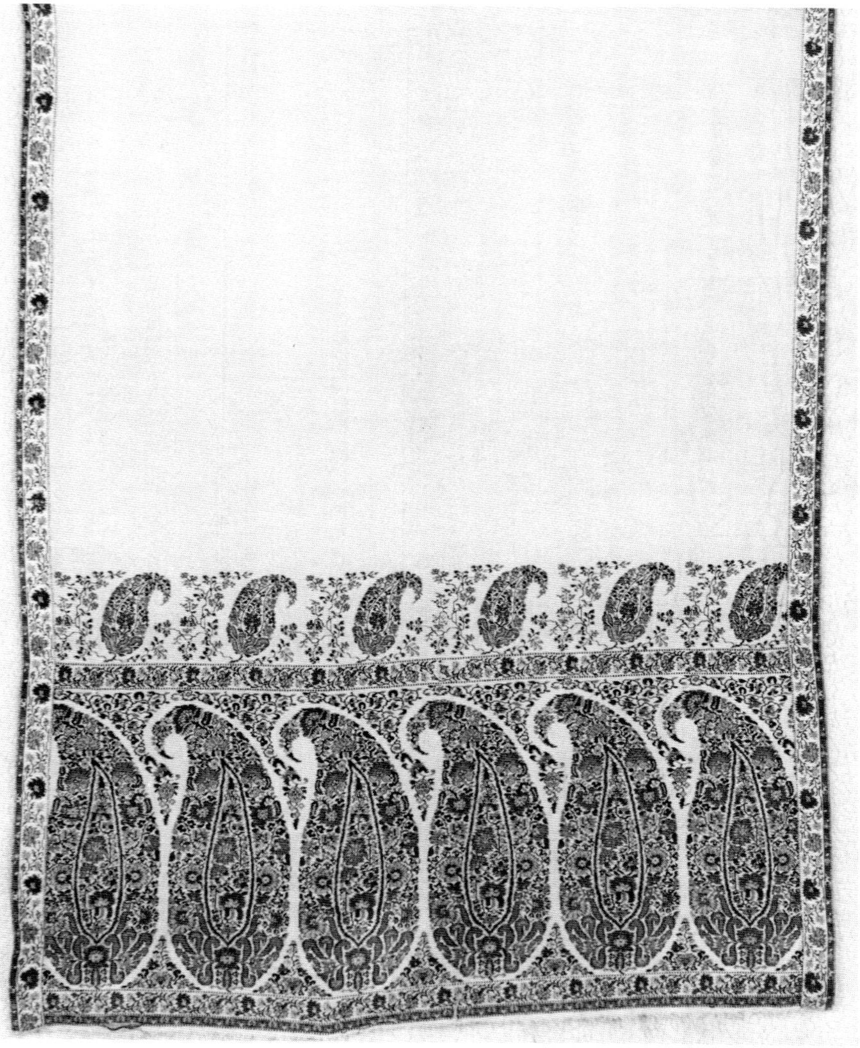

FIG. 3. A contemporary Paisley shawl, ca. 1810. (By kind permission of the Chief Curator of Museums and Art Galleries, Paisley, Renfrewshire.)

This once was Dr. Jeffray's shop,
The famous sawbone-cutter,
But now it's let to Peter Cook,
For selling bread and butter.

He remained in office for 58 years, indeed long after his faculties had deserted him. Such was the man who had the most profound influence on Robert Carswell, an influence that was never forgotton or discounted. When Carswell's famous Atlas was at last published, it was dedicated to Professor Jeffray "as a befitting occasion on which to express my gratitude, and to acknowledge the influence you thus exercized in directing my attention, in a special manner, to the study of 'Pathological Anatomy'."

The other influence on Carswell in his youth was the local environment in which he lived. Paisley was a prosperous town with a growing population; its wealth was founded on textiles: first linen, then silk and cotton. The weavers were among the most skilled craftsmen of the time and the apogee of their craft was reached in the Paisley shawl (Fig. 3). This delicate, luxurious, and beautiful garment was famous throughout Britain and Europe, its wearing considered as haute couture in the European capitals and as a mark of good taste in England. The silk weavers were said to own their own house and loom, sometimes kept a horse, dressed like gentlemen, and had topics of conversation which "ranged from a curious medley of battlefields, theology and Tory politics" (9).

In such a community, the artistic standards were high and the interest in art considerable. One of the Lord Paisleys of the time was responsible for establishing an Institute of Art in Glasgow, and the annual exhibition of this Institute was one of the special events in the British Isles. The town itself had many additions made to it in this era and a contemporary remarked of a stall recently erected in Paisley's Moss Street: "It is 72 feet long, has a genteel front of cut stone, and is one of the neatest and most commodious of the kind in Britain. It cost the community £1,200" (1).

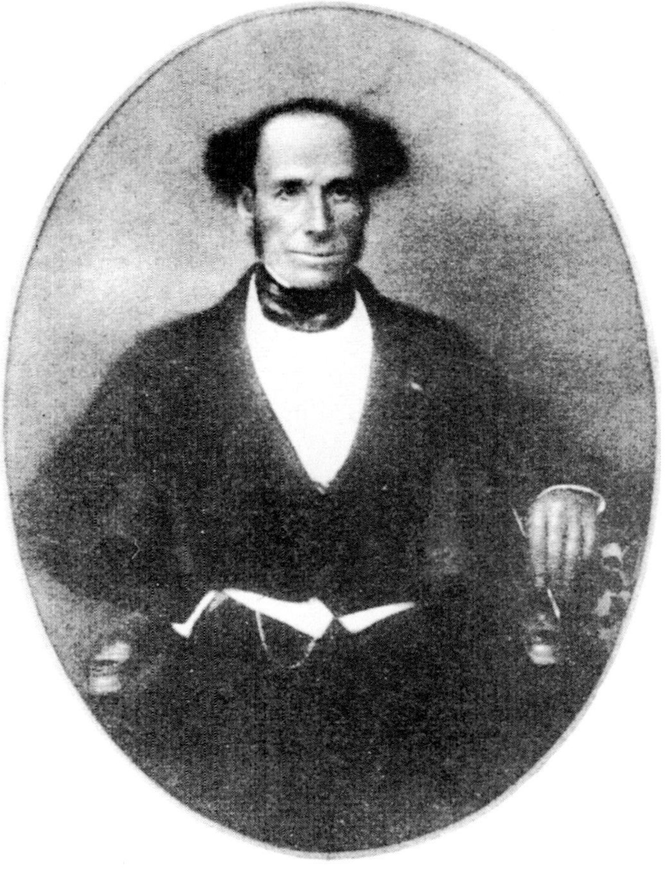

FIG. 4. Sir Robert Carswell as Professor of Pathology.

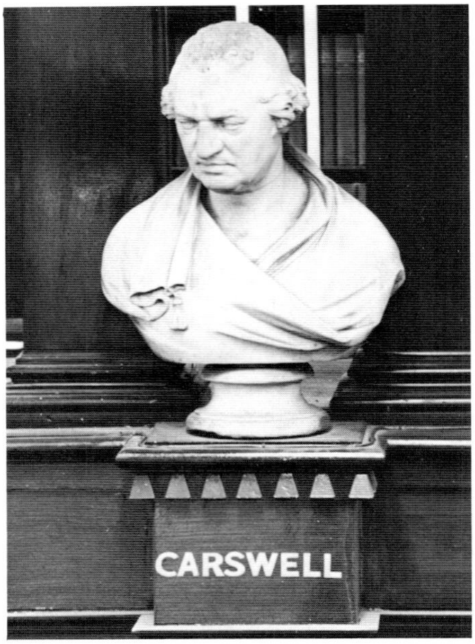

FIG. 5. Bust of Sir Robert Carswell. (By kind permission of C. R. Peacock, Esq., Chief Librarian, University College Hospital Medical School, London.)

It was in this environment that Robert Carswell remained until he was 25: He was well acquainted with the methods of the artist and was an expert at water coloring and etching. At this time in Scotland, the unique contribution of the artist was not stressed because the craftsman was expected to carry out the work as directed by his patron; Carswell, however, was not only a fine craftsman, but also gave an individual stamp to his creations, especially in his use of colors. The artistic merit of his many pathological drawings, especially those illustrating the brain, has not been surpassed.

When Robert Carswell had completed his studies at Glasgow University, he went to Edinburgh, where he stayed during the years 1821 to 1824, interrupted by two years sojourn in France, 1822 to 1823.

The foremost Edinburgh physician at this time was Dr. John Thompson, who was also Professor of Surgery and Pathology. He was much impressed by the young man and advised that he should have the best postgraduate education available. "Except in Edinburgh and Glasgow, medicine as an art and a science in British Universities hardly existed although the private anatomical academies and the embryonic schools attached to some of the London and provincial hospitals acted as minor centres of teaching" (11). Most postgraduate study was accomplished by visiting the continent, and thus Carswell divided his time between Paris and Lyons, coming under the influence of the great Louis.

He returned to Edinburgh in 1824 and received his M. D. degree from Marischal College, Aberdeen University, in 1826. The degree entry states: "'Richard' Carswell who greatly distinguished himself by his researches respecting pathological anatomy . . . on the motion of Sir James McGrigor." There is a note appended that Sir James attended the ceremony himself, a practice he was loth to do unless he considered the candidate exceptional.

Meanwhile, Carswell returned to Paris, where he had started to prepare a collection of pathological drawings. The first Chair of Pathology at University College in London was created during this period, and it was offered to Meckel, who refused it. Carswell was then approached; he accepted and the Council of University College, with commendable foresight, commissioned him to stay on in Paris, at a salary of £350 a year, to complete his collection. By 1831, he had carried out 2,000 drawings, which now are housed in University College. It is this work that forms the basis of his atlas, *Pathological Anatomy: Illustrations of the Elementary Forms of Disease* (5).

Carswell (Figs. 4 and 5) returned to London as the first Professor of Pathology and was also appointed physician to University College Hospital in 1834, the year the Hospital was opened. His salary was paid from the students' fees, of which he received two-thirds, and he also had a private practice, although this was not very successful, because most of his energy was devoted to his atlas. He was by this time suffering severely from a chronic lung disease; the atlas was published in 1838, and soon afterward he resigned the Chair and took up a position as physician to King Leopold of the Belgians, hoping that the change of climate would help him. He went to Laeken to take up his position with his wife, the former Mademoiselle Chardenot.

Carswell's main claim to fame lies in his book *Pathological Anatomy: Illustrations of the Elementary Forms of Disease* (Fig. 6). Although we are concerned here only with his contribution to neurology, he was a general pathologist, and he also made many significant observations in this field. He was a distinguished morbid anatomist and had considerable influence as a teacher, but the abrupt termination of his scientific career prevented him from taking a permanent leading place in his profession. His unique attraction, however, is that he belongs to that select group of artist physicians that flourished in those years: Richard Bright, Wilhelm His, John and Charles Bell, Thomas Hodgkin, Jacob Henle, Jean Cruveilhier, Lord Lister, James Hope, Joseph Leidy, and Alexander Auvert. Carswell's atlas appeared in 1838, four years after that of James Hope, but it became the standard work of pathology for the time and its reception easily surpassed that of Hope's. The quality of the brilliantly colored lithographs, each drawn "from nature" by the artist, opened a new vision of gross pathology to British medical eyes. The work was criticized in part because the representations were too bold or too vivid and fell a little pshort of the finer shades found in Cruveilhier's work, but the final consensus seems to be that his illustrations fall "midway in technical and textural excellence between Hope's and Cruveilhier's productions" (7). His atlas was better than that of Hope's, although neither in size nor in execution did it quite rival Cruveilhier's magnificent folios.

The organization of the atlas was according to Carswell's own concept of disease. Thus, some unusual combinations occurred, but it has to be understood that there was little knowledge of the nature of disease at that time, or of neuroanatomy. The microscope, used in the 17th century by Leeuwenhoek, Malpighi, and Swammerdam, had been neglected in the 18th century. Carswell therefore makes a distinction between "inflammation" and "pus" and between "mortification" (gangrene) and "softening." Nonetheless, his drawings of tuberculous organs, for instance, although he had profited by Laennec's veiws, were stated to "easily surpass Laennec's in their fidelity to nature" (10). His contribution to neuropathology is illustrated by the following examples.

INFLAMMATION

Inflammation was the commonest disease, in Carswell's opinion, "occurring in all the organs and almost all the tissues." He recognized the early involvement of capillaries in the process, which he thought had a primary and a secondary form. In the primary lesion, he

Pathological Anatomy.

ILLUSTRATIONS

OF THE

ELEMENTARY FORMS OF DISEASE.

BY

ROBERT CARSWELL, M. D.

PROFESSOR OF PATHOLOGICAL ANATOMY IN UNIVERSITY COLLEGE, LONDON; PHYSICIAN TO UNIVERSITY COLLEGE HOSPITAL; MEMBER OF THE ROYAL MEDICAL SOCIETY OF EDINBURGH; CORRESPONDING MEMBER OF THE ROYAL SOCIETY OF MEDICINE OF MARSEILLE, ETC. ETC.

LONDON:

PRINTED FOR THE AUTHOR, AND PUBLISHED BY

LONGMAN, ORME, BROWN, GREEN, AND LONGMAN,

PATERNOSTER-ROW.

1838.

FIG. 6. From the frontispiece of the atlas.

distinguished ramiform, capilliform, uniform, punctiform, and maculiform types. His major contribution here, however, was in the description of traumatic subdural abscess, which he was the first to describe. Hooper, 12 years previously, had demonstrated acute pachymeningitis interna, but he gave no indication of its etiology, unlike Carswell, who wrote: "these appearances are extremely characteristic of the inflammation which succeeds mechanical injuries to the head for which I have never met with them in any case of idiopathic inflammation of this membrane" (Fig. 7).

At this time, inflammation was diagnosed whenever congestion, redness, swelling, and minor hemorrhage occurred, irrespective of the cause. Thus, Carswell illustrates the surface of the pons: "presenting the punctiform and maculiform characters (of inflammation)" (Fig. 8). The identify of this lesion cannot be determined, although it is likely to be a form of inflammation. Figure 9 illustrates an example of cortical vein thrombosis associated with suppurative meningitis ("coaguable lymph").

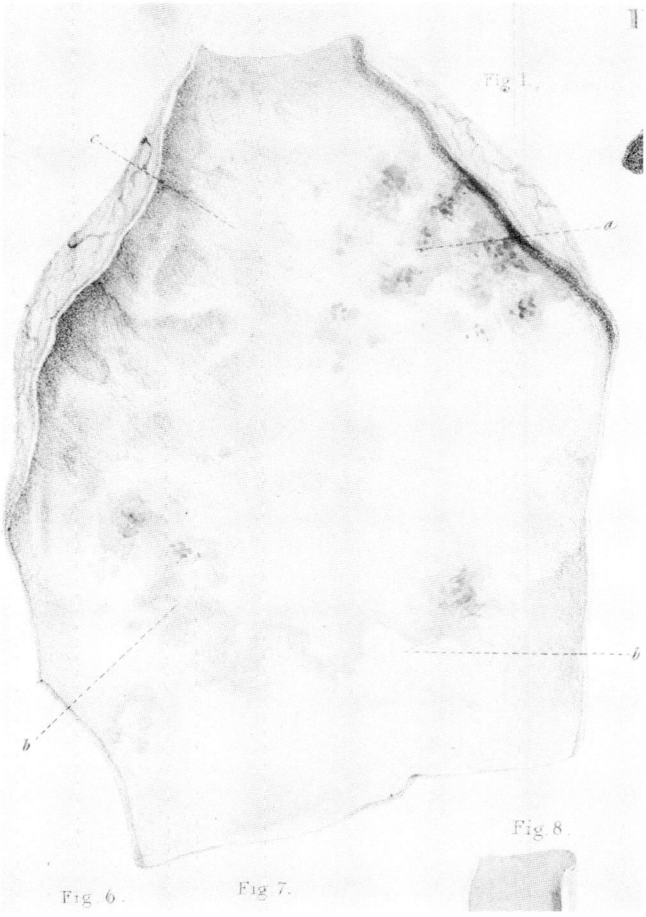

FIG. 7. Acute pachymeningitis interna.

"ANALOGOUS TISSUES"

Carswell regarded "all solid, morbid products, which resemble the natural elementary tissues of the body" as analogous tissues. Among the examples he cites are the false membranes of diphtheria, vascular thrombi, phleboliths, vegetations on heart valves, certain types of scars, adhesions, serous and dermoid cysts, and fibroids of the uterus. Fibrin clots found in the vessels after a stroke he also regards as further examples. With respect to his classification, he terms osseous transformation of the arteries of the brain an example of analogous transformation. A further example of transformation is what he terms cartilaginous transformation of the spinal cord. This, as beautifully illustrated by him, is one of the best, if not the first, examples of arachnoid plaques (Fig. 10).

ATROPHY

Descriptions of the nature of atrophy include references to "monstrosities" (i.e., congenital atrophy) defined thus: "A dimunition of bulk, or the complete disparition, soon after birth,

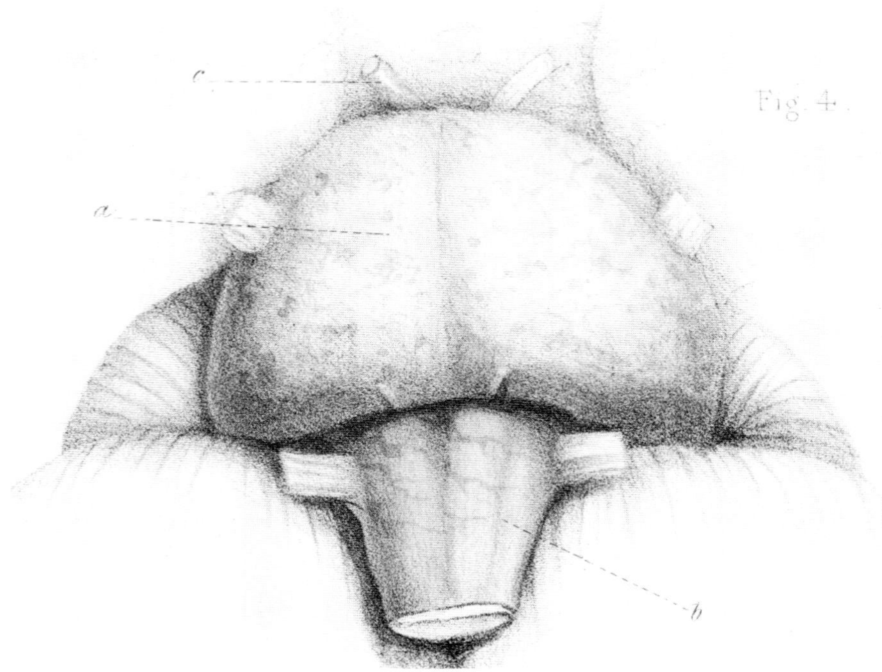

FIG. 8. Surface of pons with "punctiform and maculiform characters (of inflammation)."

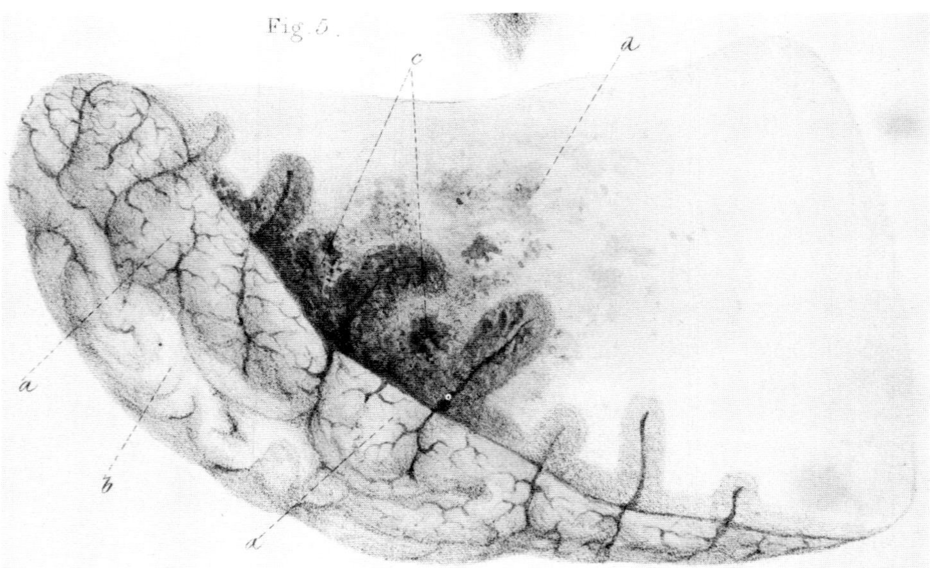

FIG. 9. Cortical vein thrombosis.

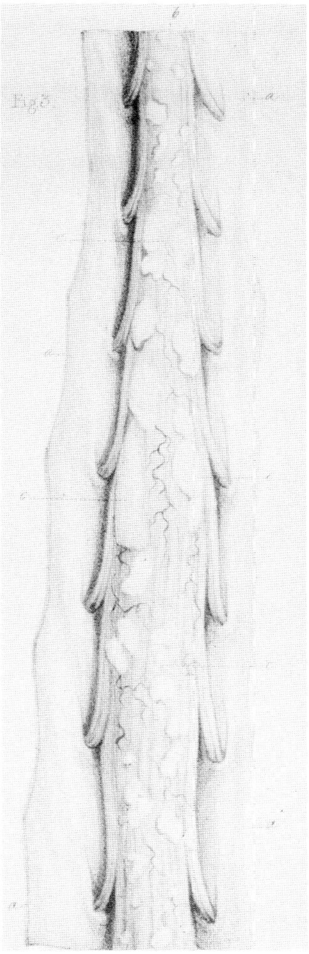

FIG. 10. Arachnoid plaques of the spinal cord.

of organs which performed functions essential to the existence of life but which are now no longer necessary to the maintenance of life, afford also interesting examples of atrophy." The examples given are the ductus arteriosus and the umbilical arteries. He also commented on the general atrophy that occurs with senescence in which organs "having attained the maximum of their development, decline after a variable period of time and tend gradually towards decay." This he terms senile atrophy and states that "the brain, spinal cord and nerves participate in the general decay of old age." The cerebellum, he observed, "remains unaltered, even at the most advanced period of life." The description of general paresis of the insane (Fig. 11) merits quotation in full:

> The accumulation of serosity in the cavity of the arachnoid, and in the pia mater between the convolutions of the brain, which occurs in the insane and in old persons affected with general paralysis, is accompanied by various degrees of atrophy of that organ, but more especially of the grey substance of the convolutions. In this form of atrophy, we find the entire brain separated from the inner surface of the cranium by a greater or less quantity of serosity, which is also accumulated in the pia mater between the convolutions. The upper,

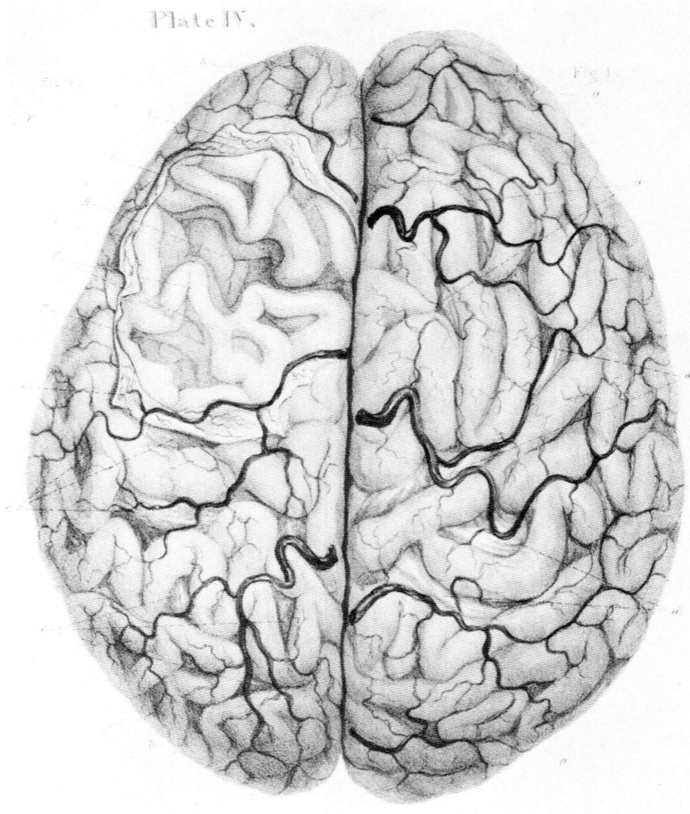

FIG. 11. Atrophy of cerebral cortex in general paresis of the insane.

lateral, posterior, and anterior surfaces of the hemisphere are the parts in which the effusion is most abundant and most frequently observed. It may be confined to the sulci of a few only of the convolutions, or occupy the greater number of them on both hemispheres; or it may be slight or partial on one hemisphere, and extensive or general on the other. The presence of the effusion, its situation and extent, are readily recognized by the peculiar colour of the membranes beneath which it is situated, which present the appearance of irregular patches of a milk-white colour. In these parts also the membranes are opaque and thickened, and are, in general, united together in such a manner that the effused fluid is retained within them as within a sac. On detaching them from the surface of the brain, the fluid, therefore, is carried away with them at the same time, and in the situation which it occupied, are perceived irregular depressions, or excavations, situated between, and extending to the bottom of, the convolutions, which are variously reduced in bulk, being more or less diminished in breadth and depth, sometimes much more in the former than in the latter direction of their dimensions. The surface of the excavations, which consists of the atrophied convolutions, present a smooth glossy aspect, and is formed by the cortical substance, the colour of which is generally paler than natural, and most frequently corresponds with an increase of its consistence. Sometimes, however, its colour and consistence are not altered, or the former may be redder than natural, and the latter sometimes diminished, either generally or in circumscribed spots. The white substance of the convolutions presents a proportionate diminution of bulk, but little alteration of its colour or consistence. This form of atrophy of the brain is met with in the great majority of cases of insanity which terminate in general paralysis. The existence of the former and the occurrence of the latter must be

> regarded in the relation of cause and effect, and in many cases which I have examined, the progressive development and degree of the one strikingly corresponded with the extent of the other.

The localized atrophy and arachnoidal thickening is well shown in Fig. 11, and is stated to be "met with in the great majority of cases of insanity which terminate in general paralysis." Although Carswell was not always able to distinguish with confidence between simple senile atrophy (i.e., Alzheimer's disease) and the atrophy which was secondary to syphilis, his descriptions leave little doubt that he suspected the types had different etiologies.

The illustration by which Carswell is best known is that of multiple sclerosis (Fig. 12). He shares the honor with Jean Cruveilhier, whom he certainly must have met since they were contemporaries in Paris and Lyons: Perhaps they had even discussed this unique lesion. Carswell's illustrations are from patients he had seen in the post-mortem room in Paris. His description, so vivid, clear, and unmistakable, is best left to himself to relate:

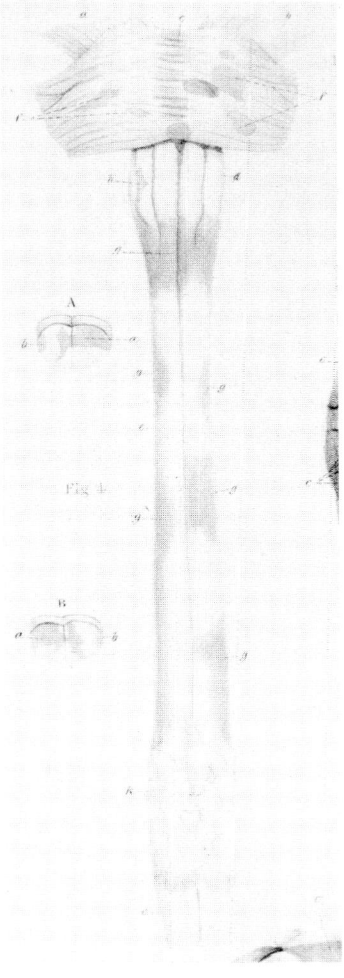

FIG. 12. Multiple sclerosis of the brain stem and spinal cord.

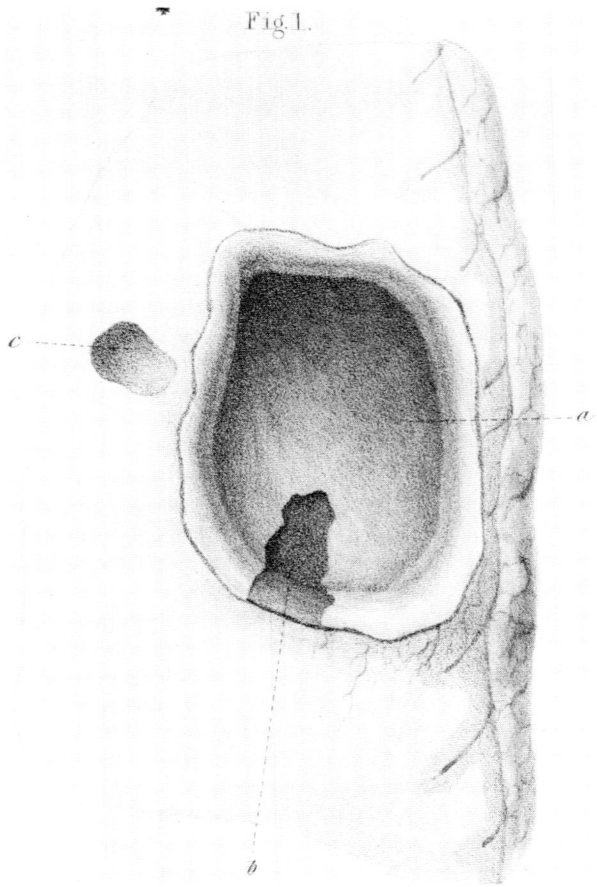

FIG. 13. Brain abscess.

I have met with two cases of a remarkable lesion of the spinal cord accompanied with atrophy. One of the patients was under the care of Mons. Louis, in the Hospital of La Pitié, the other under the care of Mons. Dhomel in the Hospital of La Charité, both of them affected with paralysis. I did not see either of the patients, but I could not ascertain that there was anything in the character of the paralysis or the history of the cases, calculated to throw any light on the nature of the lesion found in the spinal cord. I have represented the appearances observed in one of these cases in Plate IV, fig. 4, [our Fig. 12], in which the pons Varolii was also affected, and which convey an accurate idea of the physical characters of the lesion. In this case a distinct portion of the cord was affected with softening, which of itself would no doubt have accounted for the paralysis; but in the other case there was no other lesion present than that to which I allude, to which the paralysis could be attributed. The anterior surface of the spinal cord presented a number of spots, from a quarter of an inch to half an inch in breadth, of an irregular form, of a yellowish brown colour, smooth, glossy, without vascularity or any alteration in the colour or consistence of the surrounding medullary substance. The medullary substance thus affected was very firm, somewhat transparent, and atrophied. At the root of the medulla oblongata, these changes occupied the whole breadth of both the medullary fasciculus to the extent of half an inch in breadth from above downwards. Further down, they were confined to distinct spots on each fasciculus, and several of the same kind, but smaller, occupied the pons Varolii. The depth to which the medullary substance was affected in this manner varied from half a line to three or four lines, and on dividing the cord, it was seen to penetrate as far as the grey substance.

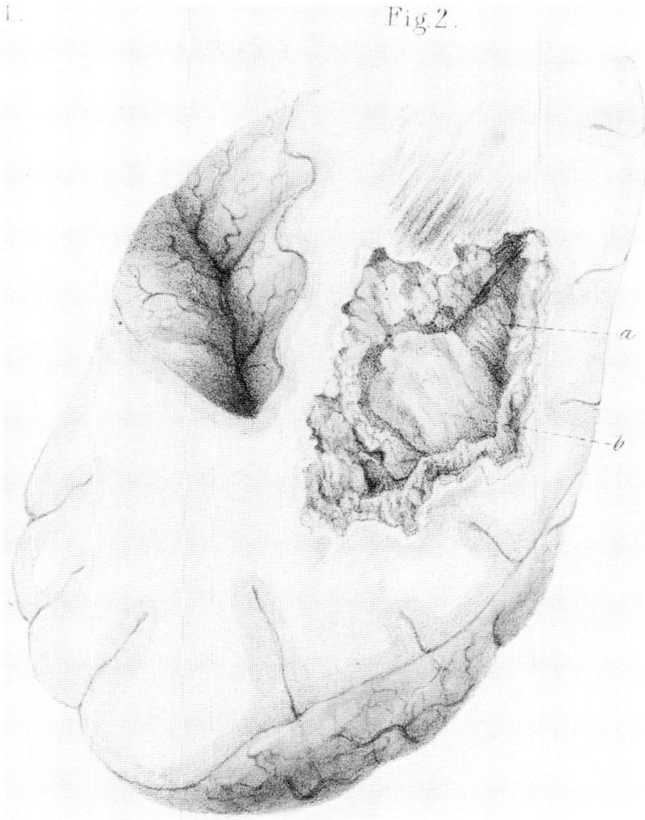

FIG. 14. Brain abscess.

One may digress here and see illustrated in Carswell's account of his third type of atrophy how he was influenced by medical and philosophical thinkers of that time. Carswell occupied himself with the form of atrophy that occurs from the diminished exercise of the function of an organ. He cites the observation of the famous French military surgeon Baron Larrey. It was that lesions of the cerebellum are apt to be followed by degeneration of the testicles. Carswell studied two young men who were given to excesses in masturbation "In each of these patients the cerebellum was the seat of a tumour as large as a hen's egg (composed entirely of the medullary sarcoma)."

Dr. Macdonald Critchley, in describing "Neurology's debt to F. J. Gall" (8), commented on the concept of the cerebellum as a sex organ. Phrenological thought had clearly been influenced by the few clinical examples that suggested that there was some relationship between the shape of the head and those given to sexual excesses. Gall himself noticed a unique shape of the head of a hypersexed widow and "designated the cerebellum as the seat of degenerative instinct, later renamed the organ of amativeness." Gall was apparently not the first to suggest the cerebellum as the center of venery: This was originally supposed by Swedenborg. In collaboration with Vimont and Broussay, Gall published a monograph on this subject. His work was mainly based on clinical cases, one of which is worth reporting: "a

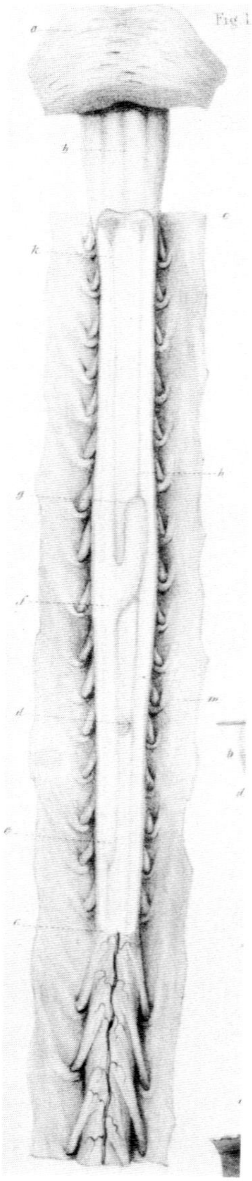

FIG. 15. Spinal cord abscess.

woman of ardent temperament with imperious sexual desires had often supported, not to say provoked, the embraces of 10, 12, or 15 men in one day. During her stay in the Salpêtrière she frequently experienced severe pain in the neck being then seized by violent sexual desires which she satisfied with masturbation 10 or 12 times a day." These examples illustrate how Carswell was influenced by the views held in his day and should make us all the more sensible of his achievements.

PUS

Here Carswell demonstrates a variety of abscesses of the brain, showing that these lesions can occur as metastases (Figs. 13 and 14): in one case, from infection of the arm. His example of an abscess of the spinal cord merits particular attention (Fig. 15).

He was one of the first to describe this lesion, which occurred as an extension of osteomyelitis of the spine, and he shows beautifully the limitation of pus to the central gray matter. Carswell was also aware that patients with paraplegia often develop pressure sores, or as he calls it, "mortification from debility."

HEMORRHAGE

His description of intracerebral hemorrhage is worth reading in his own words, and his excellent representations can hardly be bettered today. The same praise may be given to his description of subdural hematoma:

> The most remarkable of these cases occurred in a stout man, a porter, of middle age, who stumbled in the street from the effects of liquor, and struck his head against the pavement. He got up immediately, and walked home. A few days after, he felt himself less capable of making considerable exertion than formerly; he could not, as before the accident, raise a heavy load, or walk steadily under a heavy burden. This state increased, but not to such a degree as to prevent him from continuing his daily occupation for three weeks, at which period he presented himself at the Hôtel Dieu of Lyons. His general health was good; his intellectual faculties were entire; he walked and expressed himself with perfect freedom; the pulse and temperature of the skin were natural. Under these circumstances the receiving physician refused to admit him. Next day he was brought to the hospital in a state of complete coma, with stertorous breathing and general paralysis, and died during the day. We found that he had gone home and complained to his wife that he had been refused admission to the hospital because he had no fever; and that she, in order to remove this objection, had administered to him nearly a quart of hot wine containing a quantity of pepper. The result of the autopsy was interesting: at least six ounces of blood covered the superior half of the surface of the brain, but was separated from it by the arachnoid, between which and the dura mater it was enclosed. The blood was partly fluid and partly coagulated, red or almost black; and a false membrane, of the thickness of card-paper, lined the internal surface of the dura mater in contact with the blood, presenting in several points of its extent numerous vessels of new formation. The only lesion observed in the brain itself was congestion of its venous system.

SOFTENING

Carswell was aware that occluded cerebral vessels resulted in cerebral softening.

MELANOSIS

As mentioned earlier, he did not use a microscope and was influenced to a great extent by a contemporary thought, as reflected in his views on malignancy. This apart, his illustrations of lesions of the brain, under the heading of "Melanosis," are very characteristic, although he was not aware of their exact pathology. This is seen in his beautiful illustration of metastatic malignant melanoma (Fig. 16). Carswell was the complete pathologist, and showed his knowledge of comparative pathology by his reference to the fact that similar tumors occur in horses.

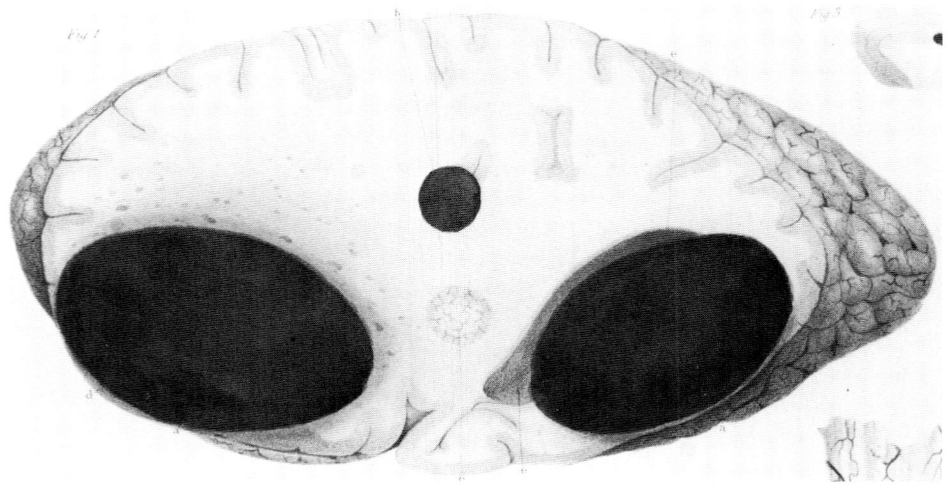

FIG. 16. Metastatic malignant melanoma.

His descriptions of carcinoma, although excellent, again reflect the ignorance of the time, in which "the contemporary practice was of classifying malignancies on the basis of their gross structure." In his work he does not mention meningiomas, although he must clearly have been aware of their presence. Cruveilhier featured them in his atlas.

TUBERCLE

What Carswell died of is unknown, but there is reason to believe he may have had chronic pulmonary tuberculosis. It is apt therefore that he should devote a whole section of his atlas to a description of this disease, with illustrations of pulmonary, genital, intestinal, and other forms. He points out the special susceptibility of the female genital tract to this infection. We are reminded of Carswell's description when we read how young Glaswegian girls, squatting on the stone floors, developed genital tuberculosis from contact with the infected sputum of their parents. His illustrations of tuberculoma of the brain are superb (Fig. 17). He was aware of the propensity of large tuberculoma to occur in the cerebellum (Fig. 18).

CONCLUSION

What is characteristic of Carswell is his intelligence, insight, expert knowledge, and ability to grasp the significance of a new observation and to record it for posterity. The description of an abscess of the spinal cord, the unmistakably clear demonstration of multiple sclerosis, spinal cord arachnoid plaques, subdural inflammation and brain abscesses, attest to his pioneering achievements. How can one surpass his drawing of a subdural hematoma, a lesion that was not fully understood until nearly 100 years had elapsed, or his description of traumatic petechial cerebral hemorrhage. His deficiencies are easy to find but are negligible when one considers the work offered and what prevailed at that time. With all the modern advances we have made, we can look back on him with a smile and be lulled into a false judgment.

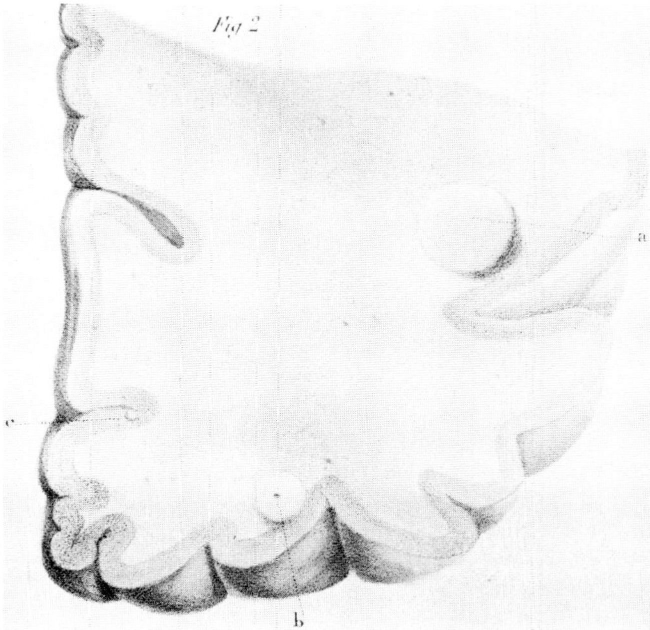

FIG. 17. Tuberculoma in the brain.

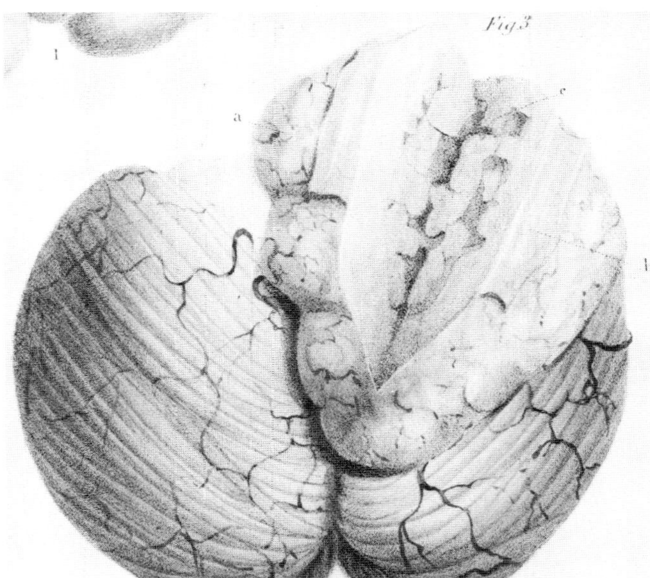

FIG. 18. Large tuberculoma of the cerebellum.

His services to Louis Philippe when in exile were rewarded with a knighthood by Queen Victoria in 1850 and by his being made Chevalier of the Order of Leopold and Chevalier of the Legion of Honour.

His later life, spent at Laeken near Brussels, was occupied in looking after the poor and in the usual official duties. He made no further contributions to the medical literature, and the earlier works (listed) in collaboration with others, remained his sole ventures into medical writing. His fame was recognized in his own time, and there is no better illustration of this than that he was summoned by Queen Victoria to attend the exiled Louis Philippe. He accompanied the King of the Belgians to England on June 24, 1841. On July 3, 1855, his name is given in a list who dined with Queen Victoria, and the *Lancet* of July 14, 1855 mentions that "Sir Robert Carswell, the eminent pathologist, has been on a visit to Buckingham Palace and has had the honour of dining with Her Majesty several times during the month."

Back in Belgium, he made one or two visits to the south in search of health. This lonely man died aged 64 on July 15, 1857, after a long and lingering illness. Lady Carswell survived him, but they had no children, and his name and memory have faded into obscurity. His name is not even mentioned in the Royal File of "Appointments of Court Dignitaries," nor in "Conventions with Physicians" of the Belgian Court. Nor, alas, is his portrait to be found among those of the numerous Court dignitaries or private physicians of the Belgian kings. Perhaps he would have been happiest to leave his atlas as the only monument, but respect dictates that his achievements should be recorded so that posterity can honor Paisley's unique physician.

REFERENCES

1. Brown, R. (1886): *History of Paisley*, Vol. II, p. 61. J. & J. Cook, Paisley.
2. Cameron, A. D. (1969): *Living in Scotland 1760–1820*, p. 107. Oliver and Boyd, Edinburgh.
3. Carswell, R. (1830): Researches on the digestion of the walls of the stomach after death. *Edinb. Med. Surg. J.*, 34:282.
4. Carswell, R. (1833): Induration, Melanosis, Mortification, Perforation, Scirrhus, Softening and Tubercle. Chapters in *Cyclopaedia of Practical Medicine*, edited by J. Forbes, A. Tweedie, and J. Connolly. Sherwood, Gilbert and Piper, London.
5. Carswell, R. (1838): *Pathological Anatomy: Illustrations of the Elementary Forms of Disease*. Longman, Orme, Brown, Green and Longman, London.
6. Carswell, R., and Cullen, W. (1824): On Melanosis. *Trans. Med.-Chir. Soc. Edinburgh*, 1:264.
7. Castiglioni, A. (1947): *A history of Medicine*, translated from the Italian and edited by E. B. Krumbhaar, p. 694. Alfred A. Knopf, New York.
8. Critchley, M. (1965): Neurology's debt to F. J. Gall (1758–1828). *Br. Med. J.*, 4:775–781. Reprinted in: *The Divine Banquet of the Brain*. Raven Press, New York.
9. Gilmour, D. (1874): *Paisley Weavers of Other Days*. Alex Gardner, Paisley. Houston & Sons, London.
10. Krumbhaar, E. B. (1962): *Pathology*. Hafner, New York.
11. McMenemey, W. H. (1960): Neurology investigation in Britain from 1800 to the founding of the National Hospital. *Proc. Roy. Soc. Med.*, 53:36–40.

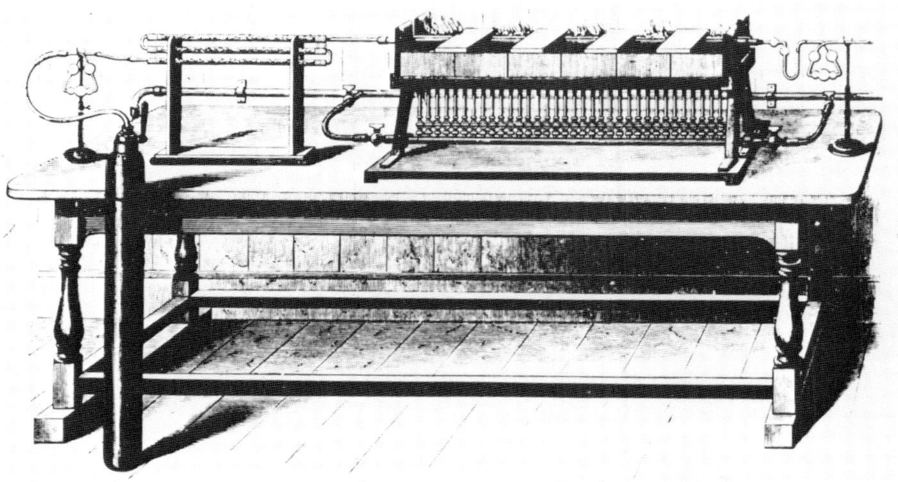

FIG. 2. Thudichum's "most valued possession"—the combustion apparatus or train, a present to him from his teacher, Liebig. The equipment is used in the accurate elementary analysis of organic compounds, and in its application Thudichum was a master. Reproduced from a proof of an original engraving. (From Drabkin, ref. 1., with permission from the University of Pennsylvania Press.)

which comprised 323 pages (11); and 10 years later, *A Manual of Chemical Physiology, Including Its Points of Contact with Pathology*, of 195 pages (12). These were standard textbooks used both in England and the United States, when medical schools hesitantly started to introduce clinical chemistry to their curricula.

All through these years (13–15), Thudichum lectured in various medical schools in London, and he received a gold medal for his original work on urochrome, the normal pigment of the urine; 25 years later, when he was 60, he published his last paper on urochrome (16). And 10 years later, when he was 70, he still struggled with the problem why some, but not all, people develop gallstones: *Ueber den chemischen Process Gallensteinkrankheit beim Menschen und in Thieren, mit neuen Versuchen* (20) was a lifelong challenge. His work on bilirubin and porphyrins is also valued by researchers who have investigated these substances (17–19).

BRAIN CHEMIST

Why did the successful laryngologist with a passion for clinical chemistry leave urine and bile and start analyzing the brain? Was it when he realized how little was known about the composition of the brain? Was it the challenge to map out an unknown continent? Or was it somebody else, who chose him? The Privy Council's chief medical officer was Sir John Simon (1816–1904); was he the initiator or merely the man who managed to allocate sizable funds to Thudichum for 17 years from 1865 to 1882?

Thudichum had his laboratory in his own house, the most advanced combustion apparatus (the gift from Liebig); he had been taught spectroscopy by Robert Wilhelm Bunsen (1811–1890), and he had a willingness to make an all-out effort, to devote his time, his spirit, and his honor. He spent his grant money and his own money on a huge platinum retort for distillation of various brain extracts and on platinum salts for chemical analysis; he casually cautioned his readers that if one is unprepared to make the sacrifice or lacked the means of obtaining such a platinum retort, one had better keep out of brain chemistry.

His aim was to describe the chemical composition of the brain. Hundreds of ox brains and dozens of human brains formed the basis of Thudichum's investigations. He was later criticized for being static, with no understanding of the dynamic qualities of the brain, and he made no contacts with those who were about to start biochemistry or neurophysiology. Were he able to answer this criticism today, he would probably just repeat what he wrote then, that he had been impressed by the glaring lack of knowledge of the chemical composition of the brain. First things first; to Thudichum, this meant chemical analysis; after that, the road would be open for a second generation of researchers.

Cephalin, phrenosine, and sphingomyelin were first isolated from the brain by Thudichum; he also isolated galactose and lactic acid from the brain, and we owe several of these names to Thudichum. He repeatedly encountered new problems; one of the substances was especially sphinxlike, so he named it sphingomyelin!

Most researchers keep their more valuable samples for some time as reference substances, but few intend to keep them forever. Hundreds of Thudichum's isolates were rediscovered in his own stable 28 years after his death, when Otto Rosenheim visited Thudichum's daughters to learn as many details as they remembered about their father (they remembered that their father tended his dahlias in the early morning—they were among the finest in all London—before he had his morning horseback ride in Hyde Park). How these brain specimens had come from his laboratory to his stable is unknown; they are now in the National Institute of Medical Research, Mill Hill, London. Thudichum had to work with macromethods, and so the rediscovered specimens are quite substantial; several have been reanalyzed, to prove that Thudichum's capacity for analysis and purification has stood the test of time.

THE FIGHTER

It is one thing to perform good research, another to get it published (26–29). Thudichum had no easy access to the relevant journals because some key editors were his deadly enemies. This delayed communication of his research, started a long time before with his urine and bile pigment findings. Hematoporphyrin was first discovered by Thudichum, who named it cruentine; it was three years later that Felix Hoppe-Seyler (1825–1895) "discovered" it and claimed priority, but his only achievement was the more catchy word, hematoporphyrin; he missed the compound's fluorescence, which Thudichum had already described. Hoppe-Seyler was from 1877 in a strong position because he had his own journal *Zeitschrift für physiologische Chemie*, commonly called, as it is today, *Hoppe-Seyler's Zeitschrift*.

On Thudichum's bile pigment studies, Hoppe-Seyler wrote:[1]

> So many morsels of research results, devious and frequently patently false (spurious), are reported by Thudichum on the bile pigments, the blood pigment and its split-products, pigments which he recovered from the urine, that it would be impossible here to present them in excerpt.

Another important biological journal in Germany was *Jahres-Bericht über die Fortschritte der Thier-Chemie*, whose chief editor was Richard Maly (1839–1891). Notwithstanding the more outspoken attacks of earlier days, it still is easy to envisage Thudichum's feelings

---

[1]"Thudichum giebt von den Gallenfarbstoffen, dem Blutfarbstoff und seinen Zersetzungsprodukten, Farbstoffen, die er aus dem Harne gewonnen hat, so viel den bisherigen Untersuchungsresultaten Abweichendes und vielfach offenbar Falsches an, dass es unmöglich wird seine Aufgaben hier im Excerpte wiederzugeben."

A TREATISE

ON

THE CHEMICAL CONSTITUTION

OF

THE BRAIN.

BASED THROUGHOUT UPON ORIGINAL RESEARCHES.

BY

J. L. W. THUDICHUM, M.D.

FELLOW OF THE ROYAL COLLEGE OF PHYSICIANS, LONDON; PRESIDENT OF THE WEST LONDON MEDICO-CHIRURGICAL SOCIETY, ETC., ETC.

LONDON:
BAILLIÈRE, TINDALL, AND COX,
20, KING WILLIAM STREET, STRAND.
1884.

FIG. 3. Title page from Thudichum's *A Treatise on the Chemical Constitution of the Brain*, ref. 23. (Courtesy of the Wellcome Trustees, London.)

when he read the following editorial annotation by Maly:[2]

> The second communication contains analyses of uncharacterized barium and iron precipitates obtained from the urine. This teaches nothing except that Mr. Thudichum's dilettantism remains uncontrolled, an epidemic plague for physiological chemistry.

Thudichum did not meekly turn the other cheek, as some of his titles show (26–29): "Offenes Sendschreiben an die kaiserliche Akademie der Wissenschaften zu Wein, Beleuchtung der Undersuchungen über die Gallenfarbstoffe von Richard Maly in Graz, Leipzig und Heidelberg"; "Ueber Indikan und das Verhältniss des Herrn Dr. Max Jaffe zum Begriff der chemischem Reinheit. I. Vom 'reinem' und 'unreinem' Indikan"; "Ueber die Eisensalze der

[2]"Die zweite Abhandlung enthalt Analysen von uncharacterisierten Ba- und Fe-Niederschlagen aus Harn, die nichts lehren, als dass Hernn Thudichum's Dilettantismus noch fortfährt, eine Landplage für physiologische Chemie zu sein."

extractiven Säuren aus Menschenharn. Mit schluss Bemerkungen betreffend Hrn. E. Salkowsky's 'Beiträge' zur Chemie des Harns"; "Abwehr der Verdächtigungen, welche Her Neubauer zu Wiesbaden betreffs der Kryptophansäure veröffentlicht hat"; "Würde under Würdigung. Antwort auf den Angriff des Herrn Drechsel." For this reason, most of his brain work from 1865 to 1883 was presented—and buried—in the Report Series of the Medical Officer to the Privy Council (22).

In 1883, the grant money was stopped for unknown reasons, and the next year Thudichum published his monumental monograph, *A Treatise on the Chemical Constitution of the Brain, Based Throughout Upon Original Researches* (23), a proud but substantiated claim (Fig. 3). The following year saw a Russian translation (24), but a German edition did not appear until 1901 (25), a few months before he died.

Many of his papers were primarily read in the "Royal Society for the Encouragement of Arts, Manufactures and Commerce," a society with wide interests, in which everything from the sewer system of London to new textbooks for the English primary schools was debated. The journal of the society was the *Journal of the Society of Arts and the Institutions in Union* (32–34,38,39,42).

When Hoppe-Seyler and Maly in his native Germany could successfully start their "own" journals, why could not Thudichum, too, since it would have ended his difficulties in communicating his findings to his fellow scientists? Consequently, in 1879 appeared the first volume of *Annals of Chemical Medicine;* editor, Thudichum; author of most of the papers, Thudichum. The second—and the last—volume appeared in 1881. Thudichum's attempt to found the first journal of biological or physiological chemistry in the English language had failed. It is noteworthy that Thudichum's premature venture took place some 25 years before the start of the first two successful ones in English: the *Biochemical Journal* (England, 1906) and the *Journal of Biological Chemistry* (United States, 1905).

PUBLIC HEALTH PIONEER

In between, Thudichum took a keen interest in the society in which he lived. He had great hopes in the health potential of the Turkish bath (31), and to gain some experience he had one built in his own house—the first in London. He published an enthusiastic pamphlet on its merits: This was not one of his major papers and was criticized in a journal, whereupon Thudichum wrote to the editor: ". . . thus biased, you construct the following sentence: 'But Dr. Thudichum was not only philosophic in his details; he was also enthusiastic in his praises of the bath. Dr. Richardson . . . happily took a more moderate view of this calorific instrument.' This sentence is not English as regards either grammar or morality; for, under the cloak of commendation, you insert the dagger which is to kill the confidence of your readers in my assertations; and this act you attempt to disguise by malversation of the language." But the editor can always have the last words: "Dr. Thudichum must take upon himself the credit or discredit which a writer will meet with who indulges in the kind of language to be found in this letter. We last week requested him to modify his mode of utterance, not for our own, but for his sake; and we can only regret that he has but so partially followed our advice."

He also wrote on the Upper Thames as a source of water supply of London with special regard to public health and security (34,35). One of Thudichum's two sons completed this part of his endeavours by becoming a sewage engineer.

There are also two papers on diseases of meat and on food adulteration, with legislative suggestions (38). As late as 1898, when 69 years old, he published a 150-page volume in

German on public health, its accomplishments and tasks (37). We can also note that he was commissioned by the "Pure Wine Association" to undertake a chemical analysis of wines, a happy task (40).

SOME PSYCHOTROPIC SUBSTANCES

Thudichum is a Renaissance figure, not only in his lust for life, his accomplishments in widely different fields, his yearning for insight, but foremost due to his integrative capacity. When Thudichum wanted to know whether or not ethanol was indeed completely metabolized in the human body, what did he do? He arranged around 1866 a garden party for a large group of students at St. Thomas's Hospital, where he was a lecturer and the first director of the laboratory of chemistry and pathology (1865–1871):

> There were 33 in number, including myself. We drank, from 2 o'clock in the afternoon till 7 in the evening, 44 bottles of wine, consisting of white and red Hungarian, Burgundy, and

A TREATISE

ON

WINES

THEIR ORIGIN NATURE AND VARIETIES
WITH PRACTICAL DIRECTIONS
FOR VITICULTURE AND
VINIFICATION

BY

J. L. W. THUDICHUM, M.D.
F.R.C.P. LOND.

LONDON
GEORGE BELL AND SONS
1896

FIG. 4. Title page from Thudichum's *A Treatise on Wines*, ref. 48. (Courtesy of the Wellcome Trustees, London.)

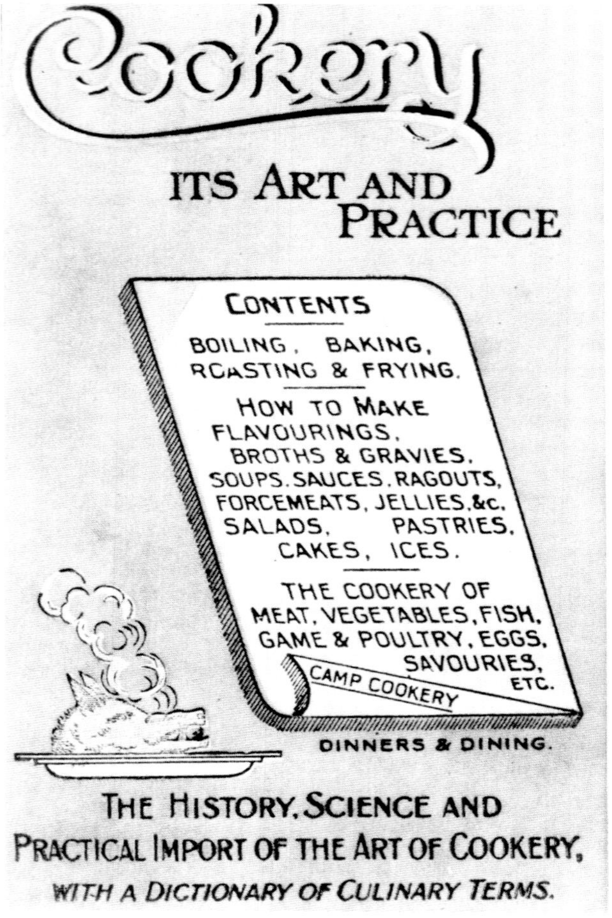

FIG. 5. Part of the title page from Thudichum's *The Spirit of Cookery*, ref. 47. (Courtesy of the Wellcome Trustees, London.)

> Sauterne. The alcoholic content of the total was aggregate of 4,000 grammes of absolute alcohol. All the urine passed from 2 o'clock til 6 next morning was collected and distilled—only 10 grammes of alcohol were collected. The rest was burned in the system.

It was not by chance but by careful selection that his students in the above mentioned experiment tasted various wines, neither was it the only time he brought samples to his lectures for the audience to test. He even carried his own wine to some parties to remain protected from the passage of inferior products over his palate.

The experience of a life of wine tasting formed the basis for two major books (Fig. 4) on wine and wine production (760 and 387 pages) (41,48). Wine had a positive influence on health, when it was used esthetically (the title of a paper from 1884) (44). Thudichum would probably not draw applause from teetotallers with the following statement:

> Compared to the benefits (rouses the higher faculties of thought, memory, and imagination, the poetical forms of all phases of the mind; it increases the zest for life and its duration) which wine confers, the harm produced by its misuse is truly insignificant; even its symbolic

> role has protected its physiological mission, and it ought to increase and secure that protection for all time to come.

And then there is a paper referring to "a new alcoholic drink made from tea" (39).

His openness and experimental desire led him to study the therapeutic possibilities of opium and cocaine (43,46). One of his research subjects for the study of physiological effects of opium smoking was one of his patients, a famous diva by the name of Maria Broma. This should be seen in the proper time perspective. It was at this same period that the respectable Sherlock Holmes let his mind wander to find light in the darkness with the help of the white powder, and years before Sigmund Freud started his year-long use of this psychoactive principle and even wrote to his fiancée to suggest the use of cocaine.

The fine wine bottles emptied by Thudichum and the opium smoke have gone with the wind, but his cigar boxes are preserved, as he used them for storing chemical specimens. Any cigar connoisseur will testify that in the field of Havana tobacco, Thudichum was without compromise; as this aspect of life would not be complete without food, so at the age of 66, Thudichum published a 700-page cookbook (Fig. 5).

EPILOGUE

Thudichum became a physician, clinical chemist, and neurochemist, but it might all have gone in another direction. His family was very gifted for music, and his father, a German headmaster, felt that young Ludwig could benefit from a good song teacher, and he obtained one of the finest Italian singers of the period, Monsignore Mario. The Italian must have been quite pleased with his pupil, as 18-year-old Thudichum (announced as "Monsignore Fiorentino") played an active role in one of Mario's public concerts in Marbach, singing duo with his teacher. All Thudichum's children played the piano and were good singers, one of his daughters, Lottie, becoming a professional oratorio singer. It was indeed a house of music.

Not until the year of his death in 1901 did Thudichum obtain recognition in his native Germany. His monograph on the brain, *Die Chemische Konstitution des Gehirns des Menschen und der Tiere* (Fig. 6) (25) was at long last published in his native language. In the preface we find his last will and testament:

> On account of the difficulty of obtaining material for study, Institutes should be set in operation in which not only infectious diseases, but those in which the diseases of the brain and nervous system can be studied, with a view toward answering chemical questions as well as the general investigation of the cellular fabric . . .
>
> I regret that I cannot present here the points of contact between the chemical constitution and its alterations under the hold of disease; they are numerous, yet complicated, and at present imperfectly established. My readers will visualize many such relationships if they are inclined to follow my presentation. I entreat them to read the entire work and especially not to pass over the technical part, so that from the demonstrated facts they can picture more correctly the meaning of the whole . . .
>
> My medical soul, to express it in poetical words, hangs grimly upon the infallibility of the chemical method. It was for me a spiritual headmaster in the agitated sea of medical conjecture, in which one so frequently sails without any compass. Together with the unfolding of the aetiology and diagnosis has the chemical method of exploration and management of disease states nourished me in the conviction that the healing art, apart from its practice, through talent (genius) and its dominion over human spirits, will develop into a consummate science capable of applicability with astronomical accuracy. Towards this end, however, as in Theology in the case of the spurious documents (attestations), so in Medicine, to use a phrase of Darwin's, the "false facts" must be rooted out and the scientific certainties estab-

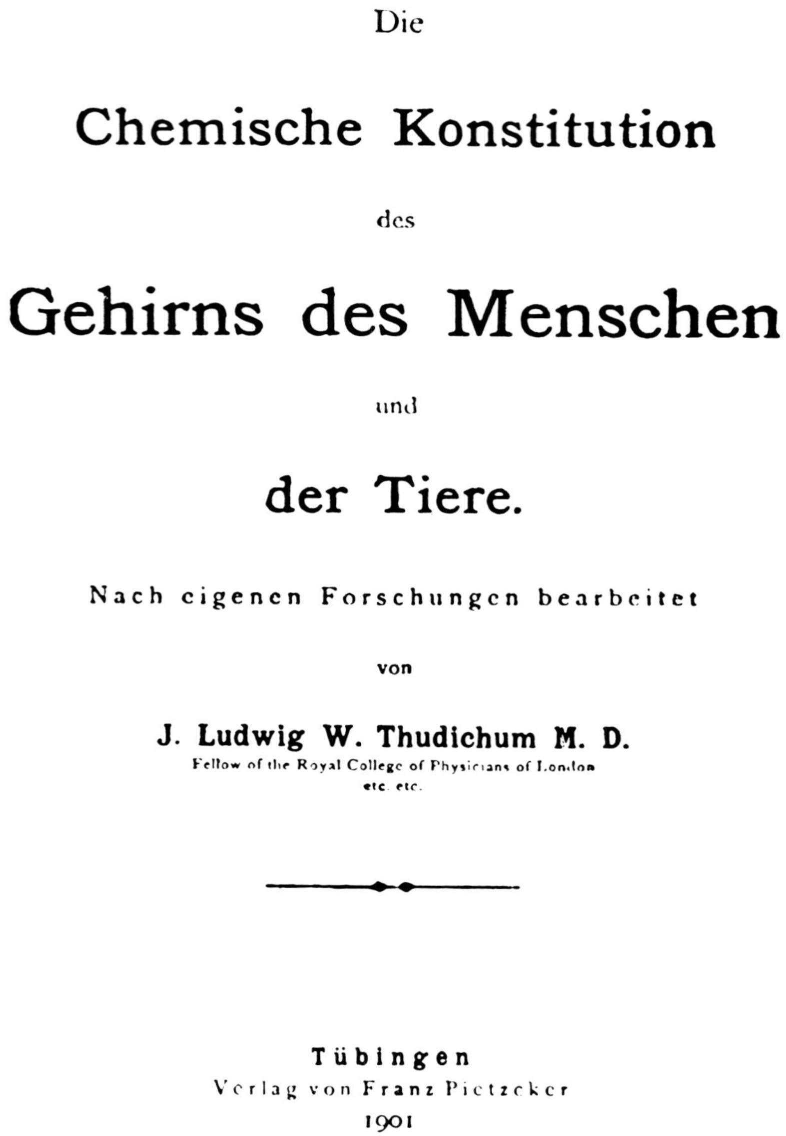

Die

Chemische Konstitution

des

Gehirns des Menschen

und

der Tiere.

Nach eigenen Forschungen bearbeitet

von

J. Ludwig W. Thudichum M. D.

Fellow of the Royal College of Physicians of London etc. etc.

Tübingen

Verlag von Franz Pietzcker

1901

FIG. 6. Title page from Thudichum's *Die Chemische Konstitution des Gehirns des Menschen und der Tiere*, ref. 25.

> lished for the discernment of all enquirers. Accordingly I hope that this small contribution will also serve in the promotion of human insight in large. (May 23, 1901, 11 Pembroke Gardens.)"

Shortly afterward, he returned to his alma mater, the University of Giessen, to receive an honorary degree on the occasion of the fiftieth anniversary of his graduation. A circle was closed (Figs. 7 and 8).

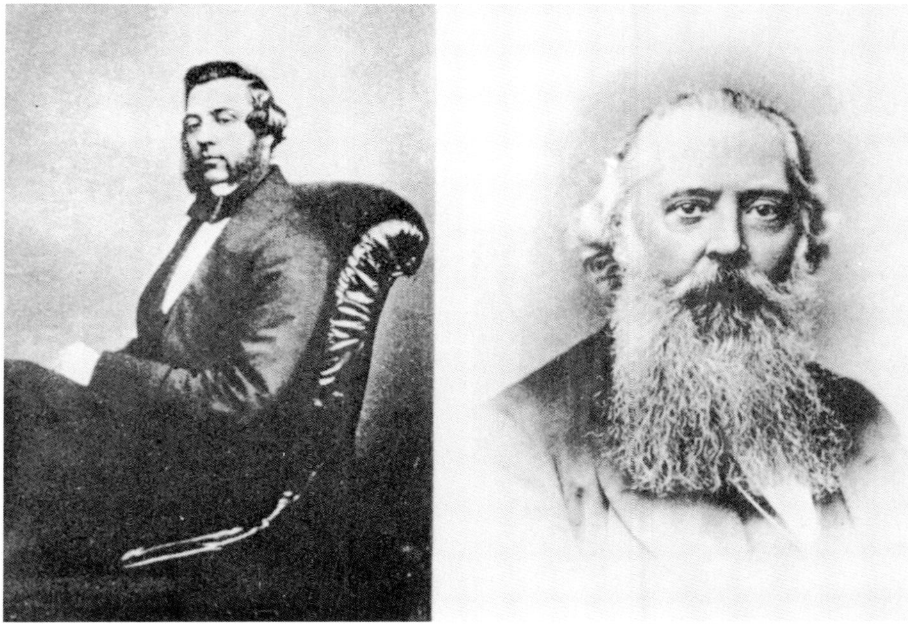

FIGS. 7,8. Johan Ludwig Wilhelm Thudichum, at age 30 (left) and in his late 60s (right). (Courtesy of the Wellcome Trustees, London.)

REFERENCES

1. Drabkin, D. L. (1958): *Thudichum—Chemist of the Brain*, University of Pennsylvania Press, Philadelphia.
2. McIlwain, H. (1958): Thudichum and the medical chemistry of the 1860s to 1880s. *Proc. Roy. Soc. Med.*, 51:127–132.
3. McIlwain, H. (1975): Cerebral isolates and neurochemical discovery (The Second Thudichum Lecture). *Biochem. Soc. Trans.*, 3:579–590.
4. Page, I. H. (1937): *Chemistry of the Brain*. Baillière, Tindall & Cox, London.
5. Page, I. H. (1955): Thudichum and the chemistry of the brain. In: *Neurochemistry—The Chemical Dynamics of Brain and Nerve*, edited by K. A. C. Elliott, I. H. Page, and J. H. Quastel. pp. 3–10. Charles C. Thomas, Springfield, Illinois.

The following references are grouped according to subject.

The Rhinolaryngologist

6. Thudichum, J. L. W. (1868): On some new modes of treating diseases of the nose. *Lancet*, 2:243, 307, 534.
7. Thudichum, J. L. W. (1869): *On Polypus in the Nose and Ozaena; Their Successful Treatment by New Methods*. Churchill and Sons, London.
8. Thudichum, J. L. W. (1888): *On Polypus in the Nose etc.; Their Successful Treatment by the Electro-Caustic etc.*, 6th ed. Baillière, Tindall and Cox, London.
9. Thudichum, J. L. W. (1888): *A Monograph on Polypus and Other Diseases of the Nasal Cavity; Based Entirely Upon Original Researches*, 7th ed. Bailliére, Tindall and Cox, London.

Clinical Chemist

10. Thudichum, J. L. W. (1858): *A Treatise on the Pathology of the Urine. Including a Complete Guide to its Analysis*. J. Churchill, London.

11. Thudichum, J. L. W. (1863): *A Treatise on Gall Stones: Their Chemistry, Pathology, and Treatment*. J. Churchill, London.
12. Thudichum, J. L. W. (1872): *A Manual of Chemical Physiology, Including Its Points of Contact with Pathology*. Longmans, Green, London.
13. Thudichum, J. L. W. (1875); Further researches on bilirubin and its compounds. *J. Chem. Soc.*, 28:1875.
14. Thudichum, J. L. W. (1877): *A Treatise on the Pathology of the Urine, Including a Complete Guide to its Analysis*, 2nd ed. Chruchill, London.
15. Thudichum, J. L. W. (1886): *Grundzüge der anatomischen und klinischen Chemie. Analecten für Forscher, Aerzte und Studierende*. Hirschwald, Berlin.
16. Thudichum, J. L. W. (1889): Urochrome, the colouring matter of urine, and its derivates. *Med. Press. Circ.*, 47:161.
17. Thudichum, J. L. W. (1895): Gall-stones: their origin, nature, and the treatment of the diseases which cause them, and those to which they give rise. Proc. W. Lond. Med.-Chir. Soc., 6:36.
18. Thudichum, J. L. W. (1898): Ueber das Urobilin. *Arch. Pathol. Anat. Physiol. u. klin. Med.*, 153:154.
19. Thudichum, J. L. W. (1898): The process of medical chemistry, comprising its application to physiology, pathology and the practice of medicine. *Med. Press, Circ.*, 66:298.
20. Thudichum, J. L. W. (1899): Ueber den chemischen Process Gallensteinkrankheit beim Menschen und in Thieren, mit neuen Versuchen. *Arch. Pathol. Anat. u. Physiol. u. klin. Med.*, 156:384.
21. Thudichum, J. L. W. (1900): Einige wissenschaftliche und etische Fragen der biologischen Chemie. *J. Frakt. Chem.*, 61:568.

Chemist of the Brain

22. Thudichum, J. L. W. : Further researches on the chemical constitution of the brain. *Report Med. Off. Priv. Council, New Series*, 1874, 1876, 1878, 1880, 1882, 1883.
23. Thudichum, J. L. W. (1884): *A Treatise on the Chemical Constitution of the Brain Based Throughout Upon Original Researches*. Baillière, Tindall, and Cox, London.
24. Thudichum, J. L. W. (1885): *Fiziologicheskaya chimiya golovnogo mozha;* translated by M. Liona, Kharkov. (Russian translation of 1884 treatise).
25. Thudichum, J. L. W. (1901): *Die Chemische Konstitution des Gehirns des Menschen und der Tiere. Nach eigenen Forschungen bearbeitet*. Pietzcker, Tübingen. (German edition of 1884 treatise).

The Fighter

26. Thudichum, J. L. W. (1876): Offenes Sendschreiben an die kaiserliche Akademie der Wissenshaften zu Wien, Beleuchtung der Untersuchungen über die Gallenfarbstoffe von Richard Maly in Graz, Leipzig und Heidelberg. *Annal. d. Chem.*, 181:242.
27. Thudichum, J. L. W. (1877): Ueber Indikan und das Verhältniss des Herrn Dr. Max Jaffe zum Begriff der chemischen Reinheit. I. Vom "reinen" und "unreinen" Indikan. *Arch. ges. Physiol.*, 15:343.
28. Thudichum, J. L. W. (1877): Ueber die Eisensalze der extractiven Säuren aus Menschenharn. Mit schluss Bemerkungen betreffend Hrn. E. Salkowsky's "Beitrage" zur Chemie des Harns." *Arch. ges. Physiol.*, 15:455.
29. Thudichum, J. L. W. (1877): Abwehr der Verdächtigungen, welche Herr Neubauer zu Wiesbaden betreffs der Kryptophansäure veröffentlicht hat. *Arch. ges. Physiol.*, 15:468.
30. Thudichum, J. L. W. (1882): Würde und Würdigung. Antwort auf den Angriff des Herrn Drechsel. *J. prakt. Chem.*, 25:190.

Public Health Pioneer

31. Thudichum, J. L. W. (1861): The physiological and therapeutic action of the Turkish bath. *Br. Med. J.*, 1:126.
32. Thudichum, J. L. W. (1863): On an improved mode of collecting excrementitious matter. *J. Soc. Arts, London.*, 11:440.
33. Thudichum, J. L. W. (1880): Discussion of H. Carr's paper on: Our domestic poisons in relations to trade and art. *J. Soc. Arts, London*, 28:159.
34. Thudichum, J. L. W. (1884): Discussion of Dr. P. Frankland's paper on: Upper Thames as a source of water supply. *J. Soc. Arts, London*, 32:556.
35. Thudichum, J. L. W. (1884): Introduction to a discussion on the water supply of London with special regard to public health and security. *Proc. W. Lond. Med.-Chir. Soc.*, 1:41.
36. Thudichum, J. L. W. (1885): *Aids to Public Health*. Baillière, Tindall, and Cox, London. 56 pp.

37. Thudichum, J. L. W. (1898): Briefe über öffentliche Gesundheitspflege ihre bisherigen Leistungen und heutigen Aufgaben. Pietzker, Tübingen.

Some Psychotropic Substances

38. Thudichum, J. L. W. (1866): On the disease of meat as affecting the health of the people. *J. Soc. Arts, London,*: 14:391. (For this the Society's silver medal was awarded.)
39. Thudichum, J. L. W. (1869–1870): On wines, their origin, nature, analysis and uses; with special reference to a new alcoholic drink made from tea. *J. Soc. Arts, London*, 18:109.
40. Thudichum, J. L. W. (1871): Report of the chemical analysis of wines of the pure wine association (For private circulation only). J. King, London.
41. Thudichum, J. L. W. (1872): A treatise on the origin, nature, and varieties of wine: being a complete manual of viticulture and oenology. Macmillan, London.
42. Thudichum, J. L. W. (1875): Discussion of W. L. Scott's lecture on: "Food adulteration and legislative enactments relating thereto." *J. Soc. Arts, London*, 23:438.
43. Thudichum, J. L. W. (1883): Über das Opiumrauchen als therapeutisches Mittel. *Verhandl. d. Congr. f. innere Med. Weisbaden*, 2:307.
44. Thudichum, J. L. W. (1884): The aesthetical use of wine and its influence upon health. W. Clowes & Sons, London.
45. Thudichum, J. L. W. (1884): Über das Opiumrauchen als therapeutischen Mittel. *Z. Therap. m. Einbzb. d. Elect. u. Hydrotherap. Wien*, 2:61.
46. Thudichum, J. L. W. (1885): *On the Coco of Peru and Its Immediate Principles; Their Strengthening and Healing Powers*. Baillière, Tindall, and Cox, London.
47. Thudichum, J. L. W. (1895): *The Spirit of Cookery. A Popular Treatise on the History, Science, Practice, and Ethical and Medical Import of Culinary Terms*. F. Warne & Co., London & New York.
48. Thudichum, J. L. W. (1896): *A Treatise on Wines. Their Origin, Nature and Varieties with Practical Directions for Viticulture and Vinifaction*. George Bell & Sons, London.

Historical Aspects of the Neurosciences,
edited by F. Clifford Rose and W.F. Bynum.
Raven Press, New York ©

Some Notes on the History of Neuroendocrinology[1]

V. C. Medvei

38 Westmoreland Terrace, London SW1V 3HL, England

I am greatly honored to have been asked to make this contribution to the volume on *Historical Aspects of the Neurosciences* in honor of Dr. Macdonald Critchley.

Many medical men, including those with a special interest in endocrinology, believe that neuroendocrinology began only in the last 40 years. Some, who are a little older, may remember the publication in 1946 of Roussy and Mosinger's great volume, *Traité de Neuro-Endocrinologie* (1), with its parts, "Le système neuro-endocrinien, le complexe hypothalamo-hypophysaire, and la neuro-ergonologie et son évolution récente." In the introduction, the authors wrote:

> Après une étape longue de plus de deux siècles, durant laquelle les disciplines morphologiques, physiologiques et cliniques ont établi leur assizes sur des bases essentiellement analytiques, la médecine s'engage aujourd'hui sur des voies nouvelles. Elle tente de rapprocher ce qu'elle avait, peut-être trop longtemps séparé. Elle cherche à aborder de plus en plus, en un esprit de synthèse et dans une vue d'ensemble, l'étude des vastes problèmes relatifs au mécanisms régulateurs de la vie normale des tissues et des organes, ainsi que leurs dérèglements au cours des processus morbides . . . Il en est ainsi de la Neurologie et de l'Endocrinologie. Ces disciplines tend aujourd'hui à se rapprocher l'une de l'autre à tel point que l'étude des régulations nerveuses et celle de régulations hormonales ce confondent de plus en plus en une science de synthèse: La Neuro-Endocrinologie . . . Puis B. Aschner, J. Camus, et G. Roussy (2) ont démontré, par des expériences devenues classiques, la possibilité de provoquer ces syndromes par des lésions nerveuses. Or, les corrélations anatomiques et fonctionelles entre l'hypothalamus—noeud vital du système neurovégétatif—et l'hypophyse, gland directrice de toutes les manifestations de la vie organique, se sont révélées par la suite extrémement étroites, en même temps que d'une grande complexité.

Roussy's studies go back to the first decade of the 20th century.

From 1928 to 1940, a great contribution to the subject was made by Berta and Ernst Scharrer, originally from Germany, and their group. In 1928, they observed large cells in the hypothalamus of teleost fishes, filled with secretory droplets, some of them multinuclear and surrounded by capillaries. They continued their studies in other fish because, as they remarked, "there is so great a variety . . . that every species must be described separately" (3,4). The varied appearances observed were tentatively interpreted as a series of stages in a cycle of formation and

[1]This chapter is based on the author's book, *A History of Endocrinology*, MTP Press Ltd., Lancaster, England, 1981.

discharge of inclusions of cells, leading to the concept of neurosecretion. Similar observations were made in other species, including man, and in insects. Such secretory granules were found to displace the Nissl-staining material to the periphery and were traced in fish and man along axons leading to the neurohypophysis (5). In the early 1950s, it was proved that the posterior pituitary lobe hormones originated from two large-celled hypothalamic nuclei. Camus and Roussy had insisted since 1913 on the predominance of the hypothalamus (6). Roussy and Mosinger recorded in 1933 the following three stages of development of opinion (7): (a) the hypophyseal, based on the work of Biedl, Cushing, and Marañon; (b) the phase of the tuber cinereum, based mainly on the work of Bernhard Aschner (8) around 1912; and (c) the final recognition of the control of the hypothalamus over the pituitary as the main neurohumoral mechanism (9), based on the work of G. W. Harris.

As early as 1919, Carl Caskey Speidel reported on "gland-cells of internal secretion" in the spinal cord of skates (10). Scharrer and Scharrer (11) mention that A. A. Berthold in his celebrated but overlooked experiment of the testicular transplant in 1849 "implicated the nervous system as a target organ." They also comment on the curious fact that Brown-Séquard, who was both a neurologist and a pioneer in endocrine research, "never seems to have become interested in possible connections between the central nervous system and the endocrine glands." F. J. Gall in 1818 (12) and J. Vimont in 1835 (13) mentioned that unilateral castration causes atrophy of the contralateral hemisphere of the cerebellum: "Toutes les fois qu'on a enlevé un seul testicule à un animal, de quelque espèce qu'il soit, le lobe du cervelet, du côté opposé, s'atrophie visiblement . . ." (12). In a like manner, A. Maestre de San Juan reported in 1856 from Spain that gonadal hypoplasia could be observed in men with agenesis of the olfactory lobes; so did F. Weidenreich in 1914, but these reports were ignored until confirmed experimentally by Scharrer and Scharrer (11). In 1913, G. Peritz referred to this state of affairs (14), posing a number of questions to which even now many of the answers are missing.

The concept of chemical transmission of nerve impulses had to face great difficulties between 1910 and 1950, before it became generally accepted. F. H. Lewy had stated in his 60-page description of the diseases of the endocrine glands that "die vegetativen Kerne im Zentralnervensystem und Hypophysenhinterlappen ein einziges zusammengehoeriges System bilden" (15) ("the vegetative nuclei in the CNS form with the posterior lobe of the pituitary a single, consecutive system").

Three of the pioneers, Sir Henry Dale, Walter B. Cannon, and Otto Loewi are now dead. Two surviving eyewitnesses, Wilhelm Feldberg and Z. M. Bacq, have written memoirs of that period (16,17). According to Feldberg, for the true beginning of his narrative, ". . . we must go back to Dale's early publication in 1914 on 'The action of certain esters and others of choline,' in which the fundamental distinction was made between two types of action of acetylcholine, a muscarine and a nicotine action. . . ." This was the true beginning of the story of acetylcholine in synaptic and neuromuscular transmission. In 1937, Dale penned a note for the Proceedings of the Physiological Society, illustrating that 60 years previously, in 1877, Du Bois-Reymond had clearly suggested a chemical transmission from motor nerve endings to striated muscle (18). "Then there was the brilliant anticipation of this mode of action," Feldberg continues, "by T. R. Elliott, who had been the first to conceive the idea of chemical transmission in the autonomic nervous system." The prediction came true, when Feldberg and Fessard published a paper in 1942 "On the cholinergic nature of the nerves to the electric organ of the Torpedo" (19). Bacq, in his historical sketch, says (17):

> The concept of a neuro-endocrine system, as W. B. Cannon defined it in the 1920s, is still valid. The most striking example is the series of catecholamines, of which some (adrenaline, noradrenaline) are real hormones secreted into the blood by the adrenal medulla during

> emotional shock, physical exercise, cold, or when the blood sugar concentration drops below the point tolerable to nerve cells. The same hormones are also the chemical mediators or transmitters, the indispensable substances for the transmission of excitation in one class of nerve fibres, which innervate the heart, smooth muscles, and glands . . . until 1930–1935, physiologists believed that it was the difference in the electric potential itself, the eddy current, which passed from the endings of the axon to the membrane of the effector cell and brought about the transmission. Today we know that, with rare exceptions, transmission of nerve impulses is effected in all tissues (smooth muscles, glands, striated muscles, heart, and nerve cells) through molecules which are stored in the presynaptic nerve endings. The electric events are naturally linked to the release of these transmitters and we therefore speak in a general way of 'electro-chemical events' that occur at the synapses. The neurone can, therefore, be looked upon as a kind of electrical device which transmits quants of very active molecules from its axon terminals whenever a nerve impulse reaches them.

In pursuing the tale, Bacq quotes "The forerunners," one of whom is E. Du Bois-Reymond (18): "Von bekannten Naturprozessen, welche nun noch die Erregung vermitteln könnten, kommen, so viel ich sehe, nur zwei in Frage. Entweder muesste an der Grenze der kontraktilen Substanz eine reizende Sekretion, in Gestalt etwa einer duennen Schicht von Ammoniak oder Milchsaeure oder einem anderen, den Muskel heftig erregenden Stoff stattfinden. Oder die Wirkung muesste elektrisch sein." ("Of the known processes of nature, which could transmit the excitation, there could be only two, I can perceive. There would have to be at the border of the contractile substance either a stimulating secretion, in form, e.g., of a thin layer of ammonia or lactic acid or of another substance, which excites the muscle vehemently, or the effect would have to be electric.")

Bacq also referred to Howell, an American physiologist, who in 1906 showed that small changes in the cation concentration of saline solutions used for studying isolated organs, produced effects similar to those which occur on nerve stimulation. He next recalled O. Loewi's fundamental experiment to prove the existence of the "Vagus-stoff," giving Loewi's own version of how he got the idea for his experiment. He further commented on Feldberg's work: "Without Feldberg, the research on chemical transmission might well have taken a very different course."

Bacq also discussed the opposition to the theory of chemical transmission, the leaders of which were Leon Ascher of Basel, several French physiologists, especially Malméjac, then in Algiers, and J. C. Eccles, who later emigrated to Australia and New Zealand. Eccles "tried to refute the solid arguments provided by Brown, Dale, Feldberg, and myself (Bacq)." It was not before 1944 that Eccles began to admit an error of misinterpretation and placed himself firmly behind Sir Henry Dale's interpretation. Specific examples of close connections between endocrine and nervous mechanisms can be found in the literature with increasing frequency from 1920, and especially from 1930 onward: von Monakow (20), Hoskins (21), Roizin (22), and Stockard (23).

It was remarkable that (Sir) Edward A. (Sharpey) Schaefer, with George Oliver, the discoverer of a specific physiological response to adrenal extract in 1893/4 (24), rejected Brown-Séquard's hypothesis of the endocrine function of the gonads. Although "removal of the generative organs" led to "marked alterations in the development of other parts of the body," Schaefer's conclusion was that "the changes are without a doubt produced through the nervous system, and are not connected with the gonads" (25). Similarly, the heated controversy between Pavlov on the one hand and Bayliss and Starling on the other, whether hormones or nerves control the gastrointestinal tract, is now resolved: Both were right (26). As several peptides seem to be able to fulfil both functions, the distinction between hormone and neurotransmitter is difficult to maintain. Regulatory peptides can be released into the blood (hormonal function) or in the axon (neurocrine function) or released locally (paracrine function); for example, cholecytokinin may carry out any of these three functions (27). Similarly, adrenaline and noradrenaline, originally described as hormones, are now regarded as neurotransmitters. By November 1979, there were 21 neuropeptides enumerated capable of ambidexterous behavior!

One of the greatest contributions to the idea of neuroendocrine function, was made between 1945 and 1971 by the late Geoffrey W. Harris of Cambridge, both theoretically and experimentally. There is not space in this chapter to discuss his great merits in this field in detail, but he was one of the few modern research workers who studied neuroendocrine development in the fetus (28). R. Zander had noted in 1890 the connection between the adrenals and other organs, especially the brain (29), and he had referred to an observation on the absence of the adrenal cortex in anencephali recorded by Morgagni (1733), Soemmering (1792), and Meckel (1802).

The most interesting ideas by far of what is now termed neuroendocrine connections were voiced in the 17th and 18th centuries, although their origins date back to antiquity. René Descartes' *Traité de l'homme*, published in 1662, may be regarded as the first textbook of physiology (30), a treatise that covered the whole field of animal physiology and that was meant to be an appendix to the "Discourse on method" (1637). He considered the brain as the organ integrating the functions of mind and body (see also his "Des passions de l'âme," published in 1649): "For the parts of the blood which penetrate even into the brain do not serve merely to nourish and maintain its substance, but instead chiefly to produce a very subtle breath or rather a very lively and very pure flame which they call the animal spirits. . . . In proportion as the animal spirits enter the cavities of the brain, they pass into the pores of its substance, and from these pores into the nerves, . . ." whence they proceed through the hollow nerves to the rest of the body; but when the spirits in the ventricles were uncertain about their proper destination, the pineal directed them "by leaning to one side or other of the middle line."

Descartes' forerunners in antiquity were Anaxagoras (500–428 B.C.) and Herophilus of Chalcedon (4th century, B.C.). Thomas Wharton described in his "Adenographia" in 1659 (31) the pituitary and pineal glands. Of the pituitary, he wrote that the function of it is "according to Bauhin, to drain off the moisture of the brain." This theory goes back to Galen and Vesalius. The latter said in "De Fabrica . . ." in 1543: "Glandula pituitaria cerebri excipiens, . . ." that the waste material excreted by the brain, "a glandular organ," passes through the infundibulum into the pituitary and from there to the nasopharnyx (32). On this theory were based the use of pills and sneezing powders "to purge the brain"; ". . . glandulae vero non ta sanguini qua nervi famulantur (the glands serve not so much the blood as the nerves) . . . aliae succum nutritium nervis ministrant, aliae secrementa eorum foras exportant, adeoque omnes nervorum ministerio incumbunt" ("some procure the nutritional juice for the nerves, others remove their secretions outside: thus all administer to the nervous system"). Wharton also gave a good description of the pineal gland and referred to Riolan, according to whom its function was that of a valve between the third and fourth ventricles.

Conrad Victor Schneider of Wittenberg, however, refuted by careful studies and by the description of "Schneider's pituitary membrane" in 1655 Galen's idea that the pituita is discharged into the nasal cavities (33). This was followed, five years later, by the proof that only the macerated ethmoid bone displays pores (34), which, in the living person, are completely filled with vessels. The pituitary, according to him, did not contain a cavity nor any liquid. Schneider also compared the relative weights of the brain and of the pituitary gland and found this quotient very low in man in comparison with that of certain other animals.

Richard Lower, in his "Dissertatio de origine catarrhi in qua ostenditur illum non provenire a cerebro . . ." (1670) (35), confirmed Schneider's views experimentally. Geoffrey Harris would regard this idea as modern in its endocrine conception. Thomas Willis, Lower's friend, for whom the latter planned and carried out the experiments, shared this view; but Hans H. Simmer feels that Willis and Lower were wrongly credited with the suggestion of pituitary hormones because the translation of one of Willis' sentences from the Latin was at fault (36). Harvey Cushing translated the first part of that sentence as follows: "The blood . . . takes some part of the superfluous serum *of* the pituitary gland, . . ." whereas the translation into English of the same passage in 1681 by S. Pordage used the word "to" instead of "of": the blood of the arterial circle "might carry away some part of the superfluous serum to the pituitary gland" (37). In Simmer's opinion, "Willis spoke indeed, of uptake by the gland and not of discharge . . ." An experiment convinced Willis of a receptive function of the pituitary. When he injected ink into a carotid artery, part of the ink appeared in the pituitary tissue. "The foregoing analysis," Simmer continues, "removes the temptation, to read into Lower's or Willis' statements the germ of the conception of internal secretion."

Nevertheless, Willis, in a later edition (1676) of "Cerebri anatome" (38), and Morgagni (1761) (39) were among the first to observe the abnormal passage of cerebrospinal fluid from the nose. The first case of a patient with communicating hydrocephalus, confirmed at postmortem, was described by C. Miller in 1826 (40). P. J. Tillaux (1877) reported the first case of rhinorrhoea, proven by chemical analysis to be cerebrospinal fluid (41). St. Clair Thompson (1899) wrote a monograph, "The Cerebrospinal Fluid: Its Spontaneous Escape from the Nose" (42), reviewing the literature then available and adding a case history of his own. Of the 21 patients reviewed with spontaneous cerebrospinal fluid leak from the nose, only nine could be substantiated. The etiology was known only in three cases: congenital hydrocephalus (43); pituitary "swelling" (44); and defects in the cribriform dura (45). H. Cairns reviewed the position again in 1937 (46), giving four etiological groups: acute traumatic, delayed posttraumatic, following nasal surgery, and spontaneous. Recently, Cole and Keene (47) reported on three such patients where CSF rhinorrhoea was due to pituitary tumor (prolactin-secreting adenoma). Thus, Galen and Vesalius might have well observed such patients.

Willis, in 1664, in his "Cerebri anatome," on page 169, suggested that the pineal gland, the epiphysis cerebri in contrast to the hypophysis, or "glandula superior" (Niels Stensen) was collecting the cerebrospinal fluid, as it was "to receive and retain within it the serous humours deposited from the arterious blood."

Humphrey Ridley put forward in his "Anatomy of the Brain," in 1695 (48), a hypothesis, which was also accepted by William Cowper in 1698 (49), that "the glandula pinealis, which we take to be a lymphatic gland, receives lymph free from the lymphducts which pass the third ventricle of the brain to the infundibulum and glandula pituitaria." This view prevailed throughout the next two centuries and to the beginning of the 20th century (50)!

G. W. Harris referred specifically to Galen in his Dale Lecture for 1971, six months before his death. He called it "Humours and Hormones," because it began with Galen's views on the function of the pituitary gland. He then mentioned Lower's idea that substances pass from the brain through the infundibulum and pituitary stalk to the gland, where they were distilled back into the blood. "It is interesting," he added, "to compare this early idea with our own views 300 years later, that neuro-secretory material, formed in hypothalamic nuclei, pass down the nerve fibers, through the infundibulum to the posterior pituitary, where they 'distil' into the blood as the octapeptide hormones, oxytocin and vasopressin, and that hypothalamic nerve terminals liberate releasing factors into the portal vessels of the infundibulum and that these are carried down the stalk to the anterior pituitary, where they evoke 'distillation' of protein hormones into the blood" (51).

Professor Solly (now Lord) Zuckerman discussed the problem in the Seventh Addison Memorial Lecture at Guy's Hospital in London in December 1953 (52). He called it: "Secretions of the Brain: Relation of Hypothalamus to Pituitary Gland." After mentioning the Aristotelian concept of the four humors, and that one of them, phlegm (or pituita), produced by the brain, escaped "by way of the infundibulum of the third ventricle into the pituitary body, and thence along the olfactory nerves through the cribriform plate of the ethmoid into the nose" (see also Galen and Vesalius), he refers to Swedenborg, who wrote ca. 1742 (53): "For the purpose of preparing the blood, the soul has established in the cerebrum an illustrious chymical laboratory, which it has arranged into members and organs and by the ministry of these it distils and elaborates a lymph animated by the animal spirit, whereby it imbues the blood with its own inmost essence, nature and life." To Swedenborg, "The infundibulum is not only a *vas deferens* or an excretory duct, but it is also a *vas secernens* or a secretory vessel. . . ."

It was not until Joseph Lieutaud, a professor of medicine at the University of Aix-en-Provence and a Foreign Member of the Royal Society of London, discovered a hypothalamo-hypophyseal connection, that a very modern twist was given to the knowledge of the functions of the brain (54). Describing in 1742 the third ventricle of the brain, he drew attention to a deep anterior fossa, the aperture of which gradually narrows as it approaches the base of the pituitary stalk. This stalk, he observed, is, contrary to usual belief, not canalized, but is a kind of cylinder, "two or three lines thick," formed of a gray substance, and covered by pia mater. Running along it are very small longitudinal vessels, which communicate with those of the pituitary gland below. "The stalk which arises from the pituitary gland, corresponds exactly with the deepest part of that pit, but it has no cavity, as has been assumed . . . one perceives very small vessels, which pass (in) along its axis, communicating with those of the gland, which receives this column or which sustains it. I have given the name 'pituitary stalk' to this part, because I believe that the term funnel would not be suitable for it. It is not difficult to demonstrate the solidity of the pituitary stalk and I shall describe the method for doing so."

Nine years later, Théophil de Bordeu, the French physician, attacked Lieutaud's theory on the function and secretions of the brain. Incidentally, it was de Bordeu who first seemed to have had a conception of hormonal action, presented in his treatise "Analyse Médicinale du Sang" in 1775 (55). Zuckerman comments: "As we now know, Lieutaud and de Bordeu were both right and wrong. De Bordeu was wrong and Lieutaud was right in suggesting that the axial-stalk vessels communicate with those of the pituitary; while de Bordeu was well justified in attacking Lieutaud's conception of the structure and function of the brain, and in doubting that a vital fluid flows from the base of the brain to the pituitary." That which Lieutaud described in 1742, what does it look like in 1980?

G. T. Popa and U. Fielding rediscovered and reported on the important anatomical link between the hypothalamus and the anterior pituitary in 1930 and 1933 (56,57), by the axial-stalk vessels described by Lieutaud 200 years ago, although their view concerning the direction of the flow has now been revised. Although they also knew that other observers before them had described the pituitary portal vessels, such as S. Lothringer in 1886 (58), they did not seem to be aware of Lieutaud's work and his controversy with de Bordeu. Recently, J. N. Henderson and P. M. Daniel in London published the results of their work on "Portal Circulations and their Relations to Countercurrent Systems" (59). They came to the conclusion that the distribution of portal circulations throughout the animal body is

> . . . commoner than is generally supposed. Most portal circulations consist of two serial capillary beds, connected by one or more larger vessels ('convergent' portal circulations, e.g., the hepatic portal, placental, hypophysial, renal, ovarian, and testicular circulations . . .). A second type of portal circulation, which is less common, consists of two serial capillary beds that are not connected by larger vessels. These we have called 'continuous' portal circulations: adrenal and pancreatic circulations are examples of this type. When a countercurrent concentrating mechanism exists in the body, it is always part of the primary or secondary bed of a convergent portal circulation, though some convergent portal circulations are not associated with countercurrent mechanisms . . . what characterizes portal circulations is that they possess two serial capillary beds (supplying different cell types) that are not separated by the heart. We will refer to the two capillary beds as 'primary' and 'secondary' respectively . . . Popa and Fielding first realized, in 1930, that the vessels running along the pituitary stalk connected two capillary beds, and formed a portal system analogous to the portal veins of the liver. These workers actually mistook the primary for the secondary bed, thinking that the blood passed up the stalk. We know now that blood flows down the stalk in the long portal vessels, carrying neurohormones from the hypothalamic nerve cells to the epithelial cells of the adenohypophysis. . . . It seems, however, that the original idea about the direction of the blood flow in the pituitary stalk was not entirely wrong, for Page et al. (60) described in 1976 portal vessels in the stalk in which blood could flow from the neurohypophysis up to the median eminence. Oliver et al. (61) have shown, in 1977, experimentally, that neurohypophysial hormones do, in fact, pass up the stalk to influence the release of hormones from the median eminence. . . . These authors make the suggestion that there is a countercurrent exchange of hormone(s) between the ascending and descending portal vessels.
>
> Such is the course of history. Soothsayers were the first serious students of the liver (59), and thought of the entry of the great vessels into the liver as the gate of the organ—the porta hepatis. Rufus of Ephesus, a Roman surgeon, described this arrangement in about 100 A. D. . . . and some time after the discovery of the capillaries in 1660, by Malpighi, it became evident that the portal vein was at least unusual in having capillaries at both ends.

And long before Popa and Fielding, Lieutaud suggested that the axial-stalk vessels communicate with those of the pituitary below, and he was responsible for the term "tige pituitaire": la tige, from the Latin "tibia," meaning stem, stalk, trunk.

REFERENCES

1. Roussy, G., and Mosinger, M. (1946): *Traité de Neuro-Endocrinologie*. Masson, Paris.
2. Camus, J., Roussy, G., and Aschner, B. (1913): *C. R. Soc. Biol. Paris*, 75:628.
3. Scharrer, E., and Scharrer, B. (1940): Secretory cells within the hypothalamus. *Res. Publ. Ass. Nerv. Ment. Dis.*, 20:170–194.
4. Scharrer, B. (1971): Histophysiological studies on the corpus allatum of *Leukophaka Maderae*. V. Ultrastructure of sites of origin and release of distinctive cellular product. *Zellforschg., Mikroskop. Anat.*, 120:1–16.
5. Gaupp, R., and Scharrer, E. (1935): Die Zwischenhirnsekretion bei Mensch u. Tier. *Z. ges. Neurol. Psych.*, 153:327–355.
6. Camus, J., and Roussy, G. (1913): *C. R. Soc. Biol. Paris*, 75:628.
7. Roussy, G., and Mosinger, M. (1933): *C. R. Soc. Biol. Paris*, 112:775.
8. Aschner, B. (1912): *Arch. Gynaekol. Berlin*, 97:200.
9. Roussy, G., and Mosinger, M. (1933): *C. R. Soc. Biol. Paris*, 112:775.
10. Speidel, C. C. (1919): *Gland-Cells of Internal Secretion in the Spinal Cord of Skates*. Carnegie Inst. Wash. Publ., No. 13, pp. 1–31.
11. Scharrer, E., and Scharrer, B. (1963): *Neuroendocrinology*. Columbia Univ. Press, New York.
12. Gall, F. J. (1818): *Anatomie et Physiologie du Système nerveux en générale et du Cerveau en particulier*, Vol. 3, pp. 108–131. Librairie Grècque-Latin-Allemande, Paris.
13. Vimont, J. (1835): *Traité de phrénologie humaine et comparée*, 2me ed. Établissement Encyclographique, Bruxelles.
14. Peritz, G. (1913): Nervensystem u. innere Sekretion, In: *Hdbuch. d. Biochemie d. Menschen u.d. Tiere*, edited by C. Oppenheimer, Ergaenzungsband, pp. 496–536. G. Fischer, Jena.

15. Lewy, F. H. (1929): Die Erkrankungen d.endokrinen Druesen. *Fortschr. Neurol., Psychiatr. u. Grenzgeb.*, 1:347–408.
16. Feldberg, W. (1977): The Early History of Synaptic and Neuromuscular Transmission by Acetylcholine: Reminiscences of an Eye Witness. In: *The Pursuit of Nature. Informal Essays on the History of Physiology*, pp. 65–83. Cambridge University Press, Cambridge.
17. Bacq, Z. M. (1975): *Chemical Transmission of Nerve Impulses. A Historical Sketch*. Pergamon Press, Oxford.
18. Du Bois-Reymond, E. (1877): *Ges Abhandl. d. allg. Muskel-u. Nervenphysiologie*, 2:700.
19. Feldberg, W. (1977): The Early History of Synaptic and Neuromuscular Transmission by Acetylcholine: Reminiscences of an Eye Witness. In: *The Pursuit of Nature. Informal Essays on the History of Physiology*, pp. 65–83. Cambridge University Press, Cambridge.
20. von Monakow, C. (1919): Psychiatrie und Biologie. *Schweiz. Arch. Neurol. Psychiat.*, 4:13–235.
21. Hoskins, R. G. (1934): Endocrinology. In: *The Problem of Mental Disorder*. McGraw-Hill, New York.
22. Roizin, L. (1936): Sensorial organs as originators of neuroendocrine-vegetative reflexes in the diencephalo-pituitary region. Thesis. Univ. Milano (in Italian). Published also in *Ras. neurol. vegetativa*, 1:348–383.
23. Stockard, C. R. (1938) : The interactions of the endocrine glands and the nervous system. *Diplomate*, 10:44–51.
24. Schaefer, A. E. (1895): Address in Physiology: On internal secretion. *Lancet*, II:321–324.
25. Schaefer, A. E. (1895): Address in Physiology: On internal secretion. *Lancet*, II:321–324.
26. Bloom, S. R. (1980): The Goulstonian Lecture 1979 to the Royal College of Physicians of London: Gut and brain—endocrine connections. *J. Roy. Coll. Physns. London*, 14:51–57.
27. Bloom, S. R. (1980): The Goulstonian Lecture 1979 to the Royal College of Physicians of London: Gut and brain—endocrine connections. *J. Roy. Coll. Physns. London*, 14:51–57.
28. Harris, G. W. (1955): The relationship between endocrine activity and the development of the nervous system. In: *Biochemistry of the Developing Nervous System*, edited by H. Waelsch, pp. 431–442. Academic Press, New York.
29. Zander, R. (1890): Ueber funktionelle und genetische Beziehungen der Nebennieren zu anderen Organen, speziell zum Grosshirn. *Beitr. pathol. Anat.*, 7:439–534.
30. Descartes, R. (1662): *De homine figuris et latinitate donatus a Florentio Schuyl*. Lugduni Batavorum, apud F. Moyardum et P. Leffen.
31. Wharton, T. (1656): *Adenographia: sive glandularum totius corporis descriptio*. Londini. typ. J. G. impens. Authoris.
32. Vesalius, A. (1543): *De humani corporis fabrica libri septem*. Basileae (ex off. Ionnis Oporini).
33. Schneider, C. V. (1655): *Dissertatio de osse cribriforme, et sensu ac organo odoratus*. T. Mevii, Wittebergae.
34. Schneider, C. V. (1660): *Liber primus de catarrhis*. T. Mevii et E. Schumacheri, Wittebergae.
35. Lower, R. (1670): Dissertatio de origine catarrhi in qua ostenditur illum non provenire a cerebro. In: *Tractatus de corde*. Londini, typ. J. Redmayne.
36. Simmer, H. H. (1974): The beginnings of endocrinology. In: *Medicine in Seventeenth Century England*, pp. 215–236. Univ. of California Press, Berkeley, Los Angeles.
37. Pordage, S. (1681): The Remaining Medical Works of that Famous and Renowned Physician Dr. Thomas Willis. London. (Facsimile published in Vol. 2 of Feindel, ed., *Willis*.)
38. Willis, T. (1676): Cerebri anatome: cui accessit nervorum descriptio et usus. In: *Opera omnia*, Amsteladami.
39. Morgagni, G. B. (1761): *De sedibus et causis morborum per anatomen indagatis libri quinque*. Venetiis, typog. Remondiniana. Liber I, cap. XV, art. 21.
40. Miller, C. (1826): *Trans. Med.-Chir. Soc. Edinb.*, 2;243–248.
41. Tillaux, P. J. (1877): *Traité d'Anatomie Topographique*, p. 56. Paris (cit. after Thompson).
42. Thompson, St. Clair (1899): *The Cerebrospinal Fluid. Its Spontaneous Escape from the Nose*. Cassell, London.
43. Leber, T. (1883): *v.Graefe's Arch.Ophthalmol.*, 29;273–292.
44. Gutsche, P. (1895): *Laryngoscope*, 11:460.
45. Mermod, G. (1896): *Ann. maladies de l'oreille, du larynx, du nez et du pharynx*, 22:337–344 (cit. after St. Clair Thompson).
46. Cairns, H. (1937): *J. Laryngol. Otol.*, 52:589–623.
47. Cole, I. E., and Keene, M. (1980): Cerebrospinal fluid rhinorrhoea in pituitary tumours. *J. Roy. Soc. Med.*, 73:244–254.
48. Ridley, H. (1695): *Anatomy of the Brain*, p. 83. London.
49. Cowper, W. (1698): In: *The anatomy of human bodies*, Table X. Oxford (?pirated from Govert Bidloo's "Anatomia humani corporis," Amsteladami, 1685).
50. Magendie, F. (1825, 1827): Mémoire sur une liquide qui se trouve dans le crâne et le canal vertébral de l'homme et des animaux mammifères. *J. Physiol. Exp. Pathol.*, 5:27–37. 7:1–29, 66–82.
51. Harris, G. W. (1971): Humours and hormones: The Sir Henry Dale Lecture for 1971. *J. Endocrinol.*, 53:ii–xxiii.
52. Zuckerman, S. (1954): The secretions of the brain: relation of hypothalamus to pituitary gland. *Lancet*, I:739–743. Part 2. *Lancet*, I: 789–795. (The Seventh Addison Memorial Lecture, delivered at Guy's Hospital, London, Dec. 16, 1953).

53. Swedenborg, E. (1882): *The Brain Considered Anatomically, Physiologically and Philosophically*, edited by R. L. Tafel, Vol. 1, London.
54. Lieutaud, J. (1742): *Essais anatomiques*. P. M. Huart, Paris.
55. de Bordeu, T. (1775): VI. Analyse médicinale du sang. In: *Recherches sur les maladies chroniques*. Paris. (1751): *Recherches Anatomiques sur la Position des Glandes et sur leur Action*. G. F. Quillau, père, Paris.
56. Popa, G. T., and Fielding, U. (1930): The vascular link between the pituitary and the hypothalamus. *Lancet*, II:238–240. (1930): A portal circulation from the pituitary to the hypothalamic region. *J. Anat. London*, 65:88–91.
57. Popa, G. T., and Fielding, U. (1933): Hypophysio-portal vessels and their colloid accompaniment. *J. Anat. London*, 67:227.
58. Lothringer, S. (1886): Untersuchungen an der Hypophyse einiger Saeugethiere und des Menschen. *Arch. mikr. Anat.*, 28:257.
59. Henderson, J. R., and Daniel, P. M. (1978): Portal Circulations and their Relation to Countercurrent Systems. *Quart. J. Exp. Physiol.*, 63:355–369.
60. Page, R. B., Munger, B. L., and Bergland, R. M. (1976): Scanning microscopy of pituitary vascular casts. *Am. J. Anat.*, 146:273–302.
61. Oliver, C., Mical, R. S., and Porter, J. C. (1977): Hypothalamic-pituitary vasculature: evidence for retrograde blood flow in the pituitary stalk. *Endocrinology*, 101:598–604.

Historical Aspects of the Neurosciences,
edited by F. Clifford Rose and W. F. Bynum.
Raven Press, New York ©

The Acromegaly of Maximinus I: The Possible Influence of a Pituitary Tumor on the Life and Death of a Roman Emperor

Harold L. Klawans

Department of Neurology, Rush-Presbyterian St. Luke's Medical Center, Chicago, Illinois

For hundreds of years, collectors of Roman coins have been aware of the distinctive, if not peculiar, profile of the Roman Emperor Maximinus I (235–238 C.E.) (Fig. 1). His coin portraiture clearly demonstrates his heavy features, prominent supraorbital ridge and markedly protruding lower jaw (prognathism). These features taken together are highly suggestive if not pathognomonic for a clinical diagnosis of acromegaly. Acromegaly comes from two Greek words: "akron," which means extremity or extreme, and "megale," which means great. This is a descriptive term that has been applied to a clinical disorder characterized by enlargement of the extremities, especially hands and feet, as well as the nose and jaw. Such a diagnosis would not only explain the peculiar facial features of this emperor but may also shed some light upon other aspects of his life.

Maximinus was from one of the semibarbarous tribes of the interior of Thrace (1). He was born in Thrace in about 173 C.E. of an obscure and barbarous family, the son of Micca,

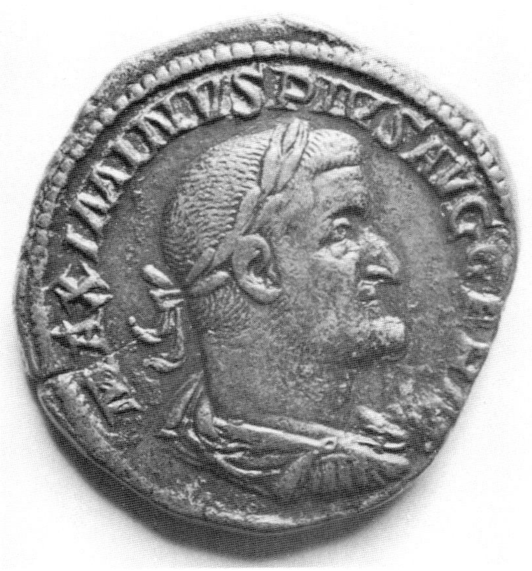

FIG. 1. Sestertius of Maximinus, MAXIMINUS PIVS AVG GERM. AVG: abbr. for Augustus, which was the most distinctive title of the emperor. GERM: abbr. for Germanicus, an honorary title given in reference to victories over German tribes. This title is often also hereditary (23).

a Goth, and of Ababa, an Alanian (2). It is clear that Maximinus was not a Roman citizen by either descent or place of birth. It appears that he must have obtained his citizenship while in the army, perhaps for service in the field under the governor of Dacia. The major features of his military career and his brief term as emperor are well known. He attracted the notice of the Emperor Septimus Severus (Fig. 2) (193–211 C.E.) because of his extraordinary size and strength, and he obtained a military commission. Under the reign of Severus (Table 1) and his son Caracalla (Fig. 3) (211–217 C. E.), Maximinus obtained the rank of centurion "with the favor and esteem of both those princes the former of whom was an excellent judge of merit" (3). Following the murder of Caracalla, Maximinus apparently left the army. Gibbon, basing his conclusions on the *Scriptores Historia Augustae*, explains Maximinus's resignation of his commission in these words (4):

> Gratitude forbade Maximin to serve under the assassin of Caracalla. [This refers to the usurper and subsequent Emperor Macrinus (Fig. 5)]. Honor taught him to decline the effeminate insults of Elagabalus [Fig. 6].

In 222 C.E., under the Emperor Severus Alexander (Fig. 7), he returned to military service.

TABLE 1. *Roman emperors during the career of Maximinus I*

Septimus Severus (Fig. 2)	193–211 C.E.
Caracalla (Fig. 3) Son of Septimus Severus	211–217 C.E.
Geta (Fig. 4) Son of Septimus Severus Murdered by Caracalla	211–212 C.E.
Macrinus (Fig. 5)	217–218 C.E.
Elagabalus (Fig. 6)	218–222 C.E.
Severus Alexander (Fig. 7)	222–235 C.E.
Maximinus (Figs. 1 and 8)	235–238 C.E.

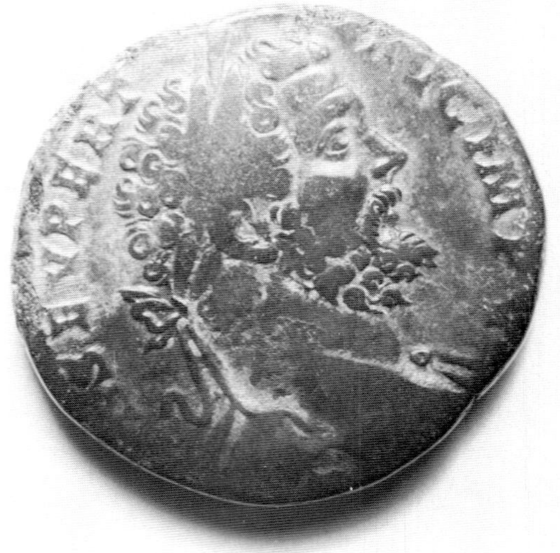

FIG. 2. Sestertius of Septimus Severus. SEV PERT AVG IMP V. SEV: abbr. for Severus. PERT: abbr. for Pertinax, predecessor of Septimus Severus as emperor. IMP: abbr. for Imperator, a title of acclamation for victories of the emperor or his subordinates.

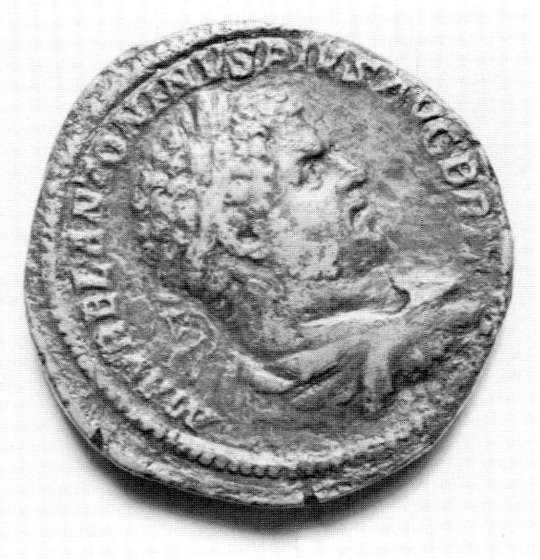

FIG. 3. Sestertius of Caracalla. M AVREL ANTONINUS PIUS AVG GERM.

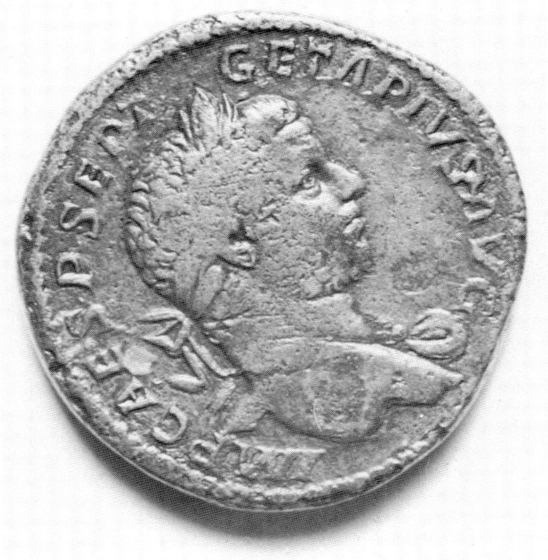

FIG. 4. Sestertius of Geta. IMP CAES P SEPT GETA PIUS AVG. CAES: abbr. for Caesar, until adopted by all emperors and given to heirs to the throne.

"On the accession of Alexander he returned to court, and was placed by that prince in a station useful to the service and honourable to himself. The fourth legion, to which he was appointed tribune, soon became, under his care, the best disciplined of the whole army. With the general applause of the soldiers, who bestowed on their favourite hero the names of Ajax and Hercules, he was successively promoted to the first military command, and had not he still retained too much of his savage origin, the emperor might perhaps have given his own sister to the son of Maximin" (5).

The reign of Severus Alexander lasted only 13 years (222–235 C.E.). This effeminate Syrian youth, who was under the thumbnail of his strong-willed mother, Julia Mamaea, became increasingly unpopular with the army, and in 235 C.E. the popular and well-loved

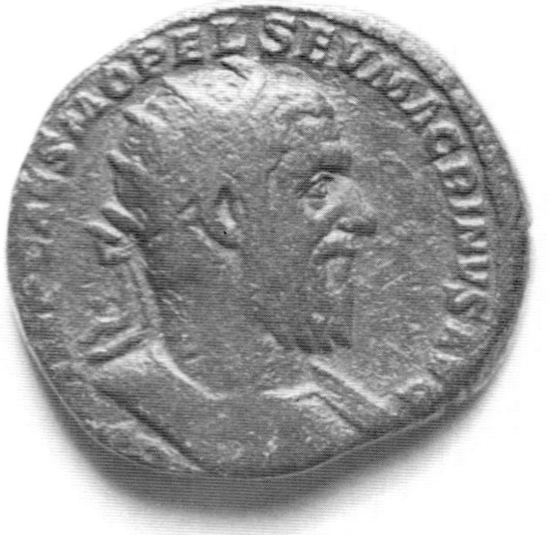

FIG. 5. Sestertius of Macrinus. IMP CAES M OPEL SEV MACRINUS AVG.

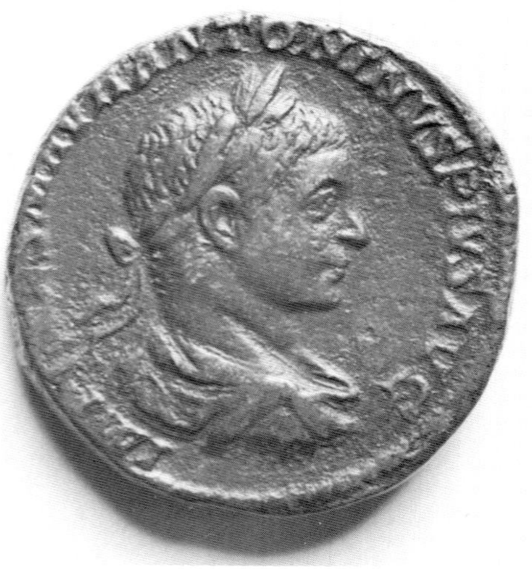

FIG. 6. Sestertius of Elagabalus. IMP CAES M AVG ANTONINUS PIUS AVG.

Maximinus was proclaimed emperor by the army and Severus Alexander was killed. Writing 1,500 years after the fact, Gibbon attributes a major role to Maximinus in engineering the entire coup and attributes a variety of motives to him including avarice and ambition (6):

> Instead of securing his fidelity, these favours served only to inflame the ambition of the Thracian peasant, who deemed his fortune inadequate to his merit, as long as he was constrained to acknowledge a superior. Though a stranger to real wisdom, he was not devoid of a selfish cunning, which showed him that the emperor had lost the affection of the army, and taught him to improve their discontent to his own advantage. It is easy for faction and calumny to shed their poison on the administration of the best of princes, and to accuse even their virtues, by artfully confounding them with those vices to which they bear the nearest affinity. The troops listened with pleasure to the emissaries of Maximin. They blushed at their ignominious patience, which, during thirteen years, had supported the vexatious discipline imposed by an effeminate Syrian, the timid slave of his mother and of the senate. It was time, they cried, to cast away that useless phantom of the civil power, and to elect for their prince and general a real soldier, educated in camps, exercised in war, who would assert the glory, and distribute among his companions the treasures, of the empire. A great army was at that time assembled on the banks of the Rhine, under the command of the

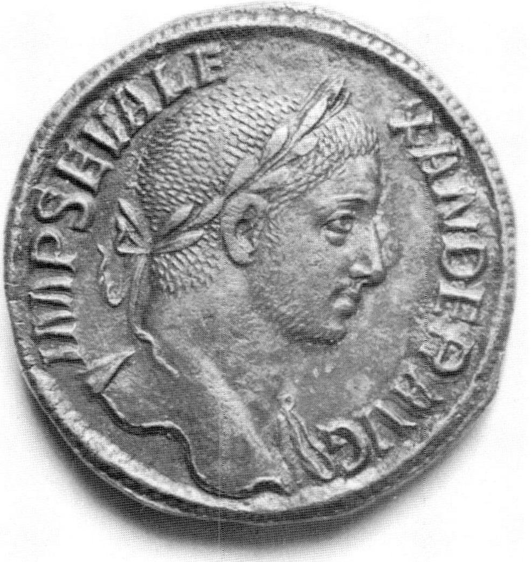

FIG. 7. Sestertius of Severus Alexander. IMP SEV ALEXANDER AVG.

> emperor himself, who, almost immediately after his return from the Persian war, had been obliged to march against the barbarians of Germany. The important care of training and reviewing the new levies was intrusted to Maximin. One day (A.D. 235, March 19), as he entered the field of exercise, the troops, either from a sudden impulse or a formed conspiracy, saluted him emperor, silenced by their loud acclamations his obstinate refusal, and hastened to consummate their rebellion by the murder of Alexander Severus.

Within three years, the once popular hero was considered to be a tyrant comparable to Caligula or Nero whose cruelty was exceeded only by his suspicious nature. Gibbon accused this once honorable man of murdering many of his benefactors and as a result leaving in characters of blood an indelible history of his baseness and ingratitude (7):

> The dark and sanguinary soul of the tyrant was open to every suspicion against those among his subjects who were the most distinguished by their birth or merit. Whenever he was alarmed with the sound of treason, his cruelty was unbounded and unrelenting. A conspiracy against his life was either discovered or imagined, and Magnus, a consular senator, was named as the principal author of it. Without a witness, without a trial, and without an opportunity of defence, Magnus with four thousand of his supposed accomplices, was put to death. Italy and the whole empire were infested with innumerable spies and informers. On the slightest accusation, the first of the Roman nobles who had governed provinces, commanded armies, and been adorned with the consular and triumphal ornaments, were chained on the public carriages, and hurried away to the emperor's presence. Confiscation, exile, or simple death, were esteemed uncommon instances of his lenity. Some of the unfortunate sufferers he ordered to be sewed up in the hides of slaughtered animals, others to be exposed to wild beasts, others again to be beaten to death with clubs. During the three years of his reign, he disdained to visit either Rome or Italy. His camp, occasionally removed from the banks of the Rhine to those of the Danube, was the seat of his stern despotism, which trampled on every principle of law and justice, and was supported by the avowed power of the sword. No man of noble birth, elegant accomplishments, or knowledge of civil business, was suffered near his person; and the court of a Roman emperor revived the idea of those ancient chiefs of slaves and gladiators, whose savage power had left a deep impression of terror and detestation.

In the end Maximinus (Fig. 8) and his son and heir Maximus (Fig. 9) were killed by the army.

The distinctive features of the life of Maximinus include the following:

1. Prodigious size and strength.
2. Honor, gratitude, and personal loyalty, and the ability to stimulate the love and loyalty of the army.
3. Unbridled ambition, cruelty, and paranoid behavior, which incurred the hatred and disloyalty of the same troops who only a few years earlier had proclaimed him emperor. There appears to be no apparent way to explain this personality change other than to attribute Maximinus with such motives as unbridled ambitions or contempt.

It is quite likely that a progressive medical condition, a hormonally active pituitary tumor, could in part account for all three of these characteristics and especially help to understand the abrupt change in his behavior.

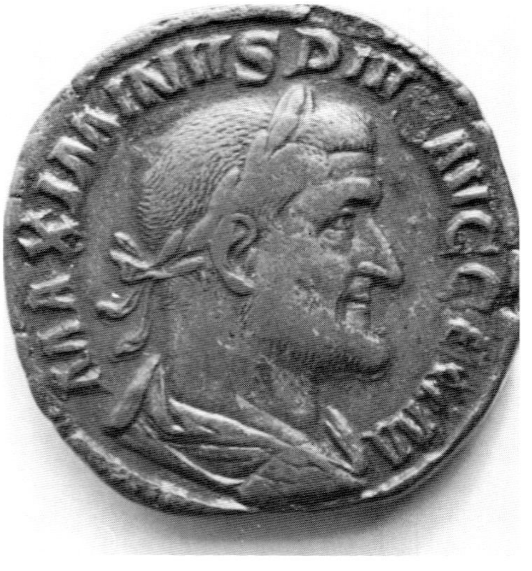

FIG. 8. Sestertius of Maximinus. MAXIMINUS PIUS AVG GERM.

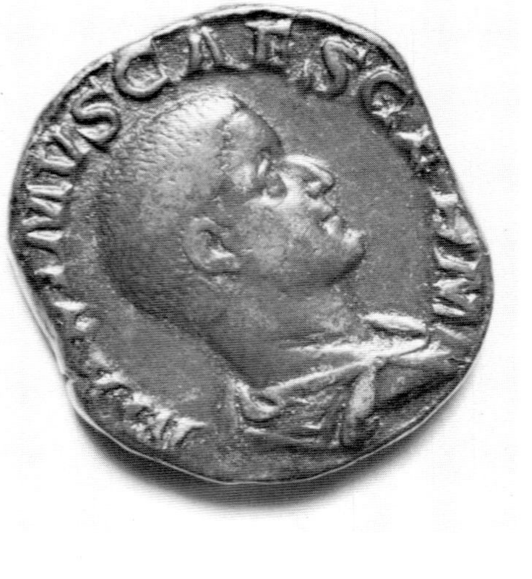

FIG. 9. Sestertius of Maximus. MAXIMUS CAES GERM.

Excessive production of growth hormone is of course usually caused by a small tumor of the pituitary and results in extraordinary overgrowth of bone and of the connective tissue of the skin and subcutaneous tissues. If the disease sets in before the age at which the growth centers of the long bones of the arms and legs have become joined, the bones grow enormously in all their dimensions, and the result is gigantism. But if the disorder begins after these centers have united, the overgrowth is confined to their ends, producing acromegaly. If the tumor begins before closure and continues active production afterward, the patient manifests both gigantism and acromegaly. Maximinus appears to have manifested both aspects.

Historical sources all agree that Maximinus was a giant, with reports of his height varying from 7′2″ to 8′6″ (8,9). As late as 1961, when the average height was certainly greater than it was in the second and third centuries, it was generally taught that among Caucasians, body height in excess of 7 feet was almost always indicative of a pituitary tumor secreting growth hormone (10). This must also have been true 1,700 years ago.

The reports of Maximinus's height are accompanied by tales of his extraordinary if not prodigious strength. Whereas acromegaly is usually associated with weakness, numerous patients have been described who were unusually strong early in the course of the disease and later gradually became weaker (11). Pierre Marie, the great 19th-century French neurologist, who first described acromegaly himself, reported one such patient (12).

It is important to note then that Maximinus is reported to have had exceptional strength, but the descriptions of this come from the period prior to his resignation from the army (217 C.E.) and mostly have to do with his initial meeting with Septimus Severus around the year 206 C.E. Gibbon retells these stories as follows (13):

> The Emperor Severus, returning from an eastern expedition, halted in Thrace, to celebrate, with military games, the birthday of his younger son, Geta [Fig. 4]. The country flocked in crowds to behold their sovereign, and a young barbarian of gigantic stature earnestly solicited, in his rude dialect, that he might be allowed to contend for the prize of wrestling. As the pride of discipline would have been disgraced in the overthrow of a Roman soldier by a Thracian peasant, he was matched with the stoutest followers of the camp, sixteen of whom he successively laid on the ground. His victory was rewarded by some trifling gifts, and a permission to enlist in the troops. The next day, the happy barbarian was distinguished above a crowd of recruits, dancing and exulting after the fashion of his country. As soon as he perceived that he had attracted the emperor's notice, he instantly ran up to his horse, and followed on foot, without the least appearance of fatigue, in a long and rapid career. "Thracian," said Severus, with astonishment, "art thou disposed to wrestle after thy race?" "Most willingly, Sir," replied the unwearied youth, and, almost in a breath, overthrew seven of the strongest soldiers in the army. A gold collar was the prize of his matchless vigour and activity, and he was immediately appointed to serve in the Horse-guards who always attended on the person of the sovereign.

There are no reports in Herodian of extraordinary physical activity when he resumed his career under Severus Alexander (222 C.E.). All reports after this date deal with his administrative ability.

The manifestations of acromegaly are very characteristic. There is a progressive enlargement of the bones and soft parts, most marked in the hands and feet, resulting, for instance, in broad, thick "ginger-bread hands." In this regard, it is particularly interesting to note that Maximinus's thumb is reported in the *Scriptores Historia Augustae* to be so thick that he used his wife's bracelet for a ring (14). Such extreme thickness of the fingers and thumb is characteristic of acromegaly. Acromegaly also has characteristic effects on the skull and face. The skull becomes enlarged and thickened, and all its bony ridges are exaggerated; the margins of the orbits, including the supraorbital ridge, the cheekbones, the external occipital protuberance, and most striking of all, the lower jaw, become enlarged. The mandible begins to jut out significantly, resulting in prognathism.

The facial features seen from the coin portraiture of Maximinus (see Figs. 1 and 8) demonstrate most of these features including: (a) marked prognathism, (b) marked supraorbital ridges, and (c) overall gross features. It is of interest in regard to his personal features that he was often compared to Ajax, Achilles, and Hercules, but never to Adonis (15). Herodian succinctly describes Maximinus as "a man of frightening appearance and colossal size" (16), a portrait that is consistent with combined gigantism and acromegaly.

According to the *Scriptores Historia Augustae*, in a single day, Maximinus could drink an amphora (about seven gallons) of wine and eat 30 or 40 pounds of meat (17). The degree of thirst (polydipsia) and hunger (polyphagia), while undoubtedly exaggerated by this anonymous but "wretched biographer," are far beyond the appetites attributed to other ancient heroes of noted strength and size. Polydipsia and polyphagia are of course two of the three cardinal symptoms of diabetes mellitus. The third is polyuria (excessive urination), which must be present in anyone who consumes anywhere near seven gallons of fluid per day. Approximately 20% to 40% of acromegalics develop diabetes mellitus due to one of two factors: (a) blockade of the action of insulin in the various tissues of the body, and (b) exhaustion of those cells in the pancreas that manufacture insulin.

It is quite possible and consistent that the increased consumption of both food and liquid that are attributed to Maximinus could be the result of acromegaly-induced diabetes mellitus. The coin portraiture again is of some help here since Maximinus's prodigious intake of food is clearly not associated with any evidence of obesity. This is of course most consistent with acromegaly-induced diabetes, in which increased appetite and food consumption result in no weight gain.

So far the only aspects of the life of Maximinus that have been attributed to his pituitary tumor are those which are a direct result of the growth hormone produced by the tumor. Such tumors can produce symptoms by a second mechanism. The progressive slow growth of these tumors can cause pressure on neighboring structures including the base of the brain, and especially the hypothalamus, which lies directly over the pituitary. It is quite possible that extension of the tumor to involve the hypothalamus could make certain aspects of Maximinus's career more understandable.

It is hard to understand how this beloved, happy, and honorable man, whose gratitude and loyalty forced him to resign from the army in 217 C.E. and who under Severus Alexander discharged his trust extremely conscientiously, earning great popularity among the troops (18), could a few years later be an ingrate with unbridled ambition. It is hard to imagine such a degree of ambition in a man who gave up his career out of a sense of loyalty and honor.

Whether or not he staged the rebellion, the troops were clearly pleased to proclaim this popular leader emperor. The army loved Maximinus despite the fact that his legion had become the best disciplined of the whole army. Armies rarely love disciplinarians unless they are fair. Three years later, he was slain in his tent on orders of the Senate by a party of Praetorian Guards. This murder was the culmination of a three-year period of cruel rages, paranoid behavior, and severe tyranny (19):

> Such was the deserved fate of a brutal savage, destitute, as he has generally been represented, of every sentiment that distinguishes a civilised, or even a human being. The body was suited to the soul. The stature of Maximin exceeded the measure of eight feet, and circumstances almost incredible are related of his matchless strength and appetite. Had he lived in a less enlightened age, tradition and poetry might well have described him as one

> of those monstrous giants, whose supernatural power constantly exerted for the destruction of mankind. It is easier to conceive than describe the universal joy of the Roman world on the fall of the tyrant.

This transition is hard to understand on purely psychiatric grounds, but such a change in behavior has been described in patients with tumors involving the hypothalamus (20). Such patients who manifest increased emotional excitability, which even builds up to severe rage attacks and aggressive behavior precipitated by paranoid ideas, have been described as having a characteristic sign of tumors involving the hypothalamus.

These patients may react to insignificant events with states of excitement and associated indiscriminant attacks against everyone who happens to be present. Some of these patients described their condition as "a feeling [as] if their rage would build up in spite of themselves until it had conquered their thoughts and left them no choice but to let it freely run its course" (21). Other patients appear to await tensely the first opportunity to release their accumulated aggressiveness.

It is easy to speculate that the pituitary tumor began to expand out of Maximinus's sella turcica and slowly impinge upon his hypothalamus and that this accounted for the vicious paranoid behavior which marked him as a tyrant and resulted in his final destruction.

Absolute diagnosis of course requires an examination of the skeletal remains of Maximinus. This will never be possible as there is no chance that his body will ever be found. After he and his son were murdered, "their bodies were thrown out for anyone to desecrate and trample on before being left to be torn to pieces by dogs and birds." The heads of Maximinus and his son were sent to Rome (22) and were further desecrated before being thrown into the Tiber. The fact that his skull is thus lost forever makes it impossible to hope for pathologic proof of the hypothesis that Maximinus represented the first proven instance of acromegaly.

NOTES AND ACKNOWLEDGMENTS

All coins illustrated here are from the collection of the author. Photography was done by Harlan J. Berk, Ltd. Rendering of coin inscription was done according to Zander Klawans (23). This work was carried out in my spare time and was not supported by a grant from anyone. The author wishes to thank Zander Klawans for his encouragement.

REFERENCES

1. Herodian (1970): *History*, translated by C. R. Whittaker, Vol. II. p. 131. Harvard Univ. Press, Cambridge, Mass.
2. (1967): *Scriptores Historiae Augustae*, translated by D. Magie, Vol. II, p. 317. Harvard Univ. Press, Cambridge, Mass.
3. Gibbon, E.: *The Decline and Fall of the Roman Empire*, Vol. I, p. 147. Random House, New York.
4. Gibbon, E.: *The Decline and Fall of the Roman Empire*, Vol. I, p. 147. Random House, New York.
5. Gibbon, E.: *The Decline and Fall of the Roman Empire*, Vol. I, p. 148. Random House, New York.
6. Gibbon, E.: *The Decline and Fall of the Roman Empire*, Vol. I, p. 148. Random House, New York.
7. Gibbon, E.: *The Decline and Fall of the Roman Empire*, Vol. I, p. 150. Random House, New York.
8. Herodian (1970): *History*, translated by C. R. Whittaker, Vol. II, p. 133. Harvard Univ. Press, Cambridge, Mass.
9. (1967): *Scriptores Historiae Augustae*, translated by D. Magie, Vol. II, p. 327. Harvard Univ. Press, Cambridge, Mass.
10. Danowski, T. S. (1962): Acromegaly and giantism. *Clin. Endocrinol.*, I:99.
11. Pickett, J. B. E., Layzer, R. B., Levin, S. R., Schneider, V., Campbell, M. J., and Sumner, A. J. (1975): *Neurology*, 25:638.
12. Marie, P. (1888–1890): *Brain*, 12:51.
13. Gibbon, E.: *The Decline and Fall of the Roman Empire*, Vol. I, p. 147. Random House, New York.

14. (1967): *Scriptores Historiae Augustae*, translated by D. Magie, Vol. II, p. 327. Harvard Univ. Press, Cambridge, Mass.
15. (1967): *Scriptores Historiae Augustae*, translated by D. Magie, Vol. II, p. 323. Harvard Univ. Press, Cambridge, Mass.
16. Herodian (1970): *History*, translated by C. R. Whittaker, Vol. II, p. 159. Harvard Univ. Press, Cambridge, Mass.
17. (1967): *Scriptores Historiae Augustae*, translated by D. Magie, Vol. II, p. 332. Harvard Univ. Press, Cambridge, Mass.
18. Herodian (1970): *History*, translated by C. R. Whittaker, Vol. II, p. 135. Harvard Univ. Press, Cambridge, Mass.
19. Gibbon, E.: *The Decline and Fall of the Roman Empire*, Vol. I, p. 161. Random House, New York.
20. Poek, H. (1968): Disorders of emotion. In: *Handbook of Clinical Neurology*, edited by P. J. Vinken and G. W. Bruyn, Vol. 2, pp. 343–365.
21. Lechner, H. (1959): *Wien Z. Nervenheilk*, 16:281.
22. Herodian (1970): *History*, translated by C. R. Whittaker, Vol. II, p. 285. Harvard Univ. Press, Cambridge, Mass.
23. Klawans, Z. H. (1977): *Reading and Dating Roman Imperial Coins*. Western Publishing Co., Racine, Wisconsin.

Historical Aspects of the Neurosciences,
edited by F. Clifford Rose and W.F. Bynum.
Raven Press, New York ©

Thomas Willis and the Foundations of British Neurology

Kenneth Dewhurst

Department of Psychiatry, University of the West Indies, Kingston, Jamaica

Thomas Willis was fortunate in his medical training. It was brief. His Oxford medical course could not have exceeded six months and was probably less; hence his bachelor of medicine degree should be regarded as a belated military honor, somewhat equivalent to a military cross, rather than an academic achievement. But the brevity and informality of his training allowed him to range more widely in his reading and contributed to his awareness of the great ferment of ideas in Commonwealth Oxford stimulated by the application of Baconian philosophy.

When the Civil War broke out in August 1642, Willis, having just taken his M. A. degree after over four years at Christ Church, was on vacation two miles away at his father's North Hinksey farm. As an ardent Royalist, he remained there to avoid conscription during the brief Parliamentary occupation. But in the spring of 1643, a combination of lack of hygiene, overcrowding, and constant troop movements caused a severe outbreak of typhus that wrought havoc in both armies and spread to the neighboring villages. One of the victims was Thomas Willis's father, who left his eldest son, a 21-year-old orphan, with the responsibility of managing a farm and supervising the education of his younger siblings (1). During the year that Thomas Willis farmed at North Hinksey, the Royalist fortunes gradually declined, but the reverse that most affected him was the occupation by Parliamentary forces of Abingdon. It was a useful base for raiding parties plundering livestock from neighboring farms, including those in the Hinksey villages. Though only two miles from Oxford, these villages, being separated from the main Royalist forces by the Thames, were difficult to defend. Willis's future brother-in-law, John Fell, confirms that it was the constant threat of raids on his farm that caused him to enlist "as a Souldier in the University Legion [where] he received Pay for some years until the cause of the Best Prince being overcome Cromwell's Tyranny afforded to this wretched Nation a Peace more cruel than any War" (2).

Undoubtedly, Willis joined one of the two auxiliary regiments formed in response to the Royal Proclamation of 1644 calling for volunteers to defend Oxford so that regular soldiers could be released for field service. It is highly likely that Willis joined the regiment recruited from members of the university commanded by the Earl of Dover. Throughout his two years of army service, Thomas Willis most probably remained with Dover's regiment in the sector near Magdalen College Grove in St. Clement's parish, defending an approach to the city that, for much of his service, came within artillery fire from a Parliamentary outpost on Headington Hill. Although we have no precise details of his military service, some likely conjectures might be made. Willis doubtlessly endured the usual hardships of military life: hunger, fear, dirt, discomfort, and boredom (3). As a tranquilizer, and to allay his hunger, he smoked a clay pipe like many of his comrades: "The use of Tobacco is not only good, but almost necessary for Souldiers or Seamen," wrote Willis (4), "where it agrees with them, in as much as it makes them both undaunted in all dangers, and able to endure hunger, cold and labour." But army life would be enlivened by the close comradeship of other scholar-soldiers, and during his service, Willis probably became better acquainted with another Christ Church graduate, John Fell, son of the Dean, who became his brother-in-law. It is known that Fell reached the rank of ensign, and Willis, having graduated a year earlier, may have reached the same rank. This couplet in his writings may have been an allusion to his army rank as it was obviously not intended to be a contribution to poetry (5):

Where Ensigns Ensigns meet
And where with Arms they one another Treat.

After the surrender of Oxford on June 26, 1646, Willis, like other Royalist soldiers, was ordered to leave the city. But when he returned there at the beginning of Michaelmas term, few changes were apparent. Under the inflexible leadership of Samuel Fell, the Vice Chancellor, Oxford was still essentially Royalist, as dons saw no justification for changing their political allegiance simply because their army had been defeated in the field. They argued, too, that it would be unconstitutional to alter university regulations without Royal assent (6). Among the most ardent university Royalists was Dr. Thomas Clayton, still Regius Professor of Physic and, in his other role as Master of Pembroke College, he had been their foremost recruiting agent. Clayton had acquired his own chair by sex-linked inheritance as, one year after "accumulating" the degrees of bachelor and doctor of medicine, he succeeded his father-in-law and began exercising the familial trait of nepotism (7). In 1642, for example, Clayton awarded a bachelor of medicine degree to his younger son six months after taking his M. A. (8), and he arranged for his elder son to succeed him as Tomlins Reader in Anatomy, although he was clearly unsuited for the post, "being possess'd with a timorous and effeminate Humour [he] could never endure the sight of a mangled or bloody body" (9). On Willis's return to Oxford, Clayton probably regarded his two years of soldiering as equivalent to "keeping terms," and in this likely event, his service would be more favorably regarded than either diligent dissertations or erudite disputation. At all events, Willis graduated and was licensed to practice on December 8, 1646 (10), having made a brief "literary" (11), rather than practical, study of medicine.

As early as 1648, Willis was referred to as "our chymist" by a Trinity College group of natural philosophers (12), and two years later, he was participating with another subgroup of eight members who shared the expense of running a laboratory at Wadham College (13). It was here that Willis analyzed vegetable, animal, and mineral bodies, including blood and urine: He prepared chemical remedies and made a special study of combustion. His research culminated in the publication of his first book, *Diatribae duae Medico-Philosophicae* (1659), wherein he set forth his chemical theory of matter consisting, he believed, of five principles. These included varying amounts of three active ones of spirit, sulphur and salt and two inert ones of water and earth, whose role was to fill in the spaces between the active principles. Whenever it suited his purpose, Willis used these five chemical principles as a substitute for the four humors, although he never completely discarded humoral pathology. He also discussed the process of fermentation in minerals, plants, and the human body. Willis regarded a fever as a form of fermentation in the blood and went on to compare the physician's role to that of the vintner as blood and humors, like wine, must be nurtured and fermented under the appropriate conditions. Thus, Willis brought together a mixture of iatrochemistry, Baconian empiricism within a setting of humoral pathology, and Harveian circulatory physiology. He often argued by using agricultural and culinary analogies based on his own observations and experience, best described as a rough and ready farmhouse empiricism. He discussed physiological, chemical, and pathological processes in terms of baking and brewing, the making of wine, cider, vinegar, mead, cheese, butter, and various broths all redolent of the brewhouse, kitchen, dairy, orchards, and stables of his North Hinksey farm.

Thirty-eight years old when his first book was published, Willis, who had married Mary Fell two years earlier, was living piously and industriously at his Beam Hall residence (Fig. 1). He had had a struggle to establish himself in Commonwealth Oxford and, as was then customary, visited the neighboring market towns in search of patients. To get there, he shared a horse with another young, struggling practitioner. Willis had several disadvantages to overcome before he could establish a successful practice: He could ill afford to mount an impressive display, and he had been on the losing side in the recent war. His appearance was unimpressive, and his stammering diffidence was unlikely to inspire confidence. John Aubrey (14) laconically described him as being of "middle stature: dark red haire (like a red pig); stammered much"; and Anthony Wood depicted him as "a plain Man, a Man of no Carriage, little Discourse, Complaisance or society" (15). Hence, while his practice was small and undemanding, Willis tended to devote much of his spare time to iatrochemistry in the company of the Oxford *virtuosi*.

At this relatively late stage in his career, there is no evidence of his interest in neurology or brain anatomy. What brought about a change in his interests? Several contributory factors may be traced. First, among the several groups of the *virtuosi* were those around William Petty (1623–1687), who had studied medicine at Leyden and Paris before succeeding Clayton as Tomlins Reader in Anatomy. He soon revolutionized the teaching of anatomy in his public lecture-demonstrations, and privately at his lodgings, where he was also interested

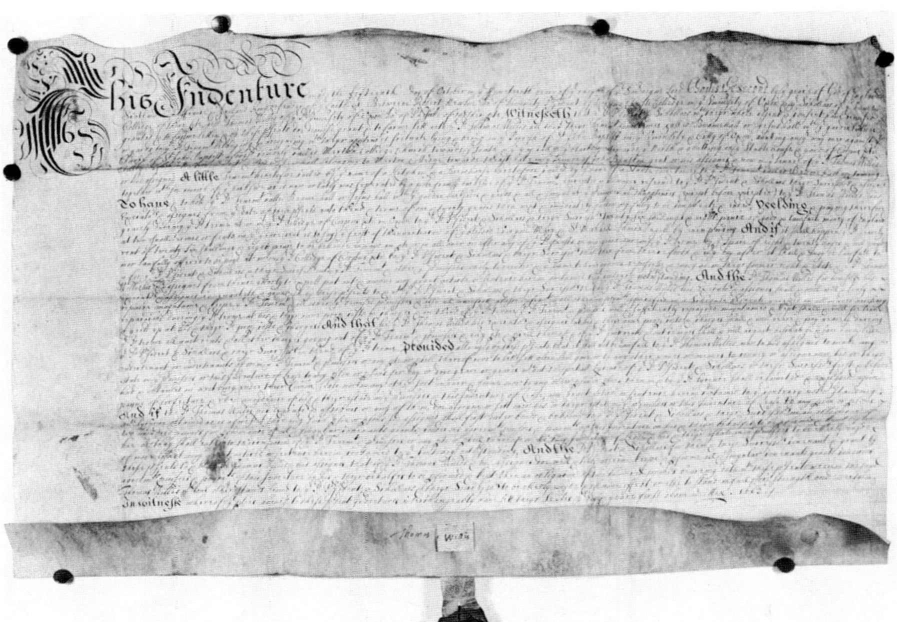

FIG. 1. The indenture for the lease of Beam Hall, Thomas Willis's Oxford residence. (By courtesy of the Archivist, Corpus Christi College, Oxford.)

in chemistry and the preparation of medicines (16). This group of natural philosophers, including Willis and Richard Lower (1631–1691), met regularly at Petty's High Street lodgings, where the biological sciences were emphasized, whereas at Wadham, there was a more mathematical or astronomical bias. The significance of Petty's circle of natural philosophers was that here Willis's interest in anatomy, and in performing necropsies, was first stimulated, and after Petty's departure for Ireland, he took over the leadership of the remnants of this group.

Another reason for Willis's interest in neurology was the fact that within four years, Oxford had been visited by several fevers with neurological manifestations. Willis was able to include accounts of three of these epidemics in his first book, acclaimed by Creighton (17) as "the first systematic piece of epidemiology written in English." In the summer of 1657, there was an epidemic of what Willis described as the "new" fever, which was probably a virus infection with gastric and encephalitic symptoms. In April 1658, there was a widespread outbreak of influenza, and in August, a third epidemic of meningococcal meningitis (18) lasted six weeks and claimed many victims, some of whom Willis examined at necropsy. Finally, in 1661, there was an outbreak of encephalitis lethargica (19), and Willis was able to study the brains of some victims, although most recovered after a prolonged convalescence. Since qualification, Willis had sought every opportunity of performing necropsies, and he soon realized that the brain was inaccurately described in the current textbooks, whose illustrations often depicted the brains of animals on the assumption that they resembled the human brain.

The most important reason for Willis's change of interest to neurology was the advent of the Restoration as that "wonderfull pacifick year" of 1660 favored Willis and other orthodox Anglican Royalists. His brother-in-law John Fell became successively a doctor of divinity, Canon and Dean of Christ Church, chaplain to Charles II, Vice Chancellor and Bishop of Oxford. On August 8, 1660, Willis was appointed Sedleian Professor of Natural Philosophy (20), and on October 30, "created" doctor of medicine (21) on the recommendation of Charles II, so that his higher medical degree may be regarded as equivalent to a distinguished service order, as is clear from the entry in the convocation register (Fig. 2). Officially, Willis owed his appointment to three electors: the Vice Chancellor, the President of Magdalen College, and the Warden of All Souls "or any two of them" (22), but in fact, he was appointed by Gilbert Sheldon (1598–1677) who, after his reinstatement as Warden of All Souls in 1659, wielded considerable influence on university affairs as, successively, Dean of the Chapels Royal, Bishop of London, and Archbishop of Canterbury. Willis acknowledged his gratitude to Sheldon in the dedication of *Cerebri Anatome* (23): "It was by your means (most Noble Prelate) that I obtained the Votes in this Famous University for the place of Sidley Professor for how small soever my Merits might seem, they were helped by the greatest and weight of your opinion." When Willis became the fourth Sedleian Professor, he succeeded to a post in which earlier incumbants had experienced rather disturbing tenures: Two had been ejected, one imprisoned, and another charged with embezzlement. His predecessor Joshua Cross had not only been expelled and charged with embezzlement, but even his very existence had been ignored, as the Vice Chancellor's register records that Willis succeeded Cross's Royalist predecessor John Edwards (24) (see Fig. 3).

It should be emphasized that Willis's appointment was not a medical one but was concerned with propagating the Aristotelian tradition. The statutes confirm that he was expected to lecture on "Aristotle's Physics, or the books concerning the heavens or the world or concerning meteoric books or the Small Natural Phenomena of the same author, or the books which treat of the soul, and also those on generation and corruption; and he is to give these

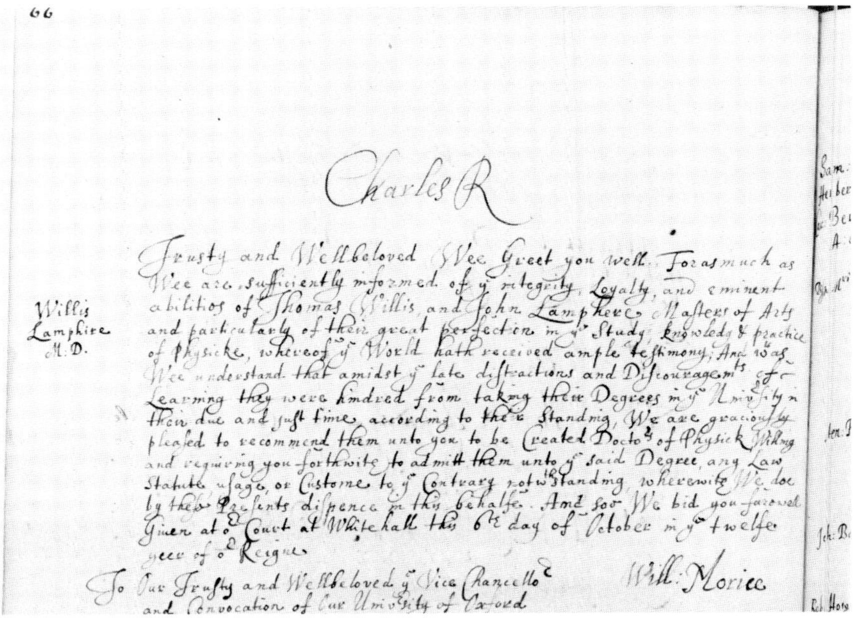

66

Charles R

Willis
Lamphire
M.D.

Trusty and Welbeloved Wee Greet you well. Forasmuch as Wee are sufficiently informed of ye integrity, Loyalty, and eminent abilities of Thomas Willis and John Lamphere Masters of Arts and particularly of their great perfection in ye Study knowledg & practice of Physicke, whereof ye World hath received ample testimony; And was Wee understand that amidst ye late distractions and Discouragemts of Learning they were hindred from taking their Degrees in ye University in their due and just time, according to their Standing, Wee are graciously pleased to recommend them unto you to be Created Doctors of Physick Willing and requiring you forthwith to admitt them unto ye said Degree, any Law Statute usage, or Custome to ye Contrary notwithstanding wherewith We doe by these Presents dispence in this behalfe. And soe We bid you farewell. Given at or Court at Whitehall this 6th day of October in ye twelfe yeer of or Reigne.

To Our Trusty and Welbeloved ye Vice Chancellor and Convocation of Our University of Oxford

Will: Morice

O.U.Arch. Conv. 1659-71. f. 66

FIG. 2. Entry in the convocation register, Oxford University, recording the award of the degree of doctor of medicine to Thomas Willis. (By courtesy of the Keeper of the University Archives.)

lectures twice every week in full term, that is, on Wednesdays and Saturdays, at eight o'clock in the morning. His audience is to be composed of the bachelors of arts, who are also to be the auditors in astronomy. The lecturer's fine, in the case of omitting to lecture, is to be ten shillings: that of a hearer who absents himself fourpence" (25). But neither the outdated university statutes nor the resurgence of Aristotelianism deterred him from defining his professional duties with more latitude. ". . . I should Comment on the Offices of the Senses, both external and also internal," he wrote, "and of the Faculties and Affections of the Soul, as also of the Organs and various provisions of all these" (26). It has been overlooked that Willis's university appointment, requiring him to lecture, stimulated the research that culminated in his greatest achievement, the publication of *Cerebri Anatome* (1664). In the earliest lectures, which have come down to us in Richard Lower's manuscripts (27) and John Locke's notebook (28), Willis mentioned that he had reiterated the "Rational Arguments" and "some not unlikely Hypotheses" of the Aristotelian formalists, but he soon realized that they were too speculative, and when "the force of Invention" was spent, he critically reexamined their observational and experimental foundations. He then compared his early lectures to the efforts of a painter who "delineated the Head of a Man, not after the form of a Master, but at the will of a bold Fancy and Pencil." And Willis concluded that he had been following "not that which is most true, but what was most convenient, and what was rather desired than what was known." As these early lectures had been based on the "received Opinions of others," he began devoting himself "wholly to the study of Anatomy," particularly "the offices and uses of the Brain and its nervous Appendix" (29). Henceforth, Willis sought every opportunity of "opening of Heads" in order to establish "a more certain Physiologie than that I had gained in the Schools on which a Pathologie of the Brain and nervous stock might be built" (30). These then were the reasons for Willis's interest in neurology: his association with Petty, his study of fevers with neurological se-

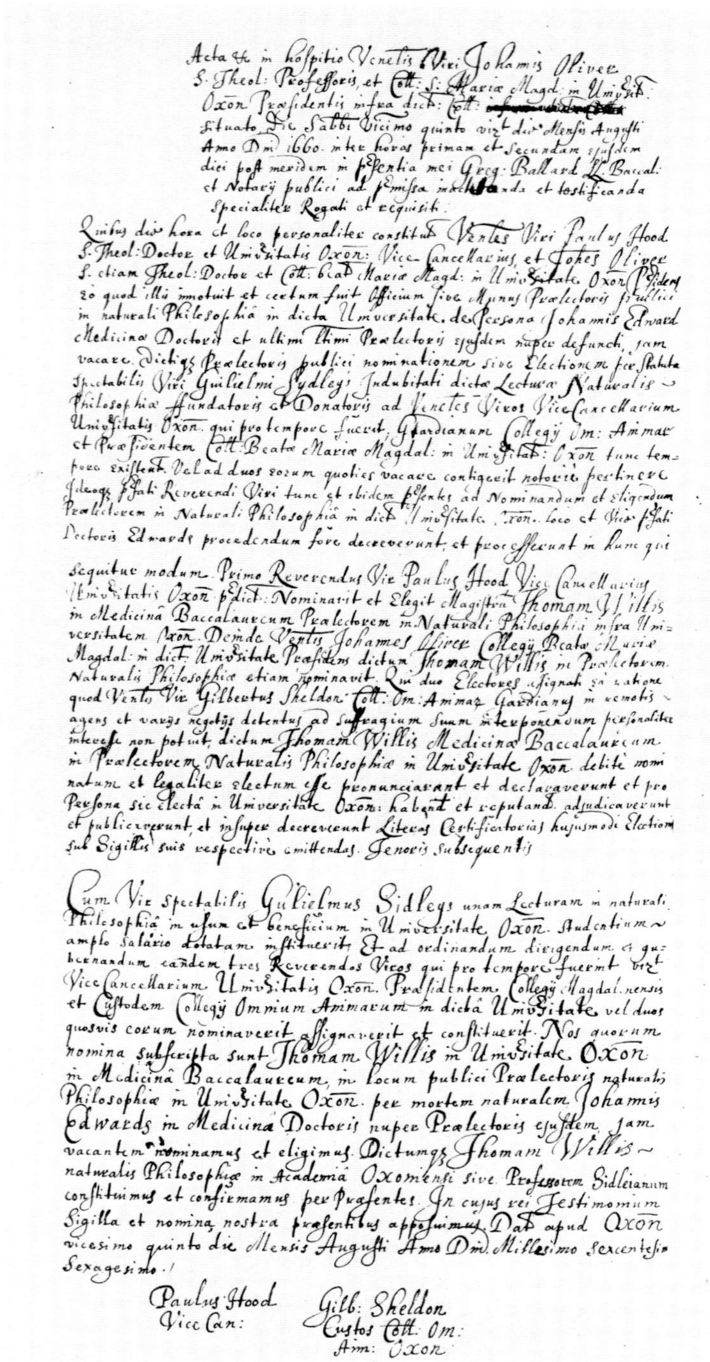

Acta &c in hospitio Venetis Viri Johannis Oliver S. Theol: Professoris, et Coll: S. Mariæ Magd. in Univsit. Oxon Præsidentis infra dict: Coll: situato, Die Sabbi Vicimo quinto vizt dict Mensis Augusti Anno Dni 1660. inter horas primam et secundam ejusdem diei post meridiem in psentia mei Greg: Ballard LL Baccal: et Notarij publici ad pmissa [illegible] et testificanda specialiter Rogati et requisiti.

Quibus die hora et loco personaliter constitut Ventes Viri Paulus Hood S. Theol: Doctor et Universitatis Oxon: Vice-Cancellarius, et Johes Oliver S. etiam Theol: Doctor et Coll: beat Mariæ Magd: in Univsitate Oxon Psident eo quod illis innotuit et certum fuit Officium sive Munus Prælectoris publici in naturali Philosophia in dicta Universitate, de persona Johannis Edward Medicinæ Doctoris et ultimi Ultimi Prælectoris ejusdem nuper defuncti, jam vacare, dictiq Prælectoris publici nominationem sive Electionem per statuta spectabilis Viri Guilielmi Sydley Indubitati dictæ Lecturæ Naturalis Philosophiæ Fundatoris et Donatoris ad Venetes Viros Vice-Cancellarium Univsitatis Oxon: qui pro tempore fuerit, Gardianum Collegij Om: Animar et Præsidentem Coll: Beatæ Mariæ Magdal: in Univsitat: Oxon tunc tempore existent. Vel ad duos eorum quoties vacare contigerit notorie pertinere Ideoqz pfati Reverendi Viri tunc et ibidem psentes ad Nominandum et Eligendum Prælectorem in Naturali Philosophia in dict Univsitate Oxon. loco et vice pfati Doctoris Edwards procedendum fore decreverunt, et processerunt in hunc qui sequitur modum. Primo Reverendus Vir Paulus Hood Vice Cancellarius Univsitatis Oxon pdict: Nominavit et Elegit Magistrum Thomam Willis in Medicina Baccalaureum Prælectorem in Naturali Philosophia infra Universitatem Oxon. Deinde Ventis Johannes Oliver Collegij Beatæ Mariæ Magdal: in dict. Univsitate Præsidens dictum Thomam Willis in Prælectorem Naturalis Philosophiæ etiam nominavit. Qui duo Electores assignat ra[illegible] quod Ventis Vir Gilbertus Sheldon Coll: Om: Animar Gardianus in remotis agens et varijs negotijs detentus ad suffragium suum interponendum personaliter interesse non potuit, dictum Thomam Willis Medicinæ Baccalaureum in Prælectorem Naturalis Philosophiæ in Univsitate Oxon debite nominatum et legaliter electum esse pronunciarant et declaraverunt et pro Persona sic electa in Universitate Oxon: habend et reputand. adjudicaverunt et publicaverunt, et insuper decreverunt Literas Certificatorias hujusmodi Electionis sub Sigillis suis respective emittendas. Tenoris subsequentis

Cum Vir spectabilis Gulielmus Sidley unam Lecturam in naturali Philosophia in usum et beneficium in Universitate Oxon. studentium ample salario dotatam instituerit, Et ad ordinandum dirigendum et gubernandum eandem tres Reverendos Viros qui pro tempore fuerint vizt Vice Cancellarium Univsitatis Oxon. Præsidentem Collegij Magdalenensis et Custodem Collegij Omnium Animarum in dicta Univsitate vel duos quosvis eorum nominaverit assignaverit et constituerit. Nos quorum nomina subscripta sunt Thomam Willis in Univsitate Oxon in Medicina Baccalaureum, in locum publici Prælectoris naturalis Philosophiæ in Univsitate Oxon. per mortem naturalem Johannis Edwards in Medicina Doctoris nuper Prælectoris ejusdem, jam vacantem nominamus et eligimus. Dictumqz Thomam Willis naturalis Philosophiæ in Academia Oxoniensi sive Professorem Sidleianum constituimus et confirmamus per præsentes. In cujus rei Testimonium Sigilla et nomina nostra præsentibus apposuimus. Dat apud Oxon vicesimo quinto die Mensis Augusti Anno Dni Millesimo Sexcentesimo Sexagesimo.

Paulus Hood
Vice Can:

Gilb: Sheldon
Custos Coll: Om:
Am: Oxon

FIG. 3. Entries in the convocation register, Oxford University, recording Thomas Willis's appointment as Sedleian Professor of Natural Philosophy. (By courtesy of the Keeper of the University Archives.)

quelae, his realization that the brain had been inaccurately described and, most important of all, the stimulus of university teaching.

What was the state of knowledge of the central nervous system when Willis began his research? This can only be briefly summarized here from the writings of others, notably Clarke (31), Clarke and O'Malley (32), Critchley (33), Meyer (34), and Clarke and Dewhurst (35). The irreverent audacity of the mechanistic Cartesian approach had already dispersed some of the aura of mystery that had for centuries shrouded investigations into the human brain. As the repository of the soul, research into the brain, and particularly investigations into psychiatric illnesses, were then in a gray hinterland between medicine and religion. In his preface to *Cerebri Anatome*, Willis combined an anticipatory sensitivity to any possible theological objections to his research, while justifying his adoption of Baconian empiricism, and flavored the whole with a dash of braggadocio. "I had resolved to unlock the secret places of Man's mind," he wrote (36), "and to look into the living and breathing Chapel of the Deity. . . ." After expressing these pretentious sentiments, he felt obliged to admit his awareness that "it hath been a long while accounted as a certain Mystery and School-house of Atheism to search into Nature" (37). Henry Stubbe (1632–1676) had criticized the restless probings of the fellows of the Royal Society on the grounds that their research would undermine the established church (38). And Thomas Sydenham (1624–1689) was opposed to the use of microscopes and the performing of necropsies, as he believed that the physician ought to confine his observations to the "outer husk of things," as God had so shaped man's faculties to perceive only the external appearance of bodies and not the minute processes of Nature's "abyss of cause" (39).

A century later, when La Mettrie (1709–1751) published his *L'homme machine* (1748) (a logical extension of Cartesianism), wherein he denied the existence of the soul and reduced mind to a function of the brain, he had to pay the penalty for outraging religious sentiments by constantly fleeing from possible imprisonment or worse. Willis took no such chances. He asserted that he intended to "look into Nature like looking into the Bible," and reassured his readers that his observations would be approved "no less by the demonstrations of Piety and Canons of the Church, than by the Rule of Experience and Knowledge" (40). He followed Pierre Gassendi (1592–1655), who claimed that animals must have souls since they show evidence of memory, reason, and similar traits. This corporeal soul, or "soul of brutes" as Willis called it, is present in man as an inferior soul subservient to the immaterial, immortal, rational soul. Thus, by concentrating on the inferior corporeal soul, Willis forestalled any possible theological objections, as he had carefully located the superior rational soul beyond the sphere of the physician's scalpel, scepticsm, or speculations. He regarded the vital portion of the corporeal soul lodged in the blood, as being akin to fire, while the sensitive portion, an immaterial aggregation of animal spirits, was coextensive with the body, and hence liable to various illnesses, including those of a psychological nature. Thus, Willis was able to concentrate on the brain itself, which was generally regarded not only as the repository of the corporeal soul but also the center of sensation, movement, and intellectual activity, although there was still some lingering support for the role of the heart in these functions. The brain was thought to vary in size according to the phases of the moon, and it was still believed that tears flowed from it. It was generally agreed that animal spirits were produced from the blood though there were wide differences as to their site of production: The lateral ventricles, the choroid plexus, the rete mirabile, and the fourth ventricle had all been suggested. Liquid waste products from the brain were thought to pass through the cribriform plate into the nose, or alternatively, by way of the infundibulum and pituitary into the nasopharynx, while gaseous effluence escaped through cranial sutures. Like the heart, the brain was believed to pulsate so that blood could be drawn into the cranium through the carotid arteries to heat it, while cooling air entered through the cribriform plate.

The cell doctrine theory with its cerebroventricular localization of function still held sway. The process was likened to that of digestion, with spirits passing through the first chamber (lateral ventricle) giving rise to judgment or common sense, then through the middle chamber (third ventricle), causing cogitation or "phantasies," and finally, the posterior chamber (fourth ventricle), where memories were evoked. With various modifications, the cell doctrine theory survived, albeit with dminishing authority, the more exacting scrutiny of the Renaissance anatomists. But when a more detailed anatomy of the ventricular system was elucidated, doubts were raised as to whether or not mental processes actually took place within it. This tendency to elevate the importance of the ventricular system had caused a corresponding neglect of the functional significance of the cerebral cortex. Thomas Bartholin (1641) had argued that as the convolutions in man were only slightly more developed than those of higher animals, they were unlikely to be associated with higher intellectual processes, and he assumed, therefore, that the cortex served to provide a protective covering for the blood vessels and the cerebrospinal fluid.

Another surviving structure from antiquity was the rete mirabile, first described by Herophilus, and subsequently incorporated into Galen's general theory of brain function. A dense mass of blood vessels of unknown function, the rete are found at the base of the brain in ungulates and carnivores; they are not present in man, monkey, or rodent, although their human presence had been assumed by the medieval physicians, and this belief survived until the 17th century. After stating in his *Cerebri Anatome* (1655) that the rete are not present in the human brain, Willis later betrayed some slight doubts and mentioned that some physicians believed that they may occasionally be found in man and signified a "slender wit or unmoved disposition," predisposing to subnormality.

These long established notions of brain function and structure were shattered during the decade between 1655 and 1665. In his *De osse cribiforme* (1655), and subsequently between 1660 and 1664, in his monumental *De catarrhis*, K. V. Schneider demolished the notion that brain excretions pass into the nose and nasopharynx. In 1658, J. J. Wepfer described the ring of arteries around the base of the brain and emphatically denied the existence of the rete in man. In 1660, Franciscus de la Boë (Sylvius) placed the production of the animal spirits in the cerebral and cerebellar cortices rather than the ventricles and thereby completely changed the emphasis of research into brain function. Two years later, Steno (1662) showed conclusively that tears come from the lachrymal glands, and as mentioned earlier, the revolutionary impact of Descartes' works between 1662 and 1664, though anatomically inaccurate, nevertheless shattered the religious mystique associated with the brain and prepared the way for a mechanistic interpretation. These were some of the most significant contributions to brain research before 1660, when Willis began his work, until its completion four years later.

Before considering Willis's contributions to brain anatomy, some confusion between past and present anatomical terms must be dispelled. The corpus callosum now refers to the white matter bridging the two hemispheres, but 17th-century anatomists included not only the bridge but all deep white matter extending to the medulla. Another deep structure, the three-legged fornix, like the corpus callosum, helped to preserve the patency of the lateral and third ventricles. The medulla oblongata differed from the present named structure: It began where the corpus callosum ended and its three parts resembled the letter Y. The two limbs of the letter formed the circular core of each cerebral hemisphere, consisting of a lateral ventricle, basal ganglia (only the thalamus had been described), and the paraventricular white matter formed the head of the medulla. In the tail of the medulla (corresponding to our brain stem) were attached posteriorly from above downward the pineal body (penis), the superior colliculi (the testes), the inferior colliculi (the nates), and the fourth ventricle or calamus scriptorius of Herophilus. The second part of the medullary tail ended at the foramen magnum, and the third part was continuous with the spinal cord. The cerebellum was attached to the second part of the medulla by the pons of Varolio, whose function was to maintain the shape of the fourth ventricle. The cerebellar peduncles had not then been described.

How much did Willis know about these recent advances and what was his own contribution? He was aware of the writings of Schneider, Wepfer, and Sylvius and also knew of the works of Descartes, although it is unlikely that he agreed with them. Willis's own neurological research is mainly embodied in *Cerebri Anatome* which, it should be emphasized, is a study in comparative anatomy, as is apparent from his dedication wherein he claimed that he had "slain so many victims, whole Hecatombs almost of all Animals, in the Anatomical Court. . . ." As well as the human brain, Willis studied those of about 15 different species, including the horse, sheep, calf, pig, dog, fox, cat, hare, rabbit, mouse, goat, and monkey, together with various fishes and fowls. He compared the size and structure of specific areas in the brains of these animals, noting their differences and similarities together with their behavior and capabilities. Another generalization concerning *Cerebri Anatome* is that despite its title, Willis did not limit himself to brain anatomy but included studies in neurophysiology and neuropathology, together with experimental and clinical neurology. When Willis became interested in brain research, he did not abandon his earlier iatrochemical interest but applied these quinary principles (41) to the neural circulation so that a deficiency of one or an excess of another or an unstable mixture of any of them may cause various diseases. Similarly, various psychiatric states may be explained in terms of a chemical imbalance in the circulating spirits or by aberrant ones taking up new pathways in different parts of the brain. Willis likened the cerebral blood vessels to a distillatory apparatus for extracting animal spirits rather like a "Chymical Elixir," and he compared the cortex to an alembic whose function he believed was to distill the spirits (42).

Willis first discussed his method of dissecting the brain, and here he was given more than his rightful share of originality. When writing to his son Edward on March 7, 1677, Sir Thomas Browne (43) mentioned that "Mr. Hobbes . . . was thought the best way for the dissection of the brayne of man, butt for sheep, etc., Dr. Willis his way was best . . ."; John Ward, his Christ Church contemporary, records that Willis's "new way of opening the Brain, is to cut them in all parts from what holds them, and so to turn them upside down" (44). There were then four methods of dissecting the brain. Galen, and later Vesalius, dissected it within the skull by making a series of transverse slices. Bartholin's method, used by Sylvius, was to expose the brain and, while *in situ*, to dissect the right and then the left hemisphere. The least popular approach was that adopted by Steno, who removed the cortex and dissected downward into the medulla. Willis followed Varolio by removing the brain, turning it upside down, and dissecting with its base uppermost.

Willis gave a good general description of the skull, meninges, and the external appearance of the brain divided into hemispheres and lobes, which he compared to "a Castle . . . divided into Towers or places of Defence, [and] is thereby made the stronger and harder to be Taken" (45). He correlated his observations with his necropsy findings in a patient with a cerebral tumor with meningeal adhesions, and thereafter he regarded meningeal irritation as one of the most serious and intractable causes of headaches. The more numerous and deeper cerebral convolutions in man, as compared to animals, signifies his "superior faculties," whereas the more flattened cerebral surfaces of cats, birds, and fishes restricts them to learning only through imitation. White matter serves for the generation of animal spirits while the gray matter is concerned with their distribution.

In his pioneering study of cerebral localization of function, Willis focused attention on the brain substance through which the animal spirits circulate while the role of the ventricles was relegated to that of a drain for removing impurities. He assumed the predominance of the cerebrum and cerebellum over the medulla: The former is the center for initiating movements and ideas, whereas the latter governs involuntary movements. His studies in comparative anatomy have revealed that the structure of the cerebellum is similar in all animals whereas the surface of the cerebrum is varied. Its surface is more orderly and constant to ensure regular control of the heart, lungs, and viscera. In the cerebellar cortex, a very pure spiritous liquor is exalted by a ferment and circulates in a regular and uninterrupted manner. Animal spirits are stored in the brain substance, and when the appetite or will is initiated, they flow downward into the corpus callosum, medulla, spinal cord, and peripheral nerves in order to stimulate movement. These spirits are refined in the thickest part of the corpus callosum, where imagination is provoked, and pass into the fornix, where "more subtil acts of Phantasie" are evoked along its narrowest strip. Connected to the corpus callosum and the medulla are the corpora striata, designated by Willis as the *sensorium commune*, or the common sensory center, with pathways for the spirits passing to and from the cerebrum and medulla. Willis came to this conclusion as he observed that the striae are almost completely obliterated in those dying after a "long Palsie", and also because he found that they are barely discernible in newly born blind puppies. Thus, sensations pass along the nerves like ripples over the surface of a liquid to the corpora striata, then to the corpus callosum, where imagination is stimulated, to reach the cortex, where they leave traces in the convolutions. Memories are evoked by a retrograde movement of the spirits peripherally along the same convolutions. Willis regarded the medulla as a highway along which spirits flow either outward toward the peripheral nerves to stimulate movement or inward to facilitate the appreciation of sensations. The corpora quadrigemina forms the anterior, and the pons forms the posterior appendix of the cerebellum. The pons act as a reservoir or storehouse for the animal spirits before passing them on from the cerebellum to the medulla. Spirits passing from the cerebrum to the medulla may be diverted through the corpora quadrigemina to the cerebellum. Thus, the corpora quadrigemina serve to convey impulses from the cerebellum to the cerebrum, where changes of mood are registered and purposeful movements initiated. Hence, emotions may influence involuntary functions, and likewise precordial sensations, such as overheating of the blood in fevers, may affect the imagination or "phantasie" through the same route. Willis is generally credited with giving the earliest satisfactory description of reflex nervous action. This may occur when sensations impinging on the corpora striata stimulate movements during sleep without any conscious initiation by the will. When these sensations reach the corpus callosum, they are immediately turned back and initiate movements designed to remove a painful or irritating stimulus (46).

It required some semantic gymnastics on Willis's part to reconcile the functional significance of this elaborate neural circulation with his own observations.[1] He had satisfied himself both anatomically and experimentally that nerves are not hollow, nor had he been able to perceive any holes in them with the aid of a microscope. He realized, too, that there are no

[1]In his Fitz-Patrick lecture, Edwin Clarke gave a most informative survey of the origin of the neural circulation (47).

connections between the brain, nose, and palate. But in order to get round this problem, he postulated that nerves consist of a "tube like substance, like an Indian Cane, [which] is every where porous and pervious" (48). And to make this alleged penetration of them easier, he likened the animal spirits to light, air, or wind. He had also injected various dyes into the pituitary but failed to find any in the nasopharynx or palate; yet he clung to the Galenic notion that the brain was purged through the excretory functions of the ventricles into the nose, palate, or through the cranial sutures. As he also believed that a defect in the circulating animal spirits may cause "horrid distempers of the Brain," Willis felt it essential to retain his belief in nasal purging, and he postulated that the unhealthy humors pass into the nose as through a cloth filter or strainer. In short, Willis was not prepared to discard basic theoretical assumptions when challenged by inconvenient empirical evidence; instead he compromised and modified rather than reject his preconceived ideas.

Of the utmost importance was Willis's description and classification of the cranial nerves, which was generally adopted for over 150 years. He gave accurate descriptions of the origins and courses of the olfactory, optic, oculomotor, trochlear, or pathetic, and was the first to describe the ophthalmic branch of the trigeminal, although he failed to mention the semilunar ganglia and included only two of its branches. He gave a good description of the sixth nerve but followed Galen by dividing the seventh nerve into hard and soft branches. Although he referred to the seventh nerve as the auditory (our eighth), he clearly distinguished it from the facial. In Willisian terminology, the eighth nerve is the vagus, and he ligated both nerves in a dog, causing convulsions and cardiac irregularities. But after cutting them, the animal survived and eventually died of starvation. Willis gave the first accurate description of the spinal accessory (our eleventh nerve), mentioning that it had "not yet been noted by other Anatomists." But when describing the ninth nerve to the tongue, and concerned with articulation and taste, Willis confused the glossopharyngeal with the hypoglossal (49).

When discussing the autonomic nervous system, Willis distinguished between the vagus complex and the sympathetic nerves or "intercostales" as he called them. He realized, too, that their involuntary function was governed by the cerebellum, and his illustrations of the peripheral autonomic nervous system were judged to be the best available until the beginning of the 18th century. He realized that in lower animals, the vagus is more important than the sympathetic, and he was the first to describe a branch going to the aortic arch and reacting to the variations in the pulse, which is the earliest reference to the depressor nerve (50).

In a scholarly survey Hierons and Meyer (51) have elucidated the priorities of the cerebral circulation. In 1561, Fallopius gave the first reasonably correct description of the basal arterial ramifications with the exception of the posterior communicating artery, which he regarded as being only indirectly connected to branches of the internal carotid through a network of small vessels. Casserio (1627) illustrated an almost complete arterial circle on one hemisphere but repeated the same error as Fallopius on the other side, and Vesling (1653) rectified this error but omitted to show the union of the anterior cerebrals. In 1658, Wepfer gave a more accurate, though unillustrated, account of this arterial circle, so that Willis's illustration was superior to those of his predecessors, and although he gave the first indisputably complete illustration of the "circle," he omitted the posterior or cerebral arteries. But more significant than the anatomical description was Willis's realization of its functional significance, which evolved from a series of sophisticated experiments and clinicopathological observations. He had, for example, injected a dye into one carotid and found at necropsy that it stained all the blood vessels, and in a dog, he ligated one carotid without any ill effects. Willis confirmed the functional significance of these arterial anastomoses at a necropsy, where he found that one carotid artery was blocked, "so that the influx of the blood being denied to this passage, it seemed wonderful, wherefore this sick person had not dyed before of an Apoplexy: which indeed he was so far from, that he enjoyed to the last moment of his life, the free exercise of his mind and animal function. For indeed, Nature had substituted a sufficient Remedy against that danger of an Apoplexy; to wit, the *Vertebral* Artery of the same side, in which the Carotidick was wanting, the bulk of the Pipe being enlarged, became thrice as big as both its Pipes on the other side . . ." (52).

Thus, in his *Cerebri Anatome*, Willis laid down the foundations of neurology, and subsequently he added two more cornerstones to them. In his earliest lectures, he explained epileptic convulsions in terms of the chemical theory advanced by Sylvius (1614–1672). The latter believed that cerebral compression and the mixing of vitriolic matter in the blood with the nervous juice caused an ebullition and fermentation. On reaching the medulla oblongata, this matter irritates the origin of the nerves, causing an upward spasm to the brain (53).[2] But in his *Cerebri Anatome*, Willis adopted an explosive theory to explain muscular contraction. The spirits in the muscular fibers, containing spirituo-saline particles, mix with arterial blood containing nitrosulphurous particles, which ignites and explodes "like the explosion of Gun-powder," causing inflation and muscular shortening. Later, Willis adopted this theory to explain all convulsive diseases in terms of a "spasmodic explosive copula," or *explosio Willisiana*. As long as explosive particles from the blood were not too numerous, they were able to mix with the spirits in the neural circulation without ill effects, but when too many accumulated, an explosion causing convulsions occurred: These convulsions might also be triggered off by reflex action from the irritation of the nervous system by worms, medicine, or acrid humors. Willis adopted this explosive theory to explain epileptic seizures. He postulated that a hereditary weak constitution of the brain was affected by a strong spasmodic copula distilled from the blood, which explodes when mixed with the animal spirits in the middle of the brain. This explosion caused the psychiatric symptoms accompanying an epileptic seizure, while other explosions throughout the body were manifest as generalized convulsions (54).

Finally, in his *De Anima Brutorum* (1672), Willis renewed his study of the anatomy of the corpora striata, which has been admirably surveyed by Meyer and Hierons (55), who rightly point out that he was the first to associate motor action and sensation with this region. He also gave the earliest description of the anterior commissure, mistaking it for an interstrial connection. Without actually so naming them, Willis clearly illustrated the internal capsule, the claustrum, and his description of the area around the third ventricle was the most accurate then available. He gently scraped the surface of the corpora striata with a penknife and unwittingly uncovered several fiber tracts. These were the sensory pathways of the medial lemnisci passing into the ventral nuclei of the thalamus, the thalamostriatal fibers, the thalamocortical pathways, and descending pathways from the cortex and the corpora striata.

How were Willis's writings received by his contemporaries? His book was favorably reviewed in the first issue of the *Journal des Savans* (1665) (56), and Thomas Birch, historian of the Royal Society, recorded that Dr. Walter Charlton, by his operations, "had found Dr. Willis's cuts in the *Anatome Cerebri*, as far as he had gone, true . . ." (57). Dr. Charles Goodall prophesied that Willis's "name as well as his writings will be advanced in our and succeeding ages" (58), and Dr. Robert Plot wrote that "his placing the Spirit to serve voluntary action in the Cerebrum and those that serve Involuntary in the Cerebellum is a viable and

---

[2]In his lectures, Willis adopted Sylvius's theory, but later in his published works, he introduced his concept of a "spasmodic explosive copula." See Dewhurst (28, pp. 79–87).

useful discovery..." (59). Dr. William Cole favored Willis's explanation that in cerebral vascular accidents, the cortex was most liable "to receive the mortifick matter," owing to its vascularity, whereas Wepfer thought that they were caused by a degeneration of the animal spirits. Cole (60) also accepted the *explosio Willisiana* as an explanation of epileptic convulsions.

In 1665, the first critical note was struck by Niels Steno, who accused Descartes and Willis of allowing speculations to intrude into their writings. In particular, he regarded Willis's attempts at cerebral localization as a modification of the theories of the ancients and expressed a healthy skepticism about the meager knowledge concerning the function of the corpora striata, as "a Man of tolerable genious may say about it whatever he Pleases." Although he drew attention to some slight errors in three of Willis's illustrations, Steno regarded the others as the best then available. Unjustly, he criticized Willis's method of dissecting the brain, as he thought that it might damage the corpora quadrigemina and the mamillary bodies. Finally, he pleaded that anatomical investigations should be designed to "tear off the glaucoma from the eyes of those who calmly accept the opinions of past ages" (61).

In England, Willis was accused by Henry Stubbe of usurping Richard Lower's anatomical skill. In his *Plus Ultra* (1670) (62), Stubbe first alleged that Willis's "discoveries" had been described earlier and then accused him of plagiarism: "... Whatsoever there is in that Piece [i.e., *Cerebri Anatome*], which is Anatomical, the glory thereof belongs to Dr. Lower, whose indefatigable industry produced that elaborate Treatise; and any man that knows the great practice of that other Doctor [i.e., Willis], will grant, that although he could not want abilities, yet he wanted leisure to attend to such painful and tedious enquiries. Dr. Willis indeed candidly doth relinquish this honour to Dr. Lower.... All that Dr. Willis contributed, that I hear, was the discourses and conjectures upon the Anatomical deductions of Dr. Lower, which as ingenious as they are, I am sure neither are, nor ever will, pass all for inventions." But in a postscript, Stubbe (63) shifted his ground and modified these strictures: "I think my self obliged to adde one thing more where I speak as if Dr. Willis had had little to do in the discoveries of Dr. Lower about Anatomy: that although the great Physician had not leisure to attend the Anatomical Inquiries yet he did propose *new matter* for *improving the discoveries*, and put Dr. Lower upon continual investigation, thereby to see if Nature and his supposition did accord: and although that many did occur beyond his apprehension: yet was the grand occasion of that work, and in much the Author."

Stubbe's pamphlet is thought to have been prompted by Dr. Baldwin Hamey who, disturbed by the growing power of the Royal Society, feared that its influence might undermine the College of Physicians. But Stubbe needed little encouragement to attack the Royal Society or to cause dissension among its fellows. It was from him that Anthony Wood (64), Willis's vindictive neighbor, quoted almost verbatim those passages favoring Lower rather than Willis. In a letter to Bishop Kennet, Willis's grandson, Browne Willis (65) mentions the cause of the dispute between his grandfather and Wood: "Some uneasiness between their servants confirmed the latter's (Wood's) Prejudices which were naturally too strong; and made him record, what he thought might under value the Family." Browne Willis, being swayed by family loyalty, must be regarded as a biased witness, but it should also be borne in mind that Wood and Lower were good friends, and it is likely that the antiquarian might favor his friend at Willis's expense. On at least one occasion, Richard Lower, though unqualified, had treated Wood (66), and there are records of them spending convivial evenings in the Oxford taverns (67).

These unsubstantiated statements by Stubbe and Wood have caused Willis's integrity to be repeatedly questioned. Hutchinson (1799) (68) criticized Willis for framing theories instead of concerning himself with observations and experiments: "Hence it is that, while his books show the greatest ingenuity and learning very little knowledge is to be drawn from them, very little use to be made of them. And perhaps no writings, which are so admirably executed, and prove such uncommon talents to have been in the writer, were ever so soon laid aside and neglected as the works of Dr. Willis." Munk (1861) (69) dismissed his contributions as "trivial," and acclaimed Lower's experimental supremacy instead. "For the anatomical as distinguished from the physiological and speculative parts of Willis's treatise 'de Cerebro'," he wrote, "and they are in fact the only portions of the work that are now of any value, it has always been understood that we are indebted to Lower."

The most severe strictures came from Foster (1901) (70), who stated that *Cerebri Anatome* was "much above the worth of the author," and he accused Willis of outright dishonesty, as his regard for the truth was "less potent than love of fame." After denouncing Willis's "rectorial mind" and his love of "words as words," Foster proclaimed that Lower should be regarded as the rightful author of *Cerebri Anatome*. With various modifications and elaborations, these strictures were repeated by Franklin (1939) (71) and Cole (1944) (72), who dismissed Willis as "the pontifical leader of a research team," while Mettler (1947) (73) regarded him as "something of a dandy." Although general opinion is now more favorably disposed toward Willis, these charges of dishonesty, plagiarism, dandyism, vanity, pomposity, and verbosity warrant a thorough investigation from contemporary sources.

While he was undertaking the research that went into *Cerebri Anatome*, Willis was simultaneously building up the most lucrative practice in Restoration Oxford. It is not, therefore, surprising that he should delegate some work to others in accordance with their interests and abilities. His contemporaries, Dr. William Petty and the Hon. Robert Boyle, both adopted a similar practice. Boyle was, in fact, the director of a laboratory employing secretaries, mechanics, glass-blowers, furnacemen, apothecaries, and doctors to carry out the less exacting tasks under his general direction. The most important contribution to Boyle's research was Robert Hooke's invention of the air pump, which enabled him to undertake his most significant experiments. John Locke (74) edited his books on the air and the natural history of blood; Boyle was also assisted by Christopher Wren and Richard Lower, yet a charge of plagiarism has never been brought against him. A nobleman, Boyle had ample means to finance his research, whereas Willis was a self-made man who, having gained admission to the university as a servant-scholar, had, with unseemly haste, become the wealthiest doctor in Oxford and the Vice Chancellor's brother-in-law. Indeed, he had begun making the transition from a professional man to that of a country gentleman when in 1663 he bought his first estate of Burlton Court in Herefordshire from John Aubrey the antiquarian (75). Willis's rapid rise to fame and fortune may well have fostered the spite and envy of the less successful.

It should be emphasized that Willis never tried to conceal the fact that his research had benefited from the help of others. On the contrary, he handsomely acknowledged their help, and here is his tribute to Richard Lower (76): "But for the more accurate performing this work as I had not leisure, and perhaps not wit enough of my self, I was not ashamed to require the help of others. And here I make use of the Labours of the most Learned Physician and highly skilful Anatomist, Dr. Richard Lower, for my help and Companion; the edge of whose Knife and Wit I willingly acknowledge to have been an help to me for that better searching out both the frame and offices of before hidden Bodies. Wherefore having got this help and Companion, no day almost past over without some Anatomical administration; so that in a short space there was nothing of the Brain, and its Appendix within the Skull, that seemed not plainly detected, and intimately beheld by us. After this, when we entered upon a more difficult task, viz the Anatomy of the Nerves, then very much appeared the plainly to be admired skill of this Man, as also his indefatigable Industry, and unwearied Labour" (Fig. 4).

Willis also expressed his gratitude to Dr. Thomas Millington and Christopher Wren (77): ". . . It becomes me not to hide, how much besides I did receive from these most famous Men, Dr. Thomas Millington, Doctor in Physick, and Dr. Chr. Wren, Doctor of Laws, and Savill Professor of Astronomy; both which were wont frequently to be present at our Dissections, and to confer and reason out the use of the Parts. . . ." He was also helped by Robert Hooke and by William Day, the leading surgeon in Oxford, whose operative dexterity was widely esteemed. Another assistant was Willis's private apothecary John Hemmings, who also acted as his amanuensis; other colleagues with whom he was closely associated were Dr. Peter Elliot and Dr. Richard Lydall, who probably helped him indirectly by allowing him to perform necropsies on their former patients. Another collaborator was Dr. Ralph Bathurst, whose biographer wrote (78): "I suspect that he [Bathurst] wrote a great part of the preface to Willis's *Cerebri Anatome*, which work he supervised before publication. The following

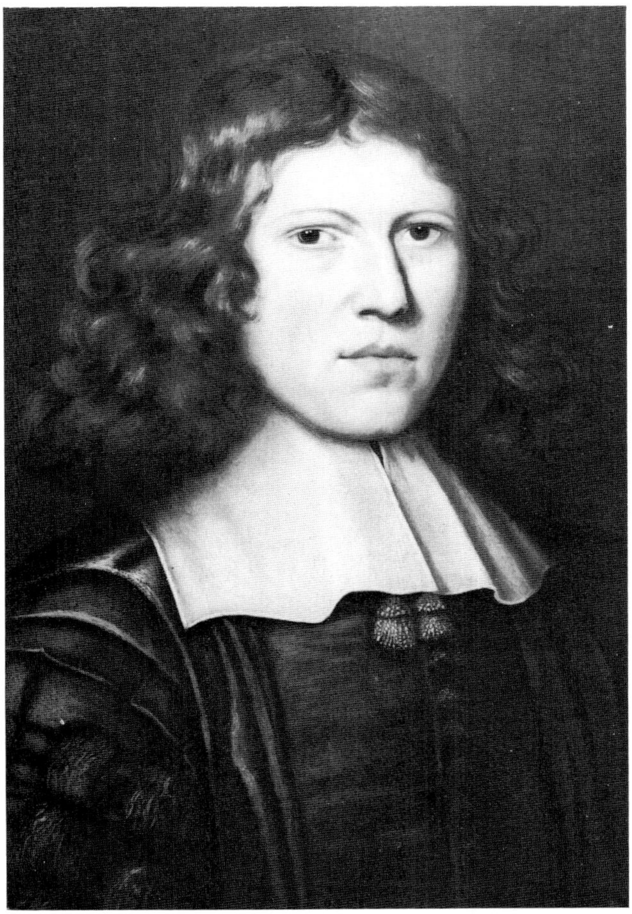

FIG. 4. Portrait of Richard Lower, attributed to the school of Jacob Huysmans. (By courtesy of the Wellcome Trustees.)

passages, in particular, are entirely in his taste and style, and much too smart for Willis. . . ." This is confirmed in Bathurst's letter of February 10, 1663/4 (79): "I have now under my review Dr. Willis's texture of the brain and nerves etc. which shortly he will be persuaded to publish as indeed they well deserve." Thus, it can be established that Willis, like Boyle, had several other helpers, apart from Lower, whose services he handsomely acknowledged.

More germane would be an inquiry into the reactions of Willis's assistants to the suggestion that he had exploited their services. All of them outlived him, several published books, two kept diaries, and the letters of others have come down to us. It is highly significant that there is not a scrap of evidence to support the allegations that he exploited their services or plagiarized their research. On the contrary, they all refer to Willis with the utmost respect. His earliest assistant Robert Hooke (80) ranked Willis alongside Harvey, Ent, and Glisson in his *Micrographia* (1665). His diary reveals that they last met in 1673, two years before Willis's death (81). Another contemporary, John Ward (ca. 1629–1681) was an Oxford medical student when Willis was carrying out his research, and among the entries in his diaries is one referring to another member of Willis's circle, Walter Needham: "Needham styles Willis next to Harvy ye glory of our English Nation" (82). The fact that Lower's first book was written in defense of Willis's *De Febribus* indicates that he bore him no ill will, and he never once criticized Willis in his later writings. When they were both practicing in London, Lower often referred patients to Willis for a second opinion.

Fortunately, there is irrefutable contemporary evidence to show that Willis completely dominated the research on the central nervous system while Lower and his other assistants were, in fact, subordinates who worked under his direction and supervision. In his letters to Boyle, Lower outlined the research culminating in *Cerebri Anatome*, wherein his references to Willis are all respectful, deferential, and free from any bitterness or recrimination. They not only throw new light on the relationship between Willis and Lower but also unfold the chronological sequence of their research better than a study of the book itself. On January 18, 1661, Lower (83) makes it clear that Willis insisted on being present at all their dissections: "The doctor [Willis] was not at leisure till of late to make these dissections of the brain, which he hoped, but at length we have had the opportunity of cutting up several, and the doctor, finding most parts of the brain imperfectly described, intends to make a whole new draught thereof, with several uses of the distinct parts, according to his own fancy, seeing few authors speak any thing considerable of it . . .".

Lower went on to discuss Willis's views on the cerebellar control of involuntary movement and described the origins and courses of the vagus and auditory nerves. He asked Willis about the nutrient properties of the nervous juice. The latter doubted that the nerves actually contained any nutritive properties, although he affirmed his belief that there was a liquor in the nerves, as he had often observed in those troubled with convulsions, epilepsies, or hysterical fits that their urine was very scanty during the fit but afterward "they make water for the like space of three or four days in very large quantity." This fluid, he believed, came from the nerves, as afterward "their heads become light and clear, which were before heavy, dull and turbulent." Lower then mentions that Willis "intends to syringe in some kind of liquors, tinctured with saffron, or other colours, into the *arteriae carotides;* the brain being first opened, just after the creature is dead, and warm, to try how the blood moves, and how the tincture may be separated in the brain. . . ." This highly sophisticated technique, known as *chirurgia infusoria*, had been introduced into Oxford by Christopher Wren in 1659 and was immediately adopted by Willis, Boyle, and Lower. It is known, too, that Willis carried out extirpation experiments on the brain of living animals as, when investigating the cerebral blood supply, he cut the cortex and medulla and blood spurted out. Boyle was interested in Willis's lectures and asked for a transcript of them. When Lower (84) sent them on November 26, 1662, he mentioned that Willis had perfected some of his anatomical observations but that he would not "be induced to publish them yet a good while. . . ." In his next letter of April 27, 1663, Lower (85) states that he had "been wholly diverted by Dr. *Willis*, whose desire it is, that I should be present at his operations, which now are very near finished. . . ." Lower was still a medical student, and as a consequence of his collaboration with Willis, he acquired a high level of experimental dexterity, which was useful when he undertook his own research.

Willis planned, and with Lower's assistance, carried out a most sophisticated experiment on the pituitary of a calf, which disposed of the old Galenic theory that cerebrospinal fluid flowed through the infundibulum into the palate. In this joint experiment they syringed milk, and later india ink, into the pituitary veins and recovered them in the jugular vein. Nothing entered the mouth. Lower mentioned it in his *De Catarrhis* (1672) without reference to Willis, who first planned it. Willis's investigations were helped by the occasional necropsy. At one postmortem, he found that the right carotid artery was obstructed and the left increased in size to compensate. This patient had never suffered from apoplexy, which led Willis to realize the functional significance of the arterial anastomoses around the base of the brain. If both carotid arteries were blocked, then the many anastomoses are "so divinely contrived inside the dura mater, before they go up into the brain (as you will see exactly described in the doctor's [Willis] scheme)," wrote Lower to Boyle on June 4, 1663 (86), "that if three arteries were quite obstructed, the fourth would convey blood into all parts of the brain and cerebellum, sufficient enough for life and motion. And to confirm this, this week we took a young spaniel, and tied both the carotidal arteries in the neck very fast and close with silk, and the dog was not at all altered by it, but continued very lively and brisk, and was so far from taking unkindly what was done to him, that within a quarter of an hour after, he got loose and followed the doctor into the town, as he visited his patients. In this pleasant humor he continued two or three days, and then we opened his head, and found all the vessels of the brain as full of blood as usually they are in other dogs, who did not suffer the same experiment. But this I might have told you in shorter time; for if one artery be syringed with any tincted liquor, all the parts of the brain will equally be filled with it at the same time . . .". On June 24, 1664, Lower (87) informed Boyle that "Dr. *Willis* will send his book of the Diseases of the Head to the press this winter . . . There is not a disease of the head, which he doth not excellently illustrate with very rare observations and cases; so that it is a pity the world should be any longer deprived of them." Thus, all the evidence in Lower's letters clearly shows that Lower's role was a subordinate one.

These letters answer most of the criticisms leveled at Willis, with the exception of his proclivity to speculation, which he obviously relished, so that the "hard sence of our already instituted *Anatomy* may be sweetened with those kind of more pleasant Speculations, as it were cloathing the Skeleton with flesh" (88). Like many of his contemporaries, Willis preferred to convey his opinions in speculative, lapidary passages rather than in dull, precise anatomical terminology. "For in truth, whatever of our Work is performed without form or beauty," he wrote (89), "may seem as the Foundations of a Building, only placed on the ground, in which no elegancy or neatness doth yet shine . . . A Superstructure indeed may be promised to be put upon this Foundation, perhaps fair and beautiful, whereby the minds of the Beholders may be pleased or instructed." Thus, when the question concerning Willis's fondness for speculation is posed, the answer must be emphatically in the affirmative: Indeed, he believed that speculations were a necessary embellishment on the foundations of neurology. Yet he speculated against a scientific background involving research into iatrochemistry, comparative neurology, clinicopathological observations, animal experiments, *chirurgia infusoria*, and anatomical and microscopical observations. What more could he have done?

ACKNOWLEDGMENTS

This research was undertaken while I held a Wellcome Senior Research Fellowship at Linacre College, Oxford. I am grateful to Lord Franks, the Wellcome Trustees, and to Mr. J. B. Bamborough, the Principal, and Fellows of Linacre College for their financial support and hospitality.

REFERENCES

1. Aspects of Willis's early life have been mentioned in the following works: *Brief Lives Chiefly of Contemporaries, set down by John Aubrey 1669–1696*, edited by A. Clark, Vol. I., pp. 302–303, Oxford (1898); DNB, Vol. 21, pp. 496–497, London (1917); *The Life and Times of Anthony Wood*, edited by A. Clark, Vol. 2, p. 326, Oxford (1892); Wood, Anthony, *Athenae Oxonienses*, 2nd ed., Vol. 2, pp. 549–551, (1721); *Biographia Britannica*, Vol. 6, Pt. 2, pp. 4291–7, London (1766); John Fell's postscript to *Pharmaceutice Rationalis*, Pt. 2, London (1675, translated by S. Pordage in "Dr. Willis's Practice of Physick," London (1684) (3 unnumbered pages after preface to reader).
2. Fell, John (1675): Postscript to *Pharmaceutice Rationalis*, Pt. 2, translated by S. Pordage in "Dr. Willis's Practice of Physick," London (1684).
3. The Civil War in the Oxford area has been discussed in the following works: Firth, C. H. (1890): A chronological summary of the Civil War in Oxfordshire, Buckinghamshire and Berkshire (1642–1646, *Proc. Excurs. Oxf. Arch. Hist. Soc.*, (New Series), 36:280–291. Clark, Sir George, Oxford and the Civil War, *Oxf. Pres. Trust. No. 1* (New Series). Varley, F. J. (1932): The Siege of Oxford. Clarendon Press, Oxford. Toynbee, Margaret, and Young, Peter (1973): *Strangers in Oxford*, Phillimore, Chichester, London. Lattey, R. T., Parsons, E. J. S., and Philip, I. G. (1936): "A contemporary map of the defences of Oxford in 1644. *Oxoniensia*, I:167.
4. Willis, T. (1674): *Pharmaceutice Rationalis*, "Of the Operations of Medicines on Humane Bodies," translated by S. Pordage, Pt. I, pp. 140–141.
5. Willis, T. (1672): *De Anima Brutorum*, translated by S. Pordage, "Two Discourses concerning the Soul of Brutes," p. 43.
6. Burrows, M. (1881): *Register of Visitors of the University of Oxford 1647–1658*, pp. lv. ff.
7. Foster, J. (1892): *Alumni Oxonienses*, Vol. IV, p. 288. Oxford.
8. Foster, J. (1892): *Alumni Oxonienses*, Vol. IV, p. 288, Oxford.
9. Wood, A. (1721): *Athenae Oxonienses*, 2nd ed., Vol. 2, p. 807.
10. Foster, J. (1892): *Alumni Oxonienses*, Vol. IV, p. 1650, Oxford.
11. Curtis, M. H. (1959): *Oxford and Cambridge in Transition, 1558–1642*, p. 153. Oxford.
12. New information on Willis and the Trinity group has been uncovered by Frank, R. G. (1973): John Aubrey FRS, John Lydall and Science at Commonwealth Oxford. *Notes and Rec. Roy. Soc. London*, 27:193–217.
13. Willis drew up a list of laboratory expenses at the end of his case book (1650–2) in Wellcome Library MS 799A ff. 48–9.
14. *Brief Lives Chiefly of Contemporaries, set down by John Aubrey 1669–1696*, Vol. I, p. 303, edited by A. Clark (1898), Oxford.
15. Wood, A. (1721): *Athenae Oxonienses*, 2nd ed., Vol. 2, p. 549.
16. Accounts of Petty are to be found in the following works: Fitzmaurice, E. (1895): *The Life of Sir William Petty*, pp. 6–21. London. Sharp, L. G. (1976): Sir William Petty and some aspects of 17th century Natural Philosophy, D. Phil. Thesis, Oxford University. Aubrey, J., *Brief Lives*, Vol. 2, p. 41. Strauss, E. (1954): *Sir William Petty. Portrait of a genius*, p. 31. Bodley Head, London.
17. Creighton, C. (1865): A History of Epidemics in Britain, AD 664–1666, Vol. I., p. 569.
18. Hierons, R. (1967): Willis's contribution to clinical medicine, *J. Neurol. Sci.*, 4:1–13.
19. Bates, D. G. (1965): Thomas Willis and the Epidemic Fever of 1661: a commentary. *Bull. Hist. Med.*, 39:393–414.
20. *Oxford Univ. Arch. Convocation Register 1659–71*, NEP/Supra/Register TA, pp. 369(v) and 370(v).
21. *Oxford Univ. Arch. Convocation Register 1659–71*, NEP/Supra/Register TA, p. 66.
22. *Oxford Univ. Statutes*, (1845): translated by G. R. M. Ward, Vol. I, p. 284.
23. Dr. Willis's Practice of Physick (1684): *The Anatomy of the Brain*, translated by S. Pordage, p. ii.
24. *Oxford Univ. Archives Convocation Register 1659–71*. NEP/Supra/Register TA, pp. 369(v) and 370(v).
25. *Oxford Univ. Statutes* (1845): translated by G. R. M. Ward, Vol. I, p. 22.
26. Willis, T. (1684): Preface to the Reader. In: *The Anatomy of the Brain*, Dr. Willis's Practice of Physick, translated by S. Pordage, p. i.
27. Roy. Soc. Lib., *Boyle Papers*, 19:ff.1–35.

28. Bod. Lib. MS Locke f.19. Published by Dewhurst, K. (1980): *Thomas Willis's Oxford Lectures*, Sandford Publications, Oxford.
29. Willis, T. (1684): Preface to the Reader. In: *The Anatomy of the Brain*, Dr. Willis's Practice of Physick, translated by S. Pordage, p. ii.
30. Willis T. (1684): Preface to the Reader. In: *The Anatomy of the Brain*, Dr. Willis's Practice of Physick, translated by S. Pordage, p. 1.
31. Clarke, E. (1968): Brain anatomy before Steno. In: *The Historical Aspects of Brain Research in the 17th Century*, edited by G. Scherz, pp. 27–34. Pergamon Press, Oxford.
32. Clarke, E., and O'Malley, C. D. (1968): *The Human Brain and Spinal Cord*, University of California Press, Berkeley.
33. Critchley, M. (1979): *The divine banquet of the brain*. Harveian Oration RCP, Raven Press, New York.
34. Meyer, A. (1971): *Historical Aspects of Cerebral Anatomy*, Oxford.
35. Clarke, E., and Dewhurst, K. (1972): *An Illustrated History of Brain Function.*, Oxford.
36. Willis, T. (1684): Epistle Dedicatory to His Grace Gilbert, Archbishop of Canterbury. In: *The Anatomy of the Brain*, translated by S. Pordage, p. i.
37. Willis, T. (1684): Epistle Dedicatory to His Grace Gilbert, Archbishop of Canterbury, etc. In: *The Anatomy of the Brain*, translated by S. Pordage, p. i.
38. Stubbe, H. (1670): *Censure upon Certain Passages contained in the History of the Royal Society; Legends no Histories;* and *Plus Ultra reduced to a Non Plus*.
39. Sydenham, T. (1848): *Works,*, edited by R. G. Latham, Vol. I, p. 102. Dewhurst, K. (1966): *Dr. Thomas Sydenham (1624–1689), His Life and Writings*, p. 64, Wellcome Historical Library, London.
40. Willis, T. (1684): Epistle Dedicatory to His Grace Gilbert, Archbishop of Canterbury. In: *The Anatomy of the Brain*, translated by S. Pordage, p. 11.
41. Reviewed by Davis, A. B. : *Circulatory Physiology and Medical Chemistry in England 1650–80*. Coronado Press, Lawrence.
42. Willis, T. (1684): *The Anatomy of the Brain*, translated by S. Pordage, p. 88.
43. Browne, T. (1836): *Sir Thomas Browne's Works*, edited by S. Wilkin, Vol. I, p. 217. London.
44. Power, Sir D'Arcy (1931): John Ward and his Diary. In: *Selected Writings 1877–1930*, p. 190. Clarendon Press, Oxford.
45. Willis, T. (1684): *The Anatomy of the Brain*, translated by S. Pordage, p. 91.
46. Willis, T. (1684): *The Anatomy of the Brain*, translated by S. Pordage, Summary of pp. 91–116.
47. Clarke, E. (1978):The neural circulation. The use of analogy in medicine, *Med. Hist.*, 22:291–307.
48. Willis, T. (1684): *The Anatomy of the Brain*, translated by S. Pordage, p. 127.
49. Willis, T. (1684): *The Anatomy of the Brain*, translated by S. Pordage, pp. 116–173.
50. Willis, T. (1684): *The Anatomy of the Brain*, pp. 147–182. See also Ackerknecht, E. H., (1974): The history of the discovery of the vegetative (autonomic) nervous system. *Med. Hist.*, 18:1–8. See also, Hierons, R., and Meyer, A. (1962): Some priority questions arising from Thomas Willis's work on the brain. *Proc. Roy. Soc. Med.*, 55:287–292.
51. Hierons, R., and Meyer, A. (1962): Observations on the history of the "Circle of Willis," *Med. Hist.*, 6:119–130.
52. Willis, T. (1684): *The Anatomy of the Brain*, translated by S. Pordage, pp. 82–83.
53. Surveyed by Temkin, O. (1971): *The Falling Sickness*, 2nd ed., pp. 205–209. Johns Hopkins Press, Baltimore.
54. Willis's views have been the subject of scholarly surveys by Hierons, R., and Meyer, A. (1968): Willis's place in the history of muscle physiology, *Proc. Roy. Soc. Med.*, 57:687–692. Idem (1965): On Thomas Willis's concepts of neurophysiology, *Med. Hist.*, 9:1–5, 142–155.
55. Meyer, A., and Hierons, R. (1964): A note on Thomas Willis's views on the corpus striatum and the internal capsule. *J. Neurol. Sci.*, 1:547–554.
56. *Le Journal des Savans* (1665–7): DL'An MDCLXV par le Sieur de Hedouville, Paris.
57. Birch, T. (1756): *History of the Royal Society*, Vol. I, p. 421. London.
58. Goodall, C. (1676): *The College of Physicians Vindicated and the True State of Physick in this Nation Faithfully Represented*, p. 90. London.
59. Plot, R. (1677): *Natural History of Oxfordshire*, p. 302, Oxford.
60. Cole, W. (1689): *A Physico-medical Essay Concerning the Late Frequency of Apoplexies*, p. 17. London.
61. Steno, N. (1665): *A Dissertation on the Anatomy of the Brain*, pp. 17–37. (Reprinted, Nit Nordisk Forlag Copenhagen, 1950).
62. Stubbe, H. (1670): *The Plus Ultra reduced to a Non Plus*, p. 95. London.
63. Stubbe, H. (1670): *The Plus Ultra reduced to a Non Plus*, p. 173.
64. Wood, A. (1817): *Athenae Oxonienses*, edited by P. Bliss, Vol. III, p. 1051. London.
65. Willis, B. (1817): Letter to Bishop Kennet. In: ref. 64, pp. 1048–1053.
66. Clark, A., editor (1892): *The Life and Times of Anthony Wood*, Vol. I, p. 428, Oxford.
67. Clark, A. (1892): *The Life and Times of Anthony Wood*, Vol. I, pp. 290, 410, 428, 473; Vol. II, pp. 2, 4, 12, 13, 30, 42, 44, and 172. Oxford.
68. Hutchinson, B. (1799): *Biographia Medica*, Vol. 2, p. 484. London.
69. Munk, W. (1861): *The Role of the Roy. Coll. of Physicians of London*, Vol. 1, p. 380. London.

70. Foster, M. (1901): *Lectures on the History of Physiology*, p. 270. London.
71. Franklin, K. J. (1939): The works of Richard Lower (1631–1691). *Proc. Roy. Soc. Med.*, 25:113–118.
72. Cole, F. J. (1944): *A History of Comparative Anatomy*, p. 222. London.
73. Mettler, C. C. (1947): In: *History of Medicine*, edited by F. A. P. Mettler, Blakiston, Toronto.
74. See Dewhurst, K. (1962): Locke's contribution to Boyle's researches on the air and on human blood, *Notes Rec. Roy. Soc. London*, 17:2, 198.
75. Willis's preliminary letters concerning the purchase have been published in Dewhurst, K. (1972): Some letters of Dr. Thomas Willis (1621–1675). *Med. Hist.*, 16:63–76; the Abstract of Title of Burlton Court in Hereford County Record Office K9/4, dated 21/22 January 1662/3.
76. Willis, T. (1684): *The Anatomy of the Brain*, translated by S. Pordage, p. i–ii.
77. Willis, T. (1684): *The Anatomy of the Brain*, translated by S. Pordage, p. ii.
78. Warton, T. (1761): *The Life and Literary Remains of Ralph Bathurst etc.*, pp. 40–41. Oxford.
79. Warton, T. (1761): *The Life and Literary Remains of Ralph Bathurst etc.*, p. 218. Oxford.
80. Hooke, R. (1665): *Micrographia*, pref., p. 10.
81. Robinson, H. W., and Adams, W., editors (1935): *The Diary of Robert Hooke (1672–1680)*, p. 47.
82. *Transcript of John Ward's Diary (1648–1678)*, Vol. IV, p. 868. Med. Soc. London.
83. Birch, T., editor (1772): *The Works of the Hon. Robert Boyle* (New Ed.), Vol. 6, pp. 462–463.
84. Birch, T., editor (1772): *The Works of the Hon. Robert Boyle*. (New Ed.), Vol. 6, p. 465.
85. Birch, T., editor (1772): *The Works of the Hon. Robert Boyle*. (New Ed.), Vol. 6, p. 466.
86. Birch, T., editor (1772): *The Works of the Hon. Robert Boyle*. (New Ed.), Vol. 6, pp. 466–468.
87. Birch, T., editor (1772): *The Works of the Hon. Robert Boyle*. (New Ed.), Vol. 6, p. 474.
88. Willis, T. (1684): *The Anatomy of the Brain*, translated by S. Pordage, p. 192.
89. Willis, T. (1684): *The Anatomy of the Brain*, translated by S. Pordage, p. 192.

Historical Aspects of the Neurosciences,
edited by F. Clifford Rose and W. F. Bynum.
Raven Press, New York ©

The Neurological Tradition of Charing Cross Hospital

T. J. Steiner, Rudy Capildeo, and F. Clifford Rose

Department of Neurology, Charing Cross Hospital, London W6, England

In 1290, Eleanor of Castile, wife of Edward I, died after a long illness at Harby, near Lincoln. The dutiful king, the "English Justinian," built in her memory a sculptured cross at every resting place of the funeral procession to Westminster. Each was of splendid design and execution, but the finest and most stately rose midway between the towns of London and Westminster at the final station, the village of Charing.

The details of the design of old Charing cross are now unknown. Withstanding poorly the passage of time and described in 1590 as an "old weather-beaten monument," it was finally sentenced in 1643 (1):

The Parliament to vote it down
    Conceived it very fitting,
For fear it should fall and kill them all
    In the house as they were sitting.

The cross now standing in the forecourt of Charing Cross station is little more than 100 years old. In 1864, when it was built, The Royal West London Infirmary and Lying-In Institution had been open for nearly 50 years. This was the origin of Charing Cross Hospital (Fig. 1), to which its name was soon changed, founded alongside some of the meanest and most squalid slums in London, the habitat of all manner of crooks, pimps, and prostitutes (3). "The full tide of existence is at Charing Cross," thought Dr. Johnson, and it still is.

The hospital has shown a greater readiness to change (Fig. 2) than many aspects of its environment north of the Strand. The Poor Law Infirmary and Workhouse that became Fulham Hospital (Fig. 3) was attached to the Charing Cross Hospital in 1957 and with it the West London Hospital (Fig. 4) to form the Charing Cross Group. The village of Charing now has neither Eleanor's cross nor its hospital, but the latter is alive and well (Fig. 5) in Fulham.

The concept of medical specialities, from which the hospital practice of neurology arose, was invented at Charing Cross by the innovative engagement of Mr. Charles Toplis as Medico-Chirurgical Electrician; this appointment of a "Gentleman of great respectability, education and science" (4) was specifically aimed to develop the uses of electrophysiology in patients, a possibility engendered by Galvani's demonstration of electrical activity in the nervous system. "The wide field for observation which this Charity presents will it is

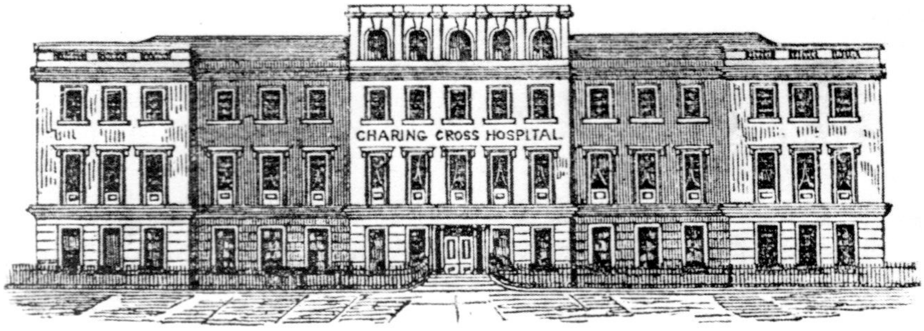

CHARING CROSS HOSPITAL,
1834.

FIG. 1. The Charing Cross Hospital, 1834. [Reproduced from Hunter, W. (1914): *Historical Account of Charing Cross Hospital and Medical School.* John Murray, London.]

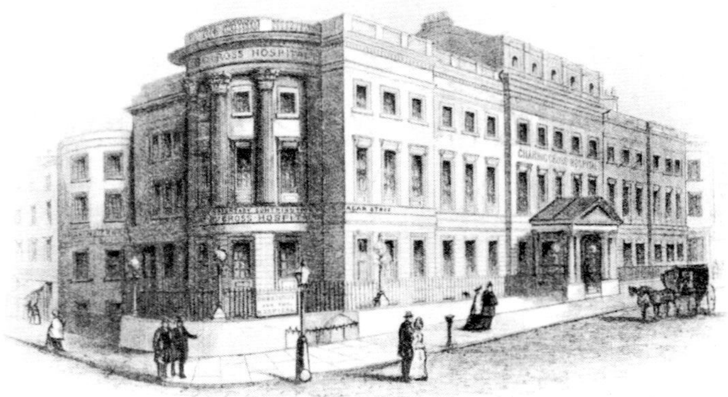

CHARING CROSS HOSPITAL, 1865.

FIG. 2. The Charing Cross Hospital, 1865. [Reproduced from Hunter, W. (1914): *Historical Account of Charing Cross Hospital and Medical School.* John Murray, London.]

presumed afford ample opportunity for ascertaining the curative instrumentality of the electrical fluid and for forming a correct estimate of its relative efficacy in the treatment of different classes of diseases and functional disarrangements" (4).

There were no true neurologists for a long time at any of the London hospitals, or elsewhere. The study of diseases of the nervous system depended upon the occasional interest of general physicians who undertook the care of those afflicted with lunacy. Charing Cross Hospital, sited as it was, offering free care to the poor from the time of its foundation, had an ideal catchment to encourage and promote the interest of committed doctors of the time, outstanding men such as Rowland and Mott.

Graduating from Edinburgh in 1827, the year that Charing Cross Hospital gained its present name, Richard Rowland was a lecturer in medicine from 1845. While at Charing

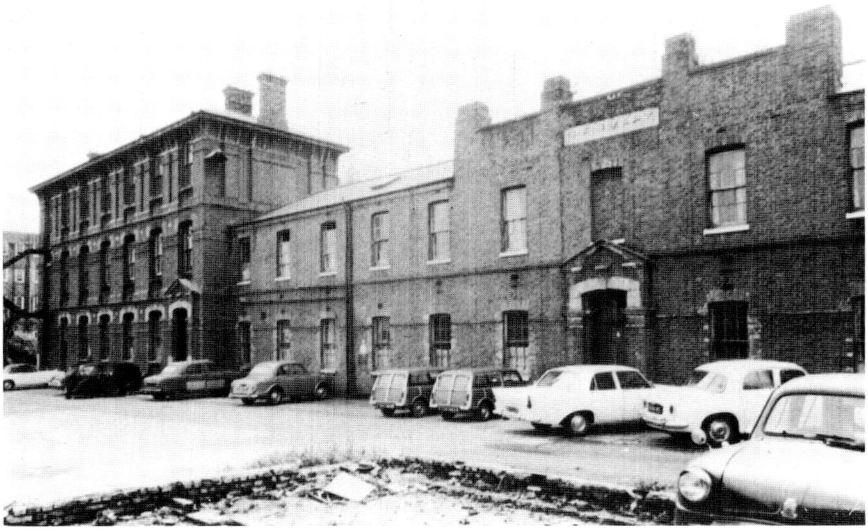

FIG. 3. The Poor Law Infirmary and Workhouse, Fulham, later Fulham Hospital.

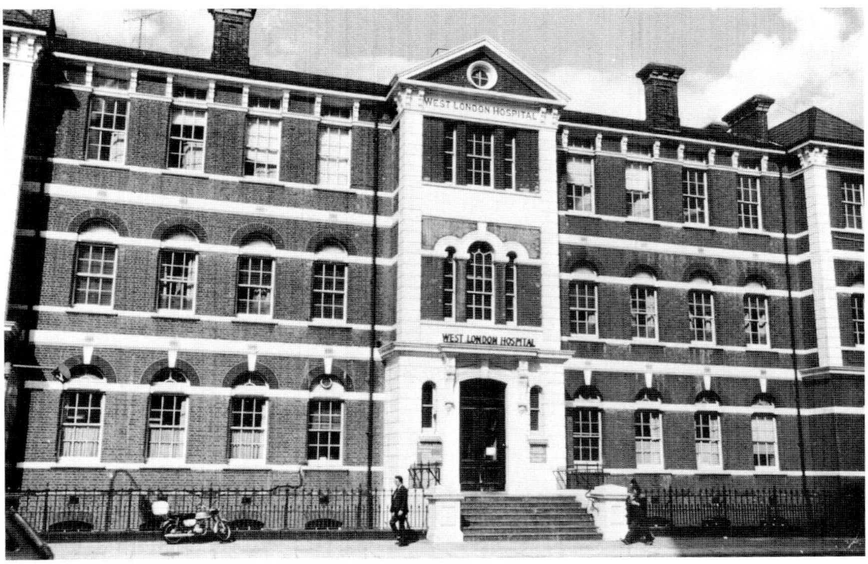

FIG. 4. The West London Hospital.

Cross, he published his treatise on softening of the brain. Sir Frederick Mott (Fig. 6), a neurophysiologist as well as clinician, worked with Sherrington on the function of the dorsal roots. Later, he studied the cerebral localization of visual pathways and the bilateral connections of the auditory pathways; he was outstanding in the study of organic dementias and the therapy of insanity, and he demonstrated the link between GPI and syphilis. Undoubtedly his achievements fostered the emergence of neurology as a discipline separate from psychiatry. He gained many honors in his lifetime apart from his Knighthood, and

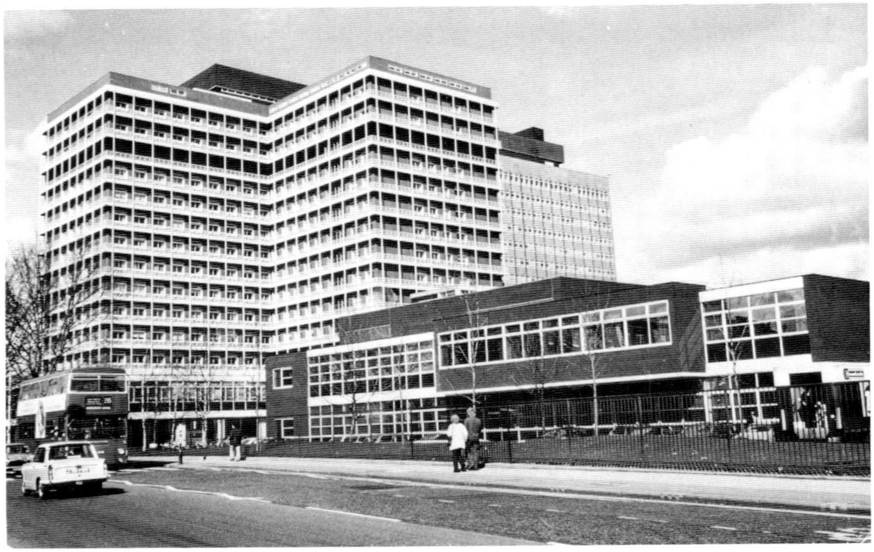

FIG. 5. The Charing Cross Hospital, 1980.

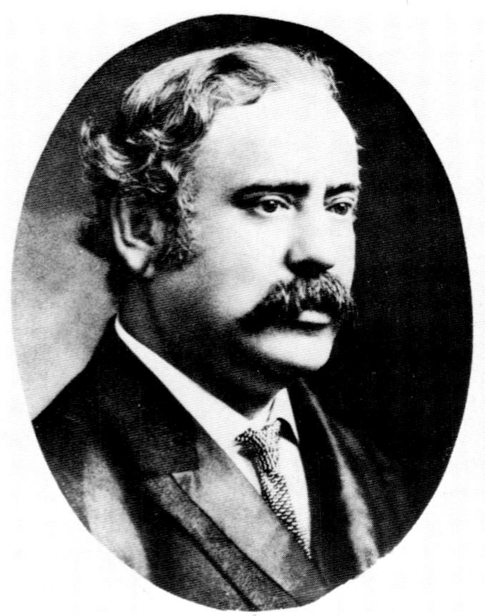

FIG. 6. Sir Frederick Walker Mott, K.B E., M.D., F.R.C.P., F.R.S. (1853–1926).

was a Fellow of the Royal Society. While Pathologist to the London County Asylums for much of the same time and Fullerian Professor of Physiology at the Royal Institution, he spent altogether 29 years of his productive life at Charing Cross Hospital, a lecturer successively on physiology, pathology and medicine and, finally, Senior Physician.

Sir David Ferrier (Fig. 7), an assistant physician to the West London Hospital early in his career, was a different sort of man. Graduating with first-class honors from Aberdeen University in classics and philosophy, he studied psychology in Heidelberg for a year before undertaking medical training at Edinburgh to qualify in 1868. His M.D. thesis on the corpora

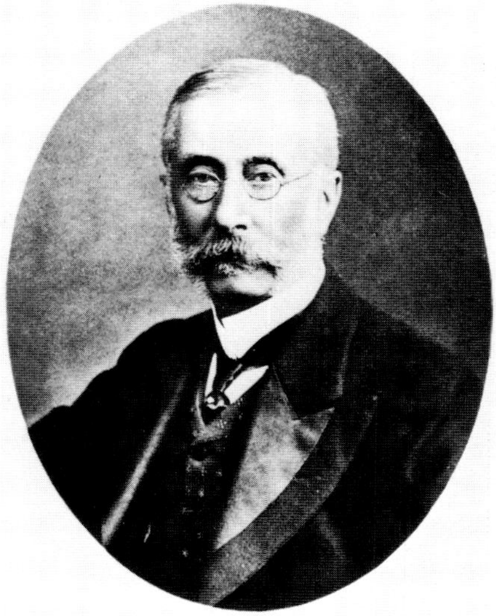

FIG. 7. Sir David Ferrier, M.A., M.D., F.R.S., F.R.C.P., F.R.C.P.I. (1843–1928).

quadrigemina was presented two years later while he worked as a general practitioner, and after that he came to London to lecture in physiology. Primarily a scientist all his life, he was never, perhaps, an outstanding clinician in those days when medicine was so much an art. Nevertheless, his patients were no doubt sufficiently impressed by the tall silk hat and black tailcoat in which he confronted them on ward rounds. Seen now as the link between Hughlings Jackson and Sherrington, Ferrier became a foremost neurophysiologist and enthusiastic experimenter on animals. His major, and possibly revolutionary, studies on cerebral localization of function were carried out during the years immediately before the Cruelty to Animals Act of 1876 became law. His own experimental accounts, in which stimulated animals somersault backwards off the operating table, do not encourage the belief that all of these could later have been repeated. At any rate, the antivivisectionists of the day brought him unsuccessfully to court in an action that gained him fame outside scientific circles.

Thomas Grainger Stewart (Fig. 8) was born a year after Sir Gordon Holmes (see Chapter 36), whose appointments included being general physician at Charing Cross Hospital. Grainger Stewart was at West London Hospital, where he was on the staff for 28 years, but the two were colleagues at the National Hospital for the Paralysed and Epileptic and, early in their careers, wrote conjointly on connections and tumors of the cerebellum—until the day they came to blows with coats off and were never friends again. Grainger Stewart's associations with the National Hospital lasted 40 years, and he was also neurologist for the Ministry of Pensions. He spent much time in shooting parties and deer stalking and was obliviously unhurried. If this was a fault, he undoubtedly shared it with Aldren Turner, with whom he published a *Textbook of Nervous Diseases* very soon after his appointment to the West London.

William Aldren Turner (Fig. 9) indeed was noted for interminable ward rounds, his juniors being instructed in every detail with punctilious care. He was assistant physician to West London Hospital from 1893 and also Medical Electrician, as Toplis had been at Charing Cross over half a century earlier. Aldren Turner had been assistant to Ferrier at King's College, London, and was later at King's College Hospital. He became an expert on epilepsy,

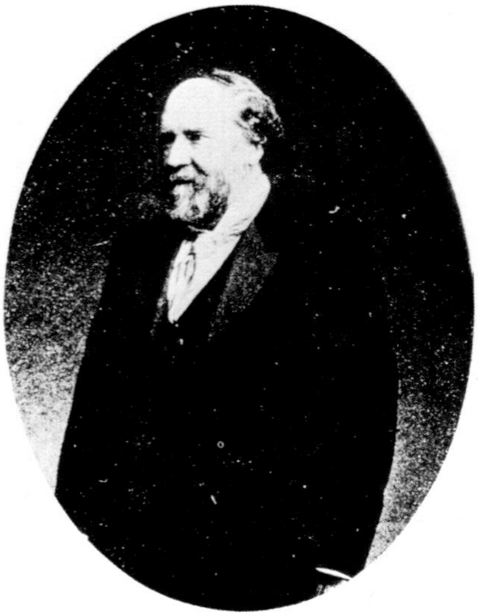

FIG. 8. Thomas Grainger Stewart, M.D, M.R.C.P.E., F.R.C.P. (1877–1957).

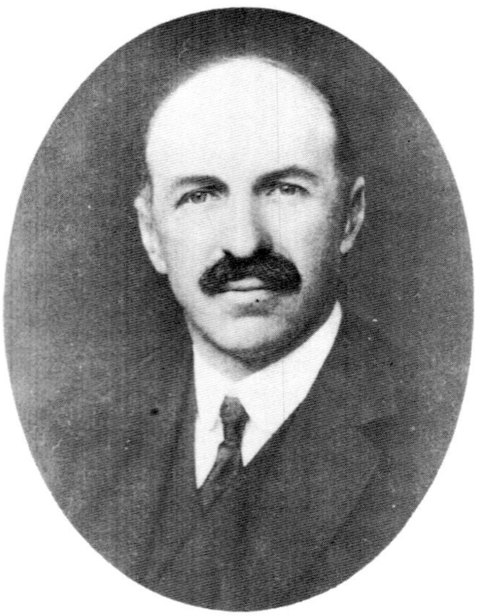

FIG. 9. William Aldren Turner, C.B., M.D., F.R.C.P. (1864–1945).

and his book on the subject, first published over 70 years ago, has been republished recently. He was neurologist to the Home Forces during the First World War, and his Bradshaw Lectures to the Royal College of Physicians of London in 1918 described his experiences of the neuroses and psychoses of war. Whereas Grainger Stewart had little merit as a teacher, Turner applied to the instruction of his students the same methodical and lucid qualities that made him, it was said, an excellent chairman of committees.

Neurological surgery was a specialty at West London Hospital even in its early days, promoted by the appointment of two assistant surgeons who had worked with the pioneer, Victor Horsley. Later to become the first President of the Society of British Neurological Surgeons, Sir Charles Ballance (Fig. 10) was appointed in 1888. Slow and extremely painstaking, Ballance was nonetheless a courageous operator. He was one of the first to

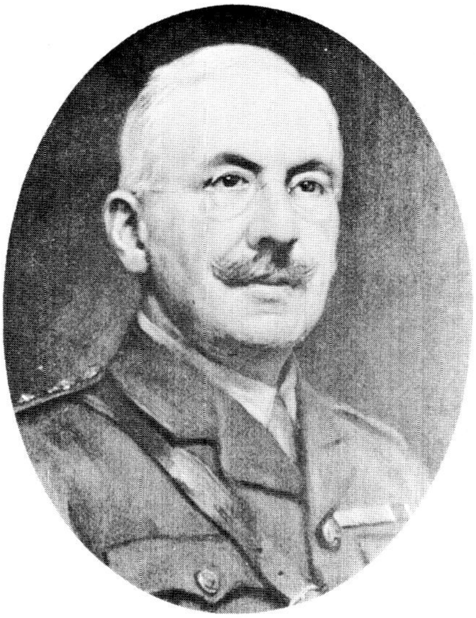

FIG. 10. Sir Charles Ballance, K.C.M.G., C.B., M.V.O., M.S., F.R.C.S. (1856–1936).

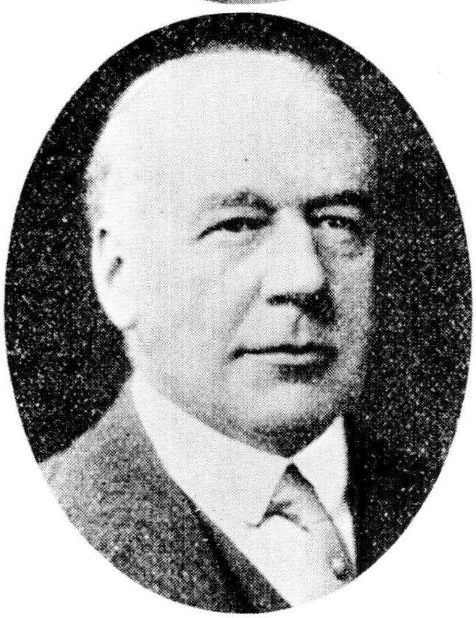

FIG. 11. Donald Armour, C.M.G., M.R.C.P., F.R.C.S. (1868–1933).

perform radical mastoidectomy with ligation of the jugular vein and also one of the first to graft the facial nerve. He had assisted when Horsley, then aged 30, performed the first operation for removal of a spinal tumor. When the lesion was not found at the expected level even after several vertebral laminae had been removed, it was Ballance who persuaded Horsley to go one segment still higher, where a benign tumor was found hiding. It is also recorded that the patient did well.

Donald Armour (Fig. 11), though appointed to West London Hospital 15 years after Ballance, had also regularly assisted Horsley and was particularly interested in surgery of the spinal cord. Later, he was surgeon and Dean of the West London Postgraduate School. Another prolific writer, with enormous energy and capacity for work, he held high office in many learned societies. In 1933, having given his official report as Honorary Treasurer at the Medical Society of London, he resumed his seat, was taken suddenly ill, and died immediately.

The son of the Chief Justice of Ontario, Armour had been one of several eminent men attracted from the colonies to Charing Cross or its associated hospitals. William Adie (Fig. 12) was born in South Australia, though it was in Edinburgh that he won the McCosh Scholarship and in Germany that he gained a gold medal for his M.D. thesis. A medical registrar at Charing Cross Hospital after active service during the First World War, he was appointed to the staff there in 1926. Adie was noted as an exceptional clinician, and teacher as well. He wrote widely on aspects of neurology before his early death at the age of 48. The syndrome of myotonic pupils and areflexia bearing his name, narcolepsy, the subject of his M.D. thesis, optic neuritis, disseminated sclerosis, pituitary tumors, and muscular dystrophy all came within his compass.

Samuel Alexander Kinnier Wilson (Fig. 13) was born in New Jersey but, like Adie, graduated in medicine in Edinburgh and continued his studies in Germany. He was a student of Babinski and of Pierre Marie. His M.D. thesis, again like Adie's, gained him a gold medal. Once he was asked by Denny-Brown for his opinion on the essential aspects of hepatolenticular degeneration. Turning up the lapels of his coat, Wilson had no difficulty replying: "Do you mean 'Kinnier Wilson's Disease'?" (2).

Wilson was at Queen Square from his days as house physician onward, the association beginning in 1904. The Guardians of Fulham Hospital, aiming to provide a panel of consultants, appointed him visiting neurologist in 1920 and paid him two guineas for each of his fortnightly sessions. Increasingly a man with little spare time, in the same year he founded and was editor of the *Journal of Neurology and Psychopathology*. He lived only to the age of 59, when cancer terminated both his huge textbook and his other distinguished writings, in which he had discoursed upon the epilepsies, disorders of motility and muscle tone, apraxia, aphasia, and epidemic encephalitis. He had been overpowering in every sense, given to skillful employment of histrionics. A patient whose signs had baffled him was peremptorily instructed to leave Kinnier Wilson his brain upon his death.

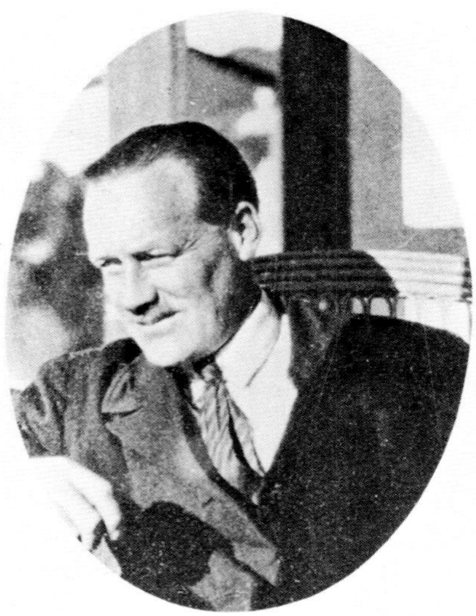

FIG. 12. William John Adie, M.D., F.R.C.P. (1886–1935).

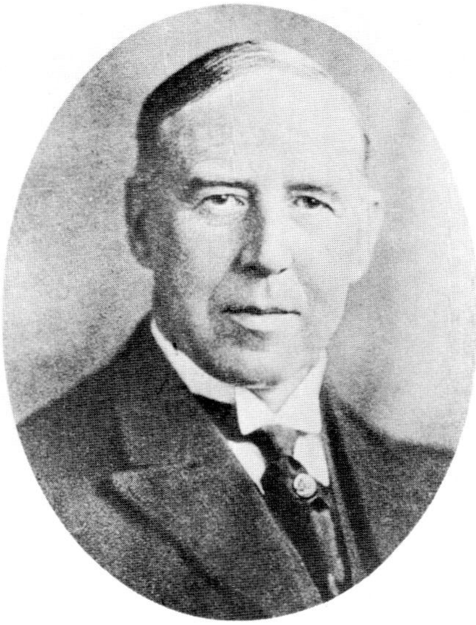

FIG. 13. Samuel Alexander Kinnier Wilson, A.M., M.D., D.Sc., F.R.C.P. (1878–1937).

Redvers Nowell Ironside, President of the Neurological Section of the Royal Society of Medicine in 1956, was neurologist at different times to both the West London Hospital and Charing Cross. Russell John Reynolds, the first radiologist appointed to the National Hospital for Nervous Diseases, Queen Square, came later to Charing Cross. The list could go on,

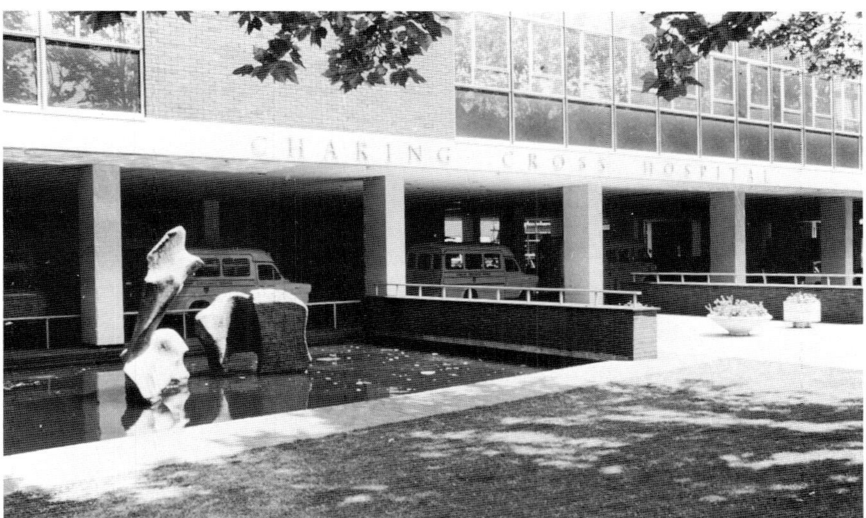

FIG. 14. The Charing Cross Hospital, 1980: main entrance.

tracing the development of neurology itself, but this can only be a brief glance at the neurological tradition of the Charing Cross Group of Hospitals (Fig. 14), founded by Dr. Benjamin Golding 165 years ago to treat the poorest sick of London.

ACKNOWLEDGMENTS

We are very grateful to the Department of Medical Illustration, Charing Cross Hospital, for their careful reproduction of some aging photographs and for providing the originals for Figs. 3, 4, 5, and 14.

REFERENCES

1. Galloway, J. (1914): *Historical Sketches of Old Charing: the Hospital and Chapel of Saint Mary Roncevall*, p. 79. John Bale, Sons and Danielsson, London.
2. Haymaker, W., and Schiller, F. (1970): *The Founders of Neurology*, 2nd ed., pp. 535–539. Charles C Thomas, Springfield, Illinois.
3. Minney, R. J. (1967): *The Two Pillars of Charing Cross*. Cassell and Co., London.
4. (1821): Minutes of the Committee of Management, Royal West London Infirmary and Lying-In Institution, Charing Cross, p. 46.

Historical Aspects of the Neurosciences,
edited by F. Clifford Rose and W. F. Bynum.
Raven Press, New York ©

Sir Gordon Holmes

B. Gerald Parsons-Smith

Department of Neurology, Charing Cross Hospital; West End Hospital for Nervous Diseases; Western Ophthalmic Hospital (St. Mary's), London, England

Gordon Morgan Holmes was born in Dublin on February 22, 1876, the first child of Gordon Holmes and his wife Kathleen (née Morgan). There were three brothers and three sisters. The Holmes family were Protestants from Yorkshire who had settled in Ireland in the mid-17th century. They lived at Dellin House, Castle Bellingham, some 40 miles to the north of Dublin. Gordon was a solitary enclosed boy whose most deeply rooted characteristic of shyness was reinforced by his grief at his mother's early death and his father's remarriage. He was happiest roaming the countryside, often on a pony, and from an early age he took a great interest in wildlife. His father, a prosperous farmer, decided that in the school holidays his son should work on the farm, and he arranged for a carpenter to teach him how to make gates, wheels, and carts, a skill he used in later life when his hobby was making furniture. For some time he was dyslexic, but he overcame this, and his village schoolmaster considered him very intelligent. He passed the entrance examination to the Dundalk Educational Institute with ease, where he completed his schooling as a boarder. Going up to Trinity College, Dublin, he intended to read classics or mathematics, but a last minute change of mind decided him on natural sciences. So it was that he became a medical student, graduating in 1897 at the age of 21 years.

In his first appointment as clinical assistant at the Richmond Asylum in Dublin, he did so well that he was awarded the Stewart Scholarship in mental and nervous disease, which enabled him to go to Germany to study neuroanatomy. But before this, he went to New Zealand, working his passage as ship's surgeon. Returning home by way of South Africa, where a crisis had developed, he volunteered to work for the British and was granted an interview with Cecil Rhodes to finalize arrangements. Fatefully, however, a few hours before the meeting was to take place, he was commanded to return instantly to his ship, which had been ordered to leave South African waters to avoid further involvement in the Boer War that had just broken out.

He spent the next two years in Frankfurt studying comparative and human anatomy under Ludwig Edinger and Karl Weigert. His start there was unpropitious. Edinger told him to make a drawing of a spinal cord section, and he spent two days on the task, but Edinger considered his finished effort to be careless and tore it up in front of him; eventually, he was successful but only at the eighth attempt. Thereafter, all went well for Holmes, and Edinger thought so highly of him that he was entrusted with the histological study of Goltz's dog without a forebrain, some 10 years after it had been killed, and Holmes's beautiful colored drawings of these sections illustrate his 1901 paper. He was now fluent in German and was offered the post of assistant neurologist, which he declined, as acceptance would have required him to take German nationality.

Edinger advised Holmes to turn to clinical neurology, recommended him for a vacancy at the National Hospital, and gave him letters of introduction to Gowers and Horsley. Holmes sent in his application and subsequently called on Gowers during his dinnertime. The interview took place in the hall. Gowers, annoyed at being disturbed and with his napkin in hand, was brusque, told him that he was not good enough, and bade him good day With only an hour or so before the boat train left for Ireland, and feeling very despondent, he called on Horsley, who could not have been more friendly. He was enthusiastic over Holmes's work in Germany, and the result was his appointment as House Physician to Hughlings Jackson, a wonderful opportunity. Many of the skills of the father of British neurology were to rub off onto the young Irishman. He learnt the necessity for careful and thorough clinical examination, something which years later he was to tell his students at Charing Cross that he had learnt from Jackson. He also practiced the examination of the eye, including ophthalmoscopy, which Jackson demanded in every neurological examination. Thirteen years later, he was appointed to Moorfields Eye Hospital.

Fortuitously at the National Hospital, Queen Square, there were several Scotsmen, of whom five were to influence Holmes in one way or another. The first was Grainger Stewart; Holmes and Stewart wrote their first paper together (1904) on the symptoms of cerebellar tumors. During that year Stewart, junior to Holmes and nearly two years younger, passed the examination of M. R. C. P. of London, a sine qua non for a consultant appointment but which Holmes did not hold. For the next few years, Holmes worked on a neuroanatomical study of the connections of the cerebellum while Stewart continued clinical work and spent considerable time away from Queen Square engaged in field sports. Among other interests in the country, Stewart was an excellent shot and became a well-known deer stalker; indeed a dangerous path high up in the tops of the Cairngorms was known as the Doctors Walk after him. Their second paper, which was dedicated to Edinger, appeared in 1908 but must have been written by Holmes, since only he possessed the neuroanatomical expertise which it required; however, the credit was shared. Shortly afterward in the same year, Stewart was elected to the staff at Queen Square, so there was every reason for Holmes to be resentful. They became quite incompatible, and a fierce mutual dislike developed, which they never resolved.

Leslie Paton, a scholarly ophthalmic surgeon who came from a cultured Edinburgh background, became a lifelong friend. He had studied botany in Berlin and at Cambridge. Of their many joint publications, their histological study of papilloedema was the most important. With another distinguished Scot, James Taylor, whom he later described as "my loyal friend," he collaborated on the nervous symptoms associated with familial optic atrophy.

Sir David Ferrier had many attributes that appealed to Holmes. A breezy dapper Scot, well established in 34 Cavendish Square with his family, he was an expert in animal neurology, a pioneer of cerebral localization, and a lover of the sea. He had written his M. D. thesis on the corpora quadrigemina while in general practice in Bury St. Edmunds. Holmes, whose own ward rounds were to last for some three hours, disapproved of Ferrier, who would rush from bed to bed not even finding the time to remove his silk top hat. Nor for that matter did he approve of Beevor's rounds, which were not considered popular as they lasted for more than four hours.

The fifth of these influential Scots was Aldren Turner, some six years older than Holmes and the son of the distinguished anatomist Sir William Turner. He had described, with Ferrier, the rhythmical tremor associated with damage to the superior peduncles. He lived at 18 Harley Street, knew London and its history well, and was an authority on the benefits, or otherwise, that might be expected from the various English and Continental spas, then used by the fashionable neurologists and cardiologists.

At the age of 30, Holmes was appointed Director of Research at Queen Square. His reputation for teaching neuroanatomy had spread to other hospitals and from them he received requests for his opinion in difficult cases; there was also some demand for a view of his complete series of sections of the human spinal cord, which he had prepared in Frankfurt. He was not afraid to voice his opinion even when it differed from those senior to him. Risien Russell, another who had been trained in Edinburgh (but was not a Scot), had studied sections from a puppy suffering from what he considered to be a degenerative process and on this account went on to conclude that the olivocerebellar fibers terminated in the dentate nuclei and not in the cerebellar cortex. Holmes explained that this was a fallacy; the disorder was not a degenerative process, and he recognized it to be a rare developmental anomaly.

He collaborated with Page May in a neuroanatomical project to determine the exact origin of the pyramidal tracts in man, monkey, and chimpanzee. The work was carried out mainly by Holmes, as May, who was an invalid, was forced to leave University College Hospital every winter for Egypt where, at Helwan on the Nile, he had built up a consultant neurological practice; the poor man died suddenly one summer in Brighton fuming with rage at seeing a carrier ill treat his horse.

A happier collaboration was that with Frederick Poynton, whose life interest was rheumatism. Their paper on the pathology of chorea was illustrated by Holmes's photographs of diplococci within the cortex of affected children. Poynton considered that this organism was the cause of acute rheumatism, a view which led to considerable controversy. Poynton was a family man, loved the country, and was at one time Senior Censor at the Royal College of Physicians. He is unique in that, after being elected F. R. C. P. when aged 34, he was subsequently elected playing captain of the Somerset Cricket Club. He was also a pioneer motorist, and Holmes, too, became a keen car owner and drove in motor trials. He eventually owned an Armstrong Siddeley Special, an elegant sports car, in which he competed in hill climbs, crashing on one occasion on the final bend but without himself suffering any damage.

Holmes's introduction to pediatric neurology came through Frederick Batten, when together they wrote a paper on ataxic dogs, another on progressive muscular atrophy of infants, and a third on the spinal cords of three children who had died of poliomyelitis. Batten was only 53 when he died in 1918. His wife, Jean, later became godmother to Gordon Holmes's daughter, Kathleen.

Holmes and James Collier knew each other well following their collaboration twice on amyatonia congenita. Both were superb artists in clinical demonstration, with a common interest in archeology and a love for travel. Collier had spent three years traveling around as a medical attendant to one of Sir William Gowers's wealthy patients, and his experiences rekindled Gordon Holmes's wanderlust. He had come to realize that there would not be a vacancy for him on the staff at Queen Square and that he had no alternative but to return to Dublin, where they wanted him. But before that, he was determined to undertake some form of overseas adventure, and his meeting with Capt. Robert Scott, the antarctic explorer, was certainly contrived. Then two chance happenings determined his future. First, he ruptured his Achilles tendon, which laid him up for several weeks and gave him the opportunity to read for his M. R. C. P. which in due course he obtained in 1908. A few months later, in December, Charles Beevor died suddenly of coronary thrombosis, at the age of only 54. Possessing the membership, Holmes was now eligible to apply for the vacancy on the staff, and was elected by a single vote. At the meeting, Hughlings Jackson, then aged 74, was too deaf to hear the committee's discussion about the candidates, and he inquired to his neighbor for whom should he vote. James Taylor wrote on a scrap of paper "HOLMES," and so a physician who was to make so many contributions to neurology was appointed to Queen Square. Having been promoted and because his work with Henry Head was not yet completed, Holmes felt impelled to withdraw from Capt. Scott's expedition. So it was with regret that he was at the quayside in 1910 to wave good-bye to the *Terra Nova* as she set sail on her journey, from which the five men who reached the South Pole never returned.

Consultants in those days gave their services free to voluntary hospitals, so without private means it was necessary for Holmes to start a private practice. After a spell in New Cavendish Street, he moved to 58 Harley Street. Starting a practice entailed a risk, and it sometimes failed. When Thomas Horder, later Lord Horder, already on the staff of St. Bartholomews Hospital, commenced at 141 Harley Street, he averaged only one patient a fortnight for a considerable time, and it was not until he had been in consulting practice for five years that he worked up to a patient a day. As it turned out, Holmes's start was more encouraging.

In Edwardian times, consultants enjoyed their leisure and took long summer holidays. Holmes always took two months away from London, which he generally spent at the family home in Ireland. There he worked on the farm, visited his many Irish friends, and acted as coach to the village tug-of-war team. In one year, his team reached the all Ireland final in Dublin, only to be beaten there by the police. Country house parties were a popular way of entertaining friends, and hostesses constantly cast their eyes around for eligible bachelors such as the tall good-looking Dr. Gordon Holmes to make up their numbers. On one weekend, Gordon and Henry Head were staying with Victor Horsley. Joined by Ernest Starling, the four of them played bowls until dinnertime, and again afterward, in an effort to develop a theory of Head's on how greater accuracy in the game could be achieved, and the game continued by the light of the acetylene headlamps of their motorcars until long after their customary bedtime.

It was Charles Beevor who had introduced Holmes to the pleasures of rowing on the Thames. Francis Walshe related that every Friday before Whitsun, Gordon would go to Oxford with three of his residents, hire a skiff at Folly Bridge, and row with them downstream to Staines, staying nights during the weekend at Wallingford and Hurley, so that he knew this stretch of the river intimately. Walshe shared these halcyon days for three successive years. They had picnics in the banks, walked across the fields to Dorchester Abbey, for which Holmes loved to act as a guide, and spent the days in wide-ranging talk as they rowed.

Gordon Holmes and Henry Head had met together weekly for five years before they published their important work in 1911 on the sensory disturbances from cerebral lesions. Holmes's contribution was his precision as an observer, which fitted in well with Head's theoretical flair and so made him an ideal collaborator. There had been one flaw in the earlier studies by Head and Rivers, namely, that the anatomical pathways essential to the system as envisaged by them had not all been provided by nature. Holmes devised the many quantitative methods of sensory testing employed, thus enabling him to link the results with his incomparable knowledge of anatomy.

By the summer of 1914, Holmes had built up a flourishing private practice. He was on the staff of four London hospitals and had, since qualification, published 55 papers, 17 of them in *Brain*. The First World War broke out in August 1914. Holmes applied for a commission in the RAMC but was rejected on account of myopia. Determined to serve in France, he and Percy Sargent, a colleague at Queen Square, joined the staff of a Red Cross hospital just behind the front line. Sargent was an experienced general surgeon with a special interest in brain surgery. He was a witty, debonaire, and generous man. Holmes described his surgical techniques as rapid and dextrous to an amazing degree. The results of their treatment of brain and spinal trauma were so successful that the War Office was aroused, revoked Holmes's disqualification, and appointed him Consultant Neurologist to the British Armies in France. He and Sargent set up their neurosurgical unit in No. 13 General Hospital, where they were to carry out the work for which they became famous throughout the medical world (Fig. 1).

Harvey Cushing, that dynamic American surgeon, described his visit to their unit in 1915 and his amazement at the overwhelming number of head and spinal wounds under their care. He considered their hospital uncomfortable, understaffed, and the medical records totally inadequate. There were 900 acutely ill soldiers, convoys of up to 300 wounded men might arrive daily, and there were only 10 doctors. The condition of the soldiers on admission was deplorable, many with trench feet brought on by standing knee-deep in stinking foul mud. Their morale was low from poison gas and from close proximity with plagues of giant bloated rats glutted with the flesh of the dead. Cushing wrote that infestation with scabies and lice was rife and observed that after lying for four days or more in rain-soaked craters, the injured heads of the soldiers became infested with maggots.

Holmes coped with all his military duties, which meant his working late every night on the neurological notes, as he had no secretary. He performed all the neurological postmortems and, in addition, this magnificent man was simultaneously engaged in three major research projects. For long periods, the weather was bitter and he had to work in an unheated room wearing his thick greatcoat, a rug wrapped around him, and his hands in mittens. Somehow he was able to handle the patients and to manipulate the smoked drum and tuning fork apparatus well enough to produce the illustrations for his paper in *Brain*, in which he assessed the effect of gunshot wounds of the cerebellum in some 70 soldiers. At the same time, he was engaged with William Lister, the distinguished ophthalmic surgeon, in an evaluation of the effect of occipital lobe trauma on vision. Together they carried out the perimetry,

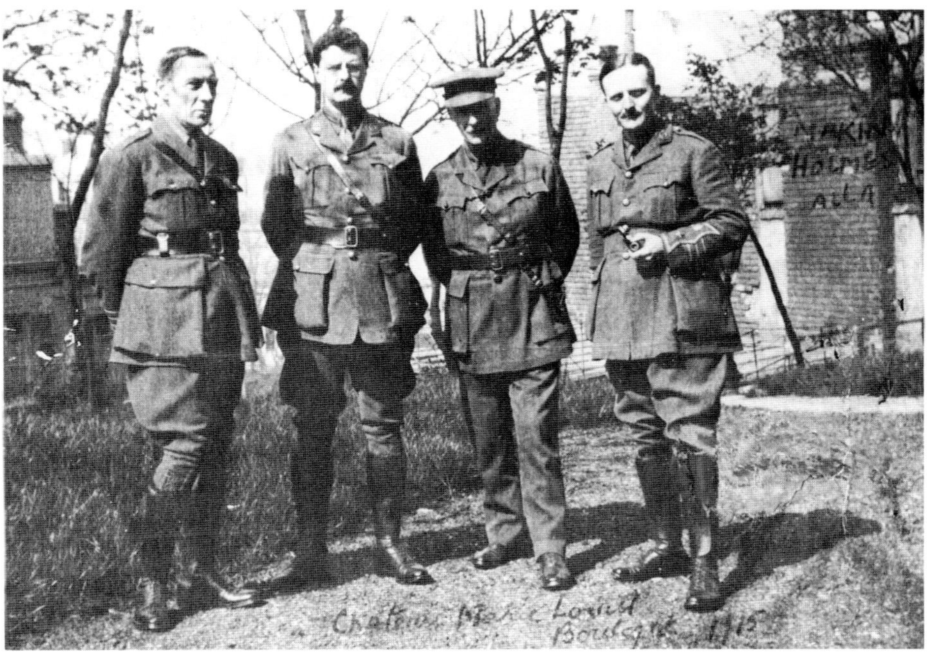

FIG. 1. Boulogne 1915. From left to right: Sir George Makins, Gordon Holmes, Wallace, and Percy Sargent.

and other tests, on hundreds of soldiers whose head injury had involved sight. Holmes's analysis of the varied neurological deficits was brilliant and can never be surpassed. Col. Lister was a modest, generous man who came from a most gifted medicoscientific family that included his uncle, Lord Lister. They had many common interests and continued to see each other when they returned to civil life.

Holmes's third research was a study of 300 soldiers who had sustained gunshot wounds of the spine, with particular reference to their bladder function, and performed all the cystograms in these cases. It is timely here to remind the reader that all these researches were done voluntarily after completing his routine duties. His physical and mental energy seemed to be inexhaustable.

To spur him on further was the influence of Dr. Jobson, another Scot. It had been love at first sight when, at the Red Cross Hospital, Gordon met Rosalie Jobson, one of the so-called Scottish Angels, a group organized by De Elsie Inglis of Edinburgh. Rosalie was a most attractive young woman who had volunteered to work in France; a top-class athlete who had represented Oxford in three sports, she was also a hockey international (Fig. 2). The attraction was mutual for when Gordon left to be commissioned, she also joined the RAMC, but unfortunately for them both, she was posted home; they met whenever Gordon could get leave. Eventually, while rowing on the Thames, they landed on a small island, where Gordon proposed and was accepted; they were wed early in 1918 in Scotland and, soon after the armistice, Col. G. M. Holmes, C. M. G., C. B. E., and Capt. R. Holmes were demobilized.

On their return to London, Gordon and Rosalie leased 9 Wimpole Street, a large house on five floors, which required a permanent staff of nine servants. Here Holmes restarted his private practice, and he and Rosalie entertained the many colleagues, overseas visitors, and students who called to see them. This was their family home, where they brought up their

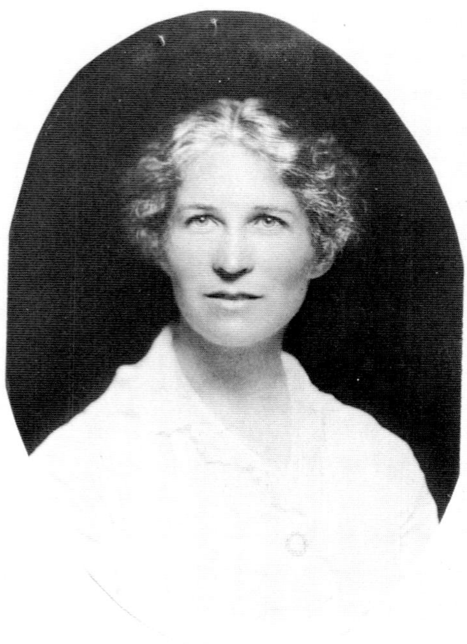

FIG. 2. Rosalie Holmes.

three daughters, Kathleen, Rosalie, and Betty. Gordon kept to a strict routine. He started every morning with a cold bath in which he invariably washed his thick hair, a habit which originated in France from the constant exposure to lice. (I knew several of his contemporaries who did likewise; indeed one, Philip Mitchener of St. Thomas's, told me 25 years later that he had shaved his head completely during the war and had not allowed it to grow again.) At breakfast, Holmes always read the *Times*. On the day he visited Charing Cross or Queen Square Hospitals, he would walk to work, but if going to The Seamans or Moorfields Hospital, he used his car. Few people knew that every Wednesday and Sunday morning, he and Rosalie drove out to Oxhey to play golf. He was very erratic, with a handicap of 20, while his wife was in single figures and generally won, which really did not bother him as he seldom kept the score, regarding golf as an excuse for a peaceful walk in the country.

Wilder Penfield tells in his diary of the many kindnesses he and others received from Gordon and Rosalie and the pleasure it gave him and his wife Helen to be invited to join them in their favorite pastime of rowing on the Thames (Fig. 3). They had three enchanting days in Oxford and were proudly shown the little island where Gordon and Rosalie became engaged. Another entry in Penfield's diary is of interest: "I danced with Mrs. Holmes," he wrote, "at the Congress ball and took her to a London theatre, both pastimes for which I have a great liking but for which Holmes found no time in his busy life." In fact, Gordon's favorite way of spending an evening was to read. He was passionately fond of Shakespeare, so much of which he had read and reread, and he loved Thackeray and Tennyson. He did enjoy the theater, but only if it was a performance of Shakespeare at the open air theatre in Regents Park and if the evening was fine. Last thing at night, he always read poetry.

Queen Square had returned to normal and, with the exception of Jackson, Batten, Gowers, and Horsley, his friends had survived. Postgraduates aware of Holmes's wartime contributions flocked to the hospital. The following excerpt from Penfield's diary will remind those who have sat at Holmes's feet of the scene in outpatients:

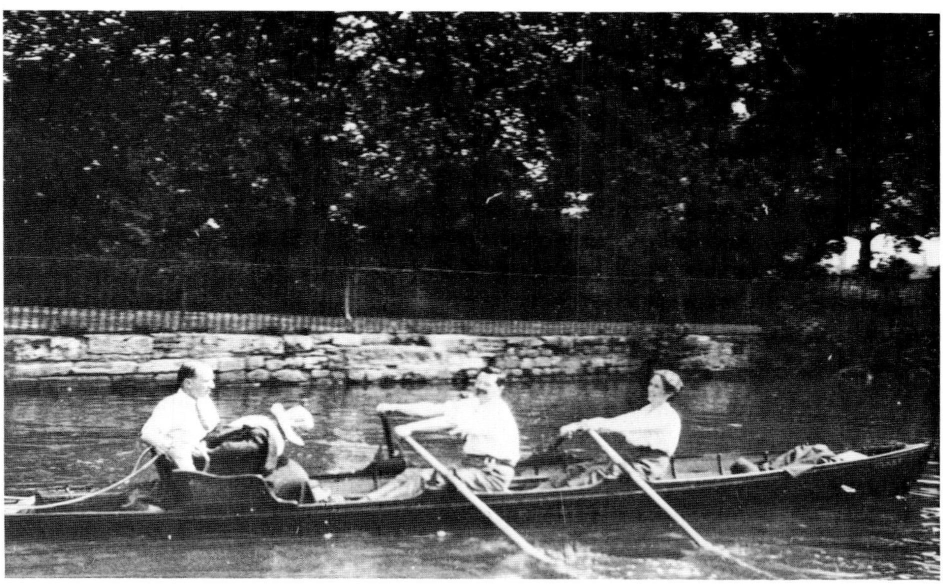

FIG. 3. Wilder and Helen Penfield, Gordon and Rosalie Holmes.

> Once a week a notice appeared on the door of the large teaching room "Dr. Gordon Holmes will examine patients at 2 o'clock." Before the hour graduate physicians from many nations crowded into the room coming as if to the mecca of Neurology to learn the art of presumptive diagnosis. They knew that Holmes was a neuroanatomist and that he would, after a few simple tests, turn to the penetrating discussion of the mysteries of the structure of the brain and spinal cord, instead of repeating the text book descriptions of various syndromes. On one such afternoon we sat waiting whilst the last arrivals filtered in to stand at the back. On the tick of two the door burst open and Gordon Holmes entered. He stood for a moment while he inspected his audience, tall and erect with black eyes and dark curly hair. When the RMO wheeled the patient into the room Holmes sat down abruptly into the single seat reserved for him in the front row.

He then proceeded to show where the lesion lay and its nature and explained his method for unraveling the symptoms and the signs.

Between the wars, at Queen Square, Holmes had two special friends, both colleagues with whom both he and his family were very close. The first was Francis Walshe. Walshe had served with distinction as a young consultant neurologist to the army in Egypt. In 1918, he published an account of 40 soldiers with multiple neuritis due to beriberi. Because of the views he expressed, he was subjected to a most vindictive verbal attack by Gowland Hopkins of vitamin fame. Walshe was deeply hurt, but Holmes stood by his old friend, encouraged him, and in 1921 welcomed him back to Queen Square on his election to the staff. Years later, it was Sir Francis who was to write the tribute to Gordon on his eightieth birthday, and then, 10 years later, in his inimitable and beautiful prose, Gordon's obituary.

The other friend was Charles Symonds, the tall, kindly, and gentle friend of so many, who died in 1978. He had had a distinguished record in World War I and then went on to his brilliant command of RAF neuropsychiatry in World War II. The two families were very close. Symonds described Holmes as the master of discipline in neurological examination and told that he never forgot one particular fault he had made in a clinical examination, which had induced Holmes to twist his arm really hard to emphasize his wrongdoing. For years, Sir Gordon had been the neurologist's neurologist, and it was Sir Charles who was to succeed him in this role.

At Charing Cross Hospital, Holmes had been appointed Assistant Physician, Pathologist, and Physician in charge of Diseases of Children, but he later shed some of these responsibilities. He enjoyed teaching students and, although they for their part feared him, they soon found that his bark was worse than his bite and came to love this large man with his clinical acumen, his patience, and his puckish sense of humor. His ward round took place behind locked doors. The nursing staff, who thought he was wonderful, saw to it that the patients lay still; they were not allowed to read a paper as the rustle might prove distracting. Only a jug of water with a glass was permitted on the locker top and, though in certain cases a vomit bowl might be provided, it was not expected to be touched; the use of a bedpan was not even to be contemplated.

Holmes had several mannerisms, such as the popping of sodamints into his mouth when his duodenal ulcer was troubling him. He might drop his glasses to the tip of his nose or hang them over one ear, and then subject one or another student to his hawklike gaze. He frequently stuck out his chest and then hooked his thumbs around his braces, aggressive maneuvers that led Charles Aring and Derek Denny-Brown to form the protective society known lightheartedly as the "Grand Order of the Braces" or "The Pants-Down Club of America." Often he would close one eye and then the other, checking the visual field in each. He might grasp a worried student by the lapels of his coat and gently rock him backward and forward in rhythm with his instructions. There was always a risk that he might spot someone new on the round. "You are new here," he would say, "Come to the front and you shall have the privilege of examining this case before anyone else does and we shall have the benefit of your opinion." If a student slipped up, he showed his disappointment brusquely but was never angry. He continually stressed the importance of careful observation, and would relate that his friend Henry Head would sometimes spend 20 hours to complete an examination compared with the usual 20 minutes.

Many cases were referred to him by other physicians. His ability to reach a diagnosis in these problem cases evoked from him the maxim that more clinical puzzles are solved by taking a new clinical history than by all laboratory tests.

The clinical part of the examination for the M. R. C. P. took place at Charing Cross Hospital during the time that he was Senior Censor at the College of Physicians. The membership candidates dreaded getting him in the clinical examination, though we had heard that, if we were shouted at, our chances were good. Sir Francis Avery Jones told me this story: On one occasion, Holmes was thought by his fellow examiner to be shouting unduly at the candidate, who was clearly discomforted, and he reproved Holmes for this. Holmes was puzzled and uneasy and then burst into a roar of laughter, saying, "He was very good, very good and I had already given him high marks when I found out he was Irish and we were having a blazing row about Dublin." Sir John Walton relates a similar story in Newcastle; Holmes and a certain well-known female candidate, regarded as being one of the brightest women in her year, were shouting at one another across the ward while she was being questioned by Sir Gordon after presenting him with the facts concerning her long case. "We were all concerned lest he decided that she was not fit to pass the examination, but when he came stumping along the ward in high dudgeon his only comment was, 'Best student I have ever examined'."

Among the staff at Charing Cross, he had two particular friends. William Adie was one of them. Adie was an Australian who had trained in Germany and then at Queen Square. He had served at an RAMC head center as a consultant in the war, and will be remembered for his pupil, for dystrophia myotonica, and for narcolepsy. A married man with a family, he was a charming, lovable character who sadly succumbed to a series of cardiac infarctions when aged 48. The other friend was Lennox Broster, a popular consultant surgeon, who was South African, a Rhodes Scholar, and Oxford rugby blue who had had a distinguished record in the army. Both he and his wife had been up at Oxford with Rosalie Holmes. He and Gordon worked up a common interest in endocrinology, particularly in the suprarenals.

Meanwhile, Holmes published many papers, contributed to several scientific meetings, and lectured on the results of his various research projects. The conclusions that he reached on cerebellar function, which were the result of study of slowly developing lesions and of acute gunshot wounds, still remain the most careful and detailed record of dysfunction of the human cerebellum.

His contribution to the understanding of the neurology of vision was immense. Before the publication of his observations, the point-to-point representation of the retina in the occipital cortex was not generally agreed upon or fully known. He made extensive studies of the effects of occipital lobe wounds on the visual fields and upon the functions of visual orientation and attention. In respect of retinal representation in the calcarine cortex, he found that the upper half of each retina is represented in the dorsal and the lower in the ventral part of each visual area. The center for macular vision lies in the most posterior part of each visual area. The macula does not have a bilateral representation. The cortical center for vision subserving the periphery of the retina he found to be situated in the anterior parts of the visual area, and the serial concentric zones of the retina from macula to periphery are represented in this order from behind forward in the visual area. Holmes found that lesions involving the lateral aspects of the hemispheres, particularly of the posterior parietal region, were associated with disturbance of high visual function, such as perception of depth and distance, and of visual orientation and localization in space, as well as of visual attention and gnosis.

Holmes received many academic honors, one of which was being elected to the Royal Society in 1933. He was also a foreign member of the Kaiserliche Akademie der Naturforscher of Germany and of the neurological societies of America, Estonia, Germany, Holland, Budapest, Paris, and Sweden. He had honorary degrees from the Universities of Durham, Edinburgh, Dublin, Fordham (New York), and the National University of Ireland. He was an honorary Fellow of the Royal Society of Medicine and its gold medallist. He held a number of important lectureships, including the Ferrier Lectureship of the Royal Society, and the Hughlings Jackson Lectureship of the Royal Society of Medicine. He gave the John Mallet Purser Lecture, the Victor Horsley Lecture and, at the old College of Physicians overlooking Trafalgar Square, the Goulstonian and Croonian Lectures. Holmes delivered the Savill Memorial Oration on local epilepsy at the West End Hospital for Nervous Diseases, one of the three neurological hospitals in London and remarkable for its attractive setting in a secluded part of Regents Park close to the Zoological Gardens. (It was completely destroyed in the Blitz on London on the very same night as its annex in Marylebone Lane was also severely damaged. Rehoused in the old Lock Hospital in Soho, it prospered again until 1972, when because of financial stringency in the National Health Service, it was closed. Its facilities were then transferred in part to Charing Cross Hospital and the rest to the Whittington Hospital.)

Gordon Holmes was more modest than most men of his standing, and he characterized himself best in his opening address at the Montreal Neurological Institute, which his friend Wilder Penfield invited him to perform in 1934. He said "If I were asked to select a motto, or a creed, for this new Institute I could do no better than copy out Francis Bacon's statement of his scientific attitude, written more than three hundred years ago.

> For myself I found I was fitted for nothing so well as for the study of truth; as having a mind nimble and versatile enough to catch the resemblance of things (which is the chief point), and at the same time steady enough to fix and distinguish their subtler differences; as being gifted by nature with desire to seek, patience to doubt, fondness to meditate, slowness to assert, readiness to reconsider, carefulness to dispose and set in order; and as being a man that neither affects what is new nor admires what is old, and that hates every kind of imposture.

In these words he revealed his own ideal.

He could not bear to hear his achievements discussed in public. On the occasion of his Presidential Address to the Ophthalmic Society of the United Kingdom, he told his old friend Leslie Paton, who was to propose the vote of thanks: "Seriously Leslie you are not to indulge in any eulogistic terms about me." Leslie obeyed. But after an address to the Charing Cross Medical School, the chairman ignored a similar request from him and proceeded to shower praise upon Holmes in such a way as to cause him visibly to squirm. Suddenly he could stand it no longer; he foiled an attempt to restrain him from leaving and, to the embarrassment of everyone present, fell off the stage and had to be helped to his feet. On another occasion, anticipating a teutonic eulogy at a formal dinner that evening, he enticed his friend Penfield to play hookey with him. They hired a double-oared rowing boat, rowed all around the Alster Lake in Hamburg, and afterward had a meal together in a pleasant restaurant. Unfortunately, he behaved like this once too often, with regrettable consequences.

It was in 1935, when as President of the 2nd International Neurological Congress, he was invited, with all the participants, to a reception at Buckingham Palace. For some reason, shyness overcame him. Never dreaming that he would be missed, he did not attend and instead did his ward round at Charing Cross. As luck would have it, King George V desired to talk with him, and he could not be found. Before this incident, many had thought that a Knighthood for him was long overdue, Percy Sargent having been knighted seven years previously, but it was not until 16 years later that he received the accolade.

The Second World War started in 1939. He joined the Emergency Medical Service and was appointed its adviser in neurology. He continued his teaching duties in the Charing Cross Hospital Medical School, which was evacuated to Ashridge. His daughters joined the services; Kathleen became a WREN, Rosalie a WAAF, and Betty a VAD. After enduring the London blitz, during which the houses on either side were damaged, 9 Wimpole Street was clearly too big for them. The Americans wanted the house as a services hostel, and regretfully, Gordon and Rosalie decided to move to Farnham, Surrey.

As Sir Gordon and Lady Holmes, they were content and happy enjoying their retirement in the country. He continued to see patients in Harley Street until his late seventies. They both continued with their regular games of golf together. The family visited them regularly, and many of their old friends would come down to spend the day with them. Gordon wrote several more papers and two books, *An Introduction to Clinical Neurology* and *The National Hospital, Queen Square*, which brought the total number of his publications to 174. He spent a lot of time looking after some four acres of garden and woodland. He propagated plants in his greenhouse, pruned the roses, and had a prolific kitchen garden, which included an asparagus bed. He felled and sawed up trees and was known to have blown up some stumps. He was enormously pleased with the events that were organized at Queen Square by way of homage to him at the time of his eightieth birthday, and grateful. He particularly treasured a 10-dollar gold piece sent to him by his boys of the "Grand Order of the Braces," or "Pantsdown Club in America." He was 87 when Rosalie's heart failed; she had had difficulty with her breathing for some while. Very grieved, he was helped to carry on by his daughter Kathleen, who ran the home and was a constant loving companion to him.

I last talked with him at the Winchester meeting of the Association of British Neurologists when he was in his ninetieth year. We sat in a corner out of the wind by the college cricket ground, where he asked me about the plans for the new Charing Cross Hospital at Fulham. He reminisced quietly about this and that, and then he talked about France in the First World War. I was astonished at his memory of events of 50 years before, of amusing incidents, and of the warm and generous memories he had of his special friends out there, among whom he numbered my father. It was getting cold and Kathleen thought that we should all go indoors. Before we parted, he made me promise to see him regularly to keep him informed about the building of the new hospital.

For the next few months, he continued with his golf nearly every day with three old cronies, and he worked in his garden. He had a happy Christmas, with his daughters, sons-in-law and grandchildren all staying with him. Shortly afterward, he died in his sleep in the early morning of December 29, 1965.

A memorial service for Sir Gordon was held at the National Hospital, Queen Square on February 4, 1966. Sir Francis Walshe, who gave the address, spoke of him as a man of integrity in his life and in his work, unself-seeking, without malice, forceful in thought and action, and in speech sometimes to the point of brusqueness. He was generous and helpful to all younger men once he found them willing to work hard and eager to add something to knowledge but impatient with the idle or the careless. He was not overtly religious, yet not irreligious, and with a natural and dignified reticence about himself. But as a clinical teacher, both by example and by precept, he was unsurpassed in his day. Sir Francis considered that he was perhaps the last representative of that remarkable group of medical men, peculiar to these islands in their day, who while wholly dependent upon the private practice of medicine, without the allure of university status or recognition, became notable teachers and had the gift and the immense energy to become contributors of the first order to new knowledge. Supremely fortunate and happy in his family life, a man of warm human feelings, his home became a place of pilgrimage, where his old students were always assured of a warm welcome from him and from that most lovable of women, his wife. Sir Francis Walshe concluded that there were other sides to him; his love of poetry—it was Holmes who had introduced him as a young man to the poetry of Francis Thompson, his deep interest in ecclesiastical Gothic, and his abiding love of a garden and working therein, which he did to the end.

Sir Gordon Holmes has bequeathed a golden heritage of neurology. He formed the minds of a generation of neurologists, and they in their turn have passed on the discipline they imbibed from him to others in many parts of the world. Professor Charles Aring in a brilliant tribute portrayed Gordon Holmes as a revered founding father of neurology in the United States. Dr. Denny-Brown, writing in the same vein, considered that by Holmes's own pioneering studies he had become the great master of what might be called inductive clinical analysis, which has since become part and parcel of American neurology. A splendid tribute to the man who had edited *Brain* for 17 years has been made by the Guarantors in the volume *Selected Papers of Gordon Holmes*, which has been compiled and edited for them by Charles Phillips. It contains reprints of several of his classical papers, 23 in all: on cerebellar function; on the cortical representation of the visual fields; on visual orientation, stereoscopic vision, and attention; on epilepsy, spinal trauma, and neuroanatomical research. It is an outstanding contribution to the history of British neurology.

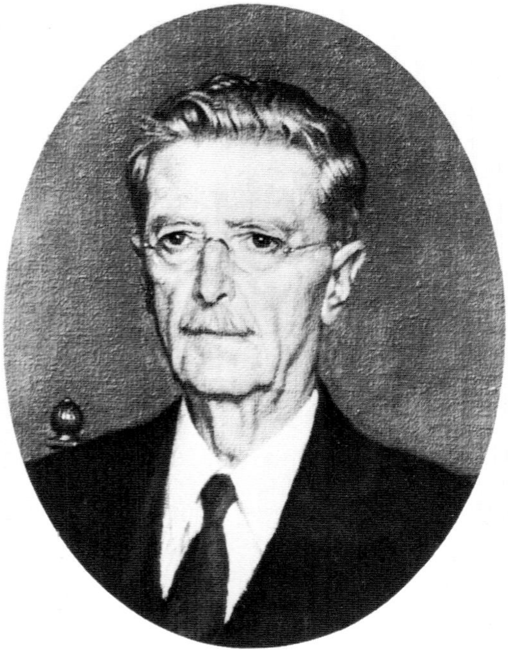

FIG. 4. Sir Gordon Holmes.

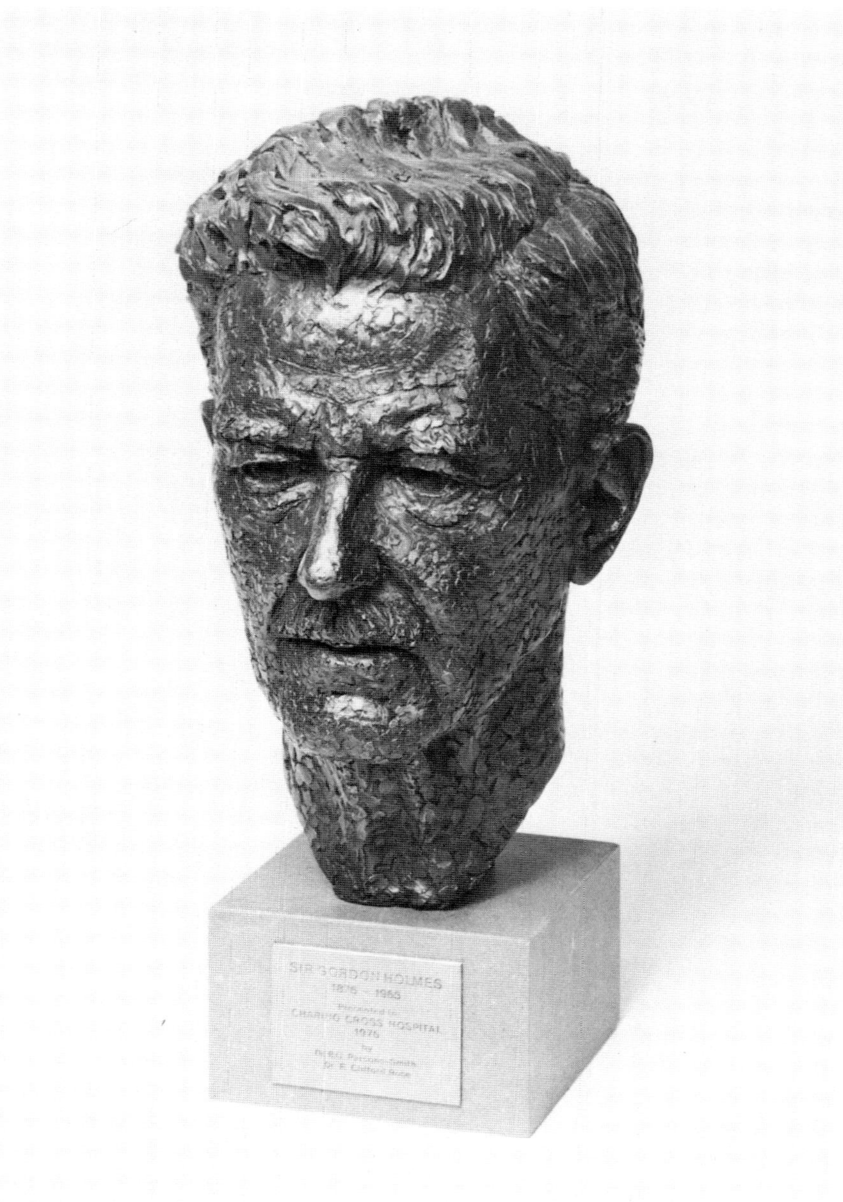

FIG. 5. The bronze head of Sir Gordon Holmes.

The centenary of the birth of Sir Gordon Holmes was celebrated at the new Charing Cross Hospital in March 1976. Neurologists from many parts of the world, who included several of Gordon's most illustrious friends and associates, took part in a four-day scientific meeting based on the theme "The Physiological Aspects of Clinical Neurology." Some 40 papers were delivered by physicians and surgeons from Australia, Canada, Eire, France, Germany,

Japan, Norway, Switzerland, and from many centers in Great Britain. Miss Kathleen Holmes unveiled a bronze portrait of her father, which had been commissioned by the neurologists at Charing Cross; this had been sculpted by Ian Hanson and the remarkable likeness that he had achieved using 10 old photographs (Fig. 4) literally took her breath away when it was revealed (Fig. 5). The participants to the meeting visited the Department of Neurology, in which we have named one ward "Gordon Holmes." The symposium culminated in a sumptuous dinner held at the Worshipful Society of Apothecaries, which was graced by H. R. H. The Princess Margaret, Countess of Snowdon, and chaired by the Emeritus President of the World Federation of Neurology, Dr. Macdonald Critchley. The events of the enjoyable evening completed the personal homage of many like-minded men and women from all over the world to the memory of a good and great physician.

ACKNOWLEDGMENTS

I am grateful to Dr. William Feindel for permission to quote from Dr. Wilder Penfield's diary *No Man Alone*, and to Little, Brown & Co. to quote from Cushing's *From a Surgeon's Journal*, 1915–1918. I am indebted to Mrs. S. Godbolt and Mr. Paul Morrell of the Medical School Library at Charing Cross Hospital for all their help. This life story of Gordon Holmes was only made possible by the many hours of conversation and research that I have enjoyed with Kathleen Holmes, whose memory, like her father's, is prodigious.

BIBLIOGRAPHY

1. Aring, C. D. (1965): A tribute to Sir Gordon Holmes: An appreciation. *J. Nerv. Ment. Dis.*, 141:497–502.
2. Brown, G. H. (1955): *Munk's Roll. Lives of the Fellows of the Royal College of Physicians of London. Volume 4, 1826–1925*. Royal College of Physicians, London.
3. Cushing, H. (1936): *From a Surgeon's Journal, 1915–1918*. Little, Brown, Boston.
4. Denny-Brown, D. (1965): The special contribution of Gordon Holmes. *J. Nerv. Ment. Dis.*, 141:502–504.
5. Holmes, G. M. (1954): *The National Hospital Queen Square 1860–1948*. Livingstone, Edinburgh.
6. Holmes, G. W. (1956): *Selected Papers;* compiled and edited by F. M. R. Walshe. Macmillan, London.
7. Horder, M. (1966): *The Little Genius*. Duckworth, London.
8. Obituary (1966): Gordon Morgan Holmes. *Lancet*, 1:101.
9. Obituary (1966): Sir Gordon Holmes. *Charing Cross Hosp. Gaz.*, 64:75–77.
10. Obituary (1966): Sir Gordon Holmes. *Lancet*, 1:158.
11. Obituary notice (1966): Sir Gordon Holmes. *Br. Med. J.*, 1:111–112.
12. Penfield, W. (1977): *No Man Alone*. Little, Brown, Boston.
13. Phillips, C. G. (1979): *Selected Papers of Gordon Holmes*. Oxford University Press, Oxford.
14. Rose, F. C. (1977): *The Physiological Aspects of Clinical Neurology*. Blackwell, Oxford.
15. Sir Gordon Holmes (1963): *Charing Cross Hosp. Gaz.*, 61:80–84.
16. Symonds, C. P. (1970): *Studies in Neurology*, Oxford University Press, Oxford.
17. Trail, R. R. (1968): *Munk's Roll. Lives of the Fellows of the Royal College of Physicians of London. Volume 5, to 1965*. Royal College of Physicians, London.
18. Walshe, F. M. R. (1966): Gordon Morgan Holmes, 1876–1965. *Biogr. Memoirs Roy. Soc. London*, 12:311–319.
19. Walton, J. N. (1980): A Memorable Neurologist (Book Review). *Br. Med. J.*, 1:706–707.

Historical Aspects of the Neurosciences,
edited by F. Clifford Rose and W. F. Bynum.
Raven Press, New York ©

Charles Edward Brown-Séquard

William Gooddy

National Hospital for Nervous Diseases, London, England

As long ago as 1960, at the time of the Centenary Celebrations of the National Hospital, Queen Square, Dr. Macdonald Critchley, then Senior Physician, commanded me and several other neurologists, then in their "salad days," to produce a suitable sketch of some former member of the Hospital staff. I chose Brown-Séquard merely because I knew his name (though I could not then have accurately recalled the details of his famous syndrome). I little thought then that I was to embark on a long course of medical detective work, which is what I now set down 20 years later. It is a moment of special pleasure in my life to be writing in honor of Dr. Macdonald Critchley, to whom neurology and neurologists personally owe so much.

Those who are not in medicine may never have heard the name of Dr. Charles Edward Brown-Séquard, and even medical men may have no knowledge of the man except that he was responsible for describing what happens when the spinal cord is cut in half—a matter to be remembered for exams but not commonly remembered, nor appreciated, for its deduction of genius that the pathways for pain and the pathways for touch were along separate routes in the spinal cord. It is not generally known that he was a founder-physician of the National Hospital, Queen Square, nor that in addition to being a neurologist, he was a pioneer in endocrinology.

We are prone to consider an abstract of a man's published works without asking ourselves what may have caused that man to do what he did or how his background and personality caused him to have the career that history may later reveal. I wish to make a brief attempt to explain the circumstances and intellectual forces that molded and directed this important man in the history of medical science, and this chapter presents, not an outline of the more than 500 published works of Brown-Séquard, but a study in space and time to link us today with the time of nearly 200 years ago, to the year of 1784, the year Dr. Samuel Johnson died, about the time of the start of the French Revolution and the drafting of the Constitution of the United States, when the younger Pitt was Prime Minister for George III, himself an involuntary patient in Queen Square, London, possibly because of porphyria. We find ourselves in Philadelphia for the birth of an American boy, to be named Charles Edward Brown. This boy grew up to be a seaman and to serve in the armed and mercantile forces of the United States.

Next we move many thousands of miles across the world to Port Louis in Mauritius in the year 1787. You may nowadays visit Mauritius on a package tour, but then it must have been a very remote island. In the details of the marriage license between Pierre Paul Séquard and Marie Elizabeth Nativel, Séquard is described as a trader from Port Louis, and hailing from Marseille, and Miss Nativel as living in the island of Bourbon (Réunion), the daughter of M. André Nativel, "who had been an officer in the national forces." One year later, in 1788, a daughter was born of this marriage, Henriette Charlotte Perrine Séquard, her birth having been registered in 1790. "The Godmother was Madame Desmoulins, who declared she did not know how to sign." Charlotte Séquard grew up in Mauritius, probably never suspecting that she was destined to be the mother of an important figure in the history of medicine, to be early widowed from an American husband, or that she would die in Paris in 1842 at the age of 54.

Our next point in time is a marriage between an American sea captain (the boy from Philadelphia), now aged 29, in 1813, and Miss Séquard (the girl from Réunion), who thus became Mrs. Brown, and it is in 1817 that we reach an important date, that of the birth of their son, Edward Charles Brown, who later became known by the names of both his parents, with an American father, a Mauritian-French mother, and British citizenship—yet dying, 74 years later, in Paris, with French nationality. By the time of his birth, his father, Captain Brown, had been lost at sea on a venture to India to bring back food during hard times, having been either captured by pirates or lost in a cyclone.

When young Brown was 21, he left Mauritius with his mother for Paris with the intention of making a literary career; but he was advised that his literary chances were slim, so he then chose to study medicine. His fees were paid by his mother, who made a living as a boarding-house keeper. Four years later, Mme. Brown died in 1842. Her son, then aged 25, added his mother's name to his own, and though he later stated that he did so according to custom, it seems equally likely that he was aware of his debt to his mother, that he was shocked and grieved by her death, and that he wished her to have some memorial, as indeed she does, by a linkage of name. He obtained his Paris doctorate at the age of 29 in 1846. He had a few medical appointments but devoted most of his time to experimental physiology "under the most harassing condition of extreme poverty." In 1852, he left France because of strong Republican opinions and went to New York, where he gave lessons in French and took midwifery cases at $5 a time.

In 1853, he married for the first time and then returned to France. The following year, he returned to Mauritius hoping to settle in practice but, finding an epidemic of cholera there, he took charge of the hospital and used the treatment method of opium, as suggested by Magendie. Ever the experimentalist, he swallowed the vomit of cholera patients. When he felt he had caught cholera, he took a huge dose of laudanum and was found semiconscious in his room, curled up in a corner, strong enough only to signal for coffee.

He decided that he wished to continue with experimental work and accepted in May 1854 the Professorship of the Institutes of Medicine and Medical Jurisprudence at the newly founded Medical College of Virginia in Richmond. Brown-Séquard was no lover of slavery, and his colleagues were no lovers of animal experiment without anesthesia nor of Brown-Séquard's so-called "asthmatic" unintelligibility of address. Within a few months of his appointment at Richmond, he disappeared without warning and returned to Paris in 1855.

We see in all these frequent and profound changes (which continued through his life, though in milder form with the passing years), a profound restlessness and recurrent dissatisfaction, which in lesser men might have resulted in bitterness and cantankerous failure. These personality traits must have had some origins in his ancestry and the background of his youth, with its uncertainties and privations. But they were offset by a degree of industry, intellectual concentration, and originality of tremendous power, together with a feeling for the future benefit of humanity and a gentle unassuming manner, which endeared him very generally. We have a glimpse of him thus in the account of Judge Condé-Williams of Mauritius: "A small dark man with a smile full of kindness."

In writing to the President of the Royal College of Surgeons of England, Brown-Séquard says: "My dear Sir, You treated me with so much kindness . . . a hospital shortly to be founded in your metropolis for the treatment of the paralysed and epileptic." I have recently discovered his original application to the Governors for the post of "Physician to the Hospital for Paralysis and Epilepsy." It contains 17 paragraphs listing good reasons why he should be chosen for the post (for which one candidate was offering the inducement of £1,000 in his own support). Brown-Séquard was appointed to the National Hospital, Queen Square, in December 1859 (see below).

In London he had an immediate success, beginning the clinical history of the National Hospital in the company of Dr. Ramskill, and lecturing at the Royal College of Surgeons in London, Edinburgh, Glasgow, and Dublin. His *Lectures on the Physiology and the Pathology of the Central Nervous System* was published in 1860 (1). In the same year, he became a Fellow of the Royal College of Surgeons, and of the Royal Society, thus obtaining within two years of arriving in England the highest distinction in science that this country confers. Among the names of his supporters was the famous surgeon, James Paget, who was a constant friend and correspondent, and to whom Brown-Séquard dedicated a journal; the then President of the Royal College of Surgeons of England whose aid Brown-Séquard had enlisted in support of his National Hospital application; Sibson, another surgeon whose name is familiar to all students of human anatomy; and William Carpenter, the first person to suggest a brain-stem activating system. In the list of Fellows of the Royal Society, Brown-Séquard appears in the same column as Lord Lister and Francis Galton, and in the company of three Bishops and a banker.

Details of his appointment to the National Hospital are scarce. The first entry in the records of the hospital shows:

> *29th December 1859*
> It was resolved and carried unanimously that E. Brown-Séquard, MD etc, be and is hereby elected a Physician to the Hospital.

Some interesting details of the medical way of life may be noted:

> *19th April 1860 (Furnishing Committee)*
> It was Resolved that the Physicians having applied through Dr. Brown-Séquard for instruments they secure such as are necessary at an expense not exceeding Twenty Pounds.
> *26th April 1860*
> Dr. Brown-Séquard intimated that he would give Clinical Lectures every Monday and his first would commence on 14th May at 3:30.

(By a curious coincidence, I later was to continue this practice of outpatient teaching on Monday, a practice with a continuous history now of 115 years.)

> *7th June 1860*
> Dr. Ramskill was also present and read a note from Dr. Séquard. It was Resolved that the names of the Physicians shall not be published nor allusion made to their cures in future advertisements.

There are further notes about rowdy and undesirable patients; about a row with a recalcitrant house surgeon, ending in his resignation; and the provision of a gymnasium.

We find also, in a minute of May 1862, the name of the man destined to become the most famous historical figure in British neurology, Hughlings Jackson. Dr. Jackson was elected Assistant Physician, with the duties of attending the National Hospital twice a day and seeing the outpatients in their home, for which extra service he was to be allowed the remuneration of £50 per annum.

In a minute of July 15, 1863, we find:

> This Committee have learned with infinite regret the intention of Dr. Brown-Séquard to retire from practice in this country and that he has in consequence tendered his resignation as one of the Physicians of this Hospital.

With this note, and his appointment as Honorary Physician, Brown-Séquard disappears from the daily life of the National Hospital, although his name still heads a list of its eminent staff on a wall tablet.

It is supposed by some that Brown-Séquard decided to leave London on an impulse provoked by seeing from his consulting-room window a line of carriages belonging to his fashionable, and no doubt, exacting, patients. He first lived at 82 Wimpole Street but soon moved to 25 Cavendish Square. The house no longer stands but an adjoining one may still be seen. Who were these "fashionable patients"? There is a letter from one of them, the Duchess of Argyll, wife of the scientific Duke of Argyll, who rocked Darwin's theory of evolution by pointing out that the human race should have perished because of the singular unfitness of its infants. A letter from Charles Darwin to Brown-Séquard, asking for a favorable review of his *Origin of Species*, reads:

> My dear Sir
>
> I cannot resist the opportunity of thanking you for your kind message through Miss Pennington. I am extremely much gratified to hear that you intend noticing my Book in some French Periodical.
>
> Whether you agree with me at all I do not know, as for anything like an approach to perfect agreement, it is out of the question in so complex a subject. But I shall be truly glad to read any criticisms from one who stands so very high in one of the very highest branches of Science, as you stand. Therefore would you have the great kindness to tell me some time where and when you publish any little notice on the subject . . . Just at present I am the more glad of any notice in France, as a French Translation will appear very soon. I daresay you do not remember it, but a year or two ago I was introduced to you at the Philosophical Club and had some little, to me interesting, conversation with you. . . .
>
> Pray believe me, my dear Sir,
> With sincere respect,
> Yours very faithfully
> Charles Darwin
>
> I do not know which edition of my "Origin" you may have seen; but the 3rd edition is in some respects considerably improved, and it is this edition which is now being translated into French.

Another indication of the fashionable circles in which Brown-Séquard may have moved, perhaps a little reluctantly, is a letter from James Paget, asking Brown-Séquard to attend an important dinner with the Prince of Wales, later King Edward VII. It is clear that Brown-Séquard was held in the greatest esteem by many of the famous figures of his time. His correspondence shows he knew, in addition to Darwin, such figures as T. H. Huxley, Jean-Martin Charcot, Agassiz, Oliver Wendell Holmes, and Louis Pasteur. Pasteur's regard is shown in his address of "Cher Grand Maitre."

There is no need now to expound in any great detail the remainder of Brown-Séquard's professional career, interesting and important though it is, except for the results of a small piece of historical research that I have been able to carry out. Briefly, Brown-Séquard, on leaving London, took the post of Professor of Physiology and Pathology of the Nervous

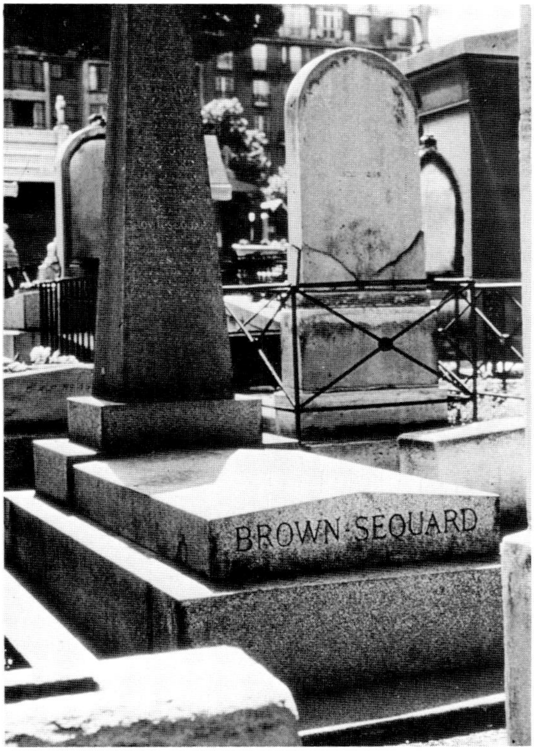

FIG. 1. Brown-Séquard's resting place in the cemetery of Montparnasse, Paris, France.

System at Harvard. On the death of his wife, he returned to Europe via Dublin to Paris. In 1872, he went back to New York, settled in practice, and married again. He moved once more to London but took a post in Geneva.

In 1878, on the death of his friend and colleague, Claude Bernard, he took on the chair of Experimental Medicine at the Collège de France, where he stayed to the end of his life, becoming a member of the Academy of Sciences in 1886. He became a French citizen at that time. He died in 1894 after a cerebral thrombosis with hemiplegia and visual field loss.

In 1961, I went on a pilgrimage to Paris to visit the grave of Brown-Séquard in the cemetery of Montparnasse. At the central office of the cemetery there was at first some doubt whether or not Brown-Séquard was indeed buried there; but eventually documents were produced, and I was able to note that the upkeep of the grave was maintained by a Mrs. McCausland of Bouverie Road, Folkestone, in England. I was escorted to the grave by a huge Negro whose philosophy was equal to his stature. As we counted along the rows of graves, he must have felt my emotion, for he said, "Never mind—for it happens to everyone—and all are equal here." Figure 1 shows where Brown-Séquard rests beside his mother. Figure 2 shows Brown-Séquard aged about 40, while Fig. 3 shows a photograph from the National Hospital records, with his autograph.

I thought I might get to know more about Brown-Séquard if I made contact with Mrs. McCausland. I knew that Brown-Séquard's daughter had married an Irish surgeon named McCausland, so I wrote to the address in Bouverie Road but had no reply; the detective trail had gone cold. It was not for some years that I discovered that Mrs. McCausland, the daughter of Brown-Séquard, had died ten days before my letter arrived. About a year after

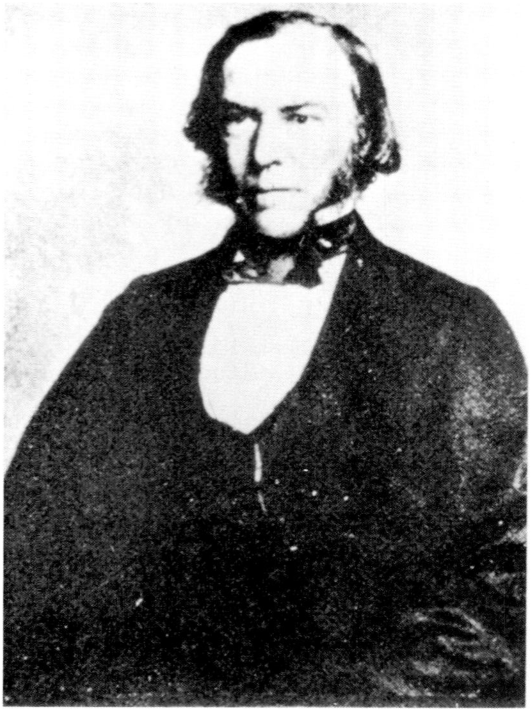

FIG. 2. Brown-Séquard at about the age of 40.

my visit to Paris, I was casually glancing through the record of old boys from my former school (Winchester), looking to see how many medical men there might be. I came across, in this very unlikely place, the name of two McCauslands, one a doctor with the initials "C. E." and an address in Folkestone. These two men proved to be Dr. McCausland, the grandson, and Maj. McCausland, the great-grandson of Brown-Séquard. It was not long before I made the first of several visits to Folkestone, where I learned a great deal more about Brown-Séquard. We even dined off plates with the Brown-Séquard monogram. Dr. and Mrs. McCausland came to a dinner at the National Hospital almost exactly 100 years after his grandfather had started work there. Dr. McCausland died in 1967 after a long life of medical practice in Folkestone.

On my first visit to Dr. McCausland's home, I was told that there were some old boxes of papers connected with Brown-Séquard; but the family was on the point of consigning them to the corporation dustcart, as they only took up space and collected dust. This collection of neglected papers proved to be a treasury of 19th-century historical documents. It is from this collection that I have been able to select many of the documents already mentioned in this chapter.

Eventually, the whole collection was acquired by the Royal College of Surgeons in London through the good offices of Mr. Leonard Payne, the Wellcome Librarian, and with the support of the late Lord Rosenheim, then President of the College. The collection is large and is still being catalogued. There is more than enough material there to keep students busy for many years.

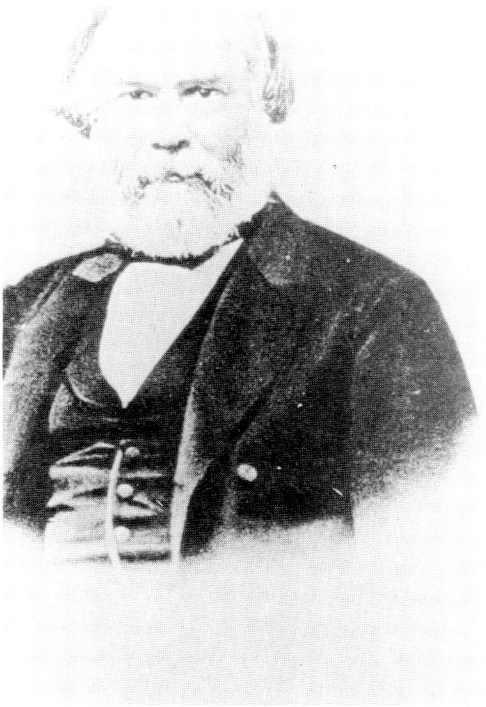

FIG. 3. A photograph of Brown-Séquard from the National Hospital records, with his autograph.

It would take another chapter at least to give you even an outline of the scope and importance of the detailed scientific work of Brown-Séquard. You will recall his spinal cord syndrome and his great discovery that there were separate pathways in the spinal cord for pain and temperature and for touch and position sense; that he spent much time on epilepsy; his concern with infectious diseases; and you may have heard some rumors of his interest, later in life, in extracts of tissues that he himself tried by intramuscular injections—this work often being regarded as representing a decline in his truly scientific investigations. But I now realize why he was so interested in putrefaction and cadaveric rigidity (the title of his six Goulstonian Lectures), and why, on learning of what we now call Addison's disease of the suprarenal glands, he immediately began, in 1856, to discover experimentally what happened if these glands were removed from animals. To quote Olmstead (2):

> The striking phenomenon which Brown-Séquard had discovered and reported to the Academy of Sciences, August 25, was that the lower animals died, usually within 12 hours, after extirpation of the suprarenal bodies. The symptoms appearing after their removal were gradual muscular weakening, which became very marked before the end; more rapid respiration at first, which later became notably diminished, irregular and gasping; a heartbeat enfeebled but more rapid than the normal state; and a fall of body temperature. In the last moments of life there were vertigo, rolling over and convulsions. Blood from a healthy animal injected into the veins of an animal deprived of its suprarenal bodies caused the latter to survive several hours longer than it would otherwise have done . . . His final conclusions were: (i) these organs are essential to life . . . ; (ii) ablation of them leads to death even more rapidly than removal of both kidneys; (iii) these organs have numerous relations with the cerebro-spinal centres. . . . The work is a classic landmark in the history of endocrinology.

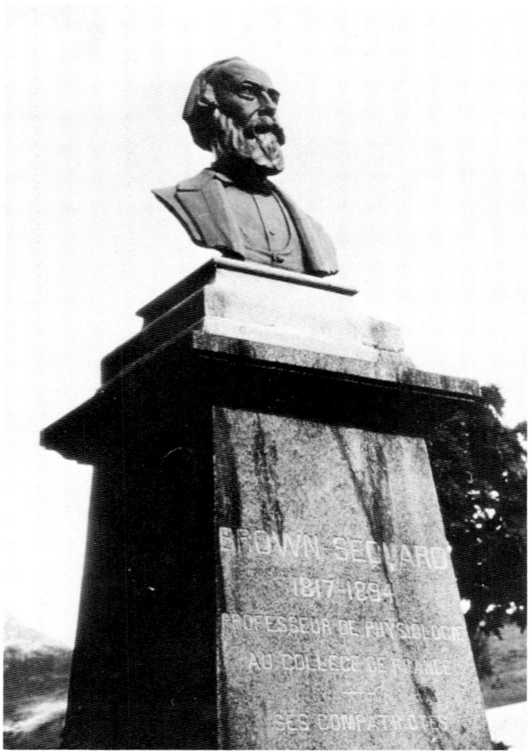

FIG. 4. Bust of Brown-Séquard in the Public Garden in Port Louis, Mauritius.

He had therefore found his elixir and was encouraged to continue in a search for further similar potent humoral agents. Clearly he had discovered cortisol. His only error was to have discovered it about a hundred years before its time. I end with the words that you may see written on the pedestal of the bust in Port Louis (Fig. 4):

> HERE TRULY WAS A MAURITIAN OF WHOM HIS COMPATRIOTS MAY WELL AND JUSTLY BE PROUD—A MAN TO WHOSE CHARACTER SELFISHNESS AND SELF-ASSUMPTION WERE UTTER STRANGERS, A NOBLE LIFE OF HIGH GIFTS AND POWERS OF INTELLECT AND RESEARCH DEVOTED ABSOLUTELY AND UNSPARINGLY TO THE WELFARE OF MANKIND IN AGES YET TO COME.

REFERENCES

1. Brown-Séquard, C. E. (1860): *Lectures on the Physiology and Pathology of the Central Nervous System*. J. B. Lippincott, Philadelphia.
2. Olmsted, J. M. D. (1940): *Charles Edward Brown-Séquard: A Nineteenth Century Neurologist and Endocrinologist*. Johns Hopkins Univ. Press, Baltimore.

Historical Aspects of the Neurosciences,
edited by F. Clifford Rose and W. F. Bynum.
Raven Press, New York ©

Houston Merritt

Arnold P. Friedman

Neurological Associates of Tucson, Tucson, Arizona 85712

The contributions of Dr. H. Houston Merritt to American neurology are reflected in the growth of neurology as an independent specialty. He understood the early relationshop of neurology to psychiatry and the pragmatic aspect of combining psychiatry and neurology into one specialty board. His teachings emphasized that neurology originated in general medicine, with neuropathology, physiology, and anatomy as its foundation. His contributions extended into so many areas that he is properly regarded as the founder of modern neurology in North America. His death on January 9, 1979, just three days before his seventy-seventh birthday, ended an era of neurology.

As a fellow in neurology at the Harvard Medical School, I observed his emphasis on the essential importance of precise observations of the patient. I was awed by the speed with which he analyzed a clinical problem, assessing the essentials and arriving at a diagnosis. At postmortem checks, it became apparent that the accuracy of his diagnoses far exceeded that of his colleagues. His past experience with comparable cases and almost instant recall, combined with unusual intelligence and intuitive insight into the problem, accounted for this unerring ability. His influence on students and house officers is apparent, as today more than 30 of them head neurology training programs in the United States.

He was a popular teacher, most appreciated by the more knowledgeable medical students and house officers. In discussion of a problem or in daily conversation, he was a happy example of linguistic economy. His speech was laconic and at times barely audible several yards away. Those who listened carefully were rewarded with "gems" of knowledge.

Merritt's contributions to neurology are legion and are recorded in 215 papers and five books on cerebrospinal fluid, epilepsy, neurosyphilis, headaches, stroke, multiple sclerosis, and genetic diseases. His book on cerebrospinal fluid, coauthored with Frank Fremont Smith, is still today the basic reference about this subject. His studies of cerebrospinal fluid in the 1930s were among the first important clinical investigations in neurology. In 1939, he collaborated with Dr. Tracy Putnam in the discovery of phenytoin (Dilantin) as an anticonvulsive agent. This was the first of over 100 compounds he tested, which established the principle that the anticonvulsant and sedative properties of a drug could be separated. Equally important, the experimental method they designed became the basis for other drugs, several of which were molecular modifications of phenytoin. A monograph on neurosyphilis, coauthored with Raymond Adams and Harry Solomon in 1946, led the way for a better understanding of syphilitic infections involving the central nervous system, including both diagnosis and treatment of this disorder. His textbook of neurology is regarded as the standard text throughout the neurological world. He completed its sixth edition late in 1978.

He was an authority on almost every phase of neurology, including cerebrovascular disease, muscle disease, multiple sclerosis, and genetic disease. Although Merritt encouraged specialty clinics in neurology, he was unhappy about the poorly trained physician who used these clinics for personal gain, rather than aiding in the treatment of patients and research of the problem or subject.

I had the privilege of collaborating on nine published papers and coauthoring a textbook on headache with Dr. Merritt. His ability to cover a wide range of subjects and work was extraordinary. One Sunday I drove to his home in Bronxville, in Westchester County, N.Y., to write up our findings for publication on ophthalmoplegic migraine. I knew that he was an ardent sports fan, but I was surprised to find him in his den observing two television sets, each with a different football game. I brought out the material, and he proceeded to reedit and revise the text, at the same time following the progress of both football games, commenting on the quarterbacks' calling of plays or details of the line plays. Before either game was over, the paper was ready for final typing.

Dr. Merritt, Charles Brenner, and myself established the first full-time headache clinic at Montefiore Hospital in New York in 1945. Establishment of the headache unit at that period was of some importance, in that it paved the way for continued research and study of this common symptom. It also showed the feasibility of specialty clinics within a Neurology Department, which have proved effective in training physicians, treating patients, and facilitating research.

Merritt skillfully played a part in establishing the National Institute of Neurological Disease and Blindness (now the National Institute of Neurological and Communicative Disorders and Stroke). Through its sponsorship, the training of residents and fellows in neurology, including electrophysiology, pharmacology, biochemistry, virology and immunology, was stressed. He continued to recognize the importance of neuropathology, as evidenced by the presence of a Senior Neuropathologist always participating in the Neurology Conferences at the Neurological Institute. Emphasis on neuropathology, neuroanatomy, and physiology were still maintained, and courses in these subjects were part of all residency training programs. He recognized that for neurology to grow, it was important for the physicians to work with the lay population in volunteer agencies. He felt that neurology could not depend solely on the federal government. It was through the lay population and other agencies that Dr. Merritt, Pierce Bailey, and several other neurologists enlisted the support of Congress to establish the National Institute of Nerve Disease and Blindness, of which he served on the Advisory Council from 1950 to 1964. Through these sources and agencies, he was able to establish individual groups to influence research and patient service programs in muscle dystrophy, multiple sclerosis, cerebral palsy, parkinsonism, and epilepsy.

Merritt's effect on neurology during the past 40 years was both broad and profound. He was Chief Editor of the *Archives of Neurology* from 1962 to 1971, President of the American Neurological Association in 1957, the American Board of Psychiatry and Neurology in 1950, and the Association for Research of Nervous and Mental Diseases in 1952, and the American Neurological Society in 1960. He was sought after as an advisor and mediator with many other organizations concerned with neurology, including the National Academy of Science special and IH committees on epilepsy, stroke, and multiple sclerosis, the Veterans Administration, Army, Navy, Atomic Energy Commission, and he was Trustee of the Association for Research in Mental Disease for over a quarter of a century.

Organizations concerned with medical research, education, or the general health field sought his services, including the World Health Organization, the National Fund for Medical Education, the Public Health Research Institute of the City of New York, the Matheson Foundation, the Josiah Macy, Jr., Foundation, and St. Luke's Hospital Center.

Merritt's honors and awards suggest the esteem in which he was held. His work for so many committees and organizations was truly remarkable. Of course, he did more than assume titles; he accepted responsibilities, many of them simultaneously, and yet he was always able to analyze the situation and give appropriate advice. He was Vice President of the Sixth Annual Congress of Neurology in Brussels back in 1955, and he was President of the Ninth Congress in New York in 1969, Honorary President of the Pan-American Congress of Neurology in 1963, as well as Honorary Member of numerous neurological societies, including the Philadelphia Neurological Society, the Royal Society of Medicine (London), the French Neurological Society, Argentine Society of Science, Neurology, Psychiatry, and Neurosurgery, etc.

His awards include the Max Weinstein Award of the United Cerebral Palsy Association in 1962, the George W. Jacoby Award of the Bronze, Hope Chest Award of the National Multiple Sclerosis Society (1966), the Lenox Award of the American Epilepsy Society (1967), Golden Anniversary Medal of the Association for Research in Nervous and Mental Diseases for Outstanding Achievement in Neurology (1970), Awards of Merit of the Parkinson Disease Foundation, Distinguished Service Award of the National Multiple Sclerosis Society, the Thomas Salmon Distinguished Service Award in Psychiatry and Mental Hygiene (1973), and the United Cerebral Palsy Distinguished Service Award (1973).

Merritt was called into consultation to attend many national leaders including a president of the United States, a well-known Russian official, and a dictator of Portugal, the latter conferring upon him its highest honor, the title of Grand Officer of the Order of Santiago. Whether his patients were distinguished or ordinary, he treated them with equal skill, interest, and devotion.

Merritt's academic record was of the highest. He received his medical degree from Johns Hopkins University in 1926. He later received honorary degrees from Harvard University, New York Medical College, and Columbia University. After training in medicine at New Haven Hospital, in neurology at Boston City Hospital, and in neuropathology in Germany, he moved in 1944 from Boston, where he had the academic rank at Harvard of Associate Professor of Neurology, to become Professor of Clinical Neurology at Columbia University and Chief of the Division of Neuropsychiatry at Montclair Hospital. Four years later, he became Professor of Neurology and Chairman of the Department of Neurology at Columbia, and Director of the Neurological Service at the Neurological Institute of the Presbyterian Hospital in New York. These academic and clinical titles he maintained even when he became Dean of the College of Physicians and Surgeons and Vice President for Health Affairs of the university in 1958. At that time, he was named the first Henry and Lucy Moses Professor of Neurology in 1963, and under his direction the Neurological Institute became a major center for neurological training and research. He adroitly led the college through major changes in curriculum and in the composition of the student body during the 1960s, a time of considerable unrest in the universities. Throughout this period, his sense of humor proved invaluable; he could relieve a tense situation with a witty remark or humorous story.

Under his direction, the Neurological Institute erected the William Black Research Building in 1960, which demonstrated the school's emphasis on biomedical research. A short time later, the medical school affiliated with the Harlem Medical Center, both events under his aegis. Thus, his university demonstrated its commitment to research, teaching, and the care of the not so fortunate. He retired as Chairman of the Department in 1967 and from the Deanship in 1970, but he continued to hold his weekly conferences and have keen interest in neurology and the Neurological Institute.

In memory of his achievements, a Merritt Chair in Neurology was established in 1970, a new conference room was named for him in 1971, and the H. Houston Merritt Clinical

Research Center for Muscle Dystrophy and Related Diseases was established with the aid of the Muscle Dystrophy Association in 1974. He was given the Distinguished Service Award of the College of Physicians and Surgeons of Columbia University in 1977 on his seventy-fifth birthday. More than 100 of his former students participated in this symposium to honor Dr. Merritt.

In his Presidential Address in 1957 at the American Neurological Association, Dr. Merritt summarized his thoughts about neurology, and those thoughts of some 23 years ago are applicable to the neurology of today. He said:

> The prospects for the future of neurology are indeed bright, particularly with regard to research and training. Our specialty has not, however, taken its proper role in clinical practice. This deficit will be remedied in the coming years if the members of this Association, and the leaders in the field, see that our young men are properly trained in all aspects of neurology, particularly in therapy.

He was a man of consequence and one of the giants in American neurology.

Historical Aspects of the Neurosciences,
edited by F. Clifford Rose and W. F. Bynum.
Raven Press, New York ©

Charcot in the 80s

Rudy Capildeo

Department of Neurology, Charing Cross Hospital, London W6, England

> Now and again there is given a man whose life and work make an enduring impression and who, escaping the thralls of nationalism becomes a teacher and leader.
>
> Sir William Osler
> (From the Obituary on Jean-Martin Charcot, September 1893)

Even with the benefit of hindsight, looking back from the 1980s to the 1880s, it is difficult to appreciate the breadth and depth of Charcot's contribution to medicine and to neurology in particular. This is not necessarily due to our innate myopia or to the passage of time, since a new student listening to the famous professor in 1883 would have had the same difficulty. Surely the Friday morning lectures, brilliant in conception and dramatic in presentation, must have always existed at the Salpêtrière. Yet the amphitheater, like the student, was new. Before Charcot, there had been no attempt at a systematic classification of the neurological diseases, no "Neuro-pathological Institution" (Charcot's term), no "Clinical Chair of Diseases of the Nervous System." For these reasons, Charcot has been rightly called the "Founder of Neurology," but the legacy he left behind was greater than even this title implies, as will be discussed in this chapter.

EARLY YEARS

Jean-Martin Charcot was born in Paris on November 29, 1825. His father was a carriage builder, employed by his wife's father, and it was the eldest of Jean-Martin's three brothers who was to inherit the family business. His two other brothers joined the armed forces, a longing that his own son was to share in the years to come. Charcot was quiet and introspective as a youth, enjoying reading and drawing. His skills as an artist taught him the importance of observation, and he used these with great effect in his teaching and scientific work. It appears that it was his own decision to become a physician, and he finished his secondary school in 1844 to become a hospital extern. In 1848, he was successful in the competitive examinations for hospital internship at the Salpêtrière and was very fortunate in having Rayer, who was physician to Emperor Napoleon III, as his teacher and mentor during these early years. In 1862, a chair in comparative pathology was created for Rayer, who later became Dean of the Faculty of Medicine in the University of Paris.

In 1853, Charcot successfully defended his doctoral thesis, in which he differentiated the symptoms and signs of gout from those of chronic rheumatism, an original piece of work.

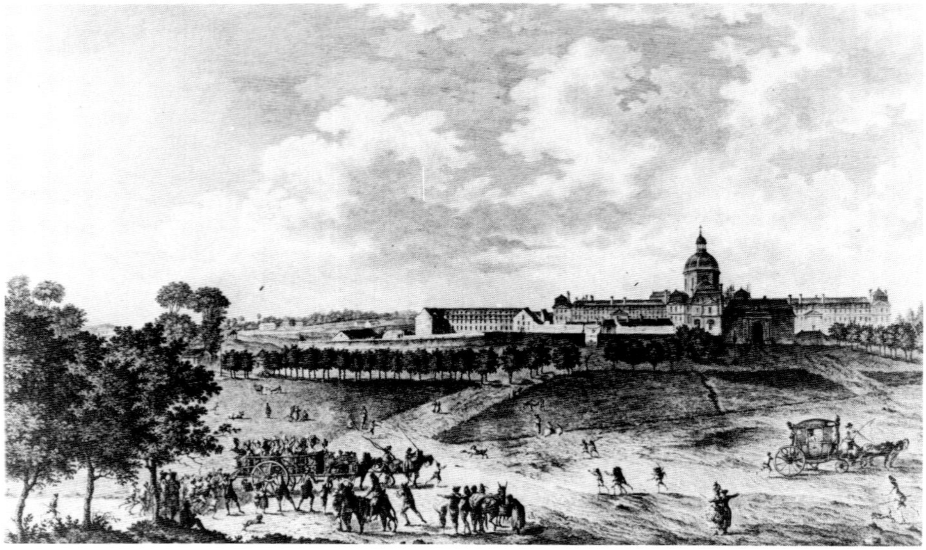

FIG. 1. La Salpêtrière, 18th century.

He afterwards became Chief of Clinic in the Faculty of Medicine, an internal appointment, and set up a small office for private consultations. Professor Rayer suggested to one of his richest patients that Charcot should accompany him as personal physician while on a health tour of Italy. Charcot filled several sketch books on the trip and was fond of describing his impressions in the years to come of Pisa, Siena, Perugia, Rome, Naples, and Florence, where the medical library was a particular favorite. In 1856, Charcot was appointed as "Physician to the Hospitals of Paris."

The competitive examination known as the "Agrégation" has been a center of controversy for many years, being a formidable stumbling block with only a few successful candidates. The title of "Professor Agrégé à la Faculté de Médécine" is an academic appointment, but without it, the highest appointments are not possible, and Charcot failed at his first attempt in 1857. His thesis was entitled "The Expectations of Medicine," probably an unwise subject to discuss with medical superiors at any stage of one's career. It is possible that Hartley's *Observations on Man, His Frame, His Duty and His Expectations* (1749) may have been his source book for this topic. Professor Pierre Janet was to recall many years later that, when visiting Charcot, he was presented with a copy of the book, which Charcot had annotated from front cover to back. When Charcot retook the examination in 1860, Rayer was determined to sit on the committee. Charcot's first subject, "Intestinal Hemorrhages" was below par, but on the "Chronic Pneumonias" he triumphed. Without Rayer, the story might have been very different.

THE SALPÊTRIÈRE

Charcot's name is inextricably linked with that of the Salpêtrière. When he first went there as a young intern, there were more than 5,000 inmates and in previous times, the number had approached 8,000. The Salpêtrière (saltpeter) was constructed as an arsenal

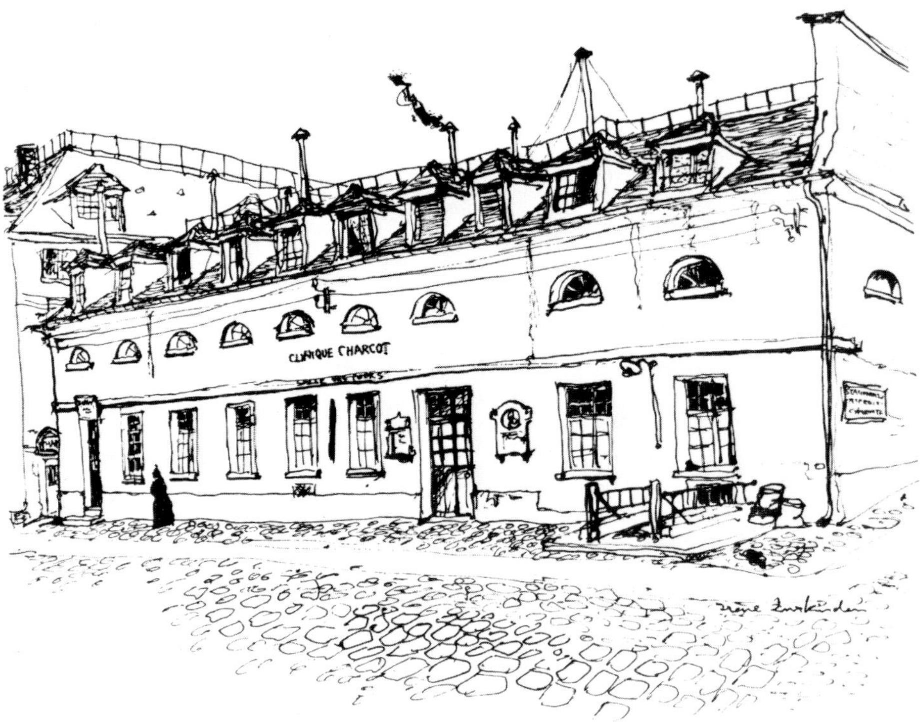

FIG. 2. Charcot's clinic.

on the Left Bank of the Seine in 1565. Previously, a small arsenal had been sited on the opposite bank within the confines of the old city, but repeated explosions so alarmed the local residents that eventually Louis XIII acquiesced to the demands of the petitioners to have the building moved. Civil strife throughout France in the middle of the 17th century resulted in a large migration of peasants to Paris. Without work and poverty stricken, they added to the large numbers of beggars already in the city. A number of charitable organizations were created, the most famous of which was led by Vincent de Paul, who managed to persuade Cardinal Mazarin, Richelieu's successor, to place the Salpêtrière at his disposition, uniting it with other hospitals in the Paris area to form the "Hospice Général." Under the royal edict of 1656, the hospitals would be used "for the confinement of beggars, unwanted womanhood and the infirm," the Bicêtre being reserved for men, the Scipion for pregnant women, and the Salpêtrière for women and prostitutes. In 1680, new buildings were constructed, which included the infamous Prison de la Force, and the Salpêtrière became the largest asylum in Europe.

During the second half of the 18th century, a general infirmary was constructed, which included a maternity ward (Fig. 1). A school and workhouse were also added for the poor children, many of whom were born and died within its confines. It is small wonder that Charcot called the Salpêtrière "this great asylum for human misery." With the new infirmary, the first medical resident was appointed and one of the most famous of these early residents was Pinel (1758–1827). During the first half of the 19th century, many famous

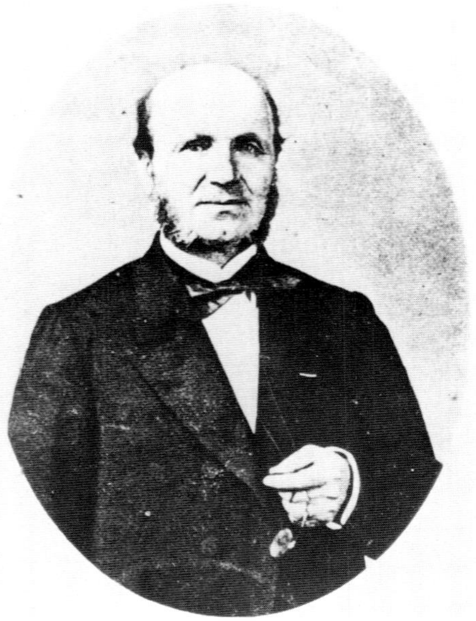

FIG. 3. Armand Duchenne (1806–1895).

physicians worked at the Salpêtrière: Baillarger, Magendie, Cruveilhier, and Lasègue, to name but a few. After his appointment as "Physician to the Hospital" in 1862, when he was 37 years old, Charcot spent the rest of his professional life there (Fig. 2).

THE YEARS OF DISCOVERY

Charcot and Alfred Vulpian were appointed to the Salpêtrière at the same time, and although Vulpian was eventually overshadowed by Charcot, the two remained the greatest of friends; together they surveyed all the patients in all the wards and in all the buildings, classifying and cataloguing the cases into clinical types. It is tempting to speculate that Charcot had foreseen the immense wealth of clinical material that already existed during his years of internship at the Salpêtrière. In his inaugural lecture in 1882, referring to the teaching and investigation of diseases of the nervous system, he said: "Where is there to be found, I asked, so much material specially adapted to this kind of study." Reviewing Charcot's early work, which included chronic rheumatism, gout, diseases of the aged, intermittent claudication, painful paraplegia of neoplastic origin, decubitus ulcers, exophthalmic goiter, lung diseases, etc., one finds no clear indication of an early interest in the diseases of the nervous system. How did it develop? The probable answer was that he was influenced by Duchenne of Boulogne, who entered his service in 1862.

Years later, Charcot was in fact to call Duchenne his master in neurology (Fig. 3). Duchenne, also a great collector of clinical material, was born in 1806, studied medicine in Paris from 1826 to 1831, after which he settled in Boulogne. In 1835, he became interested in the electrical stimulation of muscles, publishing a book on its "application to pathology and therapeutics in 1855." Dr. P. Guilly has written the definitive biography on Duchenne (1936). Duchenne joined Charcot at a time when his personal circumstances were very low, his wife having just died and his "in-laws" preventing his access to his only son. Returning to Paris, he was shunned by all the hospitals, and his work was ridiculed. Charcot helped

Duchenne in every way possible, providing him with research facilities and access to patients. With Joffroy, Charcot taught Duchenne histology and the importance of pathological anatomy. In return, Duchenne taught Charcot photography and discussed his ideas and the results of his research. Never did Charcot take any of this work for his own, and to my knowledge, there is no Charcot-Duchenne disease. Duchenne died following a stroke in September 1875 at the age of 69 years. Charcot had been his close and trusted friend to the end.

In his biography, *Jean-Martin Charcot, His Life—His Work*, Guillain states: "I can affirm, and neurologists have not pressed this point enough, that it was during a period of only eight years between 1862 and 1870 that Charcot structured his magnificent masterpieces by his description of multiple sclerosis, the tabetic arthropathies, amyotrophic lateral sclerosis, and the localisation of lesions of the spinal cord." The reason for the abrupt cessation of his work in 1870 was the Franco-Prussian War, a catastrophe followed by an even greater one, the Commune of Paris in 1871, which witnessed the spectacle of Frenchman fighting Frenchman yet again in an attempt to ensure that the new regime, headed by Thiers, would become an effective republic. The method employed to achieve this end, namely an attempt to relive the "glories of the French Revolution," had disastrous social consequences. Charcot was too busy caring for the sick, fighting typhoid and smallpox, to be concerned with research into the diseases of the nervous system. During this time, he sent his family over to England. He crossed the barricades daily to reach the Salpêtrière. Between 1870 and 1880, Charcot energetically pursued his research, and his works on cerebral localization and aphasia have been considered some of his best. The third phase of his research after 1880 was to include hysteria and the neuroses.

In his early years at the Salpêtrière, Charcot had few students. Charcot used an old, disused kitchen, which he adapted for teaching purposes. He instigated a course of free lectures on diseases of the aged and diseases of the nervous system, which were subsequently published. It was his superb ability as a teacher that was to attract eventually students to his clinic from all over the world. He devised the "anatomo-clinical method of teaching," the equivalent of our clinico-pathological demonstrations, and it was his delight to unravel slowly the complexities of a neurological case, to lead the student to discover one salient point after another, and then to "reveal all" on the blackboard using colored chalks to simplify the anatomical correlations that he did so brilliantly. "Where is the lesion, and what is the lesion, and how is the lesion linked with the clinical findings?" This is, after all, the way that we still try to teach our students the principles of neurology and, like Charcot, we recognize our limitations in attempting to explain why the lesion has occurred.

Charcot stressed the importance of observation to his students, and his slow, systematic scrutiny of the patients was exemplified by the "mysterious silence of Charcot," as described by his old pupils Meige and Souques, his last Chief of Clinic. Charcot might look at the patient for several minutes without saying a word; then he might ask a question or ask for a reflex to be checked or sensory examination repeated, each activity being punctuated by a period of silence (Fig. 4). Charcot said: "It is the mind which is really alive and sees things, yet it hardly sees anything without preliminary instruction." He also appreciated the narrowness of our comprehension: "In the last analysis, we see only what we are ready to see, what we have been taught to see. We eliminate and ignore everything that is not part of our prejudices."

With few students and a private practice that was yet to attract patients from all over the world, Charcot spent a lot of time with his interns and became personally very close to them, directing and supervising their activities and suggesting research projects for them. He set up a simple laboratory, equipped with microscopes, and soon filled the benches with

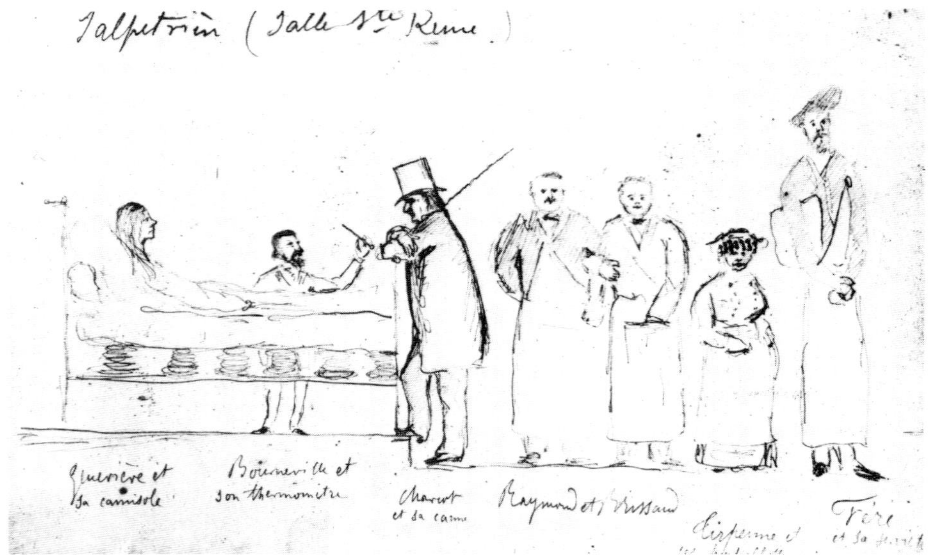

FIG. 4. The ward round.

anatomical specimens. To his students, each year appeared to herald a different discovery or different disease. Hence, they would say, "the year of the tabetic arthropathies, the year of miliary aneurysms, the year of poliomyelitis," and so on. Charcot was remarkably sanguine on this aspect of his work: "How is it that, one fine morning, Duchenne discovered a disease which probably existed in the time of Hippocrates?" (on "pseudohypertrophic muscular dystrophy").

PROFESSOR OF PATHOLOGIC ANATOMY

Alfred Vulpian was appointed to this post in 1867 as Cruveilhier's successor. Cruveilhier (1791–1874) had been the most outstanding pathologist of his day, although confining himself to macroscopic examination. Rudolph Virchow (1821–1902) and his colleagues were making enormous progress through the use of light microscopy. In 1872, Vulpian, who sought to redress this balance, was promoted to Professor of Experimental Pathology, and Charcot was nominated as his successor to the Chair of Pathologic Anatomy, which he was to occupy for 10 years, during all of which time he served as President of the Anatomic Society. His contribution to the anatomy and physiology of the spinal cord was outstanding, as demonstrated by his lectures in 1873. He used the atlases that had been so carefully prepared by Cruveilhier and Carswell for his teaching. He continued to work with Vulpian, and Bouchard joined him.

Charcot did not confine himself to neuropathology. His lectures on diseases of the liver and kidneys were published later (1887) as a book of 380 pages and translated into English and Russian. His work on chest diseases was outstanding, and he demonstrated the histological structure of the tubercle, which he considered, before Koch, to be the essential lesion of pulmonary tuberculosis. At a conference held by the British Medical Association, Charcot was surrounded by distinguished physicians, who tried to persuade him that pulmonary tuberculosis was not one disease but many. He would always listen attentively to those who expressed contrary opinions and "would lift his hands and shoulders with a little expressive gesture and would quietly say, 'It may be so'." On this occasion, however, he calmly put his hands on his drawings of the pathological and histological appearances and repeated, "Yet it is all *one process*," a truth later verified by Koch.

In the aftermath of the Franco-Prussian War and the Commune of Paris, his family returned from England. Charcot's fame rapidly increased, and his lectures began to attract a wide audience, with students coming from many different countries. In Charcot's laboratory, Kozhevnikov demonstrated that in amyotrophic lateral sclerosis, the nerve degeneration could be followed up to the motor cortex.

In his inaugural address in 1882, Charcot quoted Claude Bernard:

> Pathology should not be subordinated to physiology. Quite the reverse. Set up first the medical problem which arises from the observation of a malady, and afterwards seek for a physiological explanation. To act otherwise would be to risk overlooking the patient, and distorting the malady.

Charcot felt that at the Salpêtrière, "we are in possession of a sort of living pathological museum whose resources are almost inexhaustible." He outlined his approach to these resources as follows:

> The method most suitable to the explanation of the vast domains of pathology can be described as *nosological*. It is, in fact, the traditional method, for it is the one which, ever since medicine has existed, has been employed to investigate morbid states, to determine their characteristics, their causation, their correlations, and the modifications which they undergo by the influence of therapeutic agents. And facts of this kind, gentlemen, I beg you to observe, necessarily constitute the very foundation of every scientific construction in pathology, and without this basis, the physiology of disease would be but a vain phrase.

Charcot also predicted that neuropathology would one day become a separate specialty.

CLINICAL CHAIR OF DISEASES OF THE NERVOUS SYSTEM

In July 1881, the French Parliament voted a sum of 200,000 francs for the establishment of a new professorial chair in diseases of the nervous system, an appointment created specifically for Charcot. In his inaugural address on January 2, 1882, he "eagerly embraced the opportunity to thank the Municipal Council of the City of Paris and also the Administration of Public Assistance whose prompt and liberal aid has rendered possible a scheme without which it would have encountered obstacles well-nigh insurmountable."

It was clear from his address that this support came first, and only afterwards the support of his colleagues, as he goes on to say: "Thanks to their help, which really took place prior to the approval of the University, we are already in possession of appliances and conveniences that form a veritable Neuro-pathological Institution." Charcot had seen that:

> To make this department perfect and complete, it yet required space within the Infirmary where certain of the patients, who come to us from outside, could be temporarily admitted as in-patients. This concession we asked for many times, and at length the difficulties in the way of its achievement were surmounted. Happily for our cause it met with the support of the Director of the Public Assistance. All the obstacles were one by one removed, and now we have wards for the temporary admission of cases. They contain eighty beds—forty for women and forty for men.

It may be pertinent to recall Charcot's first wealthy private patient, with whom he traveled to Italy, an introduction made by Charcot's chief, Professor Rayer, who had the very highest of government support. The patient was Monsieur A. Fould, a rich banker who was later to become Minister of Finance. Charcot certainly had important connections with the French Government and acted as a diplomat for them on a number of occasions as did his successor, Fulgence Raymond.

On August 19, 1893, the *Lancet* published a short notice on the death of Charcot (which was followed by an obituary on August 26), stating that "he had many friends in this country and often came to England, and it may be remembered that quite recently he was sent on a visit to Bournemouth on a mission from the French Government."

Until his sudden death in 1893, Charcot enjoyed all the honors that his unique accomplishments merited. He was a member of every major medical and neurological society in Europe, and also in the United States. He was elected to the Academy of Sciences in 1883, the highest ranking academic body in France, sponsored by his old friend Professor Vulpian. His research interests at this time turned toward hysteria and the neuroses that, Pierre Marie pointed out, occurred almost by accident. Patients attached to the psychiatric service of Dr. Delasiaire were housed in a dilapidated building, and when these premises were evacuated, the administration at the Salpêtrière took advantage of it to separate nonpsychotic epileptics and hysterics from the insane. As Charcot was the senior physician at the Salpêtrière, this new service was assigned to him. Charcot attempted to employ the same methodology for the classification of hysteria as he had so successfully applied to diseases of the nervous system. Later, he was to investigate hypnotism as a means of trying to understand hysteria.

The controversy surrounding these years of Charcot's research has caused more misunderstanding about him and his methods than ever could have been imagined when one considers the scientific monument that he had built at the Salpêtrière. Few neurologists of this generation have ever read Charcot's works, yet the criticisms linger—partly because the battles were continued by some of his former pupils after his death. This may be the reason why it took so long before a biography was produced on Charcot's life and work. Guillain's book was published in France in 1955 and not translated into English until 1959 by Pearce Bailey, former Director of the National Institutes of Health, Bethesda, Maryland. It is significant that in the *British Medical Journal* of August 26, 1893, in the same issue that gave Charcot's obituary, a leader appeared entitled "Charcot and Hypnotism." The aims of the author were clear—to state precisely what Charcot actually said and did in this difficult field:

> No man was more opposed to quackery and to him is due the credit of helping to rescue somnambulism from the illegitimate embrace of the charlatan. Fifteen years ago only a strong man could have given the demonstrations which he gave without endangering his professional status and a few shallow visitors carped even at him; but he passed through the ordeal with impunity, and rendered it easy for others to prosecute the same studies. He left an example to other investigators of avoiding the rocks on which some of his *confrères* without his scientific instinct have foolishly run their craft and suffered well-merited shipwreck. Never did the illustrious professor at the Salpêtrière allow himself to be drawn aside from the path of inductive science. His scorn of the frauds and follies which sprang up in a credulous circle outside his own school was only equalled by that which he manifested for the incredulous ignoramuses in his own profession who sneered at phenomena which they could not understand but in which he recognised like our own Laycock, a nice source of neurological and psychological knowledge.

Charcot's health begain to fail in 1890. He suffered from attacks of angina and gave up his favorite cigars. Some of these episodes have been documented by his former pupils and colleagues, Professor Debove and Dr. Souques, and by Leon Daudet, who, like his famous father, Alphonse, was a close friend of Charcot. It was Madame Charcot who suggested to her husband that he take a vacation in August 1893. With Professors Debove and Straus, he went into the Morvan, where they stayed at an inn situated by the edge of the "lac des Settons" and on the evening of August 16, 1893 after a "gay dinner," as Professor Debove tells us, Charcot retired to his room. He wrote a long letter to his wife. At 3 o'clock in the morning, Straus found Charcot acutely dyspneic, seated in an armchair at the end of the bed, and called Debove. The dyspnea increased, and then his breathing became slower and stopped.

According to Charcot's wishes, there were no funeral speeches. The service was held in the Chapel of the Salpêtrière, and the coffin was transferred to the Cimetière Montmartre, where his son was also buried in 1936.

A PORTRAIT OF CHARCOT

We are always curious about great men, a curiosity that goes beyond the cataloguing of their achievements. Instead, we search for some clue in their characters that enabled them to attain the very peak of their profession. To get behind the facade can be difficult, but with Charcot we are particularly fortunate that so many of his former pupils published many personal accounts about their "Master" after Charcot's death.

The portraits that exist of Charcot date from the height of his fame (Fig. 5). In appearance, he has been likened to Napoleon or to an abbé, but his students called him the "Caesar of the Salpêtrière," supposedly on account of his punctiliousness. Charcot was certainly reserved, although less so than Vulpian. He did not show emotion readily, and those who did not know him thought he was cold and remote. His English colleagues considered that he was more like a typical English gentleman than their prejudiced view of the "typical" Frenchman. He spoke slowly and carefully, was fluent in English and German, and spoke five languages in all. Although a brilliant teacher, he was not a natural orator. He lectured without notes, giving the impression that it was impromptu but, in reality, he had spent hours writing and memorizing his lectures. During the summer, he would prepare his lectures

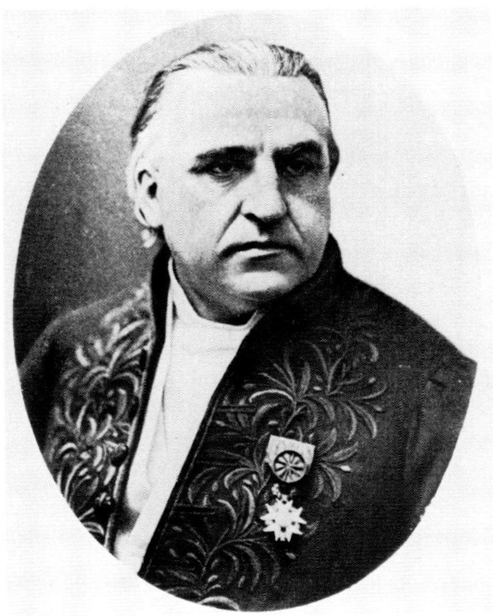

FIG. 5. Jean-Martin Charcot (1825–1893).

for the coming autumn and winter months. His students would take his lectures down in longhand and with his permission publish them. Bourneville edited many of these "Leçons," as did Guinon, which would not have been possible if the lectures had not been carefully prepared. On Tuesday mornings, he held his famous clinic, presenting patients to his students in the form of a clinical demonstration. Charcot loved to wheel in one patient after another, comparing and contrasting physical signs. The famous Friday morning lectures, looked upon as the high spot of the week's activities, were quite different. He would prepare the lecture all week, selecting patients and rehearsing the lecture the day before. Later, Charcot made the mistake of allowing nonmedical personnel to attend some of these meetings, and was criticized for turning these lectures into dramatic events.

In 1884, Charcot had moved into a magnificent house at 217, Boulevard Saint-Germain. His wife, who was a young widow with a daughter when they met, adored him, and family life revolved around him. Her father was a well-known Parisian tailor, who collected paintings as a hobby, a passion that Charcot shared, so that the new home was full of art treasures. They had two children, Jeanne, born in 1865, and Jean-Baptiste-Auguste in 1867. Although devoted to his family, Charcot did not show his affection overtly. He insisted that his son become a doctor, despite the young Jean's enthusiasm to join the Navy (as his uncle had done), and he eventually became Charcot's intern at the Salpêtrière. After Charcot's death, the love of the sea was too great for Jean-Baptiste, who later became a great man in his own right through his Arctic and Antarctic explorations. He was lost in his ship (the *Pourquoi Pas?*) in 1936, and his funeral services were held in Notre Dame Cathedral. At the time he gave up medicine, Jean-Baptiste Charcot said: "If I succeed, that would be the best way to honor the memory of my father, because the name of Charcot would be honored twice."

Charcot loved animals and, as a result of this, refused to do animal experimentation. His house always contained several, including, for a time, a monkey that sat in a child's high chair at meal times, and Charcot would roar with delight at his pet's antics. He went so far as to put a sign above one of the doors to his laboratory: "Vous ne trouverez pas une clinique des chiens chez moi."

Charcot would be at his desk in his study by 6.00 a.m. and would hire a carriage that took him to the Salpêtrière by 9.00 a.m., calling for him at noon to take him home. In the afternoons, he would see private patients in his study which, remembering his favorite Italian journey, he had modeled after the Medici Library in Florence. To this he added stained-glass windows. The effect on his private patients, seeing Charcot seated at his desk at the end of the imposing room, can only be imagined! The young Pierre Marie, who had also been intern to Paul Broca, acted as Charcot's private assistant for a number of years, taking the history, examining the patient, and presenting the case to Charcot who would then verify the findings. Charcot would diagnose the complaint and offer guidelines for treatment but generally left prescribing to the patient's own physician. His English colleagues felt that he was not particularly interested in treatment, but the probable explanation was that Charcot realized more clearly how little physicians had to offer in the way of treatment for the diseases of the nervous system. For example, Sir William Osler states that after years of study on hypnotism "Charcot became less and less hopeful as to its value as a therapeutic measure." It is doubtful whether or not Charcot ever actually hypnotized anybody, leaving it to his interns. He certainly was never deceived by his patients in the way that Luys had been at the Charité. Charcot's fee for a consultation was 40 francs, which Pierre Marie collected from the patient. Guy de Maupassant, writing at this time, tells us in one of his short stories that 20 francs would buy one silk umbrella!

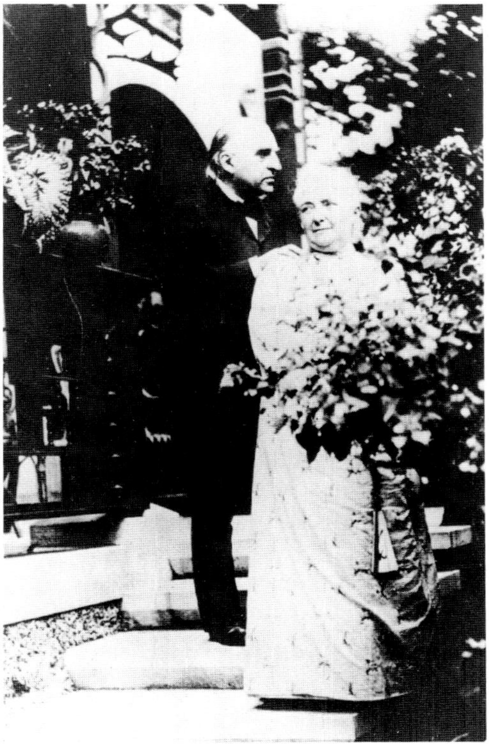

FIG. 6. Jean-Martin Charcot and his wife in his summer home at Neuilly-sur-Seine.

Every summer he took his family to Neuilly-sur-Seine, originally in the country, to a rented villa, which he eventually bought and where his son was born (Fig. 6). During the autumn and winter months in Paris, Professor and Mrs. Charcot held their famous Tuesday evening soirées, with the best food and wine, and the children and guests dressed in their finery. Charcot's favorite pupils, interns, and colleagues would sit alongside famous people from other walks of life. Among them was the Emperor of Brazil, Don Pedro d'Alcantara, who apparently played billiards with Charcot. These were glittering occasions at which Charcot, the man of learning, reigned supreme, but he refrained from discussing politics, apart from the occasion when he strongly criticized Virchow for using his scientific eminence for political ends. Charcot firmly believed that medicine and science were for the benefit of all mankind and not to be used for the claims of national superiority. Charcot was not deeply religious although he was extremely tolerant in these matters, as Professors Debove and Straus commented after his death.

Charcot showed genuine concern for his patients, and they certainly respected him as the "Master." His clinic at the Salpêtrière was a total contrast to the magnificence of his study at home. It was bare-walled apart from a signed portrait of Hughlings Jackson (Charcot suggested the term "Jacksonian epilepsy") and painted black. After becoming Professor in 1882, he preferred to have patients brought to the clinic from the wards rather than perform ward rounds. He was upset by the realities of familial diseases, to which the children would also eventually succumb. When describing the disease named after him, "the Amyotrophy of Charcot-Marie" (now called Charcot-Marie-Tooth Disease), he would quote a favorite

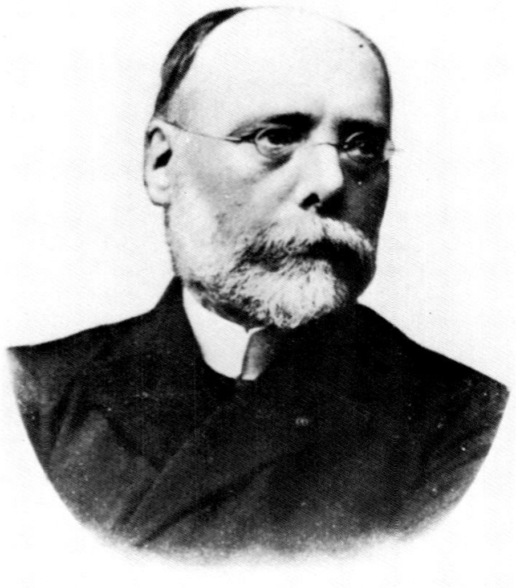

FIG. 7. Charles Bouchard (1837–1915).

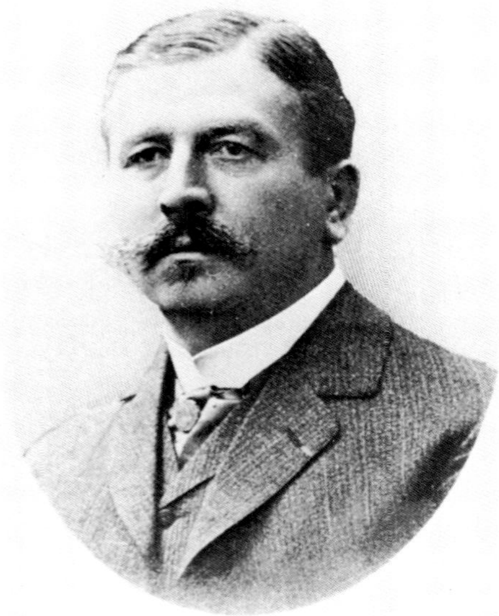

FIG. 8. Joseph Babinski (1857–1932).

expression: "What have we done Oh! Zeus! to deserve this destiny? Our fathers were wanting, but we, what have we done?"

Frequent mention has been made of his close relationship with many of his pupils and former interns, and he was particularly sad and deeply hurt when Charles Bouchard (Fig. 7) turned against him, but he never spoke about it. It was not a question of priority over the Charcot-Bouchard aneurysms, as Bouchard himself later admitted when he formally acknowledged Charcot, but by then Charcot was dead. It would seem that professional jealously and rivalry emerged only after Charcot had helped Bouchard to become Professor in the Faculty of Medicine, when Bouchard probably decided to compete with Charcot for

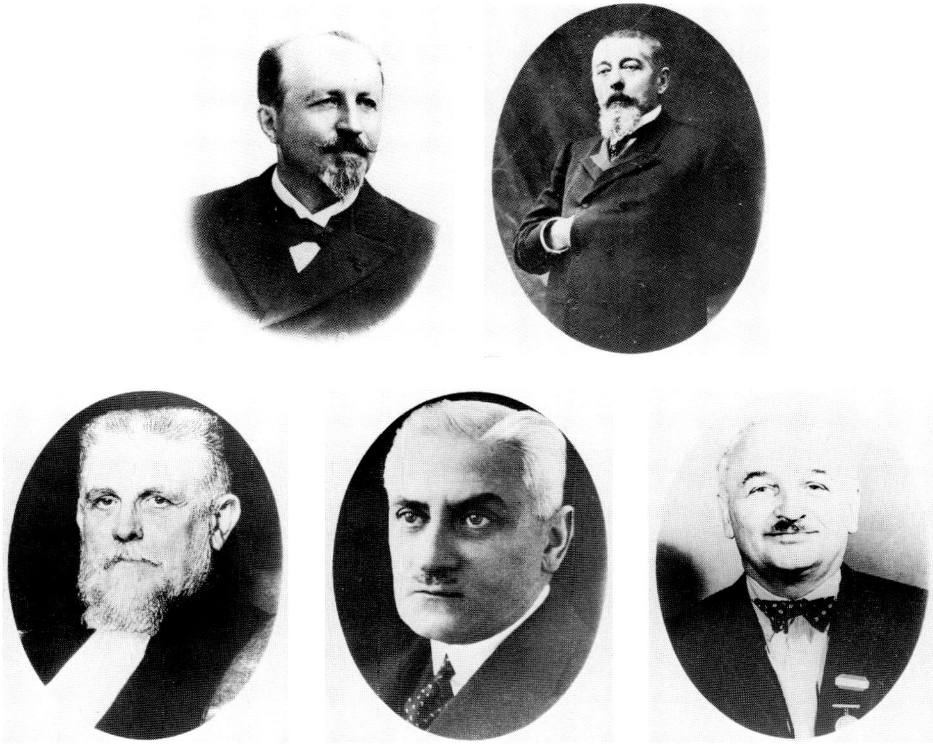

FIG. 9. From left to right: Fulgence Raymond (1844–1910); Jules Dejerine (1849–1917); Pierre Marie (1853–1940); Georges Guillain (1876–1961); Theophile Alajouanine (1890–1980).

the unofficial title of the most powerful professor in the entire faculty. Bouchard's open antagonism was to have one grave consequence. In the 1892 examinations for the Agrégations, Charcot and Bouchard were both examiners. Charcot wanted his favorite pupil, Joseph Babinski (Fig. 8). Bouchard ensured that Babinski was not nominated and pushed a candidate of his choice instead. Babinski never retook the examination and, therefore, never became a professor in the Faculty of Medicine, which deprived him of the chance to be Charcot's successor.

CHARCOT'S LEGACY

Professor Charcot created a Neurological Institute in the midst of the largest asylum in Europe. It has been said that if he had never written a word, his teaching alone would have made him famous. His artistic talents and eclectic interests are illustrated in his two books with his former intern Paul Richer. In his writing, he had the great gift of clarity and "word painting," and the neurological literature contains a large number of diseases eponymously named after him. In the years to come, his pupils carried the torch he lit, foreign students taking the new specialty of "diseases of the nervous system" back to their own countries, adopting Charcot's methods of teaching and research, and in the process becoming professors of their own departments in turn.

Professor Jean-Martin Charcot's legacy can be summarized as follows: He created the first neurological institute, he was the first professor of neurology, and he created a neurological dynasty at the Salpêtrière that stretches from the 1880s to the 1980s by virtue of the great neurologists who followed their "Master" (Figs. 9a–9e):

Fulgence Raymond	1894–1910
Jules Dejerine	1910–1917
Pierre Marie	1919–1925
Georges Guillain	1925–1948
Th. Alajouanine	1948–1954

As Dr. Wechsler wrote: "Of Charcot, it may be said with truth that he entered neurology in its infancy and left it at its coming-of-age, largely nourished by his own contributions and personal magic."

ACKNOWLEDGMENTS

I should like to thank the National Library of Medicine, Bethesda, Maryland, for all their help in the preparation of the photographs for this chapter.

BIBLIOGRAPHY

1. (1893): Obituary on Prof. Charcot. *Br. Med. J.*, 2:495–496.
2. (1893): Charcot and hypnotism. *Br. Med. J.*, 2:479–480.
3. Charcot, J. M. (1877): *Lectures on the Diseases of the Nervous System*, translated and edited by G. Sigerson. New Sydenham Society, London.
4. Charcot, J. M. (1881): *Lectures on the Diseases of the Nervous System*, second series, translated and edited by G. Sigerson. New Sydenham Society, London.
5. Charcot, J. M. (1883): *Lectures on the Localisation of Cerebral and Spinal Diseases*, translated and edited by W. B. Hadden. New Sydenham Society, London.
6. Charcot, J. M. (1889): *Clinical Lectures on Diseases of the Nervous System*, Vol. III, translated by T. Savill. New Sydenham Society, London.
7. Cushing, H. (1926): *The Life of Sir William Osler*, Vol. 1 and Vol. 2. Clarendon Press, Oxford.
8. Guillain, G. (1959): *Jean-Martin Charcot: His Life—His Work*, translated and edited by Pearce Bailey. Paul B. Hoeber, New York.
9. Haymaker, W., and Schiller, F. (1970): *The Founders of Neurology*, 2nd ed. Charles C Thomas, Springfield, Illinois.
10. (1893): Death of Professor Charcot. *Lancet*, 2:446.
11. (1893): Obituary on Jean-Martin Charcot. *Lancet*, 2:523–525.
12. Osler, W. (1893): Jean-Martin Charcot. *Johns Hopkins Hosp. Bull.*, 87–88.
13. Satran, R. (1974): Fulgence Raymond, the successor of Charcot. *Bull. N. Y. Acad. Med.*, 50:931–942.
14. Shryock, R. H. (1979): *The Development of Modern Medicine*. University of Wisconsin Press, Madison, Wisconsin.

Historical Aspects of the Neurosciences,
edited by F. Clifford Rose and W. F. Bynum.
Raven Press, New York ©

Gilles de la Tourette[1]

Paul Guilly

Ancien Interne des Hôpitaux de Paris, Ancien Chef de Clinique Neuro-Psychiatrique à la Faculté, Paris, France

Gilles de la Tourette: What an attractive surname! One that evokes a figure out of Watteau rather than the pitiful disease—fortunately very rare—to which his name remains attached. *La maladie des tics convulsifs* or *maladie de Gilles de la Tourette* is characterized by multiple abnormal and compulsive movements, accompanied by echolalia and coprolalia. Classically, the disorder progresses towards a state of increasing mental deterioration, but nowadays long remissions—sometimes apparent cures—are possible under the effect of certain drugs, such as neuroleptics of the butyrophenone type, for example, haloperidol and pimozide (a dopamine antagonist), as well as the nonbarbiturate antiepileptics valproic acid and its amide (valpromide).

It was in 1884 that Gilles de la Tourette, in the *Archives de Neurologie*, reported nine cases of convulsive tics. One of the cases was a female patient, the Marquise de Dampierre, who in 1825 was under the care of Dr. Jean Itard and who lived as recluse from childhood and "ticked and blasphemed" until the age of 80. After certain modifications in 1885, the initial description was considered "remarkably correct" by New York authorities writing in 1978.

Between 1884 and 1965, only 50 cases of this strange disease were published throughout the world medical literature, so that some began to doubt the very existence of its nosological entity. The name of Gilles de la Tourette gradually disappeared from neurological and psychiatric monographs at the same time that it faded from the most recent medical encyclopedias and books on medical history in France. The *Grand Larousse Encyclopédique*, appearing between 1960 and 1964, no longer cited a name that claimed a dozen lines in 1936 in the *Larousse du XXe Siècle*.

Besides neurologists and psychiatrists, both adult and pediatric, young French doctors did not know the name that attracted so much attention at the end of the last century; the older ones remember him only through Léon Daudet—a failed doctor—his ruthless enemy, who cruelly caricatured him through several pages of his *Souvenirs Politiques, Médicaux et Littéraires*, *Les Oeuvres dans les Hommes* and *Paris Vécu*, his best book.[2]

For nearly 80 years, theses have been written about the etiology of this disease, suggesting various types of cerebral degeneration or psychological, psychoanalytical, or psychosomatic causes. Almost all—under a deluge of words—do not explain much, but some authors have

---

[1]Translated from the French by Leslie Oliver.

[2]It is in the second volume of his *Souvenirs, Devant la Douleur*, that Léon Daudet, son of the famous novelist Alphonse Daudet, talks of Charcot, his pupils, and of contemporary medicine (1).

suggested changes in the striate bodies. The arguments changed quickly between the years 1960 and 1970, after the discovery of haloperidol, even though a certain confusion persists between the disease of "convulsive tics" and the tics of children, the latter well known by pediatric neurologists, child psychiatrists, and pediatricians as fairly common, with spontaneous recovery in the majority of cases. This is the time when Woodrow (2) jokingly stressed the number of suggested treatments for resistant tics: "going from a glass of water swallowed twelve times a day to LSD, passing by imipramine, psychotherapy and psychoanalysis, hypnosis, the antihistamines and lobotomy."

The Americans took the matter in hand with their prodigious means of scientific research, enlarging little by little the outline of Gilles de la Tourette's original description. Four research workers in New York published in 1978 a very important work entitled *Gilles de la Tourette Syndrome* (3), citing 485 cases, including 250 personal observations and a very elaborate study of 145 patients. The book involves several disciplines, including psychiatrists, neurologists, electroencephalographers, social workers, and nurses. All the conclusions converged toward a genetic etiology with familial correlations, although several points still remain obscure about this syndrome, which the authors in their publication call "a bizarre neuropsychiatric disorder." Soon "Tourette's Disease" (phonetically unpleasant) or "Gilles de la Tourette's Disease" will again be established as a true clinical entity.

In France, two child psychiatrists, P. Debray-Ritzen and H. Dubois, published in 1980 two excellent studies on infantile tics (4). In the first study, the authors only "suggest" a relationship between the disease of Gilles de la Tourette and that of infantile tics, but they commit themselves without ambiguity in their second study to favoring a common etiology. The summary of the latter is perfectly clear:

> With regard to 93 cases the clinical picture of tics of children is defined. The frequency of this condition in the infantile population is 3.3 per 1,000; it affects 4.5 boys to one girl and seems very superimposable on the disease of adult tics described by Gilles de la Tourette, the beginning of which goes back to infancy in 85 per cent of cases and which would rarely be the evolution, chronic and serious, of the disease of tics of children. A familial incidence is noted in 20 per cent of cases as well as a minimal cerebral dysfunction . . .

A scatterbrained, irrational eccentric, or, keeping to medical terminology, a hypomaniac on a basis of temperamental lack of balance, ending a short life in a state of dementia, George Gilles de la Tourette came from a family of doctors. He was born on October 30, 1857 at Saint-Gervais-les-Trois-Clochers, a large village of Poitou between Loudun and Chatellerault. It was at the college of this subprefecture that he began his studies. Very undisciplined, boisterous, flighty, his intelligence proved to be so sharp that he went through two classes in the same year, passing his *baccalauréate* at 16 years. His mother considered him to be too young for life in Paris and sent him to Poitiers, where he brilliantly completed his first three years of medical studies.

The adolescent spent long holidays with relations at Loudun, a strange little city, the roads of which, narrow and picturesque, still smell of sulphur from the devilry—under Louis XIII—of possessed nuns; "a town," wrote Sainte-Beuve, "where demons have established their stay." Loudun is also the birthplace of Dr. Théophraste Renaudot, founder of journalism in France, with his *Gazette*, and also, the initiator of a large number of social changes. As Dr. Paul Ganière[3] says so well (5):

---

[3]Dr. P. Ganière is the author of *Ils Étaient Aussi Médecins (They Were Also Doctors)*, from which the above quote is taken, an interesting book about doctors who became famous in very different branches, e.g., among the English, there are David Livingstone and Conan Doyle.

> Could it be conceived today, that a region develops without a labour exchange, pawnshop, auction rooms, dispensaries, without cultural organisations, all enterprises which Théophraste Renaudot had wanted, three centuries too soon, to give to his fellow citizens? But it is, perhaps, in the domain of social medicine that he was a forerunner with his great ideas that allowed the poor to receive the same care as the rich . . .

The endless conflicts between Renaudot—supported by Richelieu—and Guy Patin, Dean of the Paris Faculty of Medicine, remain memorable. Gilles, curious about the past, searched lofts, presbyteries, and municipal archives, finding there charts, parchments, and old papers, which allowed him, during his time as resident, to publish the first complete biography of Théophraste Renaudot and the bewildering story of *Soeur Anne des Anges*, of which the preface was written by Charcot.

From the moment of his arrival in Paris, Gilles prepared for his examinations for nomination as house physician at the age of 20 years. A contemporary speaks of him in these terms: "I have known him since the days of the residents' common room. He was a jovial and exuberant young man with a loud voice. Very ardent, but not very patient, because over-excited, he got worked up in the most minor argument. . . ." Another testimony presents him in a more displeasing light. Perhaps wishing to get himself excused because of the prefix of his name (the "de la"), he put up a wild anticlerical notice, and when carving a chicken in front of religious colleagues, he added with a laugh: "I'm carving the *heavenly pigeon*." Some took this joke very badly, and it often ended in noisy altercations.

In 1884, Gilles was house physician at the Salpêtrière in Charcot's department. He was to have other chiefs such as Paul Brouardel, the famous forensic doctor, and Alfred Fournier, whose work on syphilis of the nervous system was already authoritative. But Charcot alone became his god, the Caesar-like Charcot who then haughtily imposed his teaching and dogma on all the faculties of Europe. Gilles de la Tourette became his most enthusiastic disciple, his most efficient collaborator, his most servile praiser, as his opponents were already asserting—and they were becoming numerous—against this medical Rastignac[4] of fanatical ambition.

The last third of the 19th century saw the climax of the vogue of hysteria and hypnotism, spectacular lessons of the Master—let us leave the monumental neurological work on which his glory rests today—that attracted, in addition to French and foreign doctors, a public as heterogenous as well as numerous: philosophers, literary people, artists, men and women of the world, snobs, and simply curious people, who piled up on the seats of an amphitheater that was too small. The press, almost unanimously, gave a bad mixture of publicity to his demonstrations. The mediocre writer, Jules Claretie, collected material at the Salpêtrière for the *Amours d'un Interne (Loves of a Houseman)*, a novel that nowadays is unreadable, while a medical student, the future novelist Axel Munthe, was working in a department that, 40 years later, he would tear apart with realism in *The Story of San Michele*. Hysteria was then, as Lasègue has said, the "waste paper basket," where everything was put that could not be classified, neuroses carefully cultivated in "hot greenhouses," (old people's homes and hospitals) often ending up as theatrical presentations—"faked" according to some—sometimes outrageous and almost shocking.

Gilles presented his thesis in 1886: "Etude de la marche dans les maladies du système nerveux," applying the method of "impressions" recommended by a Polish author. He

---

[4]Translator's footnote: Rastignac was a character created by Honoré de Balzac. He was a type of elegant *arriviste* and appears, for example, in the novel *Le Père Goriot*.

popularized ideas that were not his own with great ability. A year later, he was Charcot's registrar, a post much sought after. He performed his duties with authority and with a real talent as a teacher, showing an extraordinary activity, perhaps beyond the limits of normality: large books, monographs, incessant communications on neurology and psychiatry, historical studies, scientific and literary lectures on all subjects.

He founded, with his friend Paul Richer, an artist of great talent, *La Nouvelle Iconographie de la Salpêtrière*,[5] and published it in a great number of articles, as well as in *Le Progrès Medical*, a journal then very much read by doctors, including the director, his friend Désiré Bourneville, called "Boubour" or "Bournepatte" by the house officers, the father of *sclérose tubéreuse*, and a very influential Paris town councilor. In spite of the difference in age of 17 years between the two men, they became attracted by their radical political opinions. Both wished for the departure of the nursing nuns from the hospital and recommended the secularization of all hospital staff; their enemies used to sing in the residents' common room:

> M'sieu Gilles de la Tourette
> N'est pas d'humeur facile
> Quand avec des pincettes
> On touche à Bourneville
> (M. Gilles de la Tourette
> Is not of good temper
> When with pincers
> One touches Bourneville)

We now come to the time when Léon Daudet, aged 20, a medical student, with his intimate friend Jean Charcot, the future explorer, began to attend the Salpêtrière and met Gilles de la Tourette, of whom Daudet painted this gloomy picture:

> Gilles de la Tourette was ugly like a Papuan idol with bundles of hair stuck on it. He was neither good nor bad, neither studious nor lazy, neither intelligent nor foolish, and he vacillated with his confused and malicious mind between a multitude of faults without lingering. He had a husky and worn-out voice, abrupt gestures, a strange gait. He passed for an eccentric starting an interesting subject but leaving it for another, disconcerting his masters by his queer ways which got worse and worse and became less and less amusing. . . .

We should be careful about taking Daudet's comments too literally. Daudet who distorts reality without quite contradicting himself and writes without batting an eyelid: "He was neither good nor bad, neither studious nor lazy, neither intelligent nor foolish", which strictly means nothing. As for Gilles—not without humor and with perhaps already a shade of megalomania—he declared: "I'm as ugly as a louse but I'm very intelligent." They were both wrong, as is shown by his photograph, where it can be confirmed that he was neither handsome nor ugly (Fig. 1).

Charcot, being completely skeptical about the treatment of organic diseases of the nervous system, nevertheless kept himself up to date with all the therapeutic trials in France and abroad. It is Gilles, his most receptive student, whom he asked to experiment with the bizarre treatment of locomotor ataxia by stretching the spinal cord advocated by Professor

---

[5]*La Nouvelle Iconographie de la Salpêtrière* completed three volumes of the *Iconographie photographique de la Salpêtrière*, published between 1873 and 1880 by D. Bourneville and P. Regnard with the aid of a very skillful photographer, Albert Londe, who was attached to the service of Charcot. All the volumes today are still a source of documents that one consults with curiosity and profit.

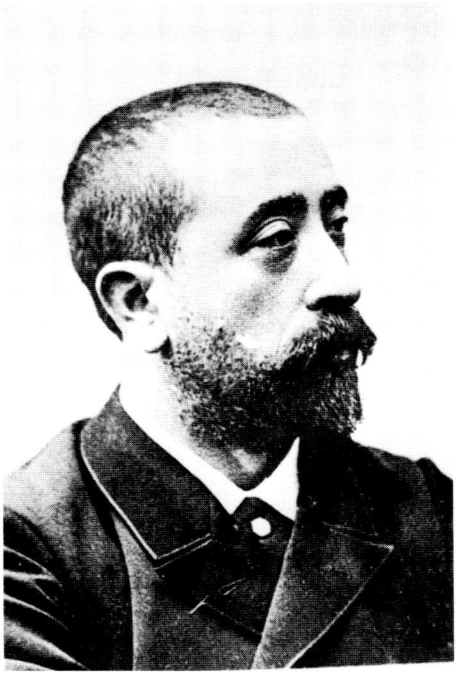

FIG. 1. Photograph of Gilles de la Tourette.

Moczutkovski of Odessa. The apparatus of Seyre of New York was used: a horizontal rod of iron with, at the two extremities, a complicated system of straps. The patient was suspended by chin and axillae for one to four minutes (Figs. 2A and 2B).

We have only one written testimony by a patient about this treatment, that of Alphonse Daudet, affected by a particularly painful advancing tabes. The novelist, in *La Doulou*, a little book published posthumously, with the moving epigraph *dictante dolore*, describes thus the pangs of a session of suspension:

> I remain up to four minutes in the air, two of which held only by the jaw. Pains in the teeth. Then when getting down when I was detached, horrible discomfort in the dorsal and cervical region, as though all the spinal cord was melting away. I am obliged to squat and get up little by little, a way—it seems—so that the spinal cord gets back into place. No appreciable effect.

And further on he adds: "Thirteen stretchings. Then spitting blood that I attribute to the congestion and fatigue caused by the treatment." A line of stops, and Daudet finishes: "Everything turns away. . . . The night swallows me up."

"A print of Goya!" wrote Edmond de Goncourt in his *Journal*, witness of a session that Macdonald Critchley recalls in his very pertinent study about the tabes of Alphonse Daudet, the origin of which he attributes to "his long liaison with the *Chien Vert* or Marie Rieu" (6). She of course was the one immortalized in his novel *Sapho*.

The suspension method of treatment, welcomed with enthusiasm, rapidly provoked many reservations: "There was no longer in France," wrote the wise Gilles de la Tourette, "a hydrotherapeutic establishment, not even a gymnasium, where it was not practiced, left most

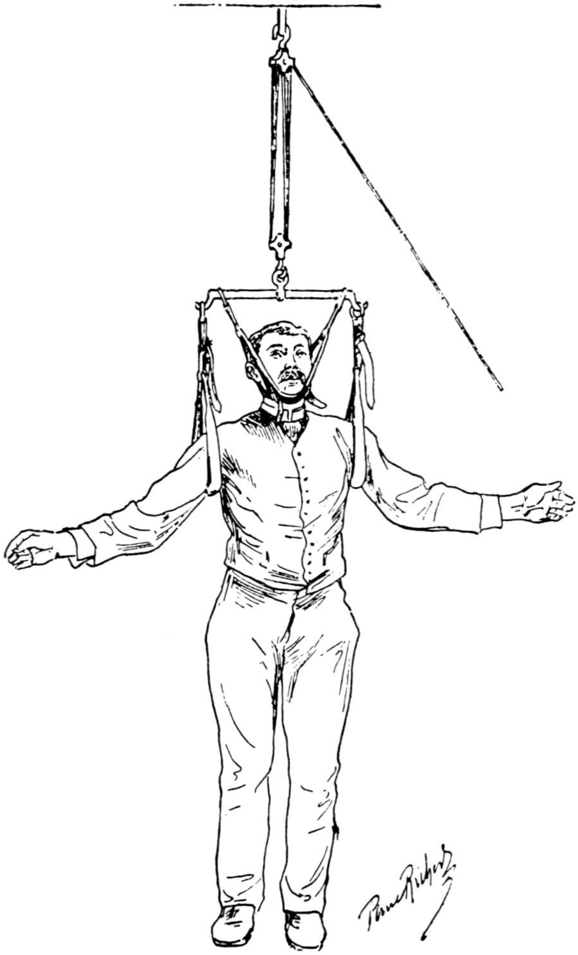

FIG. 2A. Drawing of a suspended patient.

often in the hands of the bath attendant. . . . At random, all the patients with ataxia were submitted to it, so much so that serious accidents occurred, even cases of sudden death."

Gilles and his friend, the surgeon Anthony Chipault, showed by anatomical research on cadavers that vertical traction did not produce any appreciable lengthening of the spinal cord. On the contrary, the authors state: "flexion of the spine allowed a true lengthening, measurable with a tape measure, of the spinal cord and its roots." They had constructed a portable low table, having at its posterior end a back to which was attached straps connected to a traction apparatus passing between the legs of the patient (Fig. 3), a technique now only of historical and anecdotal interest.

If Gilles de la Tourette did not accept the syphilitic origin of general paralysis—suspected already by his master Fournier—he ended up by recognizing, after much reticence, the specific nature of tabes, treating it by means of codeine and mercurial inunctions.

From tabes he went on—his brain in constant activity—to the vibratory technique, recommended 20 years earlier in London by Mortimer Grandville, who employed it for certain neuralgias. Charcot, having noticed that long journeys in a car or train relieved patients

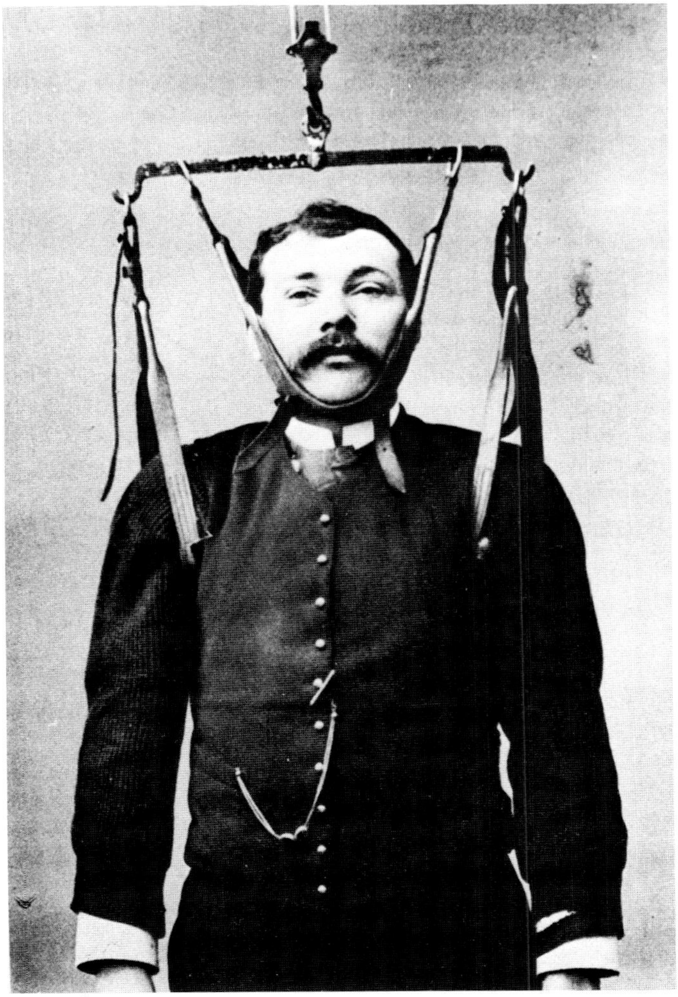

FIG. 2B. Suspended patient.

suffering from paralysis agitans, had constructed a vibrating chair (Fig. 4), a more modern adaptation of the "dancing chair" or "post-chaise seat" proposed in the 18th century for too sedentary people and which Voltaire praised in a letter to Comte d'Argental. Gilles invented a vibrating helmet (Fig. 5), an apparatus worked by electric batteries producing only mechanical vibrations; it was effective, according to him, in neurasthenia, certain types of facial pain, and vertigo.

He worked at a tremendous pace, so that only a small part of his work can be recalled here. One year after his thesis, Gilles, working with extraordinary energy, published a large book on *l'Hypnotisme dans les états analogues*. He was inspired to write on this subject by Charcot himself, who was very upset to see his dogmas on hypnosis disputed by the Nancy School, of which the leader was Bernheim. The latter had published in 1884 *De la Suggestion et de ses Applications à la thérapeutique*, giving suggestion a primary role in hypnotic manifestations. The Salpêtrière school took the completely opposite view, that

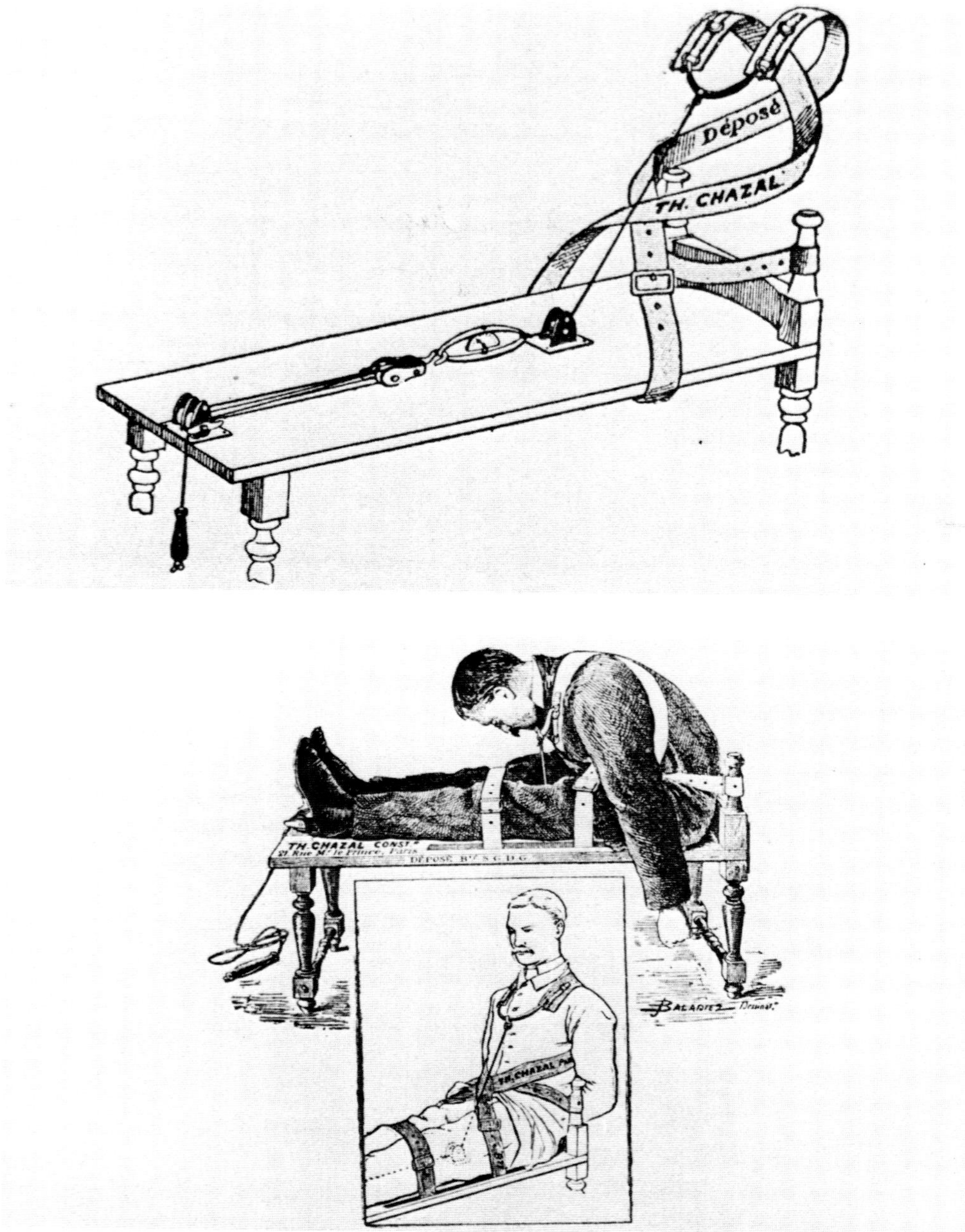

FIG. 3. Extension harness with patient sitting.

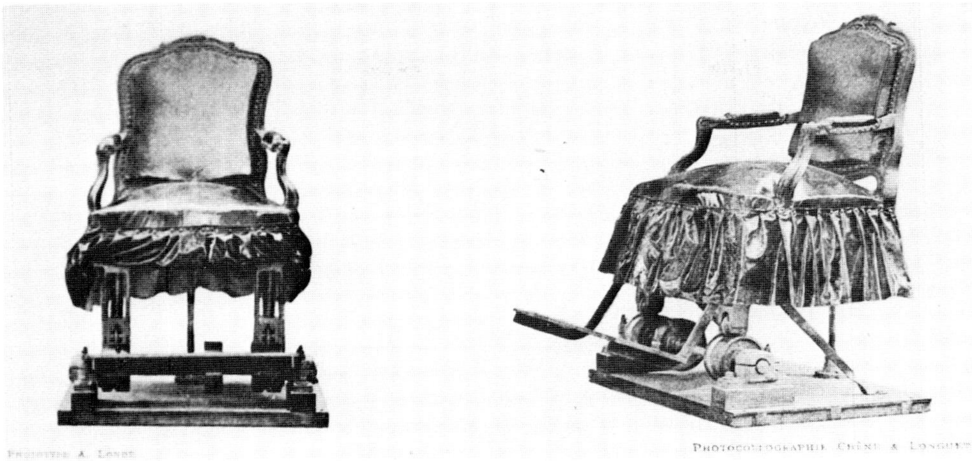

FIG. 4. "Trépidant" (trembling) armchair used at the Salpêtrière in treating what is now known as Parkinson's disease.

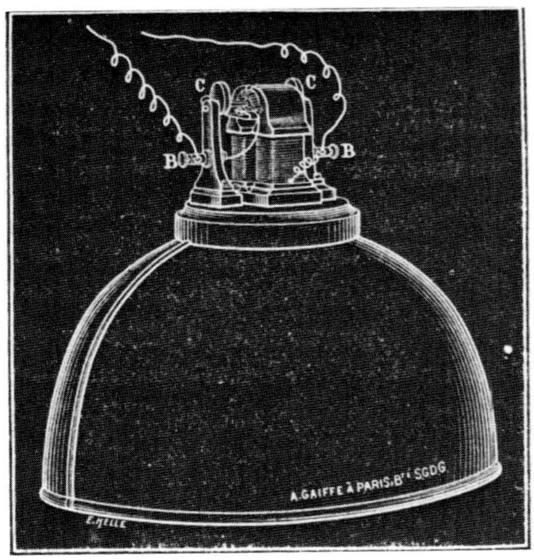

FIG. 5. Vibrating helmet.

hypnotic states were an hysterical neurosis with three successive stages: lethargy, catalepsy and somnambulism. We shall not here recapitulate the endless polemics—often lively, always passionate, and sometimes discourteous—which went on for a long time between the rival schools, but will limit ourselves to those episodes in which Gilles de la Tourette played a part.

His book on hypnotism (8) was a success and was reprinted in 1889, the great year of the Universal Exhibition, the year of the Eiffel Tower, so criticized at the beginning, especially by a capital again rich and brilliant, and completely restored at last after the disasters of 1870. There were many artistic and cultural demonstrations and, a little in the background and without too much publicity, the first International Congress of Experimental and Therapeutic Hypnotism took place.

Among the Presidents of Honor were Charcot, Brouardel, and Brown-Séquard. The paper by Bernheim, defending his ideas, was very much welcomed. But there were rare, scathing opponents, especially Gilles de la Tourette, who expressed himself with his usual fervor:

> I should like to reply to Mr. Bernheim, but the task is difficult and I do not find in his very academic paper true arguments. . . . I admit to having quite a different idea about hypnotism and its perfectly verifiable and established laws.

In the auditorium, but passing unobserved, was a man of 30 years, not very tall, with black moustache and beard, carefully dressed and with a marvellous and unforgettable expression; he was Sigmund Freud, who had worked with Charcot towards the end of 1885 and during the beginning of the following year. He soon became Bernheim's friend and translated his book into German, after returning to Vienna.

If Gilles de la Tourette's treatise on hypnotism is today obsolete, some chapters can still be read with interest and a certain amount of approval. In the pages about the *Viol dans l'hypnotisme*, he judiciously insists on the extreme practical difficulty of setting the medicolegal problems. "It is important," he wrote, "to control the application of hypnotism, as has been done in the case of medicines."

Gilles fought against the exploitation of magnetism, "every day for gain by thousands of individuals. . . ." In a passage, amusing as well as disquieting, without sparing his time or his money, "under the cover of anonymity," he himself carried out an investigation among innumerable societies of magnetism and spiritualism, consulting the more articulate sleepwalkers. He reproduced one of the prospectuses that clairvoyants distributed at that time to caretakers (of flats) and wine merchants (Figs. 6 and 7), as well as their *Diplôme de Magnetiseur*—obtained from the *Chaîne Magnétique*—"the most popular of these associations exploiting the public credulity." What good sense sometimes came from this "crazy" doctor!

This versatile man, with perhaps the potential of the great journalist, tackled the most varied subjects, often in unexpected directions. For example, risking diplomatic complications with Chancellor Bismarck, he studied the *Hystérie dans l'armée Allemande*; he went to England to report on the Floating Fever Hospitals on the Thames, which were used for the isolation of particularly contagious smallpox victims; and he recalled with emotion the detestable hygienic conditions in which the fishermen of Pen'march and of the Baie d'Audierne lived, destroyed by alcoholism, smallpox, and tuberculosis. He wrote about military hygiene and the parasites in army biscuits, and on many other themes.

At the same time, in a literary periodical, the *Revue Hebdomadaire*, Gilles wrote under the pseudonym Paracelsus about the *cas du Music-Hall mathematician Inaudi*, *Guillotine et Electricité*. He analyzed the mental state of the anarchist Ravachol, taking the opportunity to demand that insane criminals be put in asylums for penal servitide, as was the English system.

Like Charcot and Richer, who had just published their abundantly illustrated book about the *Démoniaques dans l'art*, Gilles criticized with zest and ironical style many works of art. Let us cite at random: *Tobie rendant la vue à son père*, *Le Masque de Pascal*, *Un Buste d'Eveque guérissant les écrouelles. La Mort de Charles IX*, in collaboration with Brouardel, is remarkable. His comments about the caricatures of Mesmer, his pet hate, are irresistably funny.

Charcot, getting old, became more and more attracted to his student, whose competence and permanent availability he appreciated (Fig. 8). He took him for some months as secretary and bestowed on him a singularly distinguished honor of the heavy task of writing up his

SÉCURITÉ — PROGRÈS — SCIENCE

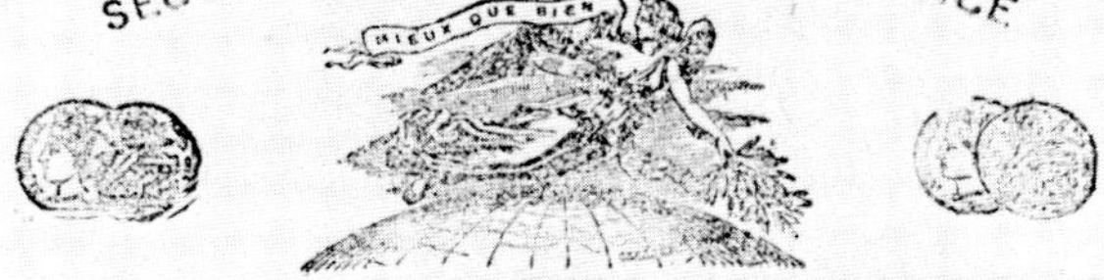

MME CHARLES

Somnambule de naissance de premier ordre

Membre et médaillée de l'Institut électro-magnétique de France,
Membre de plusieurs Sociétés savantes et humanitaires,
Propriétaire de plusieurs Médailles d'honneur de France et de l'Étranger,

A l'honneur de prévenir les personnes qui voudront bien l'honorer de leur confiance, qu'elles trouveront chez elle tous les renseignements utiles et nécessaires à leurs positions. Toutes les séances sont personnelles et données avec une grande sécurité. Cette dame, après 20 ans de succès, a su conquérir une réputation justement méritée dans toutes les grandes villes d'Europe, et principalement à Paris et dans sa banlieue, qu'elle habite six mois de l'année.

Quoique ce travail soit étranger au tirage des cartes, cette dame se charge, pour les personnes qui le désirent, de la cartomancie, et se met entièrement à leur disposition. Elle lit également sur la physionomie et les lignes de la main, travail qui lui a valu plusieurs mentions honorables.

SÉANCES EXCEPTIONNELLES SUR LA PHRÉNOLOGIE

Séances endormies à toute heure, à prix réduit

Au Salon de Mme CHARLES, l'on voit la personne que l'on aime et celle de qui l'on est aimée (sic)

CETTE DAME SE REND A DOMICILE SUR DEMANDE

CONSULTATIONS A PRIX MODÉRÉS

Mme CHARLES fait savoir au public qu'elle rentre dans sa propriété à ....., rue d'Orléans (Seine-et-Oise), et qu'elle donnera des séances tout l'hiver, jusqu'au mois de mars, époque de son départ pour Paris.

LE PUBLIC EST PRIÉ DE NE PAS CONFONDRE

L'Équipage-Salon de Mme CHARLES est pavoisé de Diplômes et de Certificats.

VENEZ VOIR Mme CHARLES ET VOUS SEREZ SATISFAIT

FIG. 6. Facsimile page from the original edition of Gilles de la Tourette's book *l'Hypnotisme dans les états analogues.*

410 L'HYPNOTISME ET LA LOI.

On voudra bien remarquer que madame Marie est diplômée. Qu'a-t-elle fait pour cela? Pas grand'chose. En prenant un abonnement d'un an à la *Chaîne magnétique* on a droit à un « magnifique diplôme » de magnétiseur.

Dechambre a raconté [1] que, moyennant 600 francs, il eût pu faire son domestique docteur de Philadelphie ; moyennant 6 francs la *Chaîne magnétique* vous sacre magnétiseur, et

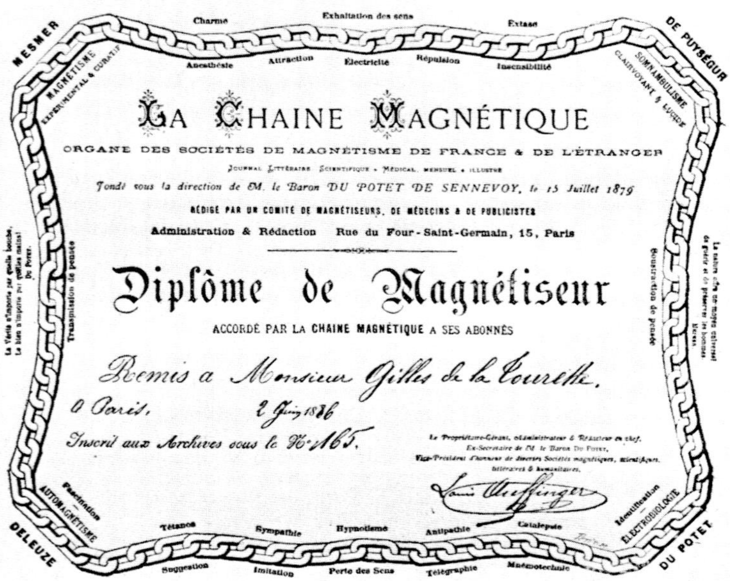

vous pouvez désormais suspendre le précieux talisman aux murs de votre appartement, entre un tableau cabalistique et une tête-système de Gall, accessoire obligé de tous les cabinets somnambuliques qui se respectent.

Nous avouons que ce n'est pas sans quelque émotion que

[1] Voy. BROUARDEL, *De l'exercice et de l'enseignement de la médecine*, 1873, p. 19.

FIG. 7. Facsimile page from the original edition of Gilles de la Tourette's book *l'Hypnotisme dans les états analogues.*

lessons and notes, the text *ne varietur* of the huge *Traité clinique et thérapeutique de l'hystérie d'après l'enseignement de la Salpêtrière*. The first volume appeared in 1891, and Charcot, who did not make friends easily and who did not easily give praise, wrote in the preface: "On reading Monsieur Gilles de la Tourette's manuscript I have several times been surprised to find in it ideas of my own that have never been expressed or which anyway had not previously been published."

The following year, an examination for teaching posts was presided over by Professor Charles Bouchard, a difficult, ambitious, independent person. An old house physician of Charcot's, he was at variance with his head of department, who had refused him his vote at the Institute. Charcot naturally campaigned for Joseph Babinski and his indispensable Gilles de la Tourette, but they were both eliminated in favor of candidates supported by Bouchard. Babinski never applied again but it is doubtful whether or not this is a matter for regret since the heavy duties of day-to-day teaching might well have diverted the innovator from a work that "resounded softly with a revolutionary accent." The great pontiff of the Salpêtrière did not have time to see the complete publication of the treatise. He died suddenly, during the night of August 15/16, 1893, from a heart attack during an archeological journey in the middle of France, accompanied by three of his students (see Chapter 39).

Gilles, the previous week, had been invited to a meal with Charcot in the little country house in Neuilly, where the neurologist spent the summer with his family. The master and the disciple then corrected together some proofs of the book. The sudden death of his venerated chief upset Gilles. He had great difficulty in pulling himself together and only succeeded by taking on more work. After several failures, due to his lack of knowledge of general pathology, he eventually succeeded to the medical staff, not in neurology, but in forensic medicine, much helped by Brouardel.

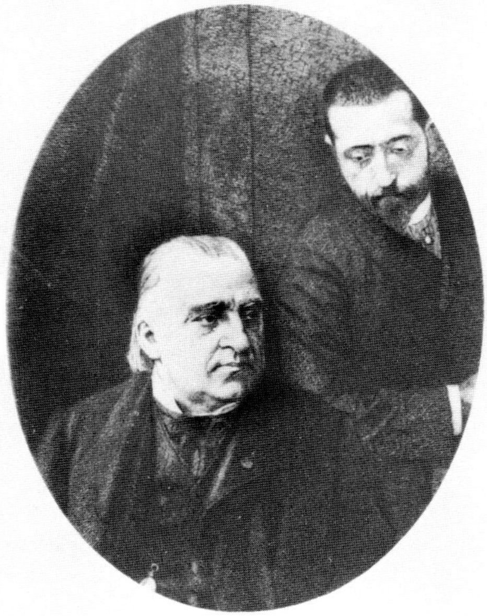

FIG. 8. Charcot and Gilles de la Tourette.

His great enterprise was to finish the publication he had undertaken. The third and last volume appeared at the end of 1895, a few weeks before Babinski, at the Société de Biologie on February 22, 1896—a memorable date—gave his paper, "Sur le reflexe cutané plantaire en extension dans certaines affections organiques due système nerveux," 34 lines that were going to change the face of neurology and count for more than the 1,800 pages of the three enormous volumes on hysteria, which lie, tarnished with time, unread.

This time of success for Gilles was also one of early disappointments. A young woman, with persecution mania and already twice confined to a mental hospital, shot him in his private consulting room three times; one bullet hit him in the occipital region. It was a superficial flesh wound, and the bullet was easily removed by the young surgeon, Pierre Delbet, and he was convalescent within a few days. But the popular press gave extensive publicity to the attack, each paper commenting according to its style and political opinions, and one hack writer, short of copy, even reproached the unfortunate neurologist for having sought, after the incident, publicity to increase his practice. Soon afterwards, he suffered the loss of a grown-up child and this shock, following on the head injury, had a deleterious influence on his already precarious nervous equilibrium.

Many of Gilles's communications at the end of the century are very disturbing. For example, *Manifestations hystériques après une chute de 17 métres de haut (!)*, *Un cas d'hémorragie cérébrale d'origine hystérique*, *Nature hystérique de la tétanie des femmes enceintes*, *Description de la diathèse vaso-motrice*, leaves us very puzzled. Even more peculiar was his theory trying to explain a biological substratum for grand mal attacks: lowering of the urea level, inversion of the calcium-phosphate ratio, and other biochemical anomalies. Inexhaustible, he found time at the end of 1896, after violent arguments with the public authorities, to have erected a statue in honor of Théophaste Renaudot. The monument was inaugurated in the Place du Marché aux Fleurs with great pomp, by the President of the Council of Ministers and Professor Brouardel.

That same year, thanks to sound political support (Bourneville and Alexandre Millerand, then revolutionary socialist member of Parliament, his old friend of the Latin Quarter), Gilles de la Tourette was appointed Chief Medical Officer of the Universal Exhibition of 1900, a difficult post full of responsibility and risks. To the surprise of many, he revealed himself as an excellent organizer, establishing a surgical service well in advance of its time, while at the same time giving appointments to his friends. Created "Officier de la Légion d'Honneur," he supported a rosette "as big as an artichoke's heart," as one of his detractors wrote. The exhibition site, with the inevitable occupational accidents, gave him the opportunity to study the posttraumatic syndrome thoroughly.

On a literary level, Gilles undertook the *Critique de l'état mental* of theater characters (*L'Arlésienne*, *Frou-Frou*, etc.) arguing, often aggressively, with their authors, theater managers, critics, and even the public. It was during a talk at the Odéon that, suddenly, he got his notes mixed up, began to stammer, and had to leave the theater amidst shouts from the audience.

The International Congress of Medicine during the Universal Exhibition gave him tremendous success, particularly in the brilliant Section of Neurology. All the great names of neurology were there: Sir Charles Sherrington and Sir David Ferrier from London; Paul Flechsig of Leipzig; von Monakow of Zurich; Pick of Prague; Georges Marinesco from Bucharest; Jendrassek from Budapest; Vladimir Roth from Moscow. France was represented by Fulgence Raymond, Jules Dejerine, Pierre Marie, Babinski, and others; Gilles de la Tourette registered at the Congress but did not read a paper.

Seven years after the death of Charcot, his famous dogmas regarding hysteria almost daily lost ground. Reports and communications were nearly all oriented toward the physiology of the nervous system and the physical signs of organic lesions of the nervous system.

With phases of depression and hypomania, Gilles de la Tourette continued to produce some publications, including in 1900 one *Traité pratique de l'épilepsie*. This monograph is well written, clear, and without any fault that could lead to any suspicion of mental deterioration. Was he perhaps helped by one of his assistants? We do not know.

At what period then should the anecdotes told by Léon Daudet be placed? Probably after 1900, but there is no clear answer. Suffice it to quote the author of *Morticoles (Saw-Bones)*[6]:

> One day in an examination, Gilles asked a candidate: "What disease begins by bleeding from the left nostril?" and received the answer: "Typhoid fever, Sir." Gilles shook his head but, at the end of five minutes silence, solemnly said: "It's typhoid, you have scored no marks, I'm going to fail you."
>
> The second story, even more surprising, is typical of a highly developed megalomania. Gilles questioned another candidate: "Who are the three greatest doctors of the 19th century?" The student reflected and replied: "Laennec, Duchenne de Boulogne and Charcot," because he knew that Gilles had been the pupil of the third one. "No, you don't know. They were my grandfather, my father and me, Coco! That's why"—Gilles then put his own hat on the amazed young man—"that's why they will erect a statue of me made of potassium bromide!"

This story, somewhat embellished each time it was told, was for 30 years the delight of the students' common room.

At the beginning of 1902, when Gilles was still physician at the Sainte-Antoine Hospital, his behavior, becoming more disturbed, forced the Public Assistance Administration to put him on indefinite leave for health reasons. His family put him in a clinic at Lausanne, where he died in June 1904. One obituary notice was so critical that a friend of Gilles's had to ask another paper to publish a rebuttal entitled: *Respect aux morts (Respect for the dead).*

It seems certain that Gilles had GPI, even if there is no absolute pathological proof. Léon Daudet, who in *Devant la Douleur* talked of his own syphilitic pain, wrote some years later in *Les Oeuvres dans les Hommes* that Gilles must have died of ill-determined madness. But Daudet, who wrote in a masterly manner with only one draft and without subsequent correction, often contradicted himself.

Doctors are familiar with the variability of syphilitic meningoencephalitis, which comes in bursts, like very long ebbs and flows, with paroxysms of delirium when the most aberrant episodes alternate, often over the course of years, with remissions of fairly normal behavior. Guy de Maupassant has left us a classical and sad example. From the publication of *Le Horla* in 1887 until his death in 1893, he went from hypomanic periods to peaceful remissions, allowing him to write two works of great talent and several short stories, for example, *l'Inutile Beauté*. Many authors, doctors, and others have laid stress on his tragic story, but among neurologists, the most pertinent essay has been by Macdonald Critchley (6).

A judgment on Gilles de la Tourette can only be at present an incomplete summary, as sources are too fragmentary and we know nothing of his family life besides the death of his child. Are any of his descendants still living? Our investigations on this point, although not

---

[6]*Morticoles*, a novel by Léon Daudet, was a violent satire à la Swift on doctors generally.

exhaustive, have remained negative, but does someone possess any of his private correspondence?

His political commitment and religious sectarianism make the interpretation of evidence left by his contemporaries difficult, since some were too laudatory, while others were more or less violently hostile. Between the violent "execution" of a Léon Daudet and the long biographical account—very eulogistic—of his friend Paul le Gendre (8), there are without any doubt more subtle shades. His case history, fairly strange, is worth further investigation and should tempt a student who is in search of a subject for a thesis and interested in the history of medicine. We feel that there remains much to be found here and there, Gilles being worth perhaps more than his uncertain reputation, albeit detestable to many.

If this biographical summary, itself critical about the adequacy of the man, his religious intolerance, his haughtiness or, to use a word of the period, his indulgence in *cabotinage* (histrionics), seems to excuse his many peculiarities and irresponsibility, it is because these are possibly due to constitutional nervous weakness. To his credit, he was much liked by his masters, pupils, and friends, to whom he was always loyal. When, after Charcot's death, his disciples quickly deserted their Master, who was often tyrannical, Gilles was almost the only one to defend Charcot, to whom he owed his career.

In the pleiad of the last pupils of Charcot—in which, at its zenith, Babinski always shone—Gilles de la Tourette was only a very secondary dim star. It seemed to be extinct until American investigators, perhaps fascinated by this uncommon name, have with enthusiasm restored to Europe[7] the man who during his lifetime had seemed a grotesque personality.

"Pauvre diable, de Gilles de la Tourette!"—an exclamation not ours but that of Léon Daudet, who wrote it in *Devant la Douleur*, at the end of a paragraph that we cite in its entirety:

> Some time before his death as I was leaving my home in rue de l'Université, Gilles de la Tourette, whom I had lost sight of for several years, saw me, and coming up to me threw his arms around me. I was amazed with such a demonstration of affection that nothing in our past relationship, I ask you to believe this, justified. He said in a jerky voice: "My dear Daudet, I like you enormously. For a long time I have wanted this formal reconciliation . . . ." Then taking a step backwards, he repeated: "Formal reconciliation . . . ." He was red in the face with large tears in his eyes. I guessed at once what was the matter. The diagnosis was not difficult. . . . Poor devil, this Gilles de la Tourette!

We do not know if Gilles had had the troubled end of Jules de Goncourt[8] who was for a long time vaguely aware of his decline, so well analyzed in *Le Journal* by his brother Edmond, and who acknowledged just a short time before his death that he was "dans les espaces vides" (up in the clouds); or the long suffering of Guy de Maupassant who, between two periods of relative lucidity, held the most megalomanic ideas, refusing to pass urine "in order not to lose the millions of diamonds that he had in his stomach," ending his life in status epilepticus; or the relatively calm death of a Nietzsche, in "The Night of the Spirit," for 10 years admired and cared for by his sister in Weimar.

We do not know, and doubtless shall never know, about the last moments of Gilles de la Tourette. There seem to be no documents, oral or written. No visitor, relative, friend, or

---

[7]We have only just learned that there exists in London an "Association for Research into the Disease of Gilles de la Tourette." Similar associations exist in the United States and Canada.

[8]The younger of the two brothers Huot de Goncourt, both well-known writers: Jules (1830–1870) and Edmund (1822–1896).

doctor has written about it, and we know that Swiss mental hospitals keep their medical secrets as rigidly as their banks respect anonymity.

REFERENCES

1. Daudet, Léon (1915): *Devant la douleur*, Nouvelle Librairie Nationale, Paris.
2. Woodrow, K. M. (1974): Gilles de la Tourette's disease. A review. *Am. J. Psychiat.*, 131:1,000–1,003. Cited by Dugas, M. et al. (1975): L'enfant tiqueur. Qui est-il? Comment le soulager? Quel est son devenir? *Rev. Praticien*, 25:47.
3. Shapiro, A. K., Shapiro, E. S., Bruun, R. D., and Sweet, R. D. (1978): *Gilles de la Tourette Syndrome*. Raven Press, New York.
4. Debray-Ritzen, P., and Dubois, H. (1980): Maladies des tics de l'enfant. *Soc. de Med. (Paris)*, 2:109–111. *Rev. Neurol. (Paris)*, 136:1, 15–18.
5. Ganière, P. (1968): *Ils étaient tous médecins*. Lib. Acad. Perrin, Paris.
6. Critchley, M.: Meeting December 4, 1968, Section of the History of Medicine, *Five illustrious Neuroluetics*. Papers on Alphonse Daudet, Heinrich Heine, Jules de Goncourt, Guy de Maupassant, and Dan Leno. Reprinted in Critchley, M. (1979): *The Divine Banquet of the Brain*. Raven Press, New York.
7. Gilles de la Tourette: *Traité clinique et thérapeutique de l'Hystérie d'après l'enseignement de la Salpétrière*, trois vol. Plon et Nourrit, Paris. T. I. Hystérie normale ou interparoxystique (1891); t. II et t. III. Hystérie paroxystique (1895).
8. Le Gendre, P. (1968): Notice biographique sur Gilles de la Tourette. *Soc. Méd. Hôpit.* (Séance du 30 déc. 1904).

Historical Aspects of the Neurosciences,
edited by F. Clifford Rose and W. F. Bynum.
Raven Press, New York ©

Some Aspects of the History of Neurology in Norway

Sigvald Refsum

Department of Neurology, University of Oslo, Oslo, Norway

LEPROSY IN NORWAY

In writing about some aspects of the history of neurology in Norway, it seems natural to start with a field in which Norwegian research has made perhaps its most important contribution to medicine on a world scale—the field of leprosy.

When leprosy first appeared in Norway is not known. According to Hansen and Lie (1) and Irgens (2), its presence about 800–1000 A.D. was linked with the raids of the Vikings, particularly to the British Isles. Toward the end of the Middle Ages, its frequency declined considerably, and the disease almost disappeared in the northern part of the continent, but on the Scandinavian peninsula, a new wave of the disease arose, peaking in Norway in about 1860. Norwegian leprosy research and the work that led to control and prevention of the disease were started in conjunction with this last wave. In some districts of western Norway, more than 2.5% of the population suffered from leprosy (2,7). A new leprosy research hospital was founded in Bergen by the government of Norway in 1849 with D. Danielssen (1813–1894) as chief physician (Fig. 1). A scientific study of leprosy had been started some time before by him in collaboration with a young doctor and member of parliament, Boeck, several careful autopsies having been performed. In 1847 appeared their first great monograph on leprosy (3), "spedalskhet," as it was called in Common Norwegian[1], in conjunction with a great atlas (Figs. 2–4). It has been said that of its kind it is still unsurpassed. It was also published in Paris in 1848 (4), received great attention, and was awarded the "Prix Monthyon." Rudolf Virchow (1821–1902), the founder of "cellular pathology," one of the greatest names in the history of pathology, and a feared critic, wrote about this work (in my translation from the German): "The precise, I would like to say, the scientific knowledge of the disease stems really from the famous work of Danielssen and Boeck on Norwegian leprosy, which in a splendid iconography has presented lucid pictures of the main changes. What we have of illustrations from earlier times possess only minor interest."

Carl Wilhelm Boeck (1808–1875) was in 1851 appointed as the first professor of dermatology at the University in Christiania (now Oslo). Bergen became a center for leprosy

[1]The word "spedalskhet" is corrupted from the word "hospital," since patients with leprosy were hospitalized

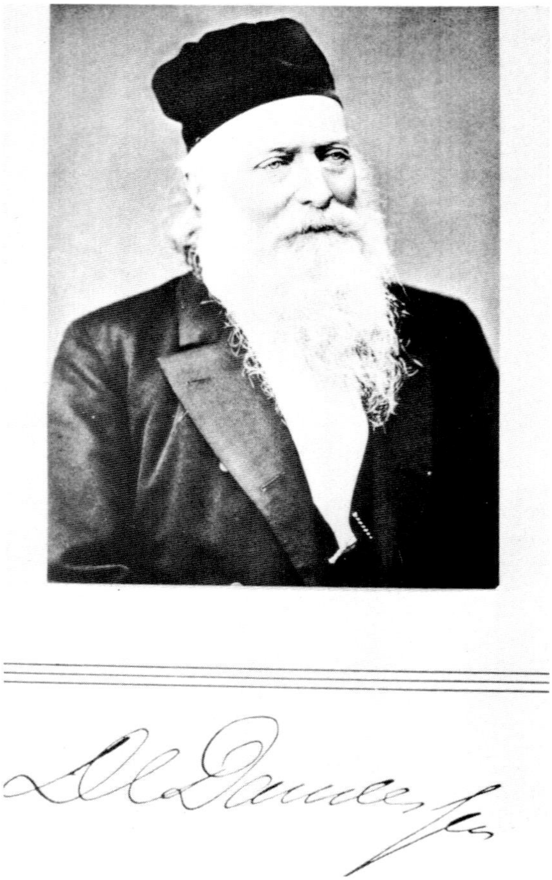

FIG. 1. Dr. D. Danielssen (1813–1894): pioneer in Norwegian leprosy research.

research. A national leprosy registry was established by Royal Decree in 1856. It was founded for the dual purpose of research and control of the disease, and was probably the first national patient registry ever established. Through the collection of detailed case histories of all leprosy patients from 1856 until the present time, the registry came to play a significant role in the control of the disease (5,7).

Leprosy also attracted considerable attention in other countries at this time, and some publications made a great impact on the discussion of etiology in Norway. In 1867, a report was published by the Royal College of Physicians of London, based on replies sent in by about 250 physicians in all the colonies of Great Britain. In 1869, there appeared a book in France by C. L. Drognat-Landré, "De la contagion, seule cause de la propagation de la lèpre." It seems that this book had a decisive influence on the young Norwegian physician, G. H. Armauer Hansen, and on his view of the etiology of the disease. From 1868, Hansen worked at Bergen's active research center (2).

In a work published in 1874 (6), which was printed in a somewhat abbreviated form in an English journal the following year, Hansen mentioned for the first time his discovery of bacteria-like formations in leprous nodes (Figs. 5 and 6). On February 28, 1873 (8), he

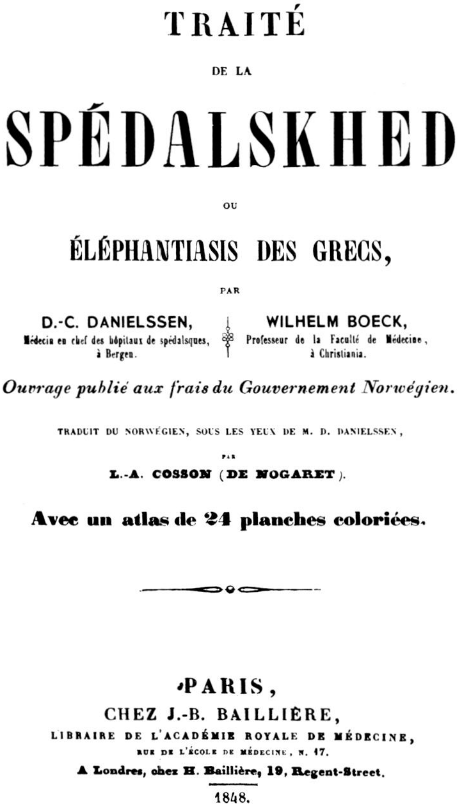
TRAITÉ

DE LA

SPÉDALSKHED

OU

ÉLÉPHANTIASIS DES GRECS,

PAR

D.-C. DANIELSSEN, Médecin en chef des hôpitaux de spédalsques, à Bergen.

WILHELM BOECK, Professeur de la Faculté de Médecine, à Christiania.

Ouvrage publié aux frais du Gouvernement Norwégien.

TRADUIT DU NORWÉGIEN, SOUS LES YEUX DE M. D. DANIELSSEN,

PAR

L.-A. COSSON (DE NOGARET).

Avec un atlas de 24 planches coloriées.

PARIS,

CHEZ J.-B. BAILLIÈRE,

LIBRAIRE DE L'ACADÉMIE ROYALE DE MÉDECINE,

RUE DE L'ÉCOLE DE MÉDECINE, N. 17.

A Londres, chez H. Baillière, 19, Regent-Street.

1848.

FIG. 2. Title page of Drs. D. Danielssen and W. Boeck's monograph on leprosy with color atlas.

examined a boy with many leprous nodules in his face. He removed one nodule from a nostril, cut through it, carefully scraped the edge of the cut with a knife, rubbed the stuff onto a glass slide, and wrote: "If one examines the specimens without adding anything, one can here and there perceive rod-like bodies either at rest or in slightly oscillating motion. . . ." Harboe (8) states that after having read Hansen's paper and repeated his classic experiments, he was free from doubt. Armauer Hansen knew that he had seen rods within the cells from leprous nodules, and his observation and description were correct. On the basis of his epidemiological studies, he developed a completely clear view that the disease was infectious, an epoch-making discovery. Hansen had demonstrated that leprosy must be a chronic, infectious disease, and this was, as emphasized by Harboe (8), the first time that a bacillus had been connected with such a disease (Fig. 7).

It was not till 1882 that Robert Koch first described the tubercle bacillus, and this background must be kept in mind in order to fully realize the epoch-making importance of Hansen's contribution. The crucial question then was whether or not the rod-shaped bodies were the direct cause of the disease. Henle had in 1840 defined the conditions that must be satisfied to prove that a microbe is the cause of a disease: (a) It must always be possible to find the microbe in connection with the disease; (b) It must be possible to isolate and study the microbe outside the animal organism; and (c) The microbe must be able to induce the disease under natural conditions when, after cultivation, it is again injected into an animal.

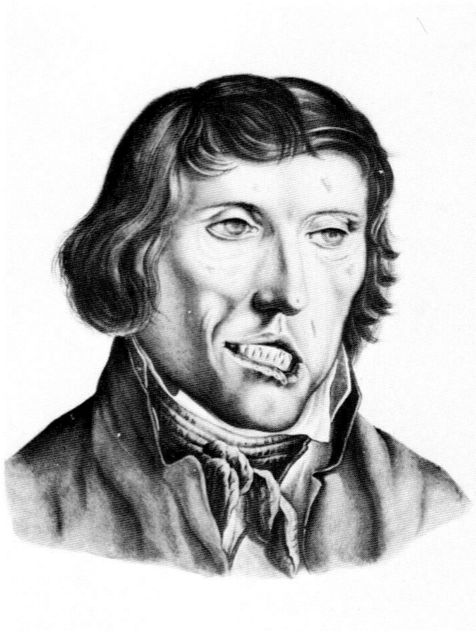

FIG. 3. Picture from the atlas on leprosy by Danielssen and Boeck. Patient with leprosy and left-sided facial palsy.

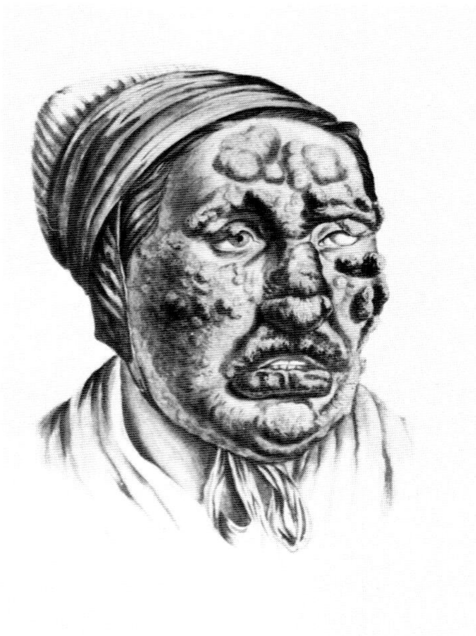

FIG. 4. Picture from Danielssen and Boeck's atlas.

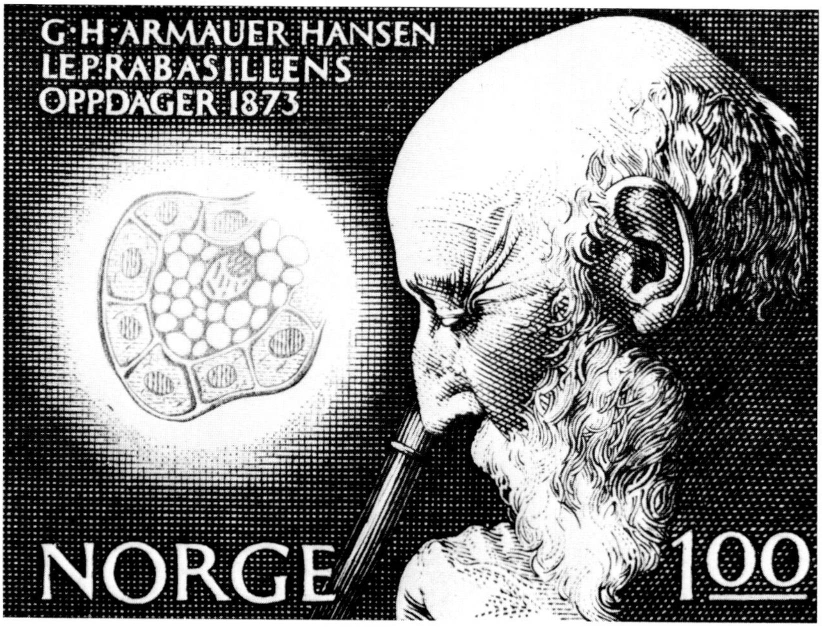

FIG. 5. Dr. G. H. Armauer Hansen (1841–1922) on a Norwegian stamp commemorating his discovery of the *lepra bacillus* in 1873.

These requirements were reformulated by Koch in 1882 and later became known as Koch's postulates (8).

Hansen carried out a long series of experiments involving cultivation and inoculation, all with negative results, and the cultivation of *mycobacterium leprae Hansen* and transmission to animals has been successful only in recent years (for short review see below).

As chief medical officer for leprosy, Hansen (1,2,5,7,8) drafted a proposal for an Act which provided that all patients with leprosy must either be isolated in separate rooms in their homes or admitted to a hospital. He was able to show, on the basis of data from the National Leprosy Register, that the number of new cases diminished most rapidly in districts in which hospitalization had been most consistently enforced; in one generation, leprosy almost disappeared from Norway.

The first official to visit Norway to study leprosy control was the English surgeon, Major H. V. Carter (1831–1897), who in 1873 was sent by the British Government from India. He found the Norwegian control program very convincing and wanted to introduce parts of it to India.

Hansen had written his previous papers in Norwegian, including the report to the Norwegian Medical Society of Christiania (Oslo) in 1874 (6), in which he described his demonstration of the bacilli in 1873. Armauer Hansen had, as reported by his collaborator for many years, H. P. Lie (9), kindly and openly shown his findings to visitors from abroad and told them his opinion about them; he had also provided them with samples of his material. These were now published using better staining methods than Hansen had had at his disposal. Robert Koch stated that he considered these bacilli demonstrated by Hansen as a particular species and the "contagium" of leprosy. Reports that might be regarded as priority claims were published, so Hansen, in 1880, published an article about his results in German journals (10a); the same article was also published in French (10b) and in English in the *Quarterly*

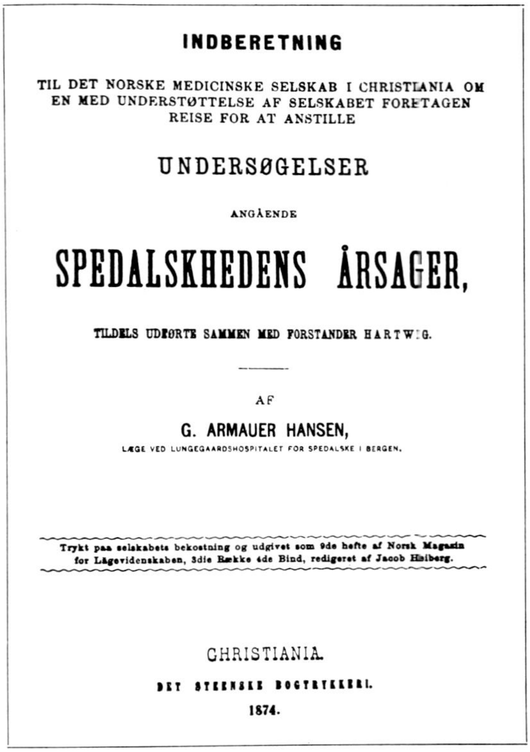

INDBERETNING

TIL DET NORSKE MEDICINSKE SELSKAB I CHRISTIANIA OM EN MED UNDERSTØTTELSE AF SELSKABET FORETAGEN REISE FOR AT ANSTILLE

UNDERSØGELSER

ANGÅENDE

SPEDALSKHEDENS ÅRSAGER,

TILDELS UDFØRTE SAMMEN MED FORSTANDER HARTWIG.

AF

G. ARMAUER HANSEN,

LÆGE VED LUNGEGAARDSHOSPITALET FOR SPEDALSKE I BERGEN.

Trykt paa selskabets bekostning og udgivet som 9de hefte af Norsk Magazin for Lægevidenskaben, 3die Række 4de Bind, redigeret af Jacob Heiberg.

CHRISTIANIA.

DET STEENSKE BOGTRYKKERI.

1874.

FIG. 6. Title page of Dr. Armauer Hansen's monograph of 1874 on the causes of leprosy.

Journal of Microscopic Science (10c), with the title "The Bacillus of Leprosy". There Hansen wrote: ". . . I feel myself called upon to announce what I have attained to, up to the present time, in my researches after the same 'contagium,' and this, partly to assert my priority with reference to this discovery, and partly in order to advance those details in research which I omitted to announce in my report to the Medical Society in Christiania, 1874, concerning my investigations into the aetiology of leprosy."

The first International Leprosy Congress was held in Berlin in 1897, with Rudolf Virchow as the president. Here Hansen was, without any opposition from anybody, pronounced as the discoverer of the *lepra bacillus*, in spite of the fact that the cultivation of the bacillus had not been successful. According to a proposal by Hansen, a resolution was unanimously passed to the effect that isolation of the patients was the best way to prevent the spread of leprosy.

To honor him, the Second International Leprosy Congress was held in Bergen in 1909 with Hansen as President. The Tenth International Leprosy Congress was again held in Bergen in 1973 to commemorate his discovery of the *lepra bacillus*, often termed *Hansen's bacillus*, 100 years earlier. The disease is, in many countries, but not in Norway, termed Hansen's disease, partly because the word leprosy carries a stigma that is best avoided.

With regard to leprosy and the nervous system, Danielssen and Boeck (3,4) in their monographs (1847, 1848) had already clearly demonstrated the marked affection of peripheral nerves. Hansen's successor as Chief Medical Officer for Leprosy, H. P. Lie (1862–1945), published in 1904 his doctoral thesis, "Lepra im Rückenmark und den peripheren Nerven,"

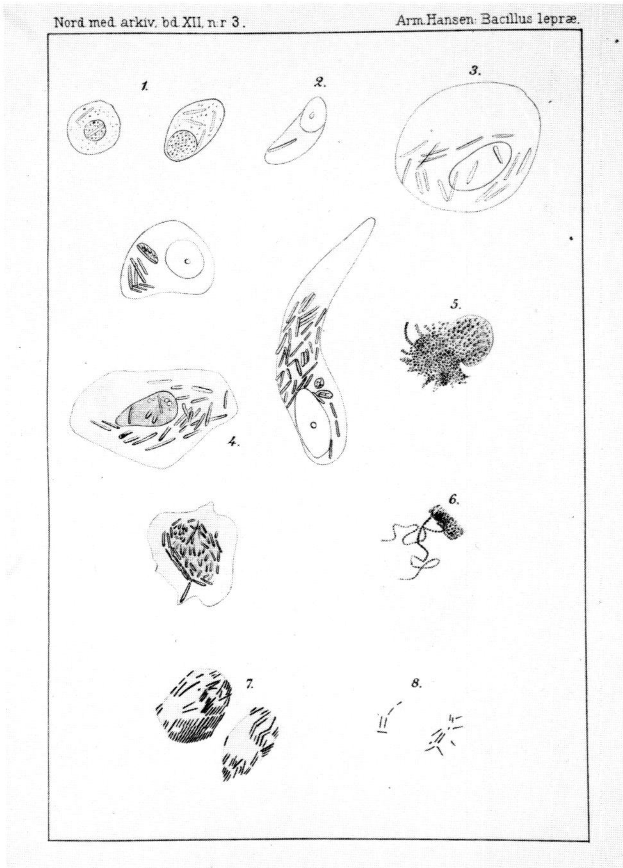

FIG. 7. *Bacillus leprae*, stained with osmic acid by Armauer Hansen.

in which it was demonstrated that the morphological alterations in the central nervous system are of a secondary, nonspecific degenerative nature (11). That all leprosy is neural leprosy, and is so from its very inception, seems now well established (12–14).

A study, *The Neurological Aspects of Leprosy ('Spedalskhet')*, was published in 1923 by my predecessor as Professor of Neurology at the University of Oslo, G. H. Monrad-Krohn (15). He was born in Bergen and had seen leprosy patients in its streets from his childhood. His book was dedicated "to the Leprosy Institutions—St. Jørgen Hospital and Pleiestiftelsen for Spedalske—of Bergen, the cradle of scientific leprosy research—and to the memory of the eminent men, who made these institutions the centre of leprosy research in this country, viz. Dr. Danielssen and Dr. Armauer Hansen." Monrad-Krohn's study was based on a clinical examination of 59 patients. One of his main conclusions was: "On the whole, I think we can safely abide by the classical opinion that the nervous manifestations of leprosy are due to a polyneuritis—and, we may add, a polyneuritis of the most peripheral kind." He underlined particularly how some twigs of the branches of the facial nerve often are involved, his monograph being a classic of the clinical neurological findings in leprosy.

As a consequence of Norwegian interest in leprosy, a humanitarian organization in Norway and Sweden, "Save the Children Federations," allotted money to an Armauer Hansen Research Institute in Addis Ababa in Ethiopia affiliated with the University of Bergen. Its first chief physician was Professor M. Harboe, who has recently reviewed the scientific work from this institute (17). Harboe emphasized that leprosy may to a great extent be considered as an immunological disease. If resistance against *mycobacterium leprae* is inadequate, the bacilli multiply with development of clinical disease. The leprosy bacillus is remarkably nontoxic and may be present in vast numbers in tissues but with very few clinical symptoms. Most symptoms of the disease are in fact caused by immune reactions against various components of the bacillus, leading in turn to tissue damage and clinical signs. *Mycobacterium leprae* is an obligate intracellular parasite. In such infections, cell-mediated immune reactions are of main importance for protective immunity.

EPONYMOUS DISEASES

Researchers who have had their names attached to a disease are in many (perhaps most) cases not those who gave the first report, but whose description has made it known to the international medical world or who have given the most lucid and comprehensive report; to evaluate priority is therefore sometimes extremely difficult or impossible. Many have claimed that all eponymous nomenclature of diseases should be abandoned, since they represent an extra burden on memory; on the other hand, without precise classification at the present time, they seem in many cases to be unavoidable. Terminology based on clinical description or particularly on biochemical mechanisms may sometimes become very cumbersome and more difficult to remember than eponymous names, and the biochemical mechanism is in very many cases unknown.

Ceroid-Lipofuscinosis—The Juvenile Form of So-Called Familial Amaurotic Idiocy (?Stengel's Disease)

In the chapter on "amaurotic family idiocy," (18), and in the chapter on the neuronal ceroid-lipofuscinoses (Batten-Vogt syndrome) (19) in the *Handbook of Clinical Neurology*, Zeman and co-workers present an historical review and give a thorough nosological analysis of this group of disorders. The nosology still remains unsolved, and the terminology is confusing. The demonstration that the lipoid accretions in the neurons of patients with the Batten-Vogt syndrome are not lipids but rather autofluroscent lipoproteins provides a compelling argument for the clear-cut nosological separation of the neuronal ceroid-lipofuscinoses from the neuronal sphingolipidoses (19).

The juvenile form of neuronal ceroid-lipofuscinoses, previously called familial amaurotic idiocy, has many eponyms attached. It has been called Mayou-Batten disease; in Germany, it is often termed Spielmeyer-Vogt disease or Spielmeyer-Vogt-Stock disease, but it was probably first reported by Stengel (20) in Norway in 1826. In the first volume of the first Norwegian medical journal, *Eyr*[2] printed in Christiania (the present Oslo) in 1826 (Fig. 8), Stengel, the physician of the Røros copper mining town in the northern part of South Norway, wrote a report on "a singular disease in four siblings" (20):

> The parents were healthy. The eldest son in the family developed normally "in somatic as well as in psychic respect" until age 6, when he started complaining about failing vision; from the 7th year his intellectual capacities gradually declined. Speech disturbances occurred and

[2]Eyr is the goddess of the art of healing in old Norse mythology.

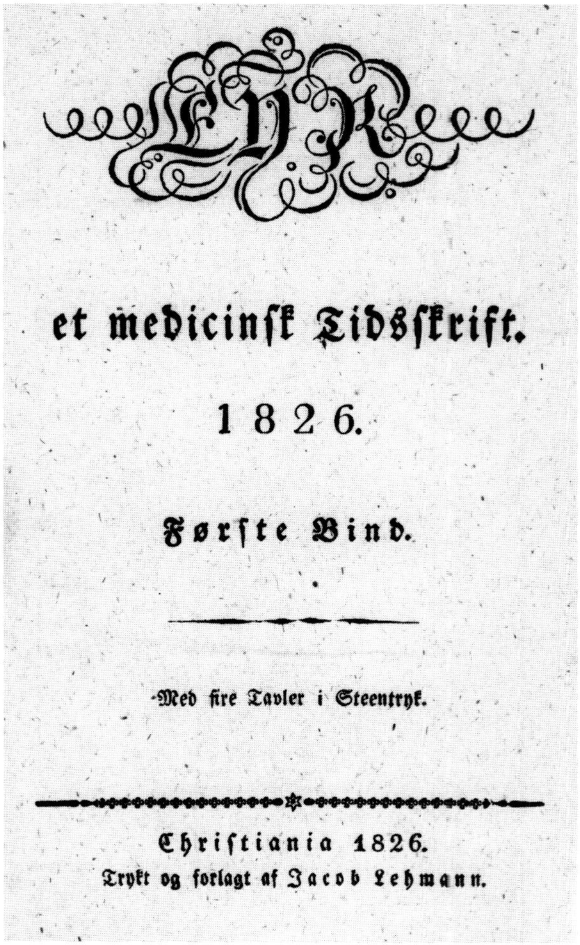

Eyr

et medicinsk Tidsskrift.

1826.

Første Bind.

Med fire Tavler i Steentryk.

Christiania 1826.

Trykt og forlagt af Jacob Lehmann.

FIG. 8. Title page of the first Norwegian medical journal, *Eyr*, first volume, 1826, in which Dr. Stengel first reported the disease later termed the juvenile form of "familial amaurotic idiocy," now commonly called ceroid-lipofuscinosis.

> progressed until his speech became almost incomprehensible. From his 9th year he became almost blind. Between the 9th and 14th year, epileptic seizures occurred with increasing severity and frequency. His behaviour had been quiet previously. From age 15, he became more and more restless, stripped off his clothes, hit out his arms, kicked in all directions and shouted and screamed incessantly. On examination his pupils were dilated and did not react to light. He died at the age of 21.
>
> A sister, born 2 years later, developed exactly the same clinical picture, starting at age 6, and died at age 20; menstruation had never occurred. A brother, born some years later, had the same symptoms and signs starting at age 6 and the course was the same as in his brother and sister; he was still alive at the age of 17 when Dr. Stengel's report was written. The last of the siblings, a girl, had the same disorder which developed at age 6.

Dr. Stengel stated that he had wanted to perform autopsies, but that he had been informed about the death of the two children only after they had been buried.

As far as I can see, this report by Dr. Stengel is the first description of the juvenile form of so-called amaurotic idiocy. The most comprehensive clinical study of this disease is given by the Swedish psychiatrist and human geneticist, Torsten Sjögren (21), whose monograph was based on studies of 115 patients from 59 families. Sjögren (21) was also the first to perform a genetic analysis based on modern statistical methods, his conclusion being that the disease is transmitted as an autosomal recessive trait. He emphasized the extrapyramidal signs and stressed that from the genetic point of view, it is entirely different from the infantile form. The condition has also been termed Spielmeyer-Vogt-Sjögren disease.

Stengel's report was, as mentioned, printed in Norwegian and seems to have been completely neglected, even in Norway. The first to have discovered this report appears to be Dr. A. Nissen in 1954 (22), who reported 10 cases in four new families, two of them from the same geographical region where Stengel had reported his cases 128 years previously. If Stengel's report had been published in English, German, or French, the eponym of the juvenile form of so-called familial amaurotic idiocy probably would have been Stengel's disease. In Nissen's cases, the neurological and ophthalmological findings were typical in all cases. In two of them, both from the same region where Stengel had reported the first patients with this disease, neuropathological studies confirmed the diagnosis. Most of the lymphocytes in the blood were vacuolated.

Available evidence on the neuronal ceroid-lipofuscinosis points to the fact that different entities are involved. Zeman (18) emphasizes that it would be unwise to speculate on these entities based on phenotypical criteria, be they morphological or clinical, but on the other hand, genetic data provide a much sounder approach to nosology. In this respect, the Spielmeyer-Sjögren type, in their opinion, may well represent a nosological entity, at least as far as the Scandinavian cases are concerned. No link between the Norwegian cases reported by Stengel (20) and Nissen (22) and the Swedish cases reported by Sjögren (21) has been demonstrated. The Swedish cases were widely distributed over the whole of Southern Sweden. Sjögren calculated the heterozygote frequency to be as high as 1%, with a tendency for accumulation in certain limited districts. In Norway, the condition seems to be much rarer; by questioning all mental hospitals and schools for the blind, only 10 cases have been found (23).

Dr. Stengel (1794–1889) (Fig. 9) has been called a German physician, but this is not correct since he was born in Holstein, which then belonged to the United Kingdom of Denmark and Norway, under a king who was also Duke of Holstein. In 1812, when 17 years old, Stengel went to Copenhagen to train as a surgeon. This was during the Napoleonic wars, and Denmark-Norway, unfortunately, was involved on Napoleon's side. There being a shortage of surgeons, Stengel was soon appointed a military surgeon and was sent in that capacity to Norway in 1814. He graduated in medicine from the Royal Frederik's University in Christiania (now the University of Oslo) in 1821 and was appointed in the same year as physician to the copper mining town of Røros, where he spent the rest of his life. On his 60-years jubilee as physician of Røros, in 1881, he was awarded the Royal Order of St. Olav "for long and meritorious activity as a physician." His son became a physician and worked in Røros for 46 years, father and son having served as physicians in Røros for 115 years.

The Norwegian veterinarian, Dr. Koppang (24), has since 1958 been able to breed English setters with ceroid-lipofuscinosis—as a possible model for human neuronal ceroid-lipofuscinosis—and aging. He bred over 500 dogs, about 300 of them being heterozygotes or homozygous normals. A controlled longitudinal morphological study revealed that the formation and accumulation of an autofluorescent lipopigment, identified as "ceroid" in the isolated state, commences *in utero* and progresses linearly with time.

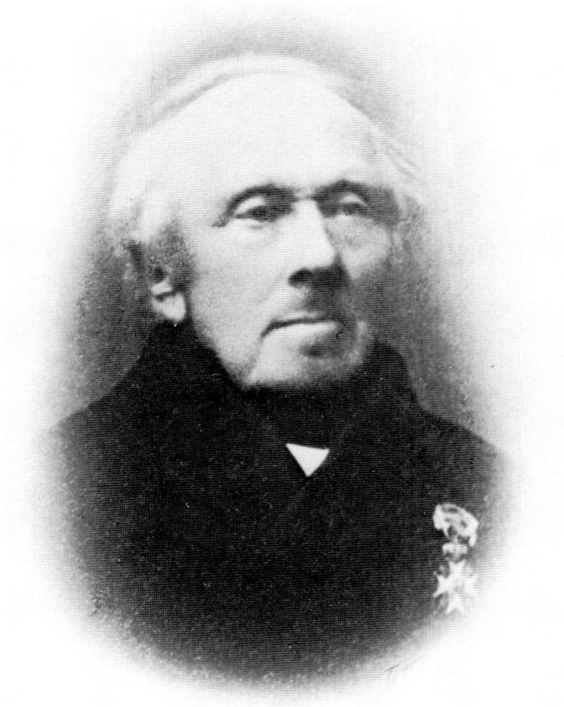

FIG. 9. Dr. C. Stengel (1794–1889).

A symposium on neuronal ceroid-lipofuscinosis, in man and in dog, was held in 1980 in Røros, the home town of Stengel, to honor his memory. Two of Dr. Stengel's great-grandsons, also physicians, were invited to the symposium. In a recent publication, the disease has been called the Stengel-Batten-Mayou-Spielmeyer-Vogt-Stock disease (25). A biography of Stengel was written in Norwegian by Kiær (26), and one has also been written in German (27).

Huntington's or Lund-Huntington's Chorea

In 1972, a centennial symposium on Huntington's chorea was held at the Ohio State University in Columbus, Ohio, sponsored by the Research Group on Huntington's Chorea of the World Federation of Neurology. The President of the Federation at that time, Dr. Macdonald Critchley, gave a review "Great Britain and the early history of Huntington's chorea" (28), Dr. Critchley having made very important studies in this field of neurology (29). An account of the history of Huntington's chorea in the United States was presented by R. N. De Jong (30), who had previously written an article about George Huntington and his relationship to the earlier description of chronic hereditary chorea (31). An extensive historical synopsis has been written by G. W. Bruyn (32) and recently by Rocatagliata (33). According to De Jong (30,31), the first description of chronic chorea in adults on an hereditary basis is that of Charles Oscar Waters, who wrote a letter to his professor of medicine, Robley Dunglison, who printed the letter in full in the first edition of his text, *The Practice of Medicine*, in 1842 (34).

An adequate description of inherited chorea as a disease *sui generis* was given as early as 1859 by Johan Christian Lund (35), district physician in Sætersdalen in Norway. Lund was unaware of Waters' report, and his account is part of a report in 1860 of the medical conditions in his district to the Ministry of the Interior (Fig. 10). It reads as follows (in my English translation):

> "As mentioned in the previous report, St. Vitus' dance appears to occur as an hereditary disease in Sætersdalen. It is most commonly called "Rykka" (i.e., "jerking disease"), sometimes also Arvesygen (i.e. "the hereditary disease"). It occurs as a rule between the ages of 50 and 60; generally starting with less conspicuous phenomena, which sometimes only slowly progress and do not become very marked, so that the patient's normal activities are not particularly hindered; but more often after a few years they increase to a considerable degree so that every kind of work becomes impossible for them, and they even have great difficulty in bringing food to the mouth by means of several detours. Their whole body, particularly, however, the head, the arms and the upper part of the body are in constant, severe jerking and flinging motion, except during sleep, when they usually are quiet. Some of the severely affected patients have in the last period of their life become *fatui* (i.e. psychotic or demented). The disease occurs in two families which are recorded below. The information is not as complete as desirable, but something to start with if the doctors in Sætersdalen will be aware of this disease in the future."

Then follow the pedigrees of the two families, in both of which the disease occurred in four generations, inherited from one generation to the next and affecting both men and women. Lund's description emphasizes the hereditary character of this form of chorea, the late onset, the progressive course, and the mental changes.

In the medical report by Lund in 1868 (36), he writes: "In a German journal the correctness of the diagnosis has been doubted; I can only answer that I don't have, and never have had, the least doubt in this respect. The clinical picture is, when the disease has reached a certain

III. Chorea Sti Viti i Sætersdalen, Uddrag af Distriktslæge J. C. Lunds Medicinalberetning for 1860.

Som i forrige Beretning anført, synes Chorea Sti Viti at optræde som en arvelig Sygdom i Sætersdalen. Den kaldes almindeligst „Rykka", tildels ogsaa „Arvesygen." Den optræder i Regelen mellem 50—60 Aars Alderen; begynder som oftest med mindre iøinefaldende Phænomener, der undertiden kun langsomt tiltage og ikke blive videre heftige, saa at Vedkommende ikke synderlig hindres i sine almindelige Beskjæftigelser, men oftere naa de efter faa Aars Forløb en ualmindelig Høide, saa at ethvert Arbeide bliver dem en Umulighed, og de endog have megen Vanskelighed med ad mangfoldige Omveie at føre Maden til Munden; hele deres Legeme, dog fornemlig Hoved, Arme og Overkrop er i stadig, heftig rykkende og slengende Bevægelse undtagen under Søvnen, da de almindelig ere rolige. Et Par af de heftig angrebne ere i den sidste Tid af deres Liv blevne fatui. Sygdommen forekommer i 2 Familier, som her nærmere anføres; Oplysningerne ere vistnok ikke saa fuldstændige, som det kunde ønskes, men dog altid Noget at begynde med, saafremt Lægerne i Sætersdalen for Fremtiden ville have sin Opmærksomhed henvendt paa Sygdommen.

18

FIG. 10. Dr. J. C. Lund's report in 1860 of a chronic, progressive hereditary chorea.

Über Ausscheidung von Phenylbrenztraubensäure in den Harn als Stoffwechselanomalie in Verbindung mit Imbezillität*).

Von

Asbjörn Fölling.

(Aus dem klinischen Laboratorium des Reichshospitales, Oslo.)

(Der Schriftleitung zugegangen am 23. Juli 1934.)

Bei Untersuchungen von schwachsinnigen Kindern habe ich eine Stoffwechselanomalie wahrgenommen, die früher beim Menschen niemals beschrieben worden ist. Die Anomalie gibt sich durch Ausscheidung von Phenylbrenztraubensäure im Harn kund, und es scheint eine Verbindung zwischen dieser Anomalie und der Imbezillität zu bestehen. Ich habe bisher 10 Patienten

FIG. 11. Fölling's first report in 1934 on phenylketonuria.

degree, characteristic." In the review of the history of Huntington's chorea in Bruyn's contribution (32) to the *Handbook of Clinical Neurology*, he states: "In all fairness it should be pointed out that Lund's excellent description 'avant la lettre' is a complete if succinct masterpiece of observation."

Lund's report remained relatively unknown because it could only be read by physicians who knew Norwegian. The description was even forgotten in Norway until it was rediscovered by Olav Hanssen (1914) (37), who traced one of the pedigrees back to about 1550. The first known case appears to have occurred in the first half of the 18th century. Hanssen in his report characteristically names the disease "so-called Huntington's chorea." In the famous *Handbook of Historical and Geographic Pathology*, edited by Hirsch (1862–1864) (38), there is an excellent German translation of Lund's report, but, unfortunately, the author concludes that Lund's cases "obviously correspond to our concept of paralysis agitans," a statement that may have contributed to the lack of recognition of Lund's contribution. Lund's original report is also reprinted by Ørbeck (39).

To assign priority to anybody for having first described a disease or syndrome is extremely difficult, or even impossible, in most cases. I agree with De Jong (30) when he writes: "In the early medical literature, it is quite difficult to differentiate chorea from other hyperkinetic disorders of both organic and nonorganic ætiology." I further agree with De Jong (30): "Thilenius in 1814 differentiated acute and chronic varieties of chorea, but his differentiation was not definite and he dealt mainly with chronic chorea in children. Some authorities, however, give him credit for first describing the inherited form of chorea. There were other physicians who described chronic forms of chorea and chorea in adults, but there is no evidence that any of these observers was aware of the presence of a chronic, degenerative, hereditary type of chorea such as that later described by Huntington." However, one of the first authors to clearly describe the disease, and perhaps the first to have recognized it as a distinct clinical entity seems, in my opinion, to be J. C. Lund, so that, in Norway, we like to call the disease Lund-Huntington's chorea.

Fölling's Disease—Phenylketonuria

While there is a great deal of disagreement about priorities as to description of diseases, with a resulting confusing abundance of eponyms, there is no disagreement about one disease, and that is phenylketonuria, or as we call it in Norway, Fölling's disease. In 1934 (40), he reported this disease in German, and its title reads in English: "On the excretion of phenylpyruvic acid in the urine as metabolic anomaly in combination with imbecility."

In a symposium on phenylketonuria, Fölling (41) reported on the original detection: "The detection and elucidation of phenylketonuria is the achievement of many scientists. I will tell of the beginning of this work as I experienced it from the first casual consultation that started it all."

> A mother sought advice because her two children were both mentally retarded. They were seven and four years old, and their unhappy mother had asked for help at many institutions. She had noticed that a peculiar smell always clung to her children. I had no real hope of being able to help her, and I examined the children mainly because I did not want to be hostile to the mother. . . . The ordinary urine analyses were also normal, but after adding ferric chloride to the urine a green colour appeared and then disappeared a few minutes later. I had never seen such a reaction, and it was not described in the literature. Urine collected a few days later, after withdrawal from the patients of all medicaments, behaved similarly. There was probably an unknown substance in the urine, and the first problem seemed to be to isolate and identify this substance.

Fölling originally termed this new abnormality *imbecillitas phenylpyrouvica*. Following a suggestion by Jervis (42), who later studied the condition among institutionalized patients in the United States, he changed the name to *oligophrenia phenylketonurica*, in jargon called P.K.U. It was stated that the disease probably showed a recessive autosomal hereditary pattern (42). With Mohr and Ruud (43), Fölling made a systematic genetic analysis of the disease, the conclusion being that it is an autosomal recessive trait. In these circumstances, it was tempting to trace the heterozygotes, and Fölling made such an attempt as early as 1937. In 1962 appeared a paper by Sydnes and Fölling (44) that described a method to detect heterozygotes for phenylpyruvic acid 2, 4, and 6 hours after administration of a dose of phenylalanine. The curve for the heterozygotes was appreciably higher than that for the control group. After Sydnes and Fölling had begun their research, a paper by Hsia et al. 45) on the same subject was published, their techniques and results being the same. As physical characteristics of the disease, Fölling noted that his patients had blond complexions with light (sometimes almost white) hair and blue eyes. Thirty-three of his 34 patients had blue or bluish eyes, but defect of pigmentation is not a constant factor of the disease, cases being observed in apparently full blooded Negroes as well as Puerto Ricans of mixed Spanish and Negro ancestry (49).

Fölling (1888–1973) was 46 years old when he reported the disease (Fig.12). In 1935, he became the first professor of clinical chemistry at the University in Oslo and head of the clinical central laboratory of the National Hospital (Rikshospitalet) in Oslo.

In 1963, a monograph on phenylketonuria was published, edited by F. L. Lyman (46). It had a foreword by the Nobel Laureate in literature, Pearl S. Buck, and the introduction on the discovery of phenylketonuria written by S. A. Centerwall and W. R. Centerwall, states: "The discovery of phenylketonuria is the story of a Norwegian doctor and a persistent, observant Norwegian mother with two retarded children."

> "If Dr. Fölling had done nothing except discover the disease which we now call phenylketonuria, his contribution to the field of metabolic disorders would have been a remarkable

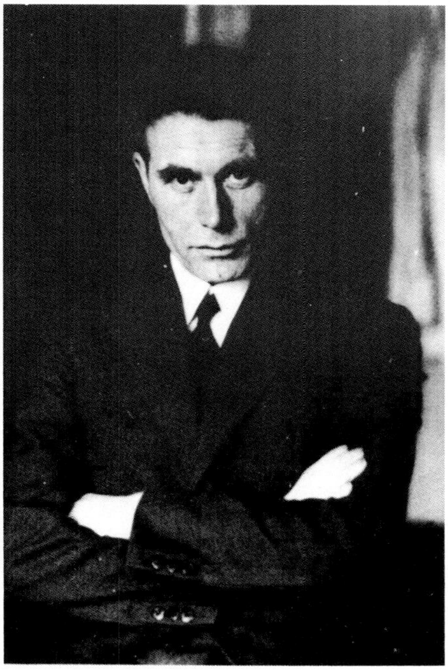

FIG. 12. Dr. A Fölling (1888–1973), age 46, when he first reported phenylketonuria.

> one. But his contribution did not stop there. He has continued to be one of the most significant contributors to the understanding of this disease. In collaboration with his Norwegian colleagues, he was the first to devise a method for measuring serum phenylalanine levels and thus the first to prove that these levels are high in phenylketonurics." He was the first to demonstrate the increased urinary excretion of certain other metabolites such as phenylacetic acid and phenylalanine (42,43).

The introductory chapter (46) ends with the following words: "The wide scope and imagination of the research Dr. Fölling had done on phenylketonuria was amazing to us. He is such a humble man that he shuns the acclaim that he justly deserves. But as one talks with him, it becomes apparent that the wealth of his knowledge and the depth of his thinking on both medical and nonmedical subjects places him rightly as one of the truly great physicians and gentlemen of his time."

We have a little story in Norway that characterizes him. Once when travelling in the United States to a medical meeting, an American colleague was sitting in the same compartment and found out that they were both going to the same meeting. The American colleague started explaining the biochemistry of phenylketonuria; Fölling listened attentively, nodding his head, and agreed with him. Finally, the American colleague asked him: "Have you ever heard about Dr. Fölling and the disease he has described?" Fölling looked down and said shyly: "I am Fölling."

In a letter to the Editor of *Lancet* (50), Letten Fegersten Saugstad reported on an association between the phenylketonuria gene and the rhesus, phosphoglucomatase-(AGM) type-1, and Kell systems. The heterozygotes are characterized by an excess of rhesus negative, Kell +, and PGM-type-1 values, which are higher than observed in any region in Norway, and which correspond to those in Ireland, Scotland, and Iceland. These three countries have the highest incidences of phenylketonuria; Saugstad therefore proposed that the Norwegian heterozygotes for phenylketonuria in her series could be descendants of an early Norwegian population with genetic structure similar to the present populations in Ireland, Scotland, and Iceland. In a study of the anthropological significance of phenylketonuria, Saugstad (51) proposed the hypothesis that the heterozygotes for phenylketonuria are descended from a completely assimilated subpopulation of Celtic origin, who came or were brought to Norway 1,000 years ago.

Norway has an incidence of Fölling's disease of one per 16,000 live births per year, which is equal to that in England, but considerably below that in Ireland, Scotland, and Iceland. The incidence in Norway and England is twice that in Sweden (52), an observation which might be related to the fact that Swedish Vikings traveled south and east and not to Britain as the Norwegians did. In Finland, Fölling's disease is very rare, only one per 250,000 live births per year. Bronze objects of western European (Scottish, Irish) origin, found in Viking graves widely distributed in Norway, have been taken as possible evidence of Vikings returning to Norway with loot (including a number of Celts as wives and slaves) from western Viking settlements. The continuity of residence since the Viking age in the most habitable parts of Norway and what seems to be a regional relationship between the sites where Viking graves contain Celtic objects and the birthplaces of grandparents of patients with Fölling's disease identified in Norway (51) lend further support to the hypothesis that the heterozygotes for the disease in Norway are descended from a completely assimilated subpopulation.

Saugstad's findings have been discussed in an editorial in *Lancet* (53), which states that they support a common ancestry for inhabitants of Ireland and Scotland and the west coast of Norway. As mentioned, Saugstad (52) suggests that this could be explained by the importation of Celts to Norway in the Viking period; an alternative explanation could be an earlier migration during the Bronze Age (53).

THE FIRST TWO PROFESSORS OF NEUROLOGY IN THE UNIVERSITY OF OSLO

Finally, I shall briefly mention the first two professors of neurology at the Royal Frederik's University in Christiania (now University of Oslo). The first was Christopher Blom Leegaard (1851–1921) who was appointed in 1895. The first professorial chair in diseases of the nervous system was established in 1882 at the Faculty of Medicine in Paris. J.-M. Charcot, who had been Professor of Pathological Anatomy since 1872, was in this year—as my predecessor Monrad-Krohn expressed it—"promoted" to the chair of clinical neurology. This was the first occasion in the entire world in which neurology was recognized as a special and autonomous discipline, and it was only 13 years later that a chair of neurology was established at the University of Christiania.

Professor Leegaard had a solid training in internal medicine at the National Hospital (Rikshospitalet) in Christiania, and he studied neurology for long periods of time at some of the centers on the continent (Vienna, Munich, Paris, Leipzig, and Heidelberg). From 1885, he was in charge of a "department of electrotherapy" at the National Hospital and taught this subject to the medical students. This became the "nucleus" of the department for nervous diseases, as the department was first termed.

Leegaard was a pioneer in the study of the epidemiology of poliomyelitis (54,55). In 1889, an epidemic occurred in a county near Oslo, where there were 54 cases, mostly in children. This epidemic was thoroughly studied and described by Leegaard, who pointed out that the epidemic spread along the main roads of communication, branching out to the sides with small groups of cases. The route of infection was supposed to occur through the alimentary tract, and the disease was pronounced contagious with a short incubation period. Leegaard proposed that the disease be subjected to public control and be made reportable to the public health authorities; he also proposed isolation for three weeks and subsequent disinfection. It has been stated that he was the first, or one of the first, to call attention to the abortive forms.

The second professor of neurology at the University in Oslo was Georg Herman Monrad-Krohn (1884–1964). In 1912, he went to England for further studies, first at the National Hospital for the Paralyzed and Epileptics, Queen Square, and he spent five years altogether in England, the first Norwegian doctor to spend so long a period of training in England.

In 1918, Monrad-Krohn wrote his thesis in Norwegian (56) on the abdominal reflexes and many of his papers deal with examination of reflexes. He was also very much interested in the disturbances of language and wrote "Dysprosody, or altered melody of language" (57) and "The Third element of speech: prosody in the neuropsychiatric clinic" (58). Monrad-Krohn's views are well summarized by N. Wertheim (59). Monrad-Krohn showed that in addition to vocabulary and grammar, one has to consider also a prosodic quality of human speech, which gives it various shades by means of variations in stress, pitch, and rhythm. There is an *intrinsic* prosody, which consists of a "standard prosodic pattern inherent in the language," a *propositional* prosody, which "serves the need of expressing various subtle shades of meaning," and an *emotional* prosody, which may convey various emotions. Disturbances of the prosody was described by Monrad-Krohn as hyperprosody, hypoprosody, and dysprosody. In the presence of dysprosody, a patient's speech may should so inexpressive that even when speaking his mother tongue, it may sound like a foreign language. Monrad-Krohn considered the dysprosodies as an after effect of aphasia, appearing during the stage of recovery so that they seem to be associated more with the function of language than with the musical faculty.

Monrad-Krohn was an astute clinical observer. It had long been known that in central facial paralysis there is often a marked dissociation between voluntary and emotional innervation, the latter being less affected than the former. This phenomenon is mentioned and illustrated in Gower's textbook of 1886. Monrad-Krohn showed and demonstrated by cinematographic registration that in central facial paresis the emotional innervation not only remains intact, but is even distinctly exaggerated on the paretic side. For this one-sided emotional hypermimia with paresis of voluntary movements of the same side of the face, Monrad-Krohn liked the term "Monrad-Krohn's sign of paradoxical hypermimia."

Monrad-Krohn wrote the textbook *The Clinical Examination of the Nervous System* in 1921; the twelfth and last edition appeared in 1964 (60). It contains a wealth of clinical observations and has become for many the first introduction to neurological examination. It was written, as he emphasized, "from the clinic for the clinic." The binding of it was blue, and it has been often referred to as "the neurologist's blue bible." It has been translated into French, Spanish, German, and Japanese.

During his whole life, Monrad-Krohn kept close contact with British neurology to which Norwegian neurology is greatly indebted. A bibliography of the works of Monrad-Krohn was printed in the *Journal of the Norwegian Medical Association* (in part in English) [*Tidsskr. f. D. norske lægfor.* (1964), pp. 479–494, edited by P. Dietrichson and B. Ranheim].

ACKNOWLEDGMENTS

I want to express my gratitude to my colleagues with whom I have had discussions on the subject of leprosy: Professor of Dermatology, N. Danbolt; Professor of Immunology,

M. Harboe; both of the University of Oslo; and Dr. med. L. M. Irgens, Institute of Hygiene and Social Medicine of the University of Bergen (also curator of the Leprosy Museum in Bergen); they have all given me valuable advice. My section on the history of leprosy in Norway is to a great extent based on the papers by Drs. Irgens and Harboe, even when personally I have consulted the original references.

I also wish to acknowledge the staff of the Medical Library, The National Hospital (Rikshospitalet) in Oslo, who has been most helpful in providing me with literature, which required considerable effort, particularly with regard to the older references, journals, and books not available in Oslo. The Department of Medical Illustrations, under the leadership of Miss Else Aarseth, has as usual rendered excellent service.

Last, but not least, my secretary, Mrs. Gerd Høye, has this time as many times before, patiently and carefully typed and retyped my manuscripts.

My heartiest thanks are due to all persons mentioned above for their kind assistance.

REFERENCES

Leprosy in Norway

1. Hansen, G. H. A., and Lie, H. P. (1909): Die Geschichte der Lepra in Norwegen. *II. Internationale wissenschaftliche Lepra-konferenz*, I Band, edited by G. H. A. Hansen and H. P. Lie, p. 52. Johan Ambrosius Barth, Leipzig; Williams & Norgate, London; Masson, Paris.
2. Irgens, L. M. (1973): *Int. J. Leprosy*, 41:189.
3. Danielssen, D. C., Boeck, C. W. (1847): *Om Spedalskhed*, Chr. Grøndahl, Christiania. (in Norwegian).
4. Danielssen, D. C., Boeck, C. W. (1848): *Traité de la Spedalskhed ou Elephantiasis de Grec.*, J.-B. Bailliére, Paris (with an atlas).
5. Irgens, L. M., and Bjerkedal, T. (1973): *Int. J. Epidemiol.*, 2:81.
6. Hansen, G. H., Armauer (1874): *Norsk Mag. f. Lægevid. 4*, Suppl., 1–88 (in Norwegian). Part of it (pp. 76–79) is translated into English: Causes of leprosy. *Int. J. Leprosy*, 23:307 (1955).
7. Irgens, L. M. (1980): *Leprosy in Norway*. An epidemiological study based on a national patient registry. *Leprosy Rev*. 51 (Suppl. 1): 1–130.
8. Harboe, M. (1973): *Int. J. Leprosy*, 41:417.
9. Lie, H. P. (1938): *Med. Rev.* (Bergen), Nr. 2, p. 49 (in Norwegian).
10a. Hansen, G. A. (1880): *Virchows Arch.*, 79:32.
10b. Hansen, G. A. (1880): *Arch. Biol.*, 1:
10c. Hansen, G. A. (1880): *Quart. J. Microscopic Sci.*, 20:92.
11. Lie, H. P. (1904): *Lepra im Rückenmark und den peripheren Nerven*. Wilhelm Braumüller, Wien und Leipzig. Enlarged special reprint from *Arch. Dermatol. Syphilis*, Vol. 73.
12. Dastur, D. K., Ramamohan, Y., and Shah, Y. S. (1973): *Int. J. Leprosy*, 41:47.
13. Dastur, D. K. (1978): In: *Handbook of Clinical Neurology*, edited by P. J. Vinken and G. W. Bruyn, Vol. 33, Part I, p. 421. North-Holland, Amsterdam.
14. Sabin, T. D., and Swift, T. R. (1975): Leprosy: In: *Peripheral Neuropathy*, edited by P. J. Dyck, P. K. Thomas, and E. H. Lambert, p. 1166. W. B. Saunders, Philadelphia.
15. Monrad-Krohn, G. H. (1923): *The Neurological Aspect of Leprosy ("Spedalskhed")*. Videnskapsselskapets Skrifter I Mat. -Naturv. Klasse, No. 16, pp. 1–78. Christiania.
16. Godal, T., and Negassi, K. (1973): *Br. Med. J.*, 3:557.
17. Harboe, M. (1980): *Int. J. Leprosy*, 48:193.

Eponymous Diseases

18. Zeman, W. (1970): In: *Handbook of Clinical Neurology*, edited by P. J. Vinken and G. W. Bruyn, Vol. 10, p. 212. North-Holland, Amsterdam.
19. Zeman, W., Donahu, S., Dyken, P., and Green, J. (1970): In: *Handbook of Clinical Neurology*, edited by P. J. Vinken and G. W. Bruyn, Vol. 10, p. 588. North-Holland, Amsterdam.
20. Stengel, C. (1826): *Eyr*, 1:347. (in Norwegian).
21. Sjögren, T. (1930–1931): *Hereditas*, Vol. 14, pp. 197–426. Genetiskt Arkiv, Lund, Sweden.
22. Nissen, A. J. B. (1954): *Nord. Med.*, 52:1542 (in Norwegian, English summary).
23. Christie Løken, Aa., and Cyvin, K. (1954): *J. Neurol. Neurosurg. Psychiatr.*, 17:211.
24. Koppang, N. (1973/74): *Mech. Ageing Develop.*, 2:421.
25. Hansen, E. (1979): *Acta Ophthal.*, 57:382.

26. Kiær, F. C. (1890): *Norges Læger i det nittende aarhundrede* (1800–1886). (Norwegian Physicians 1800–1886), Vol. 2, p. 387, in Norwegian, Cammermeyer, Christiania.
27. (1886); *Biographisches Lexicon der hervorragenden Ärzte aller Zeiten und Völker*. (Biographical Dictionary of Outstanding Physicians of All Times and Peoples), Band 5, p. 425.

Huntington's Chorea or (?) Lund-Huntington's Chorea

28. Critchley, M. (1973): In: *Huntington's Chorea*, edited by A. Barbeau, T. N. Chase, and G. W. Paulson. *Advances in Neurology*, Vol. 1, p. 13. Raven Press, New York.
29. Critchley, M. (1964): In: *The Black Hole and Other Essays*, p. 210. Pitman Medical Publishing Co., London.
30. DeJong, R. N. (1973): In: *Huntington's Chorea*, edited by A. Barbeau, T. N. Chase, and G. W. Paulson. *Advances in Neurology, Vol. 1*, p. 19. Raven Press, New York.
31. De Jong, R. N. (1973): *Ann. Med. Hist.*, 9:201.
32. Bruyn, G. W. (1968): Huntington's chorea. Historical, clinical and laboratory synopsis. In: *Handbook of Clinical Neurology*, Vol. 6. edited by P. J. Vinken and G. W. Bruyn, Vol. 6, p. 298. Horth-Holland, Amsterdam.
33. Roccatagliata, G. (1979): *Psicosi e Corea di Huntington*. Pacini Editore, Pisa.
34. Dunglison, R. (1842): *The Practice of Medicine*. Vol. 2, p. 312. Lea & Blanchard, Philadelphia. (Quoted from ref. 31).
35. Lund, J. C. (1860): In: *Report of Health and Medical Conditions in Norway in 1860 to the Ministry of the Interior*. (*Beretning om Sundhedstilstanden og Medicinalforholdene i Norge i* 1860. In Norwegian), p. 137. Printed in Christiania (1863).
36. Lund, J. C. (1868): In: *Beretning om Sundhedstilstanden og Medicinalforholdene i Norge i 1868* (in Norwegian), p. 168. Printed in Christiania.
37. Hanssen, O. (1914): *Med. Rev.* (Bergen), 31:569.
38. Hirsch, A. (1862–1864) *Handbuch der historisch-geographischen Pathologie*, II Band, p. 572. Verlag von Ferdinand Enk, Erlangen.
39. Ørbeck, A. L. (1959): *Med. Hist.*, 3:165.

Fölling's Disease—Phenylketonuria

40. Fölling, A. (1934): *Hoppe-Seylers Zschr. Physiol. Chem.*, 227:169.
41. Fölling, A. (1971): In: *Phenylketonuria and Some Other Inborn Errors of Amino Acid Metabolism. Genetics. Diagnosis. Therapy. Biochemistry*, edited by H. Bickel, F. P. Hudson, L. I. Woolf, p. 1. Georg. Thieme Verlag, Stuttgart.
42. Jervis, G. A. (1937): *Arch. Neurol. Psychiat.*, 38:944.
43. Fölling, A., Mohr, O. L., and Ruud, L. (1944): Skrifter Det Norske Videnskaps-Akademi in Oslo, I Mat.-naturv.Klasse No. 13, p. 3. *(Publication of The Norwegian Academy of Science and Letters.)*
44. Sydnes, S., and Fölling, A. (1962): *Scand. J. Clinical Lab. Invest.*, 14:44.
45. Hsia, D. Y., Driscoll, K. W., Troll, W. L., and Knox, W. E. (1956): *Nature*, 178:1239.
46. Lyman, F. L. editor (1963): *Phenylketonuria*. Charles C. Thomas, Springfield, Ill.
47. Fölling, A., and Closs, K. (1938): *Zschr. Physiol. Chem.*, 254:115.
48. Fölling, A., and Sydnes, S. (1958): *Scand. J. Clin. Lab. Invest.*, 10:355.
49. Ferriera-Fernandes, J. (1950): *Brasil-med.*, 64:225. (Quoted from Jervis, G. A., in F. L. Lyman, editor, ref. 41.)
50. Saugstad, L. F. (1973): *Lancet*, I:1255.
51. Saugstad, L. F. (1975): *Clin. Genet.*, 7:52.
52. Saugstad, L. F. (1975): *Clin. Genet.*, 7:40.
53. Editorial (1975): *Lancet*, I:1075.

The First Two Professors of Neurology in the University of Oslo

54. Leegaard, C. (1915): *Deutsche Ztschr. Nervenheilk.*, 53:145.
55. Harbitz, F. (1912): *J. Am. Med. Assoc.*, 59:782.
56. Monrad-Krohn, G. H. (1918): *Om abdominalreflexerne*. Norsk Mag. Lægevidensk. Suppl. (in Norwegian).
57. Monrad-Krohn, G. H. (1947): *Brain*, 22:204.
58. Monrad-Krohn, G. H. (1957): *J. Ment. Sci.*, 103:326.
59. Wertheim, N. (1977): In: *Music and the Brain. Studies in the Neurology of Music*, edited by M. Critchley and R. A. Henson, p. 282. W. Heineman Med. Books, London.
60. Monrad-Krohn, G. H. (1964): (in co-operation with S. Refsum): *The Clinical Examination of the Nervous System*, 12th ed. H. K. Lewis, London.

Historical Aspects of the Neurosciences,
edited by F. Clifford Rose and W. F. Bynum.
Raven Press, New York ©

Neurology in India

E. P. Bharucha

Department of Neurology, K. E. M. Hospital and G. S. Medical College, Bombay, India

Neurology in India is similar and yet vastly different from that seen in the West. Epilepsy and cerebrovascular disease have of course the same high incidence, but the latter has certain characteristics peculiar to India. Malnutrition and infection still account for much neurological illness. Infections such as tuberculosis have become uncommon in the West, though recently they have reappeared in immigrants. Sarcoidosis, on the other hand, is hardly ever seen in India, the reason for this being unclear. The demyelinating diseases are not as frequent, although they do occur.

Because the enormous birthrate of 15 million a year stretches the available economic and medical resources beyond limits, it becomes impossible to give each child the care he needs before and at birth or the food he needs to thrive; nutritional brain damage is accentuated by the ravages of infection. Since the Indian population has numerous ethnic groups, each with its own social and cultural patterns, this leads to clustering of heredofamilial disorders such as craniovertebral anomalies and certain varieties of cerebellar ataxia.

All these factors provide a background for certain clinical syndromes, many of which are peculiar to India, and the conditions discussed here include the nutritional disorders, intoxications, infections, paraplegias, and cerebrovascular disease.

NUTRITIONAL DISORDERS

B_{12} Neuromyelopathy

Many cases of peripheral neuropathy, posterolateral sclerosis, and myeloradiculopathy of obscure origin are seen in India. Because some of them were thought to be due to deficient intake or absorption of vitamin B_{12}, 42 such cases were investigated (1). The results suggested that 14 of them had evidence of malabsorption of vitamin B_{12}, two of which were true cases of subacute combined degeneration, an extremely rare condition in India.

Though B_{12} neuromyelopathy is generally believed to be due to malabsorption (10), malnutrition cannot be completely excluded, since most Indians are vegetarian from necessity, and it is known that vegetarians have a lower serum B_{12} than nonvegetarians (3). In both B_{12} neuromyelopathy and subacute combined degeneration, the marrow is megaloblastic, but there are important differences since, in acquired B_{12} neuromyelopathy, achlorhydria is not constantly present, and the symptoms consist of fluctuating mental changes, cerebellar ataxia, and sensory level and sphincter disturbances.

Neurological Disorders Accompanying B-Complex Deficiency

To determine this relationship, further studies were done on 44 suspected cases (4), all of whom were malnourished and alcoholic. The majority had pellagrous skin changes, and/or gastrointestinal disturbances. All had peripheral neuritis, essentially a sensory neuropathy, and eight had in addition a Wernicke-Korsakoff syndrome/myelopathy/posterolateral sclerosis.

The results showed that all the B vitamins were lower in patients than in controls (relatives of patients on the same diet, minus the alcohol, and without neurological symptoms). The skin changes improved with nicotinic acid, but the peripheral neuropathy required thiamine or total B complex. Mental changes improved rapidly with thiamine which, given alone, raised not only the serum levels of thiamine but riboflavin, nicotinic acid, and pantothenic acid as well. Giving nicotinic acid alone had a similar effect, so that there appears to be an interrelationship between the different fractions of the B group.

Pellagra

Pellagra has been known for centuries. (Fig. 1). In India, it occurs in the Udaipur district of Rajasthan and on the Deccan Plateau where at certain times of the year 1.0% of all admissions to general hospitals and 8 to 10% of those to mental institutions are due to pellagra (8). In Bombay, it is seen only in alcoholics.

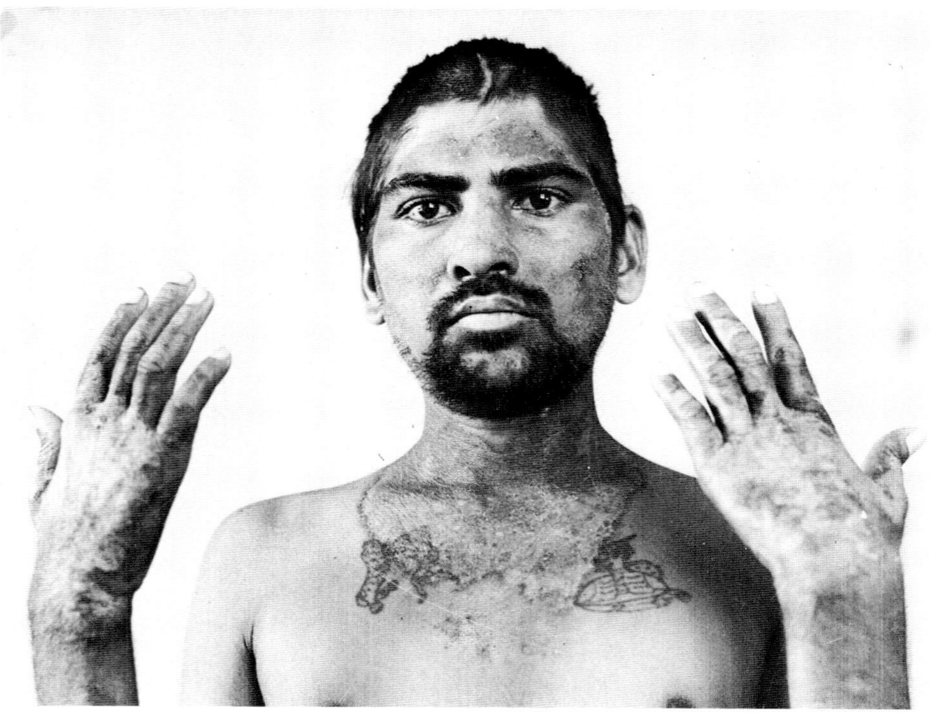

FIG. 1. Pellagra with typical skin changes. (Courtesy of S. G. Srikanthia, Director, National Institute of Nutrition, Hyderabad.)

Usually ascribed to a deficiency of nicotinic acid, pellagra is doubtful if all its symptoms are indeed due to this alone, on evidence that is mainly epidemiological. The Indian diet consists predominantly of cereal. The wheat eaters of the North and the rice eaters of the South do not have pellagra, but the populations at risk are those which subsist on maize, as in Rajasthan, or on millet, as on the Deccan Plateau. Since eating habits are difficult to change, maize and millet will continue to be eaten, so that pellagra will only be prevented by cultivating low-leucine strains and by early recognition of the disorder (14).

Protein Energy Malnutrition and the Nervous System

A deficiency of protein and calories results in kwashiorkor and marasmus, protein energy malnutrition (PEM). This has both immediate and long term effects on the nervous system. Gopalan (7,9) thinks that nearly 2% of toddlers in social class IV–V suffer from PEM. The immediate effects are apathy, irritability, weakness and wasting, hypotonia and depression of reflexes, but the long-term effects include defective intelligence and perception, which may not necessarily be irreversible (2,5,6,11–13).

INFECTIONS OF THE NERVOUS SYSTEM

The two mycobacteria, tubercle and leprosy, account for most of the chronic infectious neurological illnesses in India. The three common varieties of neurotuberculosis are cranial meningitis (TBM), spinal meningitis (Tb arachnoiditis), and tuberculoma.

In tuberculous meningitis, the infection occurs in two stages: the silent subependymal or cortical caseating Rich focus and perhaps several years later, the ravage of its rupture, a catastrophe precipitated usually at a time when the resistance is low. The clinical onset, at least in children, is fulminant, while in adults, who are being affected more and more, it is insidious. Tb lesions elsewhere in the body are seen in less than a quarter of the cases, and atypical, not to say bizarre, pictures occur frequently (19,26).

Such cases are becoming the rule, not the exception. Diagnosis from the cerebrospinal fluid (CSF) is notoriously difficult as, even at the point of death, this may be normal, and Tb bacilli, even with sophisticated techniques (Figs. 2A,2B), are found clinically in only a quarter of the cases. Guinea pig inoculation is usually negative, possibly because the Indian guinea pig seems to be a different animal in this respect (25). Other diagnostic tests are therefore constantly being sought. The labeled ammonium bromide test is one of them. After injecting labeled bromide, the blood/CSF ratio is estimated. Anything less than 1.6 is diagnostic, and from 1.9 to 1.6 is suggestive (17). Another is the test of CSF sugar after a glucose bolus. In 12 cases of TBM, it rose to 22 to 42 mg%, while in 12 controls it was only 7 to 25 mg% (15).

Tuberculomas are common in children, often located in the cerebellum, but hardly ever in the spinal cord. In adults, they affect females more than males (20).

In spinal meningitis, the exudate encircles the cord and nerve roots. It may come from an intracranial exudate or arise from the cord itself. Clinically, the acute and subacute cases present with fever, lancinating root pains in the back, chest, and limbs. Bladder paralysis is frequent. The symptoms may be confined to one level, resembling transverse myelitis, or there may be an ascending paralysis like a Guillain-Barre syndrome or ascending myelitis. The chronic form has a slow progress, resembling a neoplasm, but the involvement is diffuse. For example, pains may occur in the cauda equina, there may be a sensory level in the

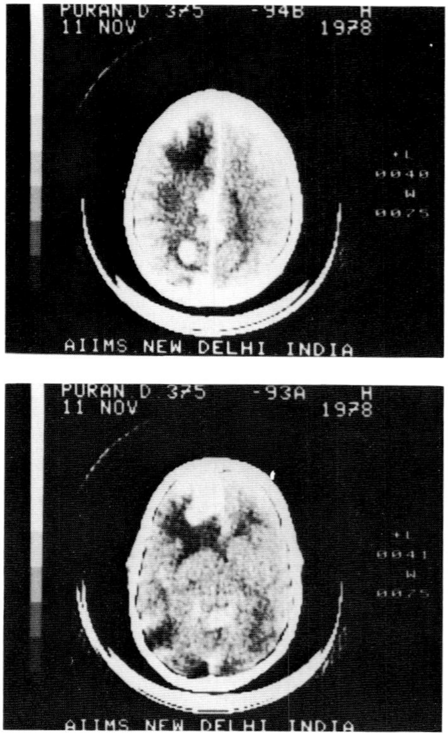

FIG. 2A,2B. CAT scans of tuberculoma. (Courtesy of Prof. S. Bhargava, AIIMS, New Delhi.)

middorsal region, and with a cervical cord lesion, there may be wasting and absent reflexes in the lower limbs.

The diagnosis is established by lumbar puncture, which shows a partial block, with very high protein and few cells. Myelography shows an irregular block, with multiple filling defects over several segments, but there is often no clinical and myelographic correlation (22).

VIRUS INFECTIONS OF THE NERVOUS SYSTEM

The enteroviruses are still common virus infections of the nervous system. In one series of unimmunized children, no fewer than 31.5% aged between six months and six years had antibodies to polio II and III, ECHO 7 and 19, and Coxsackie A-4 (23).

Poliomyelitis

Polio is still seen in epidemics in the hot wet summers. During 1971–1972, 810 cases were reported from Bombay alone, where the population was five million at that time; 62 of 82 cases had positive identification for poliovirus. Polio vaccine, which has brought polio to an end in the West, has not lived up to its reputation in India. Cases of polio are seen with distressing frequency, even after three oral doses of vaccine. They are variously ascribed to faulty storage and transport of vaccine, to unequal antigenicity of the three types of poliovirus in the vaccine, and to swallowing breast milk within an hour of taking the vaccine, since breast milk antibodies are believed to destroy the virus before it can produce gut immunity. Four doses of vaccine are now being advocated, but reverting to the old Salk vaccine may also have its advantages.

Acute Hemorrhagic Conjunctivitis

In early 1971, an epidemic of acute hemorrhagic conjunctivitis (AHC) swept through Bombay. After a latent period, which varied from two days to one month, some of these patients began to have severe pains in the back and limbs and muscle spasms, rather like early polio. There was also burning pain and hyperesthesiae, so severe as to preclude sleep. In 5 out of 10 cases, the sensory disturbances were followed by segmental paralysis, in the legs more than in the arms (16). This was dramatically sudden sometimes; for example, a woman squatting on the floor to do her housework found it impossible to stand up again, and a man strap-hanging in the bus felt his knees give way, and he folded up on the floor of the bus. In addition to lower motor neuron signs, spastic paraparesis, sphincter disturbances, and objective sensory loss were seen in some cases. The CSF showed a protein level from 60 to 110 mg %, but cells always below 10.

These cases resembled those from other parts of the world. From the conjunctiva of some cases, a virus has been isolated (24), which resembles an enterovirus. It has been injected into the spinal cord and thalamus of monkeys and produced an illness similar to the human one. Microscopically, neuronal degeneration and perivascular cuffing were seen. This enterovirus seems to produce a myeloradiculopathy, unlike poliovirus.

Japanese Encephalitis

This disease is now increasingly producing epidemics in various parts of India. The first cases were reported from around Vellore in the south (18). Since then, others have occurred in epidemics along the Eastern Seaboard, in the Krishna-Godaveri delta, in the foothills and wooded river valleys of the northeast, and in the populous northern state of U.P. Perhaps the worst epidemic was in South Central India, along the Kolar Gold Fields and adjoining districts in 1978, when over a thousand people were affected and one-third of them perished.

The virus infects wild birds, cattle, and, even more heavily, pigs. Unlike the rest of southeast Asia, India has more cattle than pigs, and so it has remained relatively unaffected till recently. The virus cycle is between egret, mosquito (culex), pig/cattle, and mosquito. Man is a tangential host, the cycle ending when the virus enters man.

The virus is partially destroyed after a mosquito bites man. What remains reaches the reticuloendothelial system and the endothelium of the capillaries. A viremia results and the virus, which is neurotropic, crosses the blood-brain barrier and enters nerve cells.

The pathological lesions are polymorphic and diffuse, as seen in a series of over 50 autopsied cases by Deshpande (21). The gray matter of the parieto-occipital cortex, thalamic nuclei, midbrain, and pons bear the brunt of the attack (Fig. 3). There are small punched-out necrotic areas or extensive necrolytic lesions, severe vascular congestion, focal subarachnoid hemorrhages, and massive edema.

Microscopically, the neurons show degeneration or necrosis. Focal aggregation of microglial cells around them produces a gliomesenchymal nodule, which is characteristic of the disease (Fig. 4). The arterioles and capillaries are directly affected by the virus, and

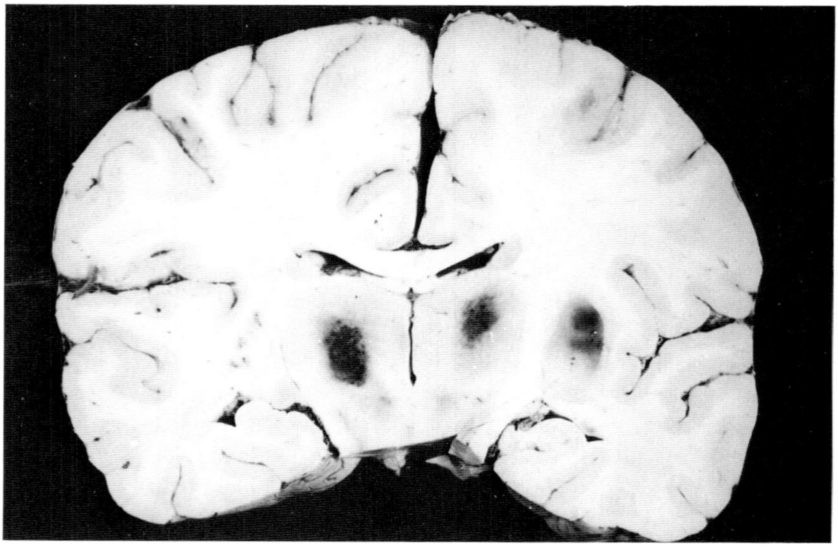

FIG. 3. Japanese encephalitis; coronal section of cerebral hemisphere. Note focal and confluent hemorrhages in both thalami and left lenticular nucleus. (Courtesy of Prof. D. H. Deshpande, NIMHANS, Bangalore.)

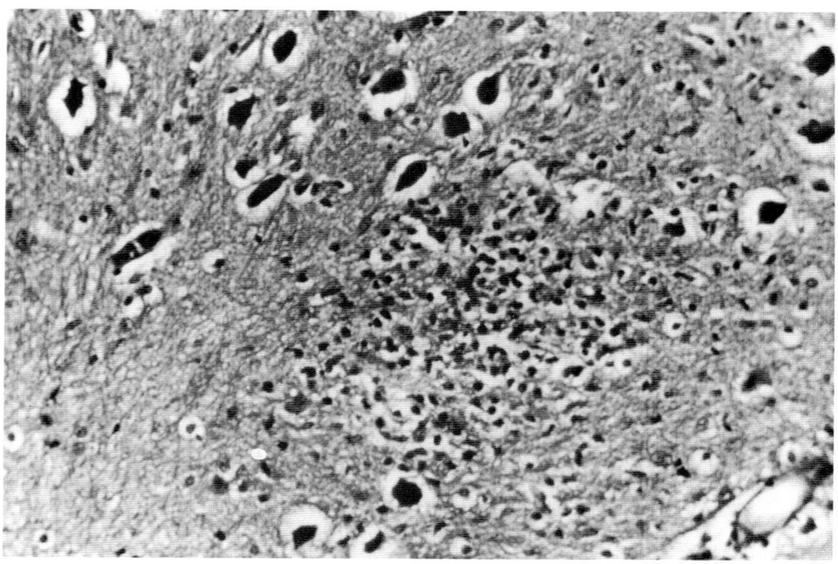

FIG. 4. Japanese encephalitis; gliomesenchymal nodule in olivary complex (medulla oblongata). (Courtesy of Prof. D. H. Deshpande, NIMHANS, Bangalore.)

there are extensive ring and ball hemorrhages. Vasospasm due to deposition of immune complexes also occurs.

The clinical features are deepening coma, convulsions, and neck stiffness. Focal neurological signs appear early, while alterations of tone and involuntary movements come later and often progress. Nearly one-third of Deshpande's fatal cases also had cysticercosis cellulosae of the brain, which may have occurred by chance. However, he quotes a report from the *Chinese Medical Journal*,where 8 out of 26 cases of Japanese encephalitis also had cysticercosis cellulosae of the brain.

The definitive tests are isolation of virus from the blood, which is difficult, or from the brain at biopsy or autopsy. Quantitative neutralization tests are also required to distinguish encephalitis from dengue.

In prophylaxis, mosquito control has not had its hoped for success, since the traditional way of living in close proximity to domestic animals still prevails in the country. Recently, success has been claimed for a vaccine made in Japan, and treatment with antiviral agents remains to be tried on a large scale.

INTOXICATIONS

Lathyrism

The term lathyrism signifies a permanent spastic paraplegia, the result of eating *lathyrus sativa*, a chick pea (Fig. 5). In India, the lathyrus is planted along with the wheat. The rains may fail and the wheat may die, but the hardier lathyrus survives and can be eaten. So lathyrism is endemic in certain parts of India, but epidemic in times of drought and famine. Lathyrism may also occur from a vetch, *vicia sativa*, a weed that may accidentally contaminate food crops.

In ancient Hindu literature, it is mentioned that a certain pulse may "make man lame and cripple and irritate the nerves." Hippocrates also knew that prolonged use of a certain pea caused paralysis. The Bible (St. Matthew, XIII, 25) says: "while men slept, the enemy came and sowed tares among the wheat." Incidentally, tares is the traditional English name for vetches, pulses, or legumes.

The neurotoxin is beta-*N*-oxalyl-amino-l-alanine (BOAA). This may interfere with the uptake of glutamate and aspartate by neural tissue. The attack rate in certain parts of rural India, in the poorer districts of M. P. and U. P., is 2,500 out of 100,000 of the population.

Clinically, the onset of paraparesis is very acute, usually coming suddenly after doing a hard day's work and/or being drenched in a downpour of rain. The patient may go to bed and wake up with spastic paraparesis; he may even develop it while sheltering under a tree during a heavy shower, and then have to crawl home on all fours. The weakness and stiffness reach a maximum in a few days and then remain stationary. There may be fever and rigor at the onset. On examination, there is marked spastic paraparesis with a scissors gait, which is permanent, the arms, trunk, and bladder usually escaping. There is no sensory loss. Autopsy reports are uncommon.

Prevention is the only hope, as there is no treatment. Lathyrism occurs only if 50% of the diet is lathyrus and if it is consumed for over six months.

Experimental evidence suggests that spastic paraparesis may be BOAA dose dependent (28), but there may also be an individual susceptibility, which is not related to HLA type (27).

Lathyrus will continue to be grown and eaten, as it is the only available food in certain areas at certain times of the year; official efforts to stop its cultivation have failed. Attempts to breed plants with a low content of BOAA have been made. Removing the toxin during cooking is also possible if the lathyrus is boiled in four times its volume of water and the water discarded.

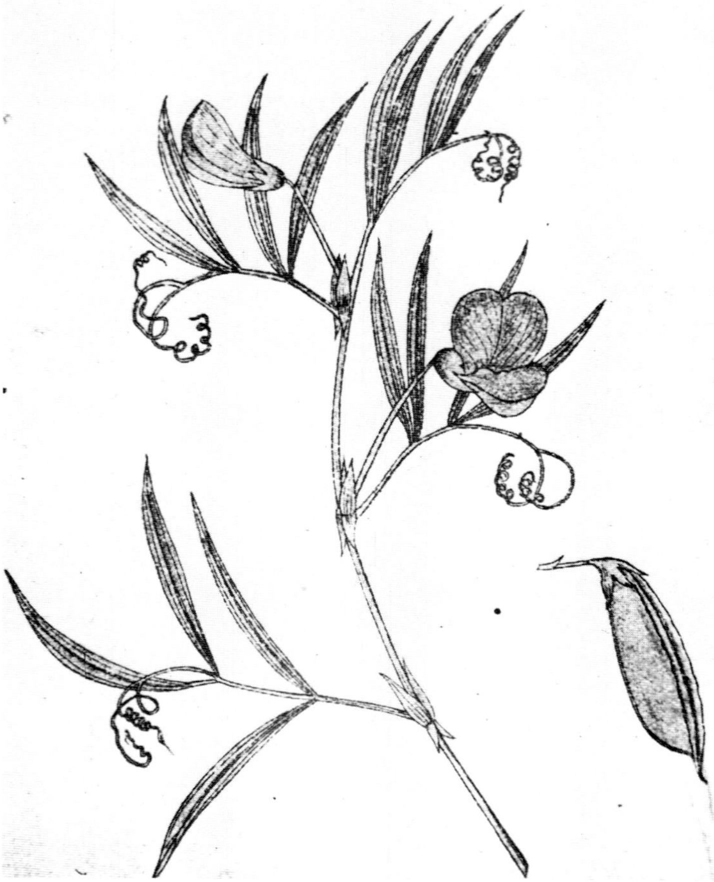

FIG. 5. *Lathyrus sativus* Linn. [From Chopra, Sir Ram Nath, Badhwar, R. D., and Ghosh, S. (1969): *Poisonous Plants of India*, Vol. 1. Govt. of India Press, Calcutta.]

PARAPLEGIA

Paraplegia in India is different from that seen in the West. Compressive lesions of the cord constitute the majority of all cases of paraplegia. Then there are regional differences in India itself. In the poorer rural areas of central India, Bihar, M.P., and U.P., lathyrism is common. From the south, T.N., and Karnataka, many cases of tropical spastic paraplegia are described. Perhaps the most fascinating (or frustrating) of all is the noncompressive paraplegia of unknown etiology, which defies all investigations, where nutritional factors have been presumed but never proven.

Compressive Myelopathy

This is present in about two-thirds of all cases of paraplegia. Combining the results of many series, these compressive lesions may be due to Tb in 12 to 20%, tumors in 12 to 14%, and the remainder to craniovertebral anomalies, cervical spondylosis, and fluorosis.

Craniovertebral anomalies are probably no more frequent than elsewhere, but their symptoms are aggravated by the prevailing custom of carrying loads on the head. Certainly, these symptoms can be relieved by surgery (30).

Fluorosis is endemic in the Punjab and on the Deccan Plateau (Fig. 6). The fluoride content of water in these areas may be as high as 25 mg/l. During the hot weather, a manual laborer may drink enormous quantities of this water, and over the years, fluoride is deposited in the vertebral column, long bones (Fig. 7), joints, teeth (Fig. 8), and even the auditory canal.

The clinical picture starts with stiffness, then weakness, wasting, and spastic paraplegia (Fig. 9). A trivial flexion injury of the neck may result in quadriparesis. Patchy numbness, paraesthesiae, and loss of bladder control also occur. Deafness is permanent. Diagnosis is made by seeing the chalky white ground glass appearance and osteosclerosis in the x-rays. The ligaments are also calcified. Prevention is possible by drinking water only from deep tube wells and by defluoridizing it with alum and magnesium oxide. Treatment by laminectomy may give relief to some cases. Metasilicate of magnesium (serpentine) 50 mg twice daily in enteric coated capsules produces an immediate and persistent increase of fluoride in the urine (36).

Noncompressive Myelopathy

In a series of 155 cases seen over a period of five years, the causes were infective/immunoallergic in 20.0%, motor neuron disease in 18.0%, heredofamilial in 14.2%, and demyelinating disease in 11.6%. But the largest group was "presumable/undetermined", and this constituted 36.2% (38).

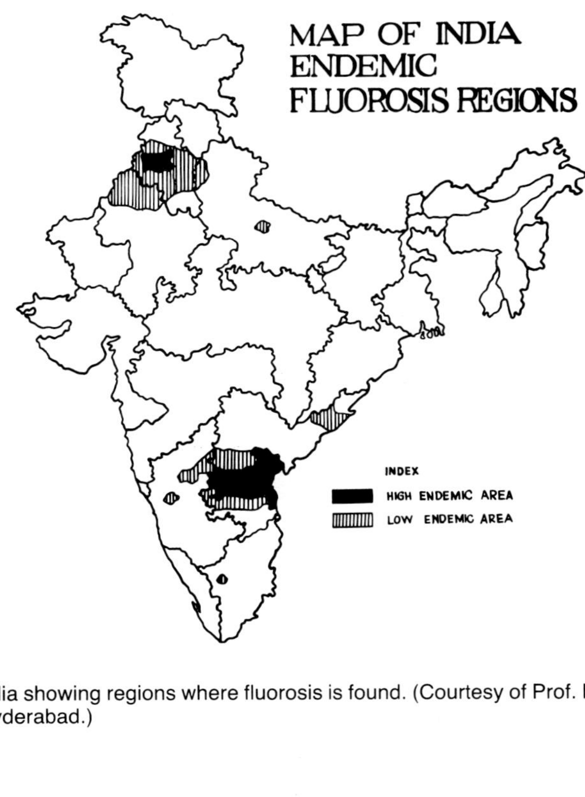

FIG. 6. Map of India showing regions where fluorosis is found. (Courtesy of Prof. D. Raja Reddy, Gandhi Medical College, Hyderabad.)

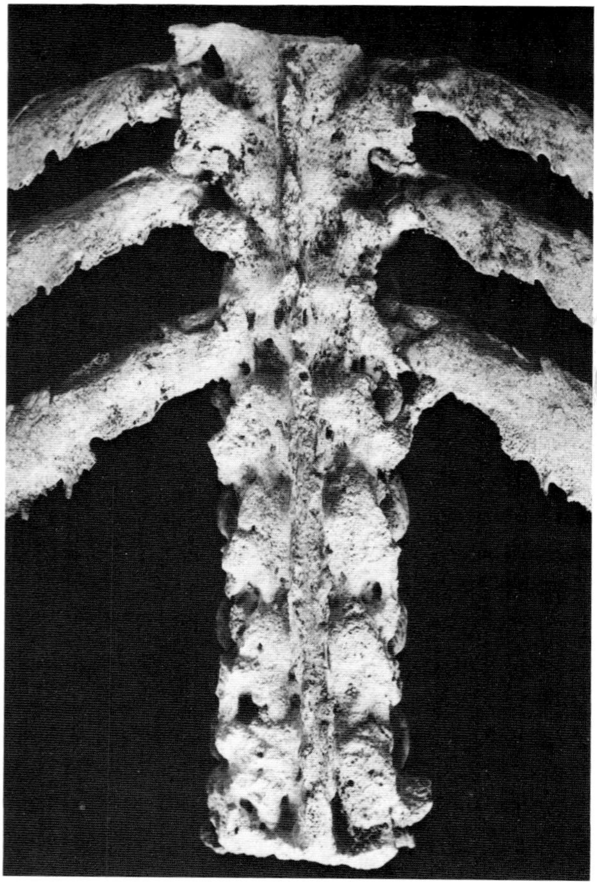

FIG. 7. Skeletal fluorosis. (Courtesy of Prof. D. Raja Reddy, Gandhi Medical College, Hyderabad.)

Motor neuron disease is seen occasionally, but spinal muscular atrophy is seen more often and at all ages in India. In many of these cases, there is no family history. A variant of motor neuron disease is seen in South India that occurs before the third decade, with wasting of the tongue, palate, face, and extremities, hyperactive deep reflexes, and deafness. It appears to be very chronic and may last for years (40).

The hereditary ataxias are among the commoner disorders of the spinal cord, producing paraplegia. There have been reports also of families with olivo-ponto-cerebellar atrophy (OPCA), with a disturbance of eye movements (41). Interestingly, one such case was shown at the Royal Society of Medicine by Ebeling and Carmichael in 1958 (32); however, this form of cerebellar ataxia is distinctly rare. In a 25-year period at the KEM Hospital, Bombay, we have seen only 11 such cases.

Multiple sclerosis (MS) is known to be rare in the tropics and subtropics, but cases are seen from time to time. A preliminary survey brought out 53 such cases from all over India (29). They were included on the basis of clinical criteria, with evidence of dissemination in time and space. Ocular disturbances, limb weakness, and sphincter disturbances were the most frequent clinical symptoms. Pyramidal, posterior column, and cerebellar signs with

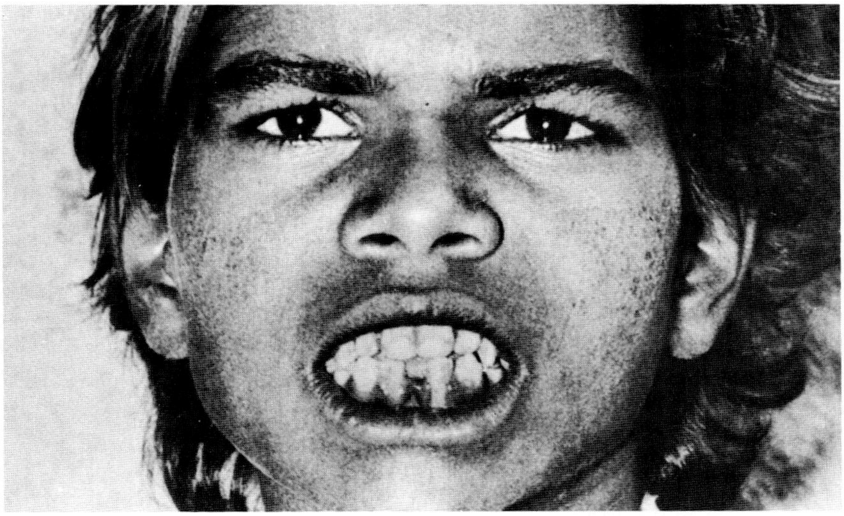

FIG. 8. Dental fluorosis. (Courtesy of Prof. D. Raja Reddy, Gandhi Medical College, Hyderabad.)

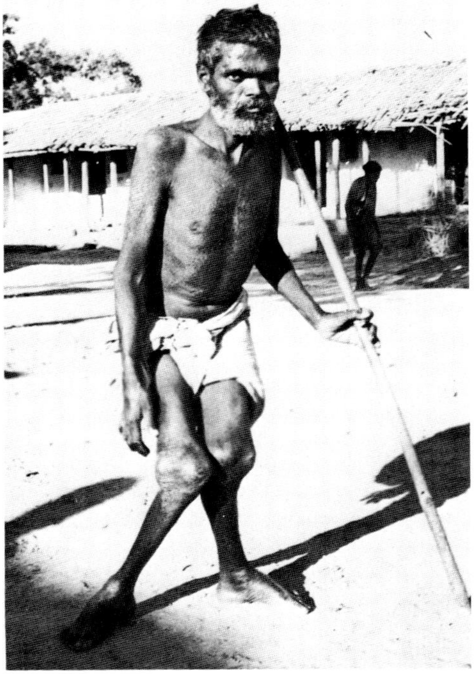

FIG. 9. Fluorotic spastic paraplegia with arthropathy. (Courtesy of Prof. D. Raja Reddy, Gandhi Medical College, Hyderabad.)

evidence of optic atrophy were usual on clinical examination. One or more remissions had occurred in 83% of these cases. The classical generalized form (paraplegia with intention tremor, nystagmus, and retrobulbar neuritis) was found in 52.77% of cases. Neuromyelitis optica was seen much less frequently in this series.

Since then, other reports have arisen. Mathew et al. (35) described 17 probable cases of MS using the criteria of Schumaker et al. (37) to identify them, and they had no cases of neuromyelitis opticas. The purely spinal type of MS was the most common. More recently, Singhal and Wadia (1975) have described 30 cases (39), two of which were proven at autopsy (31), and an additional nine cases were neuromyelitis opticas. They found a combination of optic nerve, brain stem, spinal, and/or cerebellar signs in 63% of their cases.

HLA typing has produced conflicting results. In one series (33), HLA B-12 was found to be the most common variety, whereas in our series, HLA B-3 and B-7 were frequently present. Probably the number of cases is yet too small to make any decisive comments.

Tropical spastic paraplegia, or South Indian paraplegia, is one of the many in the group of paraplegias of unknown origin. Clinically, the paraparesis starts insidiously over weeks or months. The weakness is asymmetrical and often accompanied by paraesthesiae. Objective sensory loss, when present, is confined to a loss of position or vibration sense. Bladder symptoms are present early in the disease. The course is very slowly progressive (34). Investigations, including serum B_{12}, plasma thiocyanate, and VDRL are essentially unhelpful. The protein in the CSF may be up to 60 or 190 mg%. Autopsy has been performed in two cases. In one, there was a primary demyelination of the posterior and lateral columns. In the other there was a diffuse meningomyelitis, with changes in the spinal blood vessels and secondary long tract degeneration.

CEREBROVASCULAR DISEASE

The total incidence of strokes due to cerebrovascular disease is similar in India to other parts of the world. In a series of 67,000 admissions to two teaching hospitals in Bombay, during 1959 –1960, there were 926 cases of stroke, giving an incidence of 1.4% (43). What is different is:

1. The large number of strokes in patients under 40 years of age ("young stroke").
2. The higher incidence of cerebral embolism.
3. Idiopathic occlusive disease of the aorta and its main branches.

Young Strokes

In one series of 850 strokes, 254 (about 30%) occurred in the under-40 age group (42). This is markedly different from the figures of the West. In Sweden, for instance, only 2% of strokes occurred in this age group. Why do so many strokes occur in the young in India? Is it due to premature aging? It is true that there is a high mortality in the young. In fact, 40% of the total mortality is in those under 15 years, but most of this is due to malnutrition and infection, not premature aging, so this cannot be the cause of "young strokes."

Abraham and Daniel (42) found that the chief causes in 127 young strokes of both sexes were cerebral thromboses (44.9%), cerebral embolism (13.4%), and internal carotid thrombosis (12.6%). In the 57 cases of cerebral thrombosis, the angiogram was abnormal in 19 out of 43 cases studied, the most common lesion being occlusion of the middle cerebral artery (42%). Hypertension, diabetes, high blood lipids, and syphilis were present in less than 20% of these cases. ECG abnormalities were present in only 24.5%. This and other studies indicate that cerebral thrombosis is an important cause of strokes in the young, but the etiology of this thrombosis is difficult to determine.

Cerebral Embolism

This is more frequent at all ages in India than in the West. In one series of 127 cases of stroke, no less than 20.5% were embolic (44). Figures from the West show an incidence of 15% or less (47). Moreover, many of the cases reported in India have had spontaneous clot lysis (44), something not seen in cerebral thrombosis. In Abraham and Daniel's series (42), embolism occurred most often in the third and fourth decades, the sexes being about equal. The embolus came from the heart in 87% of their cases.

Idiopathic Occlusive Disease of the Large Arteries

A disease known by many different names, such as "pulseless disease," "aortic arch syndrome," "young female arteritis," etc., Takayasu (1908) originally described this condition, observing obliterative changes in the retinal arteries (49). He made no mention of the absent pulses. Ross and McKusick (46), in a review of cases that had appeared in the world literature up to 1953 found many causes: trauma, mediastinal tumor, syphilis, etc. Sen et al. (48) described cases of stenosis of the middle aorta and its branches. For some time, they thought it was an allergic reaction to local tuberculous infection.

Since then, other reports of occlusive disease of the large arteries have appeared. Those affected are usually between 35 and 55 years of age. The aorta and the mouths of the vessels that emerge from it, especially the left subclavian, may be affected.

The pathology essentially consists of a massive proliferation of fibrous connective tissue, with fragmentation/disintegration of the internal elastic lamina. The raised intima blocks the artery, and a thrombus may occur in it and later become organized. There is no evidence of frank inflammation or atheroma (44,45).

In conclusion, though cerebrovascular disease may be broadly the same in India as anywhere else, there are certain features that make it different and interesting.

REFERENCES

Nutritional Disorders

1. Bharucha, E. P., Pimparkar, B. D., and Mondkar, V. P. (1972): Neurological mechanisms in obscure neuropathies and myelopathies. In: *Advances in Medicine*, edited by R. Viswanathan, Association of Phyns. of India, Bombay.
2. Champakam, S., Srikanthia, S. G., and Gopalan, C. (1968): Kwashiorkor and mental development, *Am. J. Clin. Nutr.*, 21:844.
3. Dastur, D. K., Quadros, E. V., Wadia, N. H., Desai, M. M., and Bharucha, E. P. (1972): Effect of vegetarianism and smoking on serum vitamin B_{12}, thiocyanate and folates in normal subjects, *Br. Med. J.*, 3:260.
4. Dastur, D. K., Wadia, N. H., Bharucha, E. P., Desai, M. M., Santha Devi, M., Quadros, E. V., Gagrat, B. M., Razzak, Z. A., Awari, F. C. R., and Irani, P. F. (1972): *Interim Report Studies on Nutritional Disorders of the Nervous System*, Tata Press, Bombay.
5. Davison, A. N. (1972): *Malnutrition and the Developing Brain*. Elsevier Excepta Medica, North Holland, Amsterdam.
6. Frisch, R. E. (1970): Present status of the supposition that malnutrition causes permanent mental retardation. *Am. J. Clin. Nutr.*, 23:189.
7. Gopalan, C. (1968): Leucine and pellagra. *Nutr. Rev.*, 26:323.
8. Gopalan, C. (1969): Possible role for dietary leucine in the pathogenesis of pellagra. *Lancet*, 1:197.
9. Gopalan, C. (1970): Some recent studies in the Nutritional Research Laboratories, Hyderabad. *Am. J. Clin. Nutr.*, 23:35.
10. Jeejeebhoy, K. N., Wadia, N. H., and Desai, H. G. (1967): Role of vitamin B_{12} deficiency in tropical nutritional neuromyelopathy. *J. Neurol. Neurosurg. Psychiat.*, 30:7.
11. Mehta, S., Teja, J. S., Wig, N. N., Thakurai, S., and Pasricha, S. (1975): PCM, a follow-up study. *Ind. J. Med. Res.*, 64:576.

12. Roy, S., Singh, N., Deo, M. G., and Ramalingaswamy, V. (1972): Ultrastructure of skeletal muscle and peripheral nerve in experimental protein deficiency and its correlation with nerve conduction studies. *J. Neurol. Sci.*, 17:399.
13. Sachdev, K. K., Taori, G. M., and Pereira, S. M. (1971): Neuromuscular status in PCM, *Neurol. Ind.*, 8:21.
14. Srikanthia, S. G., Veeraraghava Reddy, M., and Krishnaswamy, K. (1968): EEG patterns in pellagra, *EEG Clin. Neurophysiol.*, 25:386.

Infections of the Nervous System

15. Bharucha, E. P., Mondkar, V. P., and Variya, P. (1972): CSF and blood sugar curves in normals and TBM. In: *Proc. III Asian and Oceanic Congress of Neurology*, Bombay.
16. Bharucha, E. P., Mondkar, V. P., and Kulkarni, S. A. (1974): Postconjunctival myeloradiculopathy, *Neurol. Ind.*, 22:79.
17. Bharucha, P. E., Bharucha, E. P., and Da Costa, H. (1980): Ammonium bromide test in TBM, *Ind. Pediat.* 17:65.
18. Carey, D. E., Myers, R. M., Ruben, R., and Webb, J. K. (1969): Jap B encephalitis in S. India. *J. Ind. Med. Assn.*, 52:10.
19. Dalal, P. M., Rao, K. S., Khandeparkar, N. M., and Deshpande, C. K. (1973): Some observations on involvement of cerebral blood vessels in TBM in adults, In: *Tb of CNS Monograph*, National Academy of Medical Sciences, New Delhi.
20. Dastur, H. M., and Desai, A. D. (1965): A comparative study of brain tuberculoma and glioma. *Brain*, 88:375.
21. Deshpande, D. H. (1980): Japanese encephalitis, *Ind. J. Med. Res., (in press).*
22. Gourie-Devi, M., Padmini, R., and Satish, P. (1980): Hyaluronidase in spinal arachnoiditis complicating TBM. *Ind. J. Med. Res.*, 71:581.
23. ICMR Report (1972): Haffkine Institute, Bombay.
24. Kono, R., Uchida, N., Sasagawa, A., Akao, Y., Kodama, H., Mukoyama, J., and Fugiwara, R. (1973): Neurovirulence of acute haemorrhagic conjunctivitis virus in monkeys, *Lancet*, 1:61.
25. Mitchison, D. A., Wallace, J. B., Bhatia, A. L., Selkon, J. B., Subbiah, D. A., and Lancaster, M. C. (1960): A comparison of the virulence of Tb bacilli in S. Indian and British guinea pigs. *Tubercle*, 14:1.
26. Reddy, Bhaskaram, C. E., and Raghuramulu, N. (1977): Immunology response in malnourished children. *Ind. Pediat.*, 14:255.

Intoxications

27. Cohn, D. E., Streifler, M., Zamir, R., Kott, E., and Rinot, Y. (1978): HLA antigens in neurolathyrism. *Neurol. Ind.* 26:55.
28. Rao, S. L. N., Sharma, P. S., Mani, K. S., Raghunatha Rao, T. R., and Sriramachari, S. (1967): Neurolathyrism in monkeys. *Nature*, 214:610.
29. Bharucha, E. P., and Umarji, R. M. (1961): DS in India, *Int. J. Neurol.* (Montevideo), 2:182.
30. Bharucha, E. P., and Dastur, H. M. (1964): Craniovertebral anomalies, a report of 40 cases. *Brain*, 87:469.
31. Dastur, D. K., and Singhal, B. S. (1973): Two unusual neuropathologically proven cases of MS. *J. Neurol. Sci.*, 20:397.
32. Ebeling, P., and Carmichael, E. (1958): Hereditary ataxia with disordered eye movements. *Proc. Roy. Soc. Med.*, 51:16.
33. Krishnamurthy, P. R. (1980): personal communication.
34. Mani, K. S., Mani, A. J., and Montgomery, P. D. (1969): A spastic paraplegic syndrome in S. India. *J. Neurol. Sci.*, 9:179.
35. Mathew, N. T., Mathai, K. V., Abraham, J., and Taori, G. M. (1971): Incidence and pattern of demyelinating disease in India. *J. Neurol. Sci.*, 12:182.
36. Rao, S. R., Murty, K. J. R., Murty, S. V. S. D., and Reddy, S. S. (1975): Treatment of fluorosis. *Fluoride*, 8:12.
37. Schumaker, G. A. G., Beebe, G., Kibler, R. F., Kurland, L. T., Kurtzke, J. F., McDowell, F., Nagler, B., Sibley, W. A., Tourtellotte, W. W., and Willman, T. L. (1965): Problems of experimental therapy in MS. *Ann. N. Y. Acad. Sci.*, 122:552.
38. Singh, N. and Venkataraman, S. (1978): Noncompressive myelopathy. In: *Progress in Clinical Medicine in India*, edited by M. M. S. Ahuja. Atnold Heinemann, New Delhi.
39. Singhal, B. S., and Wadia, N. H. (1975): Profile of MS in Bombay region. *J. Neurol. Sci.*, 26:259.
40. Sundaram, Meenakshi, E., Jagannathan, K., and Ramamurthi, B. (1970): Clinical pattern of MND in younger age group. *Neurol. Ind.*, 8:104.
41. Wadia, N. H., and Swami, R. K. (1971): A new form of spinocerebellar degeneration with slow eye movements. *Brain*, 94:359.

Cerebrovascular Disease

42. Abraham, J., and Daniel, V. (1972): *Aspects of CVD in India*, Madras Diocesan Press, Madras.
43. Bharucha, E. P., and Umarji, R. M. (1962): CVD in India. *Neurol. Ind.*, 10:137.
44. Dalal, P. M., Shah, P. M., Aiyar, R. R., and Tikani, B. J. (1968): CVD in west central India. *Br. Med. J.*, 3:769.
45. Dalal, P. M. (1972): In: *Aortic Arch Syndrome in Tropical Neurology*, edited by J. B. Spillane, Oxford University Press, London.
46. Ross, R. S., and McKusick, V. A. (1953): Aortic arch syndrome. *Arch. Intern. Med.*, 92:701.
47. Ross Russell, R. W. (1976): *Cerebral Arterial Disease*. Churchill Livingstone, London.
48. Sen, P. K., Kinare, S. G., Kulkarni, T. P., and Parulkar, G. B. (1962): Stenosing aortitis of unknown aetiology. *Surgery*, 51:317.
49. Takayasu, M. (1908): A case with peculiar changes in the central vessels of the retina. *Acta Soc. Ophthal. Japan*, 12:554.

Historical Aspects of the Neurosciences,
edited by F. Clifford Rose and W.F. Bynum.
Raven Press, New York ©

The History of Neurology in Japan, with Special Reference to Its Postwar Period

Motoo Aki

Department of Neurology, Toranomon Hospital, 2-2-2 Toranomon, Minato-ku, Tokyo, Japan

"Will another SMON or Minamata Disease occur next year?"

The history of modern medicine in Japan began with the publication of *Kaitai Shinsho (New Book of Anatomy)* in 1774. About 200 years ago, on March 4, 1771 (Tokugawa Era), Ryôtaku Maeno (1723–1803), with his colleagues Gempaku Sugita (1733–1817) and Junan Nakagawa (1739–1786), observed the body of an executed Japanese female being dissected by an *eta* (an outcast) at Kozukaharara, an execution ground near Edo (old Tokyo). Maeno took out a book from his bosom, which he had bought in Nagasaki previously. Surprisingly, it was the same book of the same edition as the one Sugita had bought in Edo quite recently. The name of this book was *Ontleedkundige Tafelen* (Amsterdam 1734), which was the Dutch translation of the original German text, *Anatomische Tabellen von Johann Adam Kulmus* (the third edition, Amsterdam 1732).

They compared their findings, in particular, of the inner organs of the dissected human body, with the anatomic plates of this book, and they were convinced that the position and nature of these organs corresponded exactly with the description in this foreign medical text, and that the accounts in the older Chinese and Japanese books used to that day were totally incorrect. This experience made such a deep impression on them that they made a firm resolution at once to begin translating this anatomic work into the Japanese language. Actually, the next day, they began what was to have been the most wild undertaking, unprecedented in the history of Japan. Even Maeno (a brilliant scholar of this period) was said to have had only about a vocabulary of 700 Dutch words in all, and there were no grammar books nor dictionaries available. It took them four years of incredibly hard work, which Toynbee compared with the deciphering of cuneiform, reminding us of the patient ingenuity that 19th-century Western scholars were to employ. The book was at last published with the title of *Kaitai Shinsho* in 1774 and proved to be epoch making and fundamental not only in the field of medicine, but also in all branches of western science and technology in Japan. [Later Sugita wrote the most inspiring story of those days in a small book entitled *Rangaku Kotohajime*, which is translated as "Beginning of the Dutch Studies" (1).] The systematic and concrete knowledge of the nervous system was also introduced to Japan for the first time through this book.

One of the difficulties they had to meet with in translation was that they had to create many Japanese medical terms equivalent to those of the Dutch. "Shinkei" for "nerve" ("Zenuw" in Dutch) is one of these technical terms in Japanese, which has been utilized

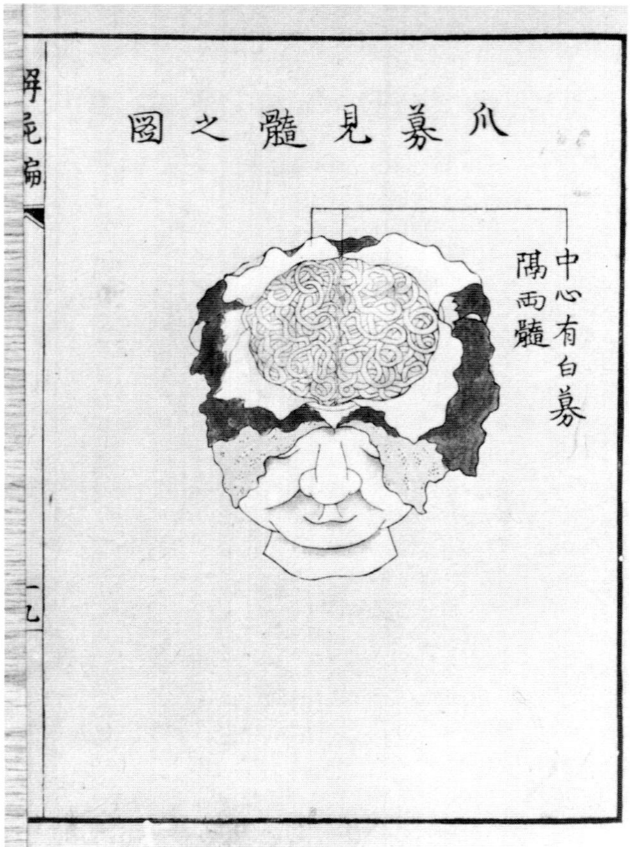

FIG. 1. A drawing of the brain, taken from *Kaishihen*, published in 1770.

even in Chinese literature since then. Another risk facing them was that publishing such a translation, with the result of introducing foreign thoughts, would infringe the laws stipulating seclusion under the Tokugawa regime. It was one year preceding the publication of *Kaitai Shinsho* that they thought it necessary to publish a preliminary document entitled *Kaitai Yakuzu (Abridged Drawings of Anatomy)*, which was their secret plan to sound out the government. Fortunately, they were not censured in the early years of their Dutch studies, but the Tokugawa regime, in its last years of power, banned all Dutch studies outside the field of medicine. Among the close successors of these students, not a few excellent Japanese devotees to Western secular science met their tragic ends before the dawn of modern Japan. For example, Choei Takano (1804–1850), who publicly urged the authorities to open Japan to foreign countries, was forced to flee from Edo and, harried by persecution, committed suicide. Today we are able to see in him highmindedness, intelligence, and the strong will to protest, which we still hold as our spiritual heritage. At any rate, since the *Kaitai Shinsho* was published in 1774, the disinterested intellectual curiosity concerning the achievements of the Western medicine intensified.

With regard to neurology, for example, Genzui Udagawa (1755–1797) translated the *Compendium medicinae* of Johannes de Gorter into Japanese (1792), and Kôan Ogata (1816–

1863) composed the *Byôri Tsuron*, the first work of general pathology (1847), through which the concept of apoplexy was distinctly introduced in Japan.

A rapid growth of medical knowledge was vividly shown in the apparent changes in the anatomical drawings of the brain. Figure 1 is taken from the *Kaishihen* (A Book on the Dissection of a Body) by Shinnin Kawaguchi (1736–1812), the second book on anatomy published in 1770, four years before *Kaitai Shinsho*. The brain was explained here as being very similar to chicken intestines. Figure 2 is taken from *Seyakuin Kaidantai Zôzu (The Anatomical Drawing of the Male)*. This work, published in 1798, 24 years after the publication of *Kaitai Shinsho*, reflects its most strong influence among many works of this period. On this occasion, Kanzen Mikumo (Seyakuin), supervised while Genshun Koishi dissected (both being physicians), and while Ranshû Yoshimura (painter) did the drawings. Moreover, Sôkichi Hashimoto, a scholar of Dutch learning, played a role in this work by labeling each organ in Japanese and partly in Dutch terms. This fact suggests strongly that they already had an excellent groundwork for the study of Western science, mainly by their Confucian tradition through the long period of the Tokugawa Era.

After *Katai Shinsho*, the clinical aspects of neurology were not sufficiently clarified. It would be safer to say that the practical side of neurology was introduced concretely by

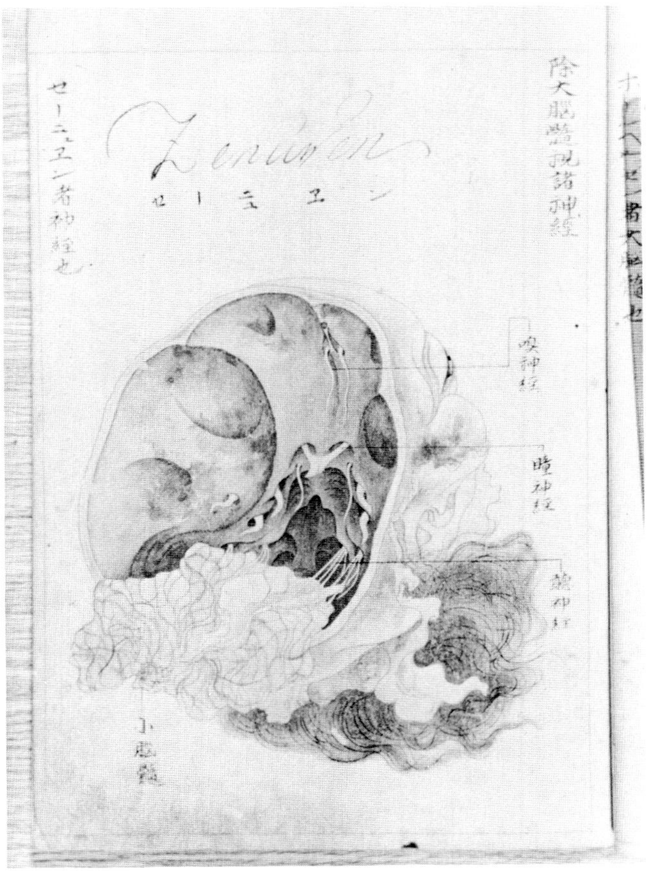

FIG. 2. A drawing of the cerebellum *in situ*, taken from *Seyakuin Kaidantai Zôzu*, published in 1798.

German physicians invited to the Tokyo Imperial University at the beginning of the Meiji Era, especially Baelz (1849–1913), who made a great contribution to the teaching of neurology as a section of internal medicine. In 1900, he published a textbook of internal medicine written in German (2), and it should be remembered that not a few of his students who studied abroad in the early years of the Meiji Era were bright enough to fully understand their foreign teachers.

Among them was S. Kitasato (1852–1931), who went to Berlin to work in Koch's Institute. He was the first to grow the tetanus bacillus and, in 1890, discovered with Behring the tetanus antitoxin. K. Miura (1864–1950) studied neurology under H. Oppenheim (1858–1919) in Berlin and W. H. Erb (1840–1921) in Heidelberg and later became a devoted student of J. M. Charcot (1825–1893) in Paris. During this time, he wrote several authoritative case reports of nervous diseases in German and French. S. Katsunuma (1886–1963), Professor of Internal Medicine at the Nagoya University, was one of his students, who later strongly supported Okinaka's effort to establish a new society of neurology.

Already an army doctor in Japan, Ōgai Mori (1862–1922) went first to Leipzig in 1884, then studied hygiene chiefly under Max von Pettenkofer (1818–1901) in Munich; he became deeply interested in public health, and not simply military hygiene. His debates with E. Neumann (a geologist, teaching in Japan from 1875 to 1885) on Japanese culture appeared in the *Allgemeine Zeitung* in 1886–1887. As an army doctor and later as one of the major literary figures in Japan, he contributed basically not only to the modernization of Japan in the Meiji Era, but also to the welfare of his country.

In the 90 years following the Meiji Restoration, Japan distinguished herself as a military power in the world. Because of this, social welfare and medical facilities were treated less seriously, along with medical education. Neurology in Japan continued to be a part of internal medicine for about 80 years, till the end of the Second World War (1945).

THE POSTWAR PERIOD

Reflection and Advance

Establishment of the Society of Neurology

Although neurology in Japan had been a section of internal medicine, the Japanese Society of Internal Medicine was established in 1903, a year after the Japanese Society of Psychiatry and Neurology. When O. Gagel (3) wrote in 1949 that "Die innere Medizin als die Mutter der Neurologie entlässt natürlich ihr früher von ihr wohlgepflegtes Kind, das sich zwar in den letzten Jahrzehnten zu eigener Selbständigkeit entwickelt hat, nur ungern aus ihrer Obhut, aber auch die Psychiatrie, die sich ebenfalls um die Entwicklung der Neurologie grosse Verdienste erworben hat, macht entsprechende Ansprüche auf die Neurologie geltend," had he considered the same circumstances in Japan? The Japanese Society of Psychiatry and Neurology has been contributing for a long time to the development of psychiatry in Japan, but neurology was left behind largely due to the dominance of psychiatrists.

In 1947, a serious and enthusiastic proposal by S. Okinaka (b. 1902) and a few of his colleagues, calling for division of this society into two mutually independent sections, was defeated decisively by a large majority of its members. It was not until after a long and difficult process of about 10 years that a new Japanese Society of Neurology was at last established in 1960.

Multiple Sclerosis

About eight years before the establishment of this new society, an argument about the existence of multiple sclerosis in Japan took place at the 51st annual meeting of the Japanese Society of Psychiatry and Neurology. On this occasion in 1953, Okinaka et al. (4) reported six clinical cases diagnosed as multiple sclerosis and insisted that physicians had always to keep this disease in mind clinically, even though at that stage there was a lack of any reliable proof by autopsy. Discussions that followed were the most heated that I had ever experienced during my whole life. Until that time, the predominant idea was that multiple sclerosis did not exist or was exceptionally rare in Japan. The opponents (mainly psychiatrists and neuropathologists) censured severely the attitude of clinicians who would diagnose it only by clinical observations. Okinaka et al. did not intend to underrate or neglect the importance of autopsy, but their purpose was only to see the advancement of knowledge and understanding of this important disease in neurology. At this point, they could not be too cautious nor too self-regarding, and they thus emphasized the responsibility of physicians in diagnosing and treating the patients as far as possible while they were still alive. In fact, only by this way could they obtain the right to stand in front of the dissecting table with pathologists.

At that time in postwar Japan, there were no teachers who were able to teach neurology and lead research activities through their own experience. Gagel (5) also wrote in the same period of West Germany (1949): "Leider besitzen wir wenige deutsche Universitäten, wenigstens in einem der Vertreter der genannten beiden Discipline (Psychiatrie und Neurologie), einen Mann, der noch in der Lage ist, das umfassende Wissensgut der Neurologie aus eigener Erfahrung und Forscherarbeit dem künftigen Arzt zu übermitteln." Indeed, physicians aspiring to be neurologists could do little but learn from their own patients and, when permitted, through autopsy.

With regard to this point, Okinaka had been the most prominent teacher who persistently held fast to the principle of clinicopathological studies, which had been established brilliantly by the Paris school in the early years of the 19th century. In his last lecture to the students in 1963, when retiring from his university, he frankly confessed that the rate of clinical diagnosis verified as mistaken by autopsy was 14.2% of cases during his 16 years as a professor, and he taught them the importance of modesty and devotion to patients. Owing to his enduring efforts, the autopsy rate in his department rose in a steady curve from 50% in 1946 to 90% in 1963 (average 86.2%) (6). At any rate, the argument about the existence of multiple sclerosis became a turning point in the progress of neurology in Japan. The famous report by Uchimura et al. (7) about "Entmarkungs encephalomyelitiden infolge der Lyssaschutzimpfung" appeared also in this period.

This problem opened a broad spectrum of international communication with many excellent scholars in other countries, where multiple sclerosis was one of the most common of neurological diseases. On the other hand, this disease began to occupy an undeniably important position in Japan as well, even though there were not so many patients as in other countries. Okinaka et al. reported cases of this disease in Japan in English three times in all (8–10). And now, we remember very well the names of the famous experienced neurologists visiting Japan during this difficult period, who kindly helped many younger neurologists to study in the same field. For example, L. T. Kurland and C. M. Poser from the United States helped greatly in the study of multiple sclerosis in Japan and supported the establishment of the Japanese Society of Neurology and later the Asian and Oceanic Congress of Neurology.

D. McAlpine from Great Britain also studied multiple sclerosis with us and gave us the most valuable suggestion regarding the mercury etiology of Minamata disease (11).

During the early 1950s, it gradually became possible again for physicians to go abroad to study medicine, among whom I cannot leave out the name of N. Yoshikura, who studied clinical neurology under R. Garçin and André-Thomas in France and acquired the spirit of these great masters deeply. He introduced in Japan the proudly cherished tradition of France through his daily practice and founded the Japanese Society of Pediatric Neurology with his young colleagues ("seven samurai") in 1970. He is now also an Honorary Member of the French Society of Neurology. It is not too much to say that neurologists of the younger generation in Japan have been awakened by his long and steady endeavors in the great tradition of clinical neurology, not only in France, but also in Great Britain, including the National Hospital, Queen Square in London.

Challenge and Response

It was just at this time of the growth in neurology that two problems occurred unexpectedly, which were of the most perplexing and difficult nature: Minamata disease and subacute myelo-optico-neuropathy (SMON). Since each of these two diseases has already been widely reported in the world literature (12–14), I do not consider it necessary to go into great detail.

SMON

A remarkable neurological syndrome following gastrointestinal complaints began to appear epidemically in Japan in the mid-1950s. It is estimated that there are at least 10,000 cases in Japan, and the overwhelming evidence points to their close association with Quinoform (clioquinol) ingestion, so that it is considered to be one of the drug-induced, iatrogenic disorders.

A study that established the name of SMON in the neurological field in Japan was reported by Tsubaki et al. (15) at the symposium on "Nonspecific Encephalomyelitis" at the 61st annual meeting of the Japanese Society of Internal Medicine in 1964. The aim was only to test the possibility of abstracting one disease entity, if any, from the complex combinations of abdominal symptoms and neurological signs, some undoubtedly of multiple etiology. The authors prudently selected the most typical six fatal cases in one district and studied them clinicopathologically. Astonishingly, these six cases revealed the same pattern in their pathological findings, and they modestly concluded that it might be possible to abstract one group of not pathognomonic, but very specific, clinicopathological characters, and they thought it appropriate to call it SMON for the time being.

I think this study should be highly appreciated, especially in the correctness of its methodology. It made a strong impression on their colleagues and at the same time gave a definite path to follow through the many difficulties at that confused stage. Without this achievement, further studies and their final conclusion would have been much delayed.

The discovery of a Quinoform derivate in the "green fur" of the patient's tongues became an important turning point. Although the epidemiological surveys were considered till then to suggest an infectious (viral) etiology, Tsubaki gave a renewed insight into this disease using the same epidemiological approach. On August 6,1970, he was the first to report to the Health and Welfare Ministry that SMON was attributable to the use of Quinoform and advised the Ministry to prohibit the sale of this drug officially. Considering the social conditions then ruling Japan and the probable repercussions, it was a courageous act as a scholar, reminding us of his master's attitude, shown at the heated argument about the existence of multiple sclerosis in 1953.

Only a month later, in September 1970, the Central Pharmaceutical Affairs Council submitted a report to the Health and Welfare Minister suggesting that the sale and use of Quinoform preparations be discontinued as long as the cause-and-effect relationship between this drug and SMON could not be refuted. The Ministry immediately issued a notice banning the sale of the drug and decided to request consumers in the whole country to stop using it; about two years later, in March 1972, the Government recognized officially the cause-and-effect relationship.

But at the same time, it cannot be denied that it had a most grave impact against the human relationship between physicians and patients, who became confused and angry; physicians suffered and became silent with remorse. Mutual confidence was maintained in some cases, but was broken in others. It was a fact that, especially after the war, Quinoform had been given, often without restriction, to patients with diarrhea, pain, and other abdominal complaints in larger doses and for longer durations in Japan than in other countries.

Irrespective of legal immunity from responsibility in this case, it again reminded physicians in practically the whole of the country of their moral responsibility. Later, when a lawsuit was started against the drug companies and the government, a few physicians who were requested by patients to certify the dose and duration of the drug used hesitated to do so, considering the risk of becoming a defendant, but most were willing to respond to these requests. But why could the physicians not find the concrete relationship between this disease and the drug much earlier? One court held that the manufacturers of the drug were responsible for its ill effects, and it ordered them to pay a compensation of some 3.25 billion yen to 119 victims for negligence in not advising them in time of the dangers of taking the drug, and the legal proceedings are still not completed.

SMON is undoubtedly the gravest warning against the general trend of too much dependence upon drugs in Japan, and I would like also to note the well-known fact that in Japan the separation of dispensing from medical practice has not yet been strictly established. In any event, the truth is that, as Schweitzer (16) said, there are great secrets we can learn only when we have come to be guilty. "Schuldig geworden sein bedeutet ein teuer bezahltes tieferes Verstehen der Dinge besitzen." May this truth be proved within ourselves!

Minamata Disease

On May 1, 1956, about 25 years ago, H. Hosokawa, the director of the hospital of the Chisso Corporation, reported four cases of an unknown disease to Minamata Health Center, Minamata Bay, Kyûshû, Japan. This was the first official recognition of so-called Minamata disease. Since then, including congenital cases, 899 cases were recognized as Minamata disease by the Kumamoto and Kagoshima Prefectural Authorities up to the end of 1959, although 3,096 patients in these districts were appealing for official recognition. Compared with Niigata-Minamata disease, which occurred in Niigata Prefecture nine years later in 1965, they encountered many difficulties from the early stage, not only medically but also socially. In fact, epidemiological, clinical, and pathological studies during the first ten years suggested the existence of many hidden and late cases of this disease, but in truth, precise data had not yet been obtained.

During these ten years, how had the patients and their families, regional practitioners, and research members felt, thought, suffered, complained, and labored? I cannot exactly imagine this. "The earliest reports of Minamata did not arouse widespread interest, although a small group of Japanese scientists and medical men did attempt to publicize the cases, in the face of official apathy and opposition from industry" (17). I can only confess now to having a feeling of deep grief and regret over this most tragic event, not only in this country, but also in the world.

M. Harada (b. 1934), a neuropsychiatrist and one of the active members of the Kumamoto University Research Team on Minamata disease, contributed several papers on this issue and published a booklet entitled *Minamata Disease* in 1972 (18). In these publications, he has shown himself as a physician to be a paragon of conscience, growing from a young psychiatrist to an expert neurologist and devoting himself wholly to his patients. Most patients with Minamata disease were poor fishermen and their families. The Chisso Corporation was one of the largest chemical companies in contemporary Japan, and Minamata City was financially supported to a great extent by the activities of this corporation. Although severely affected, the patients and their families had been neglected, solitary, and helpless for a long time, and they had even become unable to believe in each other. Among them, how powerless had Harada felt! The patients did not always have faith even with him. What was the meaning of the neutrality in his profession? What was the aim of his professional life? At last he could not help judging himself guilty. His sincere grief as a physician as well as a human is quietly appealing to everyone, even today, reminding us of the grief of St. Paul: "Oh wretched man that I am" (Romans 7:24). During these years, the government authorities were apparently on the side of the Chisso Corporation, not on the side of the patients, in this democratic society of postwar Japan. The Kumamoto University Research Team gradually concerned themselves with heavy metals and organic mercury in the effluent from the Chisso Minamata Plant; the team was requested several times by govenment authorities, including Minamata City officials, not to be hasty in naming organic mercury as the culprit and to use the utmost prudence in drawing any conclusions.

On November 12, 1959, the Food Sanitation Investigation Council (Section of the Health and Welfare Ministry) held a subcommittee meeting on Minamata disease and submitted to the Health and Welfare Ministry a report formally confirming the organic mercury theory. It was just the next day that this subcomittee (mainly composed of the members of the Kumamoto University Research Team) was suddenly ordered to disband by the Health and Welfare Minister. This signaled the government authorities' outright objection to the report just when the research team's studies had come to such a critical stage. The President of the Kumamoto University and the Director of the Department of Medicine protested and decided to continue research even without government support; their final success in identifying its cause was achieved under these circumstances.

Minamata Mediation Committee members, including the mayor and the municipal members, urged the Mutual Aid Society for the Families of Minamata Disease Patients to accept their arbitration proposal, the so-called Solution Agreement, the provisions of which said "no new indemnification claims would be lodged even if it was proved henceforth Minamata disease was caused by Chisso's effluent." Although the indemnity was an unbelievably small sum of money, ranging from 10,000 to 30,000 yen (from 30 to 100 dollars) per person annually, members of the Mutual Aid Society signed it, but with tears, on December 30, 1959. On October 7, Hosokawa (the director of Chisso's hospital) had succeeded in producing Minamata disease in experiments with cats using the effluent from the Chisso's acetaldehyde plant. The lawsuits were begun in Niigata on June 12, 1967 and later in Kumamoto on June 14, 1969. Amid strong social protest, many physicians, including neurologists, remained indifferent at first, and Harada could not help asking himself: Is it only the Chisso Corporation that should be prosecuted in court?

Japan has already established the principle, as a result of a series of court decisions between 1971 and 1973, that a polluter should compensate individuals for damages or inconvenience suffered by them. Japan has also established a system of compensation administered by the government, under which a specific polluting industry pays, where it can be indentified. But identification! How long and difficult a process that can be!

In 1971, the Environment Agency was established, which is currently promoting a comprehensive long-range environmental protection program covering seven separate types of pollution; air, water, noise, traffic, vibration, odor, and ground and soil condition. But the general impression is that the Ministry of International Trade and Industry decides important policies and may pressure its partner (the Environment Ministry). Thus, "Despite all of these efforts by the Japanese, some important long-term aspects of environmental protection remain almost completely absent from the public discussion" (19).

At any rate, as far as the problems of pollution in Japan are concerned, the exposition of J. Ui (20) is still most relevant today. Restricted only to medical treatment of Minamata disease, "no form of treatment that can favorably influence the course of the disease is yet known" (21). Minamata disease, once it has occurred, is too serious to be cured completely, a fact to be remembered by everyone.

CONSIDERATIONS

The shock dealt to Japan by the termination of the long war of 1931–1945 was profoundly great, and the early postwar years were naturally a time of great political and social, as well as economic, confusion and turmoil. The initial vision of the Occupation Authorities for Japan's future was, without any doubt, a democratic, peaceful and basically agrarian society, but the cold war forced them to revise their idealistic position. They then began gradually to rely heavily on Japan's bureaucratic and industrial leadership, so that early reforms were revised, discarded, and ignored. The economic recovery, very slow at first, began to quicken pace in the early 1950s. "In the 1950s this leadership converted into a powerful 'establishment'." It is presently firmly established in key institutions such as the Economic Planning Agency, the Ministry of Finance, the Ministry of Trade and Industry, the Bank of Japan, and the Federation of Industrial Organizations (Keidanren), which send representatives from industry to work out long term planning with the government" (22). "One of the most important factors in Japan's rapid economic growth is the special relationship between government and business. In fact, this is one of the chief differences between Japanese and American business, though it affords less of a contrast with some Western countries, such as France or West Germany. The relationship in Japan between government and business is not that of mutually suspicious adversaries, as in the United States, but of close collaborators" (23). And by the end of the 1960s, Japan had achieved the so-called economic miracle, which has made her have the third largest economy in the world.

But "During this same late 1960s period, other disadvantages and deprivations associated with economic growth had begun to attract attention." Pollution problems began to merge with others—urban crowding, health and welfare deficiencies, inflation, housing, and others, the set of problems which by 1971 had acquired the label "welfare gap" (24). SMON and Minamata disease were two nuclei of misery and disasters in this period.

Of course, it might be said that the postwar progress of neurology in Japan has been remarkable, keeping pace with the rapid economic growth of the country. But viewed from another angle, it has been only one desperate response of physicians to the grave challenges of inevitable contradictions in a country too rapidly industrialized with such efficient bureaucracy. These two diseases typify the unexpectedly remarkable changes that have been occurring over the whole range of our modernized social life, since the emergence of the two dominant social forces of the age, which appeared at the end of the war 1945 in Japan. These are the economic force of industrialization and the political force of so-called democracy, "so-called" because it does not have the same implication in Japan as in the West.

Before the end of the war, "However important these personal privileges, especially for the formation of a highly pluralistic intellectual and cultural life for modern Japan, they should not be construed as the essential feature of the Meiji constitution. The document was not aimed at confirming a democratic ethic. The privileges just mentioned, in short, were not aimed at supporting the idea of human liberty and the right to protest, but the prerogative of all to participate in the creation of a strong society" (25).

"The reasons why 'democracy' became so fashionable after the war seems to be that the Japanese found it a useful term for demeaning the old 'feudal' or 'authoritarian' pattern of the Japanese social and political systems. 'Democracy' represents a negative reaction against the operation of a pre-war system, which gave authority to a higher sector in an organization. In the Japanese system, a higher position in a hierarchial organization could hold unlimited power or privilege against the lower, since there is no clear-cut delineation of assigned roles between higher and lower. It is in this sociological and psychological soil that the imported term 'democracy' has developed its specific Japanese connotation" (26).

Nakane analyzed the structure of Japanese society from the social-anthropological viewpoint and revealed the vertical structural principle in it. Although the complex structure of society might not always permit such a one-dimensional interpretation, her theory is an important contribution. And when I read, "Thus, there is a cruelly heavy handicap against the powerless and the socially inferior" under such a vertical structure, it reminds me of the Minamata disease patients.

In 1889, Ōgai Mori (1862–1922), cited above as an army doctor and administrator with a Confucian passion for order, said: "Hygiene is essential. If hygiene is disregarded, health cannot be maintained. When health is lost, the basis of all work crumbles. Once people realize this, why cannot they progress by themselves, grasp authority over hygiene, discard their sense of dependence on officials for their health, and so take the first step towards escaping from oppression by putting hygienic methods into practice on their own?" (27)

If we let him speak in today's context, Ōgai Mori would be likely to imply the problem of pollution in "hygiene" or "public health." He also said: "If the ruler wants truly to guard public health, he should treat the poor first and the rich last. Although the rich can avert a calamity, if any, by their own property, the poor can never do so. The ruler must keep this fact always in mind" (28).

"This striking defence of the concept of public health and the duties of those concerned in its administration is typical of Ōgai. He had been brought up with the Confucian concept of cultural responsibility, and all his life was to feel the drive to educate and fight stupidity. The traditional moral demands on the ruler with respect to the ruled were not far removed from the relationship between government and people that modern public health was based on. When most of the talk in Japan was of externals, Ōgai was concerned with essentials. Modernization had to be based on a rational appraisal rather than on an emotional reaction." (29).

There are still many problems that need different approaches, but in the field of one specialized discipline of medicine, neurology, we must understand its limitations as well as its efficiency. There is a comprehensive survey, cited above, of the multifarious studies and their achievements on Minamata disease until recently, written in English, and published in

1977 (30). This book is a brilliant achievement based on strict scientific methodology, but is wanting, e.g., in social, economic, and legal aspects, that is, in a panoramic (macroscopic) viewpoint.

"Specialization alone is not enough to give us the knowledge and understanding that we are seeking. The further that specialization is carried, the more of the meaning of the phenomena is left unplumbed in the unexplored gaps between the specialists' deep but narrowly constricted borings. This method leaves critical questions not only unanswered but unasked. And they will remain unasked if the microscopic approach is not supplemented by a panoramic one. Without a combination of the two, there can be no stereoscopic vision" (31).

Of course, with regard to specialization, neurology had to be separated from the internal medicine, but specialization is not the same thing as being all-sufficient. It may mean depersonalization, i.e., it effaces the personality not only of patients but also of physicians. Is medicine essentially only a section of natural science? Is not medicine truly a part of human affairs?

Ōgai was a military doctor. So, during his long efforts to achieve true modernization, "his insistence on the independence of learning and the inevitable clash with the deeply rooted system of seniority in Japan made him few friends in the army hierarchy" (32). He must have been very much aware of the limitations under such an army hierarchy. But he had the courage to place himself in direct and bitter confrontation with his superiors and kept his uncompromising attitude to criticize sharply the medical world at that time in Japan. It would not be a different case with Minamata disease today. Indeed, Harada might have said with him: "As I have promised in the past—though my honour be besmirched and my future activities blocked, my spirit is invincible! My spirit will never be crushed!" (33).

The aim for the present must be therefore to convey the panoramic view of these unexpected accidents exactly, and to educate people to think rationally for themselves, for only by doing so can the correct balance be maintained in the reciprocal relationship of ruler (government with its strong bureaucracy and economy) and ruled (people and patients). The same can be considered with regard to SMON. "Reactionary attitudes seem to be symbolic of the whole state of Japan today. If I was a reporter of an ordinary newspaper and debated matters of politics, I have no doubt that I would be complaining of reactionary attitudes in government circles" (34).

CONCLUSION

We are now living in a beautiful country but the most polluted in the world. We are now working diligently but without any sufficient natural resources. We are now enjoying peace but between great powers armed with numerous atomic bombs. Our society is said to be constructed by the traditional vertical principle under the name of democracy. In considering modernization, we must go back to the Tokugawa Era. Success and failure were like a rope twisted during these 200 years of modernization.

Now I have a dream so far as I am standing on the ground of self-consciousness as a human, not as a part of the machines that are driven mechanically by political and economic powers. This is also a duty that many patients suffering from pollution or iatrogenic disorders have given me. I must refer here to the question that is at the beginning of this chapter. It is not a problem of probability or computerization. "No! It shall not come. It shall never come. Here is our will." This is the answer.

ACKNOWLEDGMENTS

The author is deeply grateful to Professor H. Narabayashi for his encouragement of this study and also heartily grateful to Professor T. Ogawa (Department of Medical History, Juntendo University) and Professor Y. Toyokura (Department of Neurology, Tokyo University) for their constructive comments during the preparation of the manuscript.

REFERENCES

1. Sugita, G. (1815): *Rangaku Kotohajime*. English translation by R. Matsumoto and E. Kiyooka (1969): *Dawn of Western Science in Japan*. Hokuseido Press, Tokyo. German translation by K. Mori (1942): *Monumenta Nipponica*, Vol. 5, Nos. 1 and 2. Sophia University, Tokyo.
2. Baelz, E. (1900): *Lehrbuch der inneren Medizin*, 3 Bände, Tokyo.
3. Gagel, O. (1949): *Einführung in die Neurologie*, Seite III. Springer-Verlag, Berlin.
4. Okinaka, S., Toyokura, Y., Imamura, Y., Nakamura, H., Takemoto, T., Ishikawa, T., Miwa, S., and Fujii, J. (1953): *Psychiat. Neurol. Japn.*, 55:476 (in Japanese).
5. Gagel, O. (1949): *Einführung in die Neurologie*. Seite III. Springer-Verlag, Berlin.
6. Okinaka, S. (1965): *Physician and Patients*, p. 11. University of Tokyo Press, Tokyo. (in Japanese).
7. Uchimura, Y., Shiraki, M., and Haruhara, C. (1954): *Psychiat. Neurol. Japn.*, 56:503. (in Japanese).
8. Okinaka, S., Tsubaki, T., Kuroiwa, Y., Toyokura, Y., Imamura, Y., and Yoshikawa, M. (1958): *Neurology*, 8:756.
9. Okinaka, S., McAlpine, D., Miyagawa, K., Suwa, N., Kuroiwa, Y., Shiraki, H., Araki, S., and Kurland, L. T. (1960): *World Neurology*, 1:22.
10. Okinaka, S., Reese, H. H., Katsuki, S., Ueki, K., Kuroiwa, Y., Araki, S., Shiraki, H., and Kurland, L. T. (1966): *Acta Psychiat. Neurol. Scand.*, 42(Suppl. 19):68.
11. McAlpine, D., and Araki, S. (1958): *Lancet*, 629.
12. Griffin, J. P. (1979): In: *Iatrogenic Diseases*, edited by P. F. D'Arcy and J. P. Griffin, p. 314. Oxford University Press, Oxford.
13. Christopher, A. P., and Lewis, P. D. (1974): *The Neurology of Gastrointestinal Disease*, p. 179. W. B. Saunders, London.
14. Takeuchi, T. (1977): In: *Neurotoxicology*, edited by L. Roizin, H. Shiraki, and N. Grčević, p. 235. Raven Press, New York.
15. Tsubaki, T., Toyokura, Y., and Tsukagoshi, H. (1965): *Japn. J. Med.*, 4:181.
16. Schweitzer, A. (1932): In: *Gesammelte Werke*, Bd. 5, S. 494. Verlag C. H. Bech, München.
17. Bennett, J. W., and Levine, S. B. (1976): *Japanese Industrialization and Its Social Consequences*, edited by H. Patrick, p. 461. University of California Press, Berkeley, California.
18. Harada, M. (1972): *Minamata Disease*, Iwanami Shoten, Publishers, Tokyo (in Japanese).
19. Kahn, H., and Pepper, T. (1979): *The Japanese Challenge*, p. 72. Thomas Y. Crowell, New York.
20. Ui, J. (1974): In: *Science and Society in Modern Japan*, edited by S. Nakayama, D. L. Swain, and E. Yagi, p. 290. University of Tokyo Press, Tokyo.
21. Tatetsu, S., Harada, M., Inoue, T., Tsukayama, T., Minami, R., Hattori, E., and Kabashima, K. (1977): In: *Minamata Disease*, edited by T. Tsubaki and K. Irukayama, p. 266. Kodansha Ltd., Tokyo.
22. Najita, T. (1974): *Japan, the Intellectual Foundations of Modern Japanese Politics*, p. 4. University of Chicago Press, Chicago.
23. Reischauer, E. O. (1977): *The Japanese*, p. 191. Harvard University Press, Cambridge, Mass.
24. Bennett, J. W., and Levine, S. B. (1976): In: *Japanese Industrialization and Its Social Consequences*, edited by H. Patrick, p. 461. University of California Press, Berkeley, California.
25. Najita, T. (1974): *Japan, the Intellectual Foudations of Moder Japanese Politics*, p. 85. University of Chicago Press, Chicago.
26. Nakane, C. (1970): *Japanese Society*, p. 143. University of California Press, Berkeley, California.
27. Mori, Ōgai (1889): *Complete Works* (1971–1975), Vol. 29, p. 5. Iwanami Shoten, Tokyo. (English translation of this part by R. J. Bowering.)
28. Mori, Ōgai, (1889): *Complete Works* (1971–1975), Vol. 28, p. 137. Iwanami Shoten, Tokyo.
29. Bowering, R. J. (1979): *Mori Ōgai and the Modernization of Japanese Culture*, p. 26. Cambridge University Press, Cambridge.
30. T. Tsubaki and K. Irukayama, editors (1977): *Minamata Disease*, Kodansha Ltd., Tokyo.
31. Toynbee, A. (1961): *A Study of History*, Vol. 12, p. 633. Oxford University Press, London.
32. Bowering, R. J. (1979): *Mori Ōgai and the Modernization of Japanese Culture*, p. 30. Cambridge University Press, Cambridge.
33. Mori, Ōgai (1889): *Complete Works* (1971–1975), Vol. 29, p. 334. Iwanami Shoten, Tokyo. (English translation of this part by R. J. Bowering.)
34. Mori Ōgai (1894): *Complete Works* (1971–1975), Vol. 29, p. 572. Iwanami Shoten , Tokyo. (English translation of this part by R. J. Bowering.)

Historical Aspects of the Neurosciences,
edited by F. Clifford Rose and W. F. Bynum.
Raven Press, New York ©

Leber's Optic Atrophy

G. D. Perkin

Department of Neurology, Charing Cross Hospital, London W6, England

A discussion of Leber's optic atrophy affords an opportunity to examine some recently described phenomena of the disease, said to be missing from the early accounts, and at the same time to record a contribution by Macdonald Critchley regarding the neurological syndromes sometimes accompanying the visual failure.

Though he is now credited as having provided the first description of this unique optic nerve disturbance, Leber himself (1) (Fig. 1) was aware of the earlier paper by Von Graefe (2) recording the disease in three brothers. Leber extensively reviewed the literature regarding the different forms of hereditary visual failure and added his own cases, acquired from the study of four families (Figs. 2 and 3). Complete descriptions were provided for eight cases occurring in three families (Fig. 4).

He recognized that the condition predominantly affected central vision, involved both eyes, though not always simultaneously, and predominated in men. Rather than review all

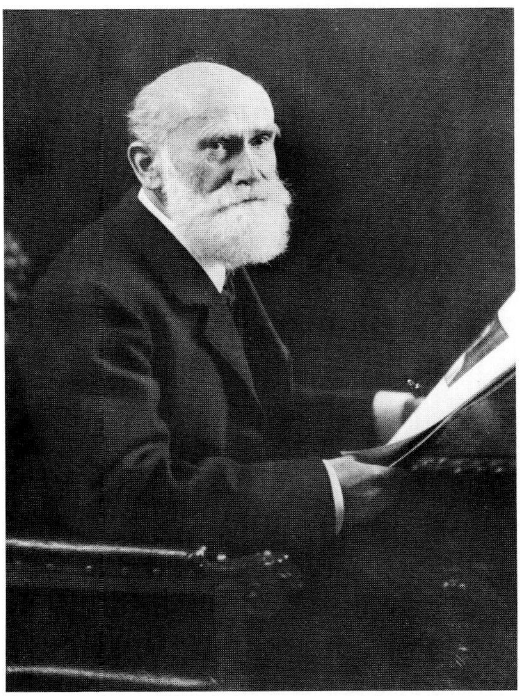

FIG. 1. Theodor Leber.

ALBRECHT VON GRÆFE'S

ARCHIV

FÜR

OPHTHALMOLOGIE.

HERAUSGEGEBEN

VON

PROF. F. ARLT IN WIEN PROF. F. C. DONDERS IN UTRECHT

UND

PROF. TH. LEBER IN GÖTTINGEN.

SIEBENZEHNTER JAHRGANG
ABTHEILUNG I.
ODER
SIEBENZEHNTER BAND
ABTHEILUNG I.

MIT HOLZSCHNITTEN UND TAFELN.

BERLIN, 1871.
VERLAG VON HERMANN PETERS.

Eine Uebersetzung in fremde Sprachen behalten sich die Verfasser vor.

FIG. 2. Frontispiece for the 1871 issue of *Archiv für Ophthalmologie.*

aspects of this condition, it seems pertinent to consider some recently described facets of this disorder, examining the claims that these had not been recognized in the early accounts.

UHTHOFF'S SYNDROME

"In letzter linie habe ich noch einer Erscheinung Erwähnung zu thun; die ich in vier Fällen beobachten konnte, wo körperliche Anstrengung mit Ermüdung eine ausgesprochene Verschlechterung des Sehens hervor brachte." (At last I have to mention a phenomenon

Ueber hereditäre und congenital-angelegte Sehnervenleiden.

Von

Th. Leber.

Während für die Retinitis pigmentosa und verwandte Affectionen die Erblichkeit und congenitale Disposition als ätiolog. Momente allgemein bekannt und gewürdigt sind,*) kennt man die auf denselben Grundlagen entstehenden Sehnervenleiden wegen ihrer Seltenheit viel weniger. Ausser einer weiter unten anzuführenden Mit-

*) Es sei gestattet, hier an die sehr interessante Beobachtung von F. Cunier zu erinnern von einer durch 5 Generationen erblichen Hemeralopie, die sehr genau genealogisch verfolgt werden konnte. (Hist. d'une Héméralopie hérédit. depuis deux siècles dans une famille, dans la commune de Vendemian près Montpellier. Gand. 1838; und Ann. d'Ocul. T. 1., p. 31.) Es handelte sich sicher um Nachtblindheit, obgleich von Himly, (Krankh. u. Missbild. II., S. 448) behauptet wird, es sei Tagblindheit gewesen, höchst wahrscheinlich also um erbliche Retinitis pigmentosa. Die Krankheit trat nicht bei allen Mitgliedern der Familie auf und ihre relative Häufigkeit nahm von Generation zu Generation ab. Es wurden nur Individuen befallen, deren Vater oder Mutter gleichfalls ergriffen waren; von der Mutter vererbte sich die Krankeit leichter. Ein anderes Beispiel erblicher Hemeralopie citirt Froriep: 2 Eltern wurden nachtblind und von ihren 7 Kindern waren es 4. (Frorieps n. Not. Bd. V., N. 3., S. 48.)

FIG. 3. Title page from Leber's 1871 paper.

which I could see in four cases, in which physical exercise together with tiring caused a marked worsening of vision.) Uhthoff's description (3) of exercise-induced visual blurring referred to patients with multiple sclerosis. In patients with that condition analyzed by McAlpine and Compston (4), a short-lived exacerbation of symptoms occurred with exercise in 33.6%, with emotional stimuli in 32.8%, and with heat in 13.6%. Such exacerbations are not unique to multiple sclerosis, having been described in patients with pituitary tumor, Friedreich's ataxia, posterior cerebral artery insufficiency and, most recently, with Leber's optic atrophy. Case 2 of Nikoskelainen et al. (5) had noticed slight blurring of vision in the left eye, especially during strenuous exercise, six months after the onset of visual symptoms. Case 3 of Lawton Smith et al. (6) experienced blurring of vision with exercise, hot baths or while drinking warm fluids, the symptom antedating visual failure. Neither of these authors indicated whether or not they had encountered similar descriptions in the literature. Taylor (7) found that one of his patients "saw best in a dull light, for example towards dusk." One of Norris' (8) cases claimed that his sight became fogged after he had been doing work sufficiently hard to cause him to perspire, the fogging gradually ceasing in about an hour's time, and another patient considered he could see better on cloudy days. Leber's second and third patients both described their vision improving in the twilight, and his sixth case "developed now also, particularly in the left eye, that fluctuation in visual acuity and

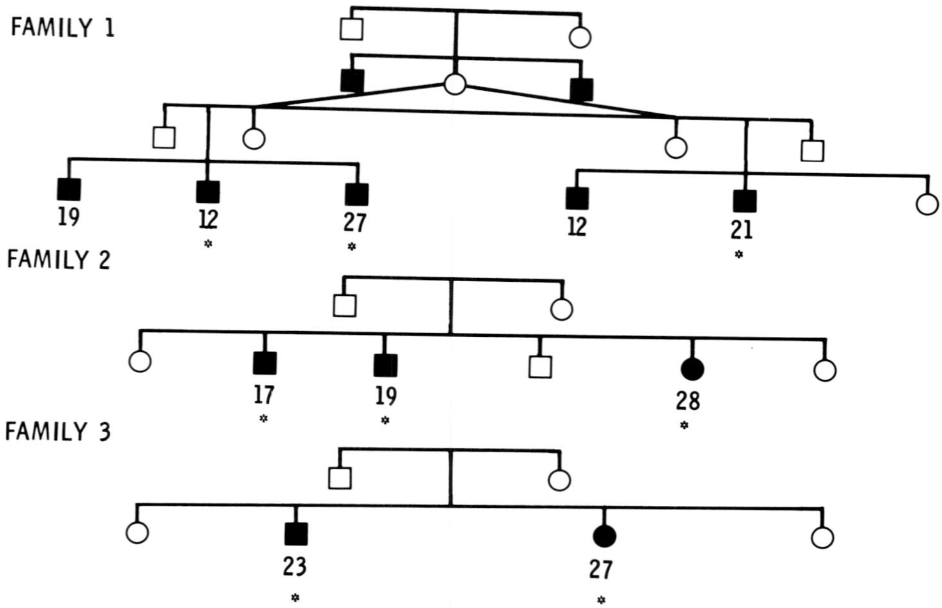

FIG. 4. The family trees of the three families studied in detail by Leber (1871). Circles represent females, squares males. Shaded symbols indicate affected members. The numbers refer to the age of onset of visual symptoms and the asterisk indicates patients either personally examined by Leber or in whom full clinical details were available. In Family 1, the disease was transmitted by an unaffected female to five of six children acquired from two marriages.

its deterioration following bodily movement and in states of emotional agitation which had been remarked earlier in the case of his sister, albeit to a lesser extent than in her case."

The phenomenon in multiple sclerosis may be explicable on the basis of the effect of heating on conduction in partially demyelinated nerve fibers (9). Optic nerve demyelination is a prominent feature of Leber's optic atrophy (10), where a similar explanation for the symptom may apply.

THE FUNDUS APPEARANCE

A unique appearance has been suggested for the optic fundus in the acute stages of the disease (6), combining opacity of the peripapillary nerve fiber layer, blurred disc margins, tortuous retinal vessels with dilatation of peripapillary and prepapillary networks together with an absence of vascular permeability on fluorescein angiography (Fig. 5). Only at a later stage does optic atrophy supervene (Fig. 6). Nikoskelainen et al. (5) concluded that original descriptions of the disorder had paid little attention to the early fundus changes. Lawton Smith et al. (6) credited Lauber (11) and Van Heuven (12) with the first descriptions. A passage from Bell's epic monograph (13) showed her awareness of the acute changes: "the main difficulty occurs in the early stages of the disease when a profound disturbance of function is already in operation and the appearance of the fundus may vary from that of complete normality to that indicative of an acute inflammatory reaction, with reddening of the nerve head, blurring of its margins, dilatation and tortuosity of the vessels and perhaps some small haemorrhages."

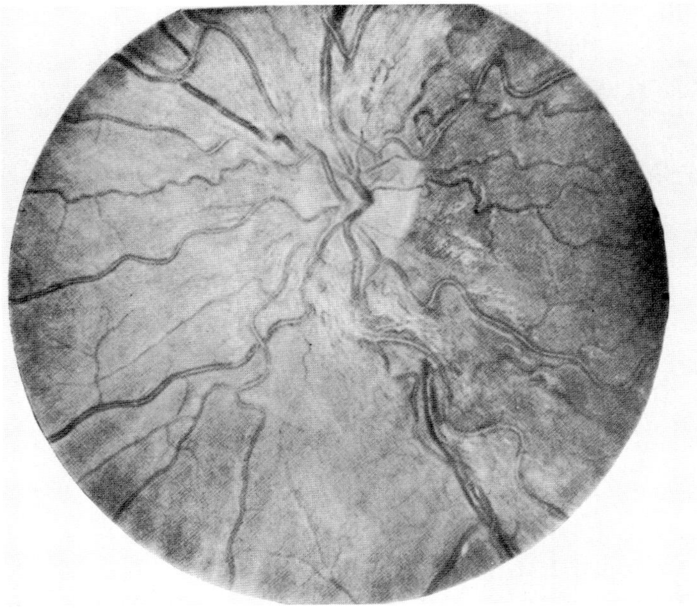

FIG. 5. Acute stage of Leber's optic atrophy.

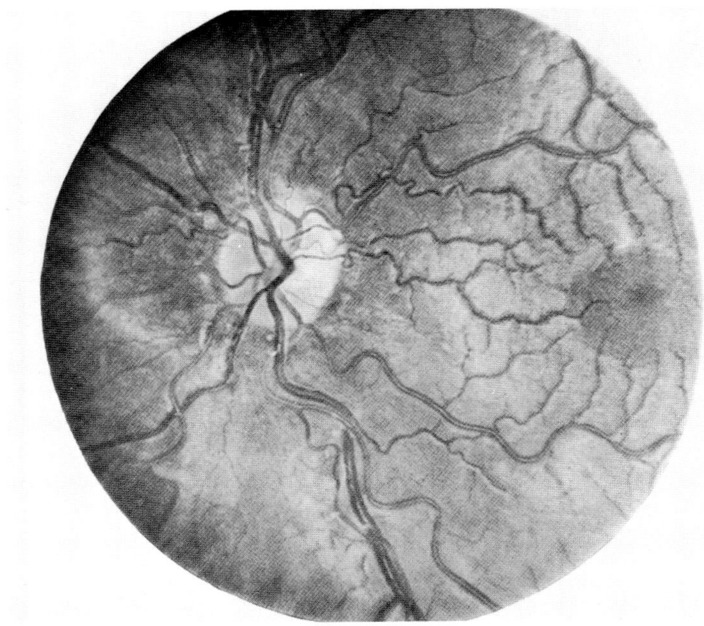

FIG. 6. Chronic stage of Leber's optic atrophy.

Curiously, Bell failed to comment on such observations by either Lauber or Van Heuven. In her resumé of Van Heuven's work (14), admittedly taken from a different paper, she simply referred to disc swelling, and her description of Lauber's finding mentioned narrowing of retinal vessels. Van Heuven's case (12) was complicated by the presence of secondary syphilis. He noted very small red spots, best regarded as very fine twisted capillaries, which he considered pathognomonic. Lauber (11) described a family with a woman of 30 and all four of her brothers affected by the disease. She presented soon after the onset of visual failure in the left eye and was found to have an indistinct optic disc with tortuous retinal veins. By the time of her admission to hospital, four weeks later, the right fundus, despite a lack of symptoms in that eye, was abnormal with indistinct margins of the optic disc, extremely tortuous vessels, and a presumed hemorrhage superotemporal to the disc. In the left fundus, a large number of extremely tortuous fine vessels were noted on the optic disc, particularly nasally. The retinal vessels were tortuous, a streaky cloudiness accompanied the upper nasal and temporal vessels, and small hemorrhages were noted inferotemporally. Surprisingly, Lauber placed little emphasis on these appearances, or that they might antedate visual symptoms. That this prodromal phase exists has been recently confirmed (5,6).

Nettleship's extensive review (15) of the disease failed to comment on the acute fundus changes, though in the same year, Batten (16) had described symmetrical retinal hemorrhages at the disc margins with "water-silk undulations of the macula." Habershon (17) concluded that, in the acute stages, there was usually some haziness of the disc margins with hyperemia. He found the vessels to be normal in size, or even enlarged, with the small retinal vessels sometimes visible. Frequently there were white lines in the course of the vessels with occasional spots and streaks of exudation accompanying or overlying them. The long sprays of retained nerve sheaths extending to variable distances out into the retina described by Norris (8) were probably the correlate of the opacity of the peripapillary nerve fiber layer. He and Batten (16) included families in whom the disease had been transmitted by males, but in other respects their cases were typical. Norris (8) divided the optic nerve appearance on fundoscopy into three stages: (a) the stage of cloudy and edematous swelling, (b) the stage of lymph reflexes, and (c) the stage of the gradual death of the nerve tissue. Higgens (18) was perhaps the first author in the English literature to appreciate the acute changes, though his description in a patient seen three weeks after the onset of symptoms in one eye, and within three days of involvement of the second eye, was limited to comments on extreme retinal hyperemia and slight blurring of the optic disc margins.

Leber's second case was seen at Von Graefe's clinic within four weeks of the onset of visual failure. A streaky appearance around the left disc was accompanied by slight dilatation of the retinal veins. Leber himself examined the patient three years later, finding white opaque streaks alongside branches of the central retinal vein. His fifth case had developed bilateral visual failure a week before being examined, preceded by pain on ocular movement, a symptom complex more reminiscent of optic neuritis. Leber observed a picture in both fundi which he described as that of a slight degree of neuroretinitis:

> . . . rather severe distension and tortuosity of the vessels, especially the veins, but also to a less extent of the arteries. Boundaries of the papillae and adjacent retina fairly severely clouded, somewhat whitish, but without apparent prominence; a few small ecchymoses on the right papilla.

The subsequent clinical course in this patient is of some interest. Two months later, in August 1870, her vision had recovered and, in the intervening period, she had noticed it to be better after resting at home than after recently going out. A relapse, in June of that year, was accompanied by similar fluctuations and by a sensation at times of a bright light observed whenever the eyes were moved. Leber suggested these were phosphenes, phenomena more often equated with optic neuritis (19,20), as Von Graefe, according to Leber, had previously observed. Recovery resulted in final visual acuities of J1 but with bilateral optic atrophy. By then, the fundal vessels appeared normal. Leber concluded:

> The ophthalmoscopic picture was only seldom quite normal; frequently there was a slight clouding of the edge of the papilla and hyperemia of the vessels, or even distinct slight neuroretinitis; frequently too there were fine white streaks along the vessels, or characteristic spots of exudate on the papilla. On one occasion there was noticed also conspicuous hyperemia of the smaller vessels of the retina, especially in the region of the macula luteum. It is to be noted that in this stage the arteries were not narrowed as is frequently the case with neuritis opt. [sic] but were found to be normal, or even enlarged.

Leber carefully separated the appearance in the acute stages from that seen later, when "there normally occurs a pronounced white or bluish white discolouration of the papilla, with or without the emergence of the lamina cribrosa, and with moderate narrowing of the vessels of the retina, particularly the arteries."

ASSOCIATED NEUROLOGICAL FEATURES

"With many of our patients there are yet other phenomena on the part of the nervous system, admittedly for the most part slight in degree, but of such a kind that the individual is to be classified as neuropathic in Griesinger's sense." Leber's "neuropathic" features included headache, migraine, with or without nausea and vomiting, and dizziness with ensuing faintness and epilepsy. Batten (16) described a case with cramps in the feet, numbness of the fingers, and tremors of the lips and chin. Taylor and Holmes (21) encountered one patient with slight lack of bladder control and weakness of the legs. Bell (13) included cases with hemiplegia and one, from the Japanese literature, with impaired memory, tremors of the lips, eyelids, tongue, and fingers, rigidity of the limbs and incoordination.

Ferguson and Critchley (22) (Fig. 7) described four siblings with the disease, three female and one male. One case had mental impairment with epilepsy, but the most conspicuous changes were encountered in the fourth member of the family. This girl developed bilateral visual failure at the age of 12, followed four years later by aching and trembling of the legs with an ataxic gait. A year afterward, peripheral pigmentary changes in the fundus were accompanied by central field defects with marked peripheral constriction (Fig. 8). The neurological findings included coarse horizontal nystagmus, mild limb cerebellar signs, a broad-based ataxic gait, brisk reflexes, and bilateral extensor plantar responses. Proprioception and vibration sense were impaired in the lower limbs. CSF examination showed 15 white cells, positive tests for globulin, and a midzone Lange curve. The authors accepted that the possibility of multiple sclerosis could not be dismissed, but they preferred to consider the case as representing a bridge between pure Leber's optic atrophy and the heredofamilial ataxias. Lees et al. (23), in discussing a similar family, suggested that this case was one of Leber's optic atrophy and associated multiple sclerosis. Wilson (10) has described a patient with optic atrophy, wasted upper limbs, generalized fasciculation, and spastic legs. The CSF contained 10 lymphocytes and showed a paretic Lange curve.

The diagnostic problems in such cases are considerable, some authors remaining reluctant to apply a label of Leber's optic atrophy. A CSF pleocytosis is not necessarily surprising,

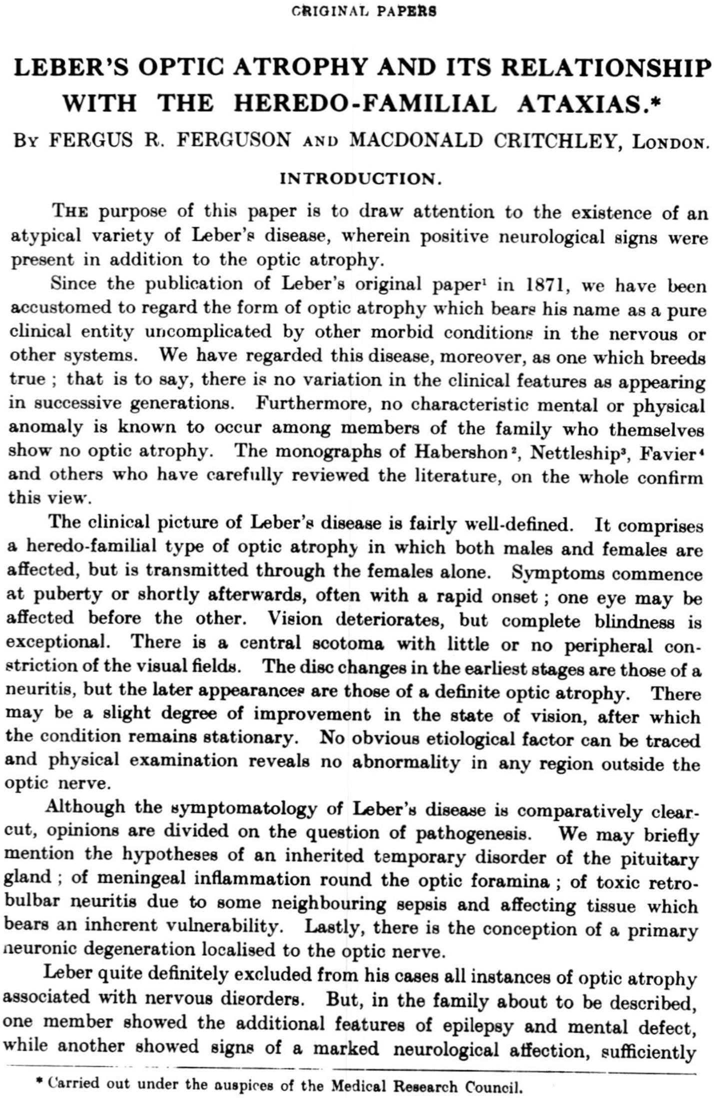

ORIGINAL PAPERS

LEBER'S OPTIC ATROPHY AND ITS RELATIONSHIP WITH THE HEREDO-FAMILIAL ATAXIAS.*

By FERGUS R. FERGUSON and MACDONALD CRITCHLEY, London.

INTRODUCTION.

The purpose of this paper is to draw attention to the existence of an atypical variety of Leber's disease, wherein positive neurological signs were present in addition to the optic atrophy.

Since the publication of Leber's original paper[1] in 1871, we have been accustomed to regard the form of optic atrophy which bears his name as a pure clinical entity uncomplicated by other morbid conditions in the nervous or other systems. We have regarded this disease, moreover, as one which breeds true ; that is to say, there is no variation in the clinical features as appearing in successive generations. Furthermore, no characteristic mental or physical anomaly is known to occur among members of the family who themselves show no optic atrophy. The monographs of Habershon[2], Nettleship[3], Favier[4] and others who have carefully reviewed the literature, on the whole confirm this view.

The clinical picture of Leber's disease is fairly well-defined. It comprises a heredo-familial type of optic atrophy in which both males and females are affected, but is transmitted through the females alone. Symptoms commence at puberty or shortly afterwards, often with a rapid onset ; one eye may be affected before the other. Vision deteriorates, but complete blindness is exceptional. There is a central scotoma with little or no peripheral constriction of the visual fields. The disc changes in the earliest stages are those of a neuritis, but the later appearances are those of a definite optic atrophy. There may be a slight degree of improvement in the state of vision, after which the condition remains stationary. No obvious etiological factor can be traced and physical examination reveals no abnormality in any region outside the optic nerve.

Although the symptomatology of Leber's disease is comparatively clear-cut, opinions are divided on the question of pathogenesis. We may briefly mention the hypotheses of an inherited temporary disorder of the pituitary gland ; of meningeal inflammation round the optic foramina ; of toxic retrobulbar neuritis due to some neighbouring sepsis and affecting tissue which bears an inherent vulnerability. Lastly, there is the conception of a primary neuronic degeneration localised to the optic nerve.

Leber quite definitely excluded from his cases all instances of optic atrophy associated with nervous disorders. But, in the family about to be described, one member showed the additional features of epilepsy and mental defect, while another showed signs of a marked neurological affection, sufficiently

* Carried out under the auspices of the Medical Research Council.

FIG. 7. Title page from Ferguson and Critchley's 1928 paper.

since lymphocytic infiltration of the meninges is sometimes a prominent finding at postmortem examination (24); indeed, it has been suggested that a primary arachnoiditis in the region of the optic nerve and chiasm underlies the visual disturbance. Similarly, abnormal globulin concentrations or colloidal gold curves would be anticipated if the infiltrating lymphocytes included immunologically competent cells.

It is over 50 years since the appearance of Ferguson and Critchley's paper. We are now more aware of the neurological conditions that may accompany the disease, and perhaps we can state more confidently that the initiating pathological process is one of primary neuronal

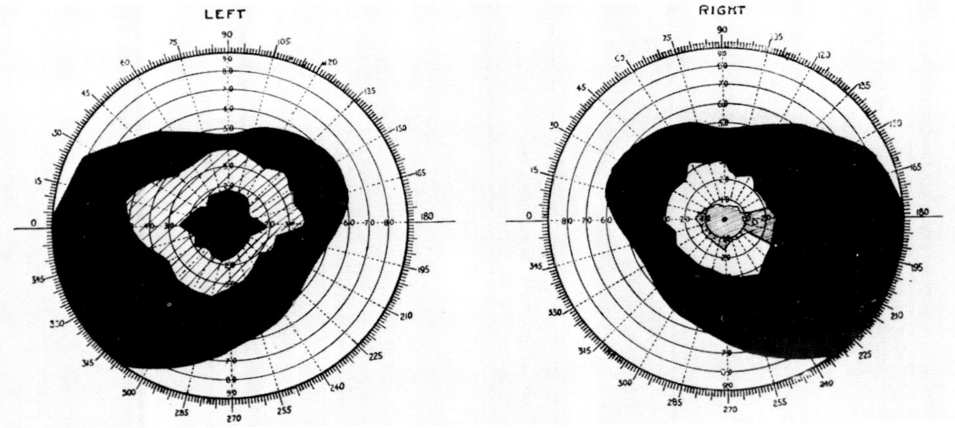

FIG. 8. Visual fields of case 4 in Ferguson and Critchley's 1928 paper.

degeneration. Many aspects of this condition remain enigmatic, not least its unique genetic expression

ACKNOWLEDGMENTS

I am indebted to Dr. C. J. Lill, who provided translations of the German texts. Figures 5 and 6 are reproduced by the kind permission of Dr. J. Lawton Smith and are taken from the *Archives of Ophthalmology*, Vol. 90, pages 349–354 (1973), Copyright 1973, by the American Medical Association. Figure 8 is reproduced by the kind permission of Dr. Macdonald Critchley and the editor, the *Journal of Neurology, Neurosurgery, and Psychiatry*.

REFERENCES

1. Leber, T. (1871): *Albrecht v. Graefes Arch. Ophthal.*, 17(2):249.
2. Von Graefe, A. (1858): *Albrecht v. Graefes Arch. Ophthal.*, 4(2):266.
3. Uhthoff, W. (1890): *Arch. Psychiat. Nervenkr.*, 21:55:303.
4. McAlpine, D., and Compston, N. (1952): *Quart. J. Med.*, 21:135.
5. Nikoskelainen, E., Sogg, R. L., Rosenthal, A. R., Friberg, T. R., and Dorfman, L. J. (1971): *Arch. Ophthal.*, 95:969.
6. Lawton Smith, J., Hoyt, W. F., and Susac, J. O. (1973): *Arch. Ophthal.*, 90:349.
7. Taylor, S. J. (1892): *Trans. Ophthal. Soc. U. K.*, 12:146.
8. Norris, W. F. (1884): *Trans. Am. Ophthal. Soc.*, 3:662.
9. Rasminsky, M. (1973): *Arch. Neurol.* (Chicago), 28:287.
10. Wilson, J. (1963): *Brain*, 86:347.
11. Lauber, H. (1902): *Wien. klin. Wschr.*, 15:1264.
12. Van Heuven, G. J. (1924): *Klin Mbl. Augenheilk*, 13:252.
13. Bell, J. (1931): In: *The Treasury of Human Inheritance*, Vol. II, Part IV. edited by K. Pearson. *Hereditary Optic Atrophy (Leber's Disease)*. Cambridge University Press, Cambridge.
14. Van Heuven, G. J., and Oltmans, G. (1924): *Ned. T. Geneesk.*, 68:1958.
15. Nettleship, E. (1909): *Trans. Ophthal. Soc. U. K.*, 29:57.
16. Batten, R. D. (1909): *Trans. Ophthal. Soc. U. K.*, 29:144.
17. Habershon, S. H. (1888): *Trans. Ophthal. Soc. U. K.*, 8:190.
18. Higgens, C. (1880): *Med. Times* (London), 1:450.
19. Davis, F. A., Bergen, D., Schauf, C., McDonald, W. I., and Deutsch. W. (1976): *Neurology* (Minneapolis), 26:1100.
20. Perkin, G. D., and Rose, F. C. (1979): *Optic Neuritis and its Differential Diagnosis*, pp. 39–40. Oxford University Press, Oxford.

21. Taylor, J., and Holmes, G. M. (1913): *Trans. Ophthal. Soc. U.K.*, 33:95.
22. Ferguson, F. R., and Critchley, M. (1928): *J. Neurol. Psychopathol.*, 9:120.
23. Lees, F., MacDonald, A.-M. E., and Turner, J. W. A. (1964): *J. Neurol. Neurosurg. Psychiat.*, 27:415.
24. Adams, J. H., Blackwood, W., and Wilson, J. (1966): *Brain*, 89:15.

Historical Aspects of the Neurosciences,
edited by F. Clifford Rose and W. F. Bynum.
Raven Press, New York ©

Brains of Dinosaurs

William Elgin Swinton

Massey College, University of Toronto, Toronto, Canada

The very title of this chapter must sound like dilettantism or it may mistakenly imply that the dinosaurs occupy a high place in the evolution of the human brain. But there is a relevance in their study. Dinosaurs, to use their popular name, were a remarkable expansion of reptilian life, were animals of greatly varying habit and of kind, and collectively occupied a great space—some 150 million years—in the evolution of the vertebrates. Some of us are today between the protagonists of the genetical inheritance school and those who, though recognizing the power of genes, recognize the power of the environment, too. Dinosaurs make ideal subjects for such studies; at the moment, their physiology is again in dispute or certainly under review.

Dinosaur bones have been found in every continent except, as yet, Antarctica. They number thousands. Complete skeletons are harder to come by, so relationships of odd bones, and even of teeth, are often difficult to determine. Skulls are occasionally complete or are sufficiently well preserved posteriorly so as to allow examination of the neurocranium. While its constitution in dinosaurs generally is not that of mammals, it does show a reduction in the number of unpaired bones. In 1935, Williston established a law relating to the evolution of skull bones in the vertebrates, and this was discussed by the great palaeontologist W. K. Gregory in the same year (1). The reduction is, of course, partly due to the specialization of the relevant areas by the disappearance of some bones and the union of others. The elements are often difficult to distinguish through the lack of clear sutures, but even in the best known dinosaur, the number of neurocranial bones appears to be 14, much more than the 8 of the human skull.

What is much more striking, and which bears no relationship to bone numbers, is the relative insignificance of the dinosaurian brain case as compared with the size of the skull. In such an advanced form as the bipedal *Anatosaurus* (Fig. 1), the length of the brain case is just less than one-fifth of the median length of the skull, and its breadth is about one-fifth at the relevant level. Dinosaurs vary so much in size and in the specialization of their skulls that no standard figure can be given or should be expected for the length, breadth, or depth of the brain case, nor would it have much meaning quantitatively or qualitatively, although its angular inclination to the skull level may be important. This statement can be clarified by pointing out that in reptiles the brain case usually does not indicate the size of the brain itself. Many studies have been made on this using endocasts. Many of these attempts at casting the difficult cavity were unsuccessful, but the use of modern flexible materials, such as latex, has greatly improved the technique without perhaps making the brain more fully studied. The dinosaur brain, like that of many other reptiles, did not fill the cavity, and it must have received the support of connective tissue. This is not new

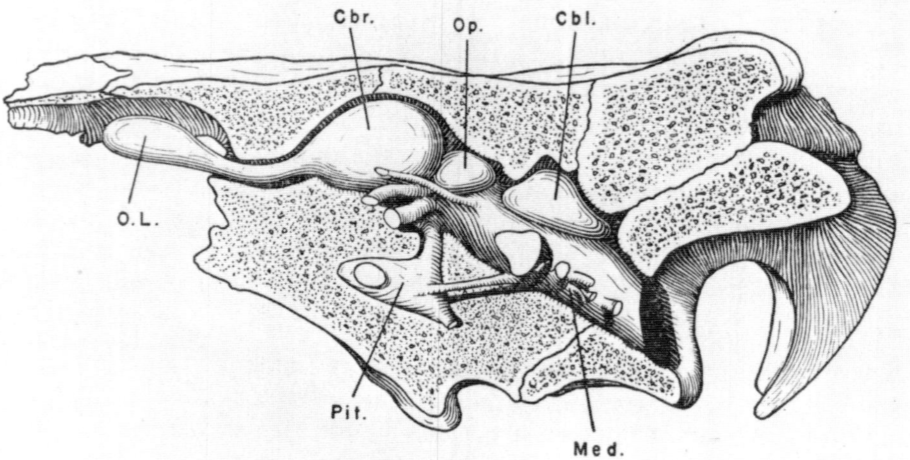

FIG. 1. Restored brain within the endocranial cavity of the skull of the hadrosaur *Anatosaurus* (From J. H. Ostrom (1961): Cranial morphology of the North American Hadrosauridae. *Bull. Amer. Mus. Nat. Hist.*, 122:33–186.)

knowledge, for classic studies of the brain of *Sphenodon*, the Tuatara, were made by Arthur Dendy in 1910 and 1911. In this case, the brain occupied only half of the space and was supported by strands of connective tissue. Since that time, Tilly Edinger, the famous palaeoneurologist, has made similar observations in alligators and turtles in her important study of fossil brains in 1929. John Ostrom has also commented on *Sphenodon*, alligators, and lizards. Recognizing the close anatomical affinity of crocodiles with the dinosaurs and their eventual origin from a common ancestor, I have been inclined to accept the crocodile brain case/brain ratio as 2 to 1. At any rate, the size of the living dinosaur brain was essentially less than was indicated by the endocasts and may have been only half the size in some forms.

This statement requires qualification, for the brain space recorded for the endocast is in most cases the cast of the dura mater with its crinkles and bulges. Henry Fairfield Osborn in 1912 (2) pointed this out for *Tyrannosaurus*, and the former presence of the brain's envelopes must be born in mind. That there are considerable differences in the quality of brain representation or simulation is, however, also well known, and brains of some carnivorous dinosaurs show apparently excellent impressions of cerebellar structures or shapes, while the Hadrosaurs, also well represented by fossils, sometimes yield excellent outlines of the cerebral hemispheres. It seems likely, as James Hopson points out in his excellent paper (3), that the forebrain is more fully represented in the endocranium. This may be associated with an observation that the brain may have been proportionately larger in young specimens and with the more certain knowledge that the olfactory region was consistently important in dinosaurs.

The brain itself, therefore, is still a largely unknown quantity. No dinosaur brain has ever been found nor is it likely to be discovered. Attempts, on my behalf, were made in 1958 by my colleague Arthur Rixon in the British Museum (Nat. Hist.) to discover any traces of amino acids by chromatic investigation in an excellent brain case of *Iguanodon*, but they yielded nothing. What then can we say of the dinosaur brain? The brain was clearly reptilian and as such shows the divisions and presumably the functions of vertebrate animals habitually breathing air in a predominantly terrestrial environment. In other words, the brain of a living crocodile (Fig. 2), which provides a probable guide to the dinosaur, has the characteristic olfactory bulbs, the paired cerebral hemispheres, the paired optic lobes, followed by the cerebellum which in turn is followed by the fourth ventricle and the medulla oblongata. This relatively simple fore-and-aft division has variations, particularly in the length of the olfactory lobes and the breadth or depth of the brain.

Although none of these actually exists in our dinosaur collections, the delimitation of areas is made possible by the size and confirmation of the regions on the casts, and the identification is made probable by the remains of, indications of, or the roots of the cranial nerves. On the whole, dinosaurs did not have specialized brains, which is consistent with the belief that they led relatively stable lives and adapted to stable environmental conditions. The size, of course, varied, mostly in relation to the size of the animals, although there are some striking anomalies.

There are also dorsal indications on some dinosaur endocasts of space for a pineal body without, however, any associated parietal opening. I know of no dinosaur with a parietal eye, such as is found in some contemporary reptiles and in the modern *Sphenodon*. The pituitary is another matter, for the depression on the cerebrocranial floor must hold both

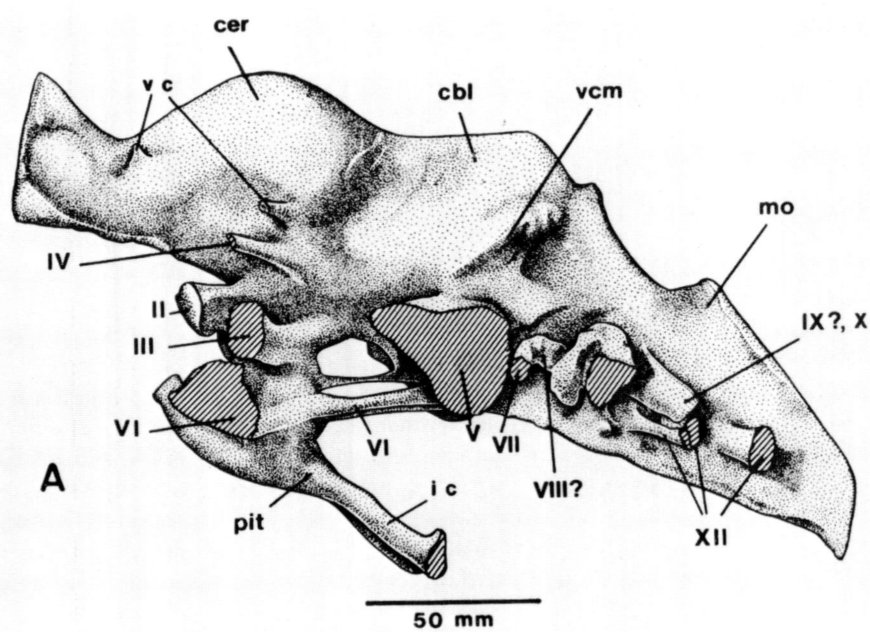

FIG. 2. Endocast of the hadrosaur *Kritosaurus Notabilis* AMNH 5350: Lateral View. (From James A. Hopson, (1979): Paleoneurology. In: *Biology of the Reptilia*, Academic Press, London.)

hypophysis and infundibulum and perhaps part of the optic chiasma. The relative use of the pituitary is of much interest. It is not always easy to identify (Marsh misidentified it in his famous figure of *Stegosaurus*), but there are instances in which I believe the signs of hyperpituitarism can be seen in the skull and body. The dinosaur brain is, however, no constant thing. Its size, its relative imprint upon the various regions of the neurocranium, and the complexity of its nerves are variable in the different kinds of animals included in the popular, nonscientific term "dinosaur," and while this is not the place to enter into the ever changing conclusions of the systematists, the conditions of the brain in the main groups can be summarized. There are two principal branches of the dinosaurian tree, distinguished by characters other than cerebral. The first great group is the Saurischia ("reptile-hips"), which is again split into the Theropoda and the Sauropodomorpha, or Sauropods. Theropods were all carnivorous bipeds; some were small (10 or 15 feet long) and others were large bipeds, like the famous *Tyrannosaurus*, with a length of nearly 60 feet, and which was the largest land-living carnivore of all time. A highly specialized group, the Deinonychids, were swift, raptorial creatures with brains that are well shown in some skulls from the late Cretaceous forms from Canada, *Stenonychosaurus* and *Dromiciomimus*. These have larger brains than other contemporary reptiles and at 37 to 45 grams are seven times larger than the brains of living crocodiles of equal size (10 feet in length). The size of the olfactory lobes, the cerebral hemispheres, and the optic development suggest behavioral patterns of considerable ability. The brain has been compared favorably with that of ratite birds, with whom they may have ancestral connections. There are indications of vascular markings on the surface of some of these endocasts. The related *Ornithomimus* (*Struthiomimus*) are toothless, birdlike dinosaurs, long known from excellent specimens in the Royal Ontario Museum. Their inadequate endocasts show a large floccular fossa and a short and deep medullary cavity.

The group of large dinosaurs (Carnosauria) includes some of the older and best-known carnivores and can be illustrated here by *Tyrannosaurus*, as it exemplifies the general characters of the closely related U.S.S.R. *Tarbosaurus* and the North American *Gorgosaurus*, as well as the earlier American *Antrodemus (Allosaurus)* and *Ceratosaurus* and the European *Megalosaurus*. The endocast here outlined is splendidly redrawn and outlined by Hopson, showing it to be a rather revolver-shaped organ in left side view, approximately 277 mm (almost 11 inches) long and of about 3 inches across the upper surfaces of the cerebral lobes. The highest part with the "horns" of the cartilaginous part of the supraoccipital and part of the filling of the longitudinal sinus give an emphasis to the cerebellum that is not justified, yet the total brain space is impressive, and it is a pity that in neither of the specimens is the complete pituitary seen. The *Tyrannosaurus'* brain has been calculated by Jenson as 270 ml and this for a body weight estimated by Colbert as 7.7 metric tons (4). The Sauropodomorphs, the large, quadruped, herbivorous forms of the Saurischia, have yielded several endocasts mainly from the Western hemisphere. These animals, renowned in popular literature, are supposed to have spent much time in water, whose buoyancy would literally take the weight from their rather elephantine feet. There are doubts about this too now, but the point is that a vegetarian life in inland waters, rivers, and pools might be expected to have effects on the olfactory region of the brain. Unfortunately, the only two endocasts known to me, that of *Diplodocus* and that of *Camarasaurus*, shed little light upon it. This is all the more regrettable because the "nostrils" in these animals were on top of the head. Both endocasts are relatively small, only some 65 mm, or 2½ inches, from back to front, as preserved, but both also show a significantly large pituitary. This is hardly unexpected, for *Camarasaurus* was 60 feet long, including the long neck and tail, of course, and *Diplodocus* had the long but rather lowly set grandeur of 87½ feet. Colbert has estimated its weight as 11.7 metric tons, and Jerison has calculated the probable brain weight as 360 ml (12 fl. oz.). The Sauropods had the advantage of a sacral booster or alleged second brain, and the effect of this is discussed below.

The second great order of dinosaurs is known also by its hips, or pelvic structure, being the Ornithischia, or birdlike pelvis. Once again the forms are well known and numerous. There were bipedal forms, though regarded as less speedy than the bipedal carnivores. Some were perhaps able to swim, for they had webbed fingers; others have remarkably long skulls; then again, there were quadrupedal forms, all of which were armoured on the head or on the body. Most were massive animals and all were herbivorous. This diversity of form and habit as regards food gathering and self-defense suggests in some cases an almost mammalian similarity, and it is therefore interesting to observe their endocasts, more especially as many of the dinosaurs were the last of their kind.

The order has the distinction of having *Iguanodon*, the first reptile to be regarded as a dinosaur in the history of the group. First found in 1822 as teeth in southern England, it has now become known by many specimens in England, Belgium, and North Africa and by footprints in Spitsbergen. Much of this Lower Cretaceous material is magnificent and has been well described. The endocast of *Iguanodon* has been depicted by several writers but shows a rather modest front to back representation with rather broad cerebral hemispheres, followed by a less broad but level hind brain and with an imperfect pituitary cast. The nerve endings on the cast are well shown [see Andrews (12)]. However, the Ornithopod brain has now been splendidly demonstrated by Hopson (3), whose reproductions of lateral, ventral, and dorsal aspects of the 250 mm (4½ inches) section show not only the main regions of the brain but a splendid array of arterial grooves, vascular canals, and all the nerves but the olfactory (where the cast is truncated) and the accessory (XI). This excellent cast and its explanation cannot, unfortunately, be adequately discussed here, for *Kritosaurus notabilis* is but one of the remarkable Hadrosaurs whose plain or hooded skulls are among the most remarkable in dinosaurs. Their way of life is still under debate as is the function of the involved premaxillaries and the enclosed passages. *Kritosaurus* had a ridged nose but was not a hooded or "helmeted" form. Its skull was 30 inches long and rather high posteriorly. Some of these bipedal herbivores of the Upper Cretaceous of North America were remarkable for the thickening of the bones above the brain case, which the dinosaurs are supposed to have used as battering rams, an idea that invokes exciting restoration pictures, but the question may still be asked about the advantage of an almost solid cranium.

The endocast of *Pachycephalosaurus* always reminds me of that of *Tyrannosaurus*, with its large pituitary bulge, but whereas *Tyrannosaurus* had a large brain for a large biped (47 feet long), *Pachycephalus* has only become known by its skull, but its relatives in peculiarity of skull have only ordinary Ornithopod bodies about 30 feet long. The writer feels that "the bony-headedness" is associated with the unusually large pituitary that can be presumed from the cranial cavities and that here we have a case of dinosaurian acromegaly (7).

This kind of suggestion is criticized by remarks made on the probable similarity that can be seen in late Cretaceous dinosaurs by Adrian Desmond in *The Hot Blooded Dinosaurs* (8), but the armored dinosaurs are often suggestive of pituitary hyperaction or senility or both. Indeed, the quadrupedal Ornithischia are all armored. Perhaps the most famous of the dinosaurs is *Stegosaurus*, the "plated reptile," with a small head close to the ground, a high body with alternating bony plates, sometimes nearly 3 feet high, and a tail with a double pair of spikes. Slow moving, vegetarian, 25 to 30 feet long, and weighing perhaps 2 metric tons, he had a brain, long pictured by Marsh as long, narrow, and calculated as weighing

100 ml or 3.4 fl. oz. The appearance of this grotesque dinosaur with its little head and small brain but with a large endosacral nerve center prompted the famous poem by Bert L. Taylor in the *Chicago Tribune* in 1912, which has done much to confuse the public view of dinosaur neurology. Part of the poem runs: *"You will observe by these remains,/The Creature had two sets of brains—/One in his head (the usual place),/The other at his spinal base,/Thus he could reason "A priori"/As well as "A posteriori."* This fact has led to much popular confusion, for the disparity between head and tail is striking. *Stegosaurus* has a "sacral brain cavity" 20 times the size of the endocranium. There are similar disparities in the Sauropods and the Hadrosaurs that have been frequently illustrated. But students of anatomy know that brachial and sacral enlargements of the spinal cord in many animals and even slight enlargements in the human cord occur. These are in no way to be interpreted as "brains" but rather as nerve centers for control of special regions. It can easily be seen that the dinosaurian hind limbs and powerful tail well deserved a "branch office" for their work, but it was not a center of intelligence.

The group that was among the last of the dinosaurs was the Ceratopsia or "horned faces"; indeed, they and the giant carnivores such as *Tyrannosaurus* were complementary if not quite compatible. The Ceratopsia, whose early Cretaceous ancestors are known from Mongolia, attained a large size with a body not unlike that of a rhinoceros, but the skull was huge, with a bony frill extending over the neck. While the whole animal might be about 25 feet long and weigh nearly 9 metric tons, the skull in *Triceratops* and *Torosaurus* might attain an overall length of 7 feet.

Within this vast head, though much was frill, lay a small chamber like a pharaoh's royal tomb in Egypt—the brain being 270 ml. This rather old measurement has been superseded now by the fine endocast of *Anchiceratops ornatus* which forms Plate XI of Lull (9). This has been clarified (and reversed) on the clearer illustration in Hopson (3). The pituitary is not large, occupying lengthwise just over one-seventh of the length from the olfactory to the truncated end of the cast just behind the roots of the hypoglossal nerve. But *Anchiceratops* was a smaller Ceratopsian with a total body length of 13 feet and a fenestrated frill to the skull (in all, 5 feet long). It may be, therefore, that the pituitary had some effect. It must be added that the plated Stegosaur's pituitary (referred to earlier) was misidentified by Marsh and even as restored by Hopson was not large in the brain, but the plates and body armament of *Stegosaurus* were on the body and dermis.

The relation of brain size to body size has been much debated, and the facts are not many. As we have seen, the endocasts help us to speculate on the brain capacity, while the body weight of even complete dinosaurs must be somewhat conjectural.

Jerison (11) points out that, all things considered, the brains of dinosaurs are right for their size. These are not his words, for he says: "The dinosaurs, including the largest, are typically reptilian with respect to gross brain size." But I find it difficult to avoid relating the slow evolution of dinosaur brains to the remarkable stability of the Mesozoic environment, and from what we know of their senses, olfaction was apparently important and good. Eyesight was good, and in some of the late Cretaceous Deinonychosauridae, it was probably very good. In some it was perhaps binocular. I have speculated elsewhere on the possibility of color vision and I will not weary you with it here. Dinosaurs have even lent us their ears, so far as evidence of semicircular canals, tympanum, and stapes are concerned.

All in all, they lived as well as they could in a world that lasted a long time. There may be something to be said for being placid, and it has already been said by Walt Whitman.

To end on another note, I must say that I do not know of any branch of vertebrate palaeontology or comparative anatomy that has developed so quickly in recent years as palaeoneurology, thanks to those whom I have mentioned in this chapter.

REFERENCES

1. Gregory, W. K. (1935): "Williston's Law" relating to the evolution of skull bones in the vertebrates. *Am. J. Phys. Anthrop.*, XX:123.
2. Osborn, H. F. (1912): Crania of *Tyrannosaurus* and *Allosaurus. Mem. Am. Mus. N.H.*, I:1.
3. Hopson, J. (1979): In: *Biology of the Reptilia. Neurology A. Paleoneurology*, edited by C. Gans, pp. 39–169. Academic Press, London.
4. Colbert, E. H. (1962): The weights of dinosaurs. *Am. Mus. Nov.*, 2076:1.
5. Swinton, W. E. (1958): Dinosaur brains. *New Sci.*, 4:707.
6. Casier, E. (1960): *Les Iguanodons de Bernissart.* Ad Gomaere Imprimeur du Roi, Bruxelles.
7. Swinton, W. E. (1970): *The Dinosaurs.* Allen & Unwin, London.
8. Desmond, A. (1977): *The Hot Blooded Dinosaurs.* Futura Pub., London.
9. Lull, R. S. (1933): Revision of the Ceratopsia or Horned Dinosaurs. *Mem. Peabody Mus. N.H.*, III:71.
10. Lull, R. S., and Wright, N. (1942): Hadrosaurian dinosaurs of North America. *Geol. Soc. Am. Spec.* Paper 40, p. 122.
11. Jerison, H. J. (1973): *Evolution of the Brain and Intelligence.* Academic Press, New York.
12. Andrews, C. W. (1897): Note on the cast of the brain cavity of Iguanodon. *Ann. Mag. Nat. Hist.* London, 6. XIX:585–591.
13. Colbert, E. H. (1961): *Dinosaurs.* Dutton, New York.
14. Edinger, T. (1968): *Neues aus der Paläoneurologie. Palaeont. Z.*, 37:49.
15. Kruger, L. (1969): Experimental analyses of the reptilian nervous system. *Ann. N.Y. Acad. Sci.*, 167:102.
16. Säve Söderbergh, G. (1947): Notes on the braincase in Sphenodon and certain Lacertilia. *Zool. Bidr. Uppsala*, 25:489.
17. Klinghardt, F. (1937): Bemerkungen über gehirne Schadel und Schädelahnliebe Bildungen. *Palaeont. Z.*, 19:162.

Historical Aspects of the Neurosciences,
edited by F. Clifford Rose and W. F. Bynum.
Raven Press, New York ©

Neurology and Art

Lawrence C. McHenry, Jr.

Department of Neurology, Bowman Gray School of Medicine of Wake Forest University, Winston-Salem, North Carolina 27103

The association between art and neurology is part of an overall relation between art and medicine. Neurology, a branch of general medicine, focuses upon the study of diseases of the nervous system. Implied in this, from an artistic standpoint, is an understanding of the anatomy and pathology of the brain and nervous system. The relationship between art and neurology can be seen in two areas. First are the methods of illustration of the nervous system, which are closely tied to the development of anatomical illustration and the history of printing. The second association is the portrayal by artists of clinical neurological disease, which, since it leads to distortions and deformities, is readily captured by the artist. Brain disease may also produce behavioral and emotional changes that are reflected in the facial expression or body posture of the patient, the realistic portrayal of which has been a goal of many artists.

Before giving specific examples of art and neurology, one should consider the fascination of art and medicine, which has been explored in the past by Choulant, Singer, Holländer, Sudhoff, Charcot, and great numbers of other physicians and surgeons. Recently, works by Herrlinger (1) and Rousselot (2) have made the relation between art and medicine more accessible. Many of the neurologically oriented illustrations in this text have appeared in the works of McHenry (3) and Clarke and Dewhurst (4).

Art and medicine are both aspects of human endeavor that have an ancient heritage. To the Greeks, the physician was an artisan, a craftsman, like a painter or sculptor. An artisan worked with his mind and his hands and applied his powers of observation to create or, medically, to heal. Another aspect is the curiosity that the professional artists have had throughout history for the pathological and abnormal. Brueghel, Bosch, Ribera, Rembrandt, and Velasquez depicted death, the plagues and portrayed lepers, dwarfs, and the physically handicapped.

NEUROANATOMY AND ART

The first known visual or artistic display of the brain is from an 11th century manuscript at Caius College, Cambridge. In the upper left of Fig. 1 is a drawing of the skull facing inwards and seen from above. The coronal, sagittal, and lambdoidal sutures are represented by double lines. The mental faculties on this diagram are "fantasia" or imagination, "intellectus" or reasoning, and "memoria" or memory. The brain is labeled cold and moist, and opposite, the heart, hot and dry. Such designations were given prominence by Aristotle and those who followed (5).

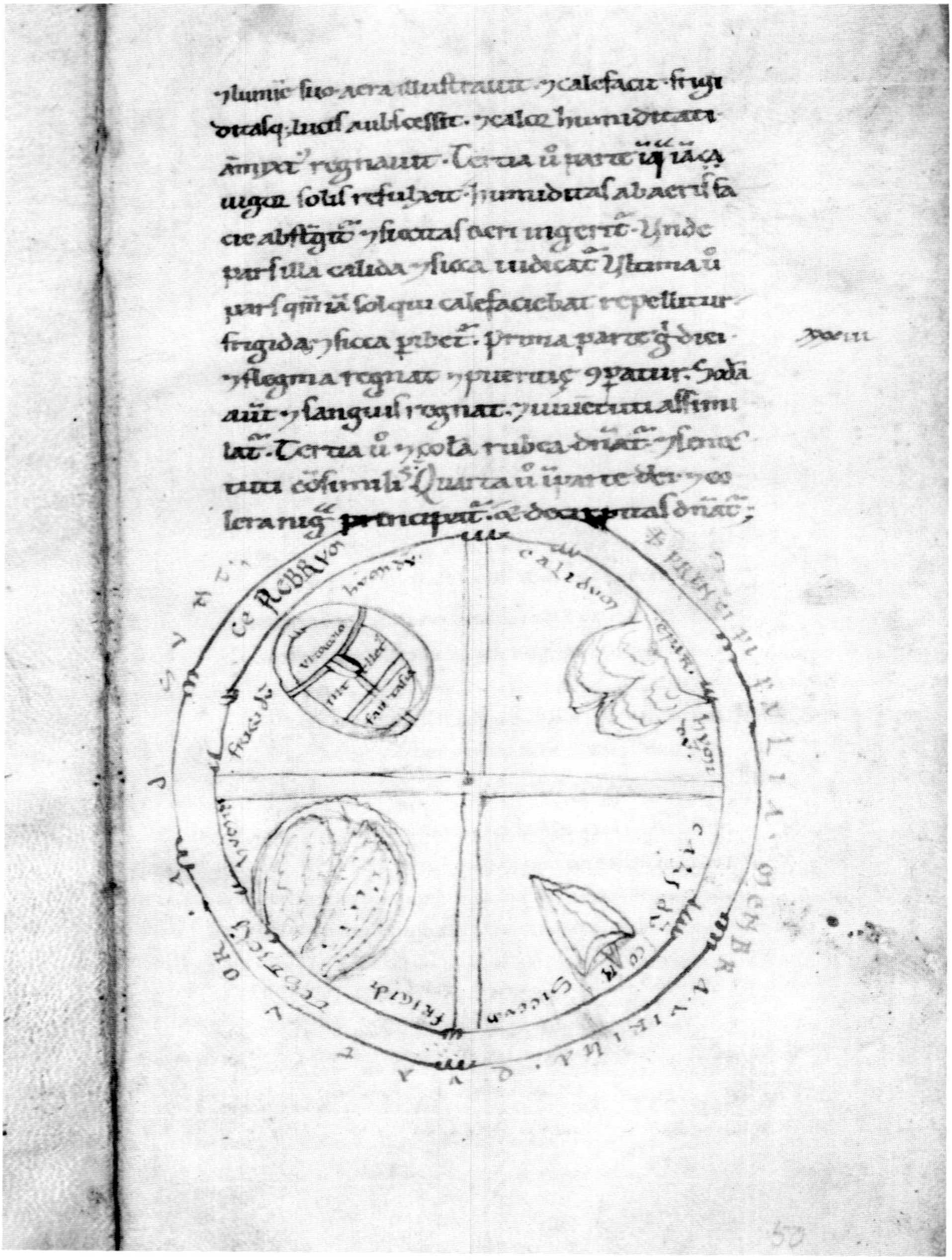

FIG. 1. Eleventh-century manuscript.

Choulant (6) has written that in two Persian manuscripts, one written about 1400 A.D. and the other a few decades later, there is a suggestion for the first time in Arabic medicine of a traditional line of anatomical drawing. These possibly spring from the same Alexandrian sources as the Western series. These manuscripts contain six pictures showing the osseous,

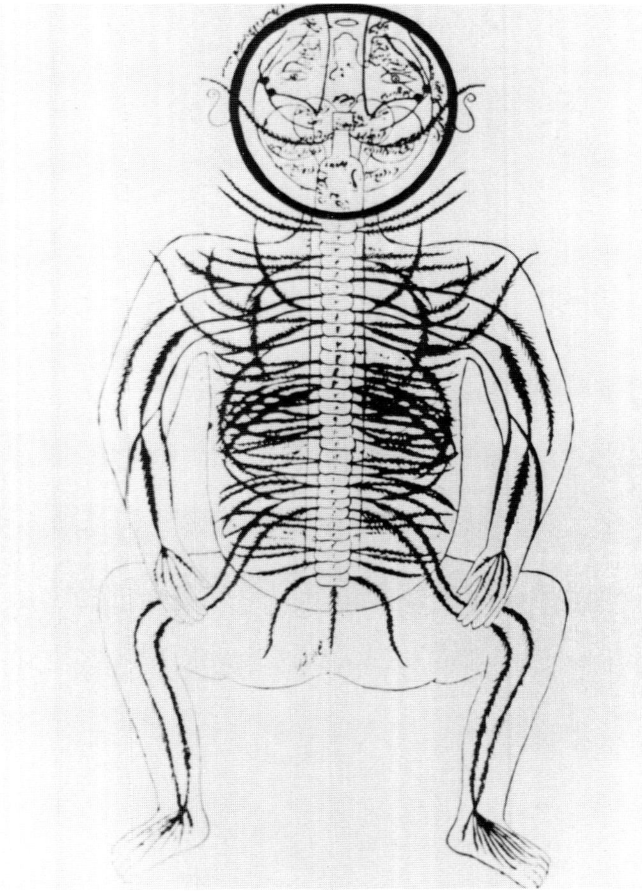

FIG. 2. Persian drawing of the nervous system.

nervous, muscular, and arterial systems and the gravid uterus. The Persian drawing of the nervous system is shown in Fig. 2.

The first possible Western illustration of neuroanatomy is in the 1345 manuscript of Guido de Vigevano. This was discovered in the Chateau de Chantilly (Musée Conde). Among the illustrations are several showing Guido's method of exposing the skull. One illustration (Fig. 3) shows the spinal cord and brain exposed together with an outline of the spinal nerves. The drawings of the figure are fairly good and the method of dissection seems quite modern, but the number of spinal nerves is only 18. The sciatic nerve, however, is shown in about the right position (6,7).

After the invention of printing in the second half of the 15th century, the reproduction of books was endlessly practiced. When the woodcut was used for illustration, there was an increase in the artistic portrayal of anatomy. Still, there was no particular demand other than for schematic anatomical representation needed for physicians who essentially followed the Galenic school. It was not desirable to represent pictorially and put before the student what up to that time had been preserved only through words and memory. It was for this reason that illustrations, although being intended for physicians, are nothing other than schematic representations.

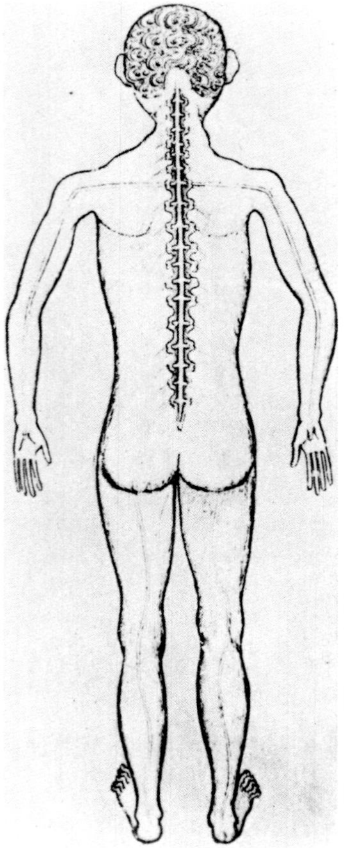

FIG. 3. Guido's dissection of the nervous system.

In the familiar woodcut from Reisch (Fig. 4), the three ventricles of the brain are shown, surrounded by what appears to be a representation of the cerebral convolutions. The medieval idea of physiological psychology is represented here. Messages from the organs of hearing, sight, taste, and smell unite in the front ventricle, forming the *sensus communis*. Here fantasy and imagination originate and pass into the middle ventricle. Between the two ventricles is the vermis, a contemporary term for the choroid plexus. Such illustrations were used by Albertus Magnus, Hundt, Versor, Ketham, Peyligk, Dryander, Leonardo da Vinci, and many others. This physiological scheme was generally accepted until the time of Descartes (5). Clarke and Dewhurst (4) have brought together in a scholarly fashion and have illustrated the history of brain function from antiquity to modern times.

The line drawings were considered by Choulant (6) as the first period of anatomical illustration, which went up to the early 1520s. During this period, only schematic representations of what had been accepted and handed down as true had been made. During the Renaissance, there were increasing facilities for scientific dissections at universities and medical colleges and toward the end of the 15th and the beginning of the 16th century, a great many discoveries regarding single parts of the human body, including the nervous system, were brought to light.

The first real advance in neuroanatomy is to be found in a marginal series of sections of the brain (Fig. 5) by Fries (8), or Phryesen, a Dutch physician who showed that engraved

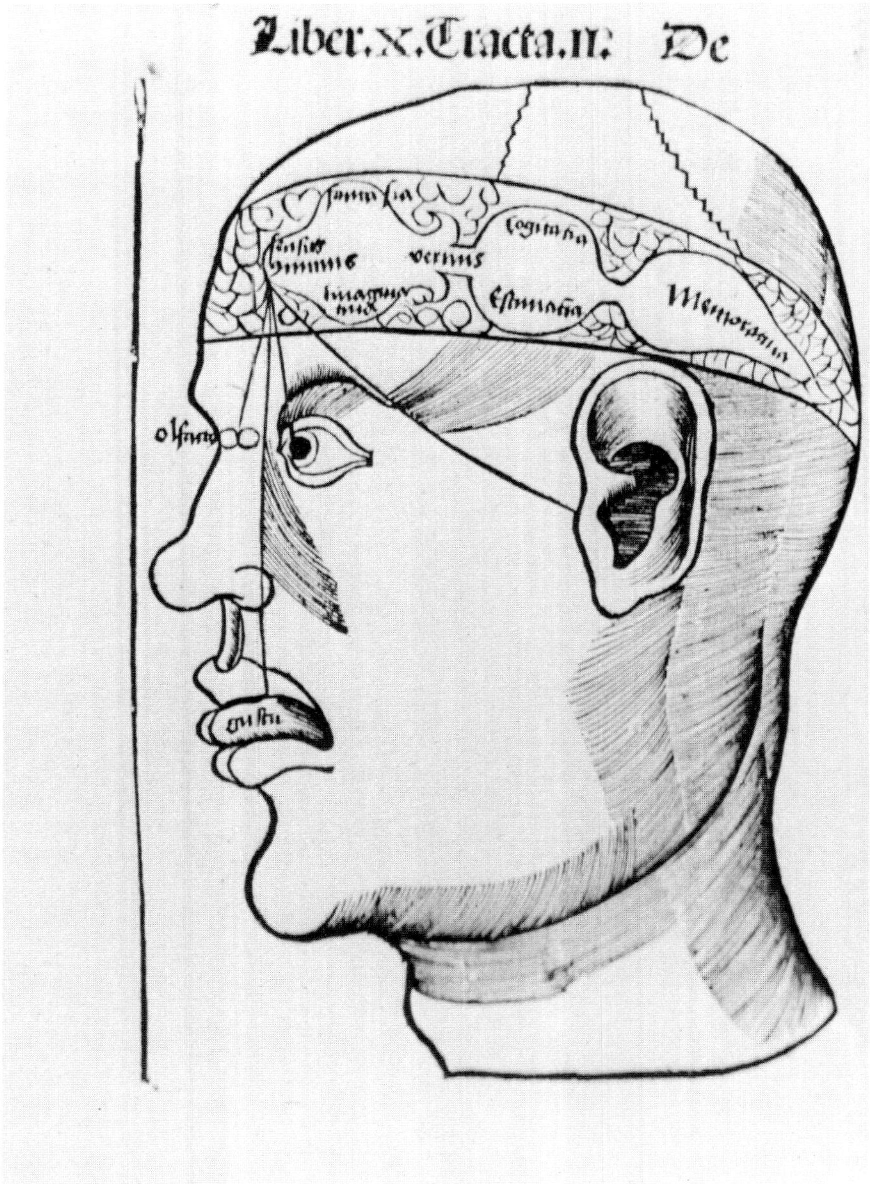

FIG. 4. Reisch's scheme of location of mental facilities.

woodcuts could be well done. The anatomy of the brain was treated in a wholly new and exceptional fashion. No one can study these drawings without a sudden sense of a leap forward in the power of anatomical observation. Against the crude artistic background of the Middle Ages, this marginal series of stages of gross brain dissection provides the first real milestone in neuroanatomy. Here is shown the optic chiasm and a crude representation of the cranial nerves. The woodcuts of Fries represent the first of six periods from the late

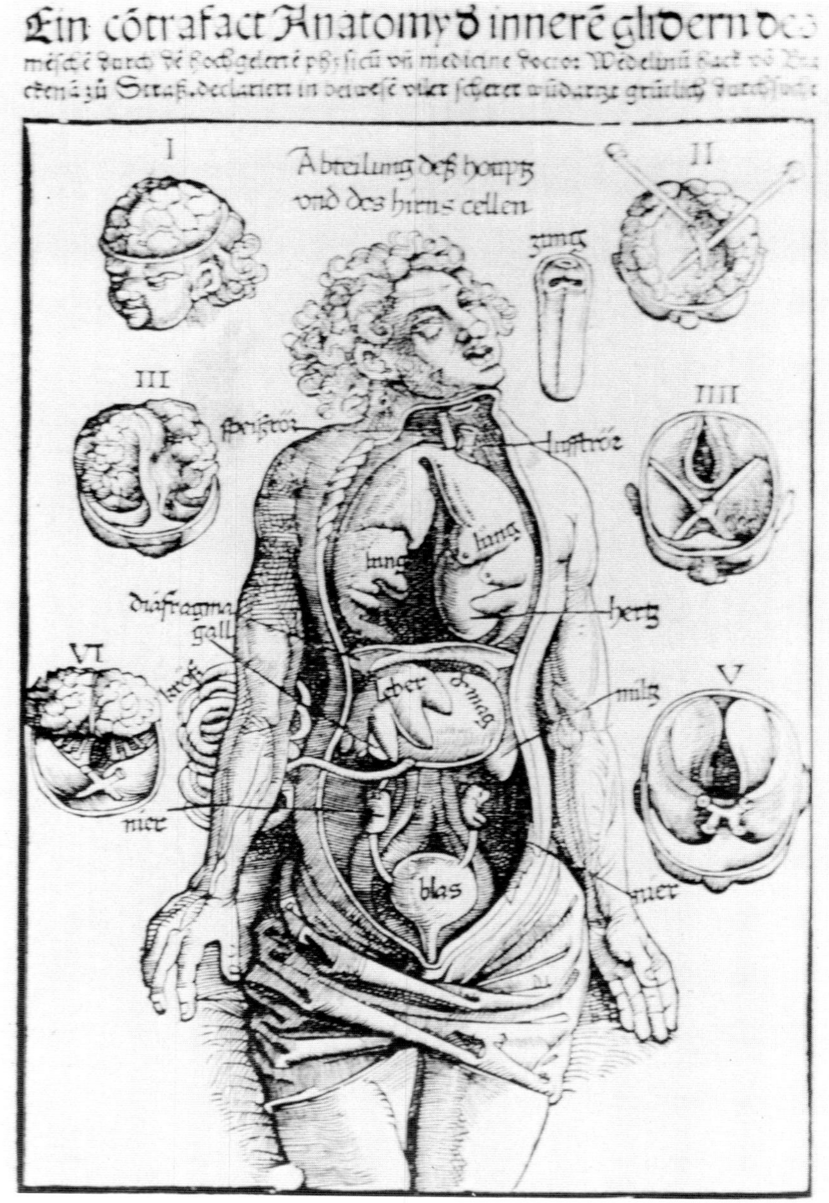

FIG. 5. Brain dissection of Fries.

15th to the early 18th centuries into which Choulant separates the history of anatomical illustration.

From a neurological standpoint, the man who made the most independent anatomical investigations and with some scientific understanding was Berengario da Carpi (9). He was himself artistically gifted. His woodcuts (Fig. 6) show the brain from above with at first one ventricle opened to show what is labeled as the vermis. This is actually the first realistic

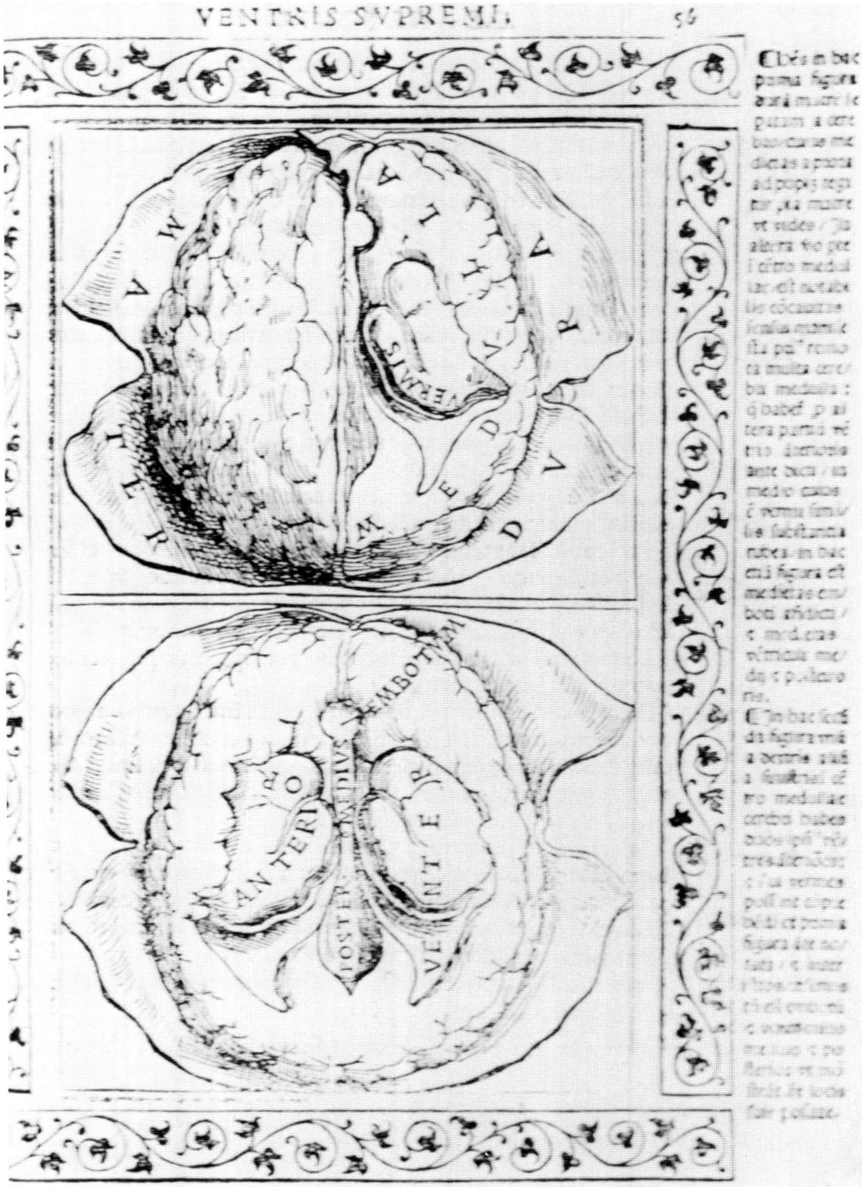

FIG. 6. Brain engraving of Berengario da Carpi.

representation of the ventricle in the cerebral hemisphere. In the lower part of the figure, both lateral ventricles and the third ventricle are exposed as well as crude representations of the basal ganglia and thalamus.

Even before this, Leonardo da Vinci (10,11), the greatest artist and scientist of the Italian Renaissance, had already studied the cross-section anatomy of the brain and different planes.

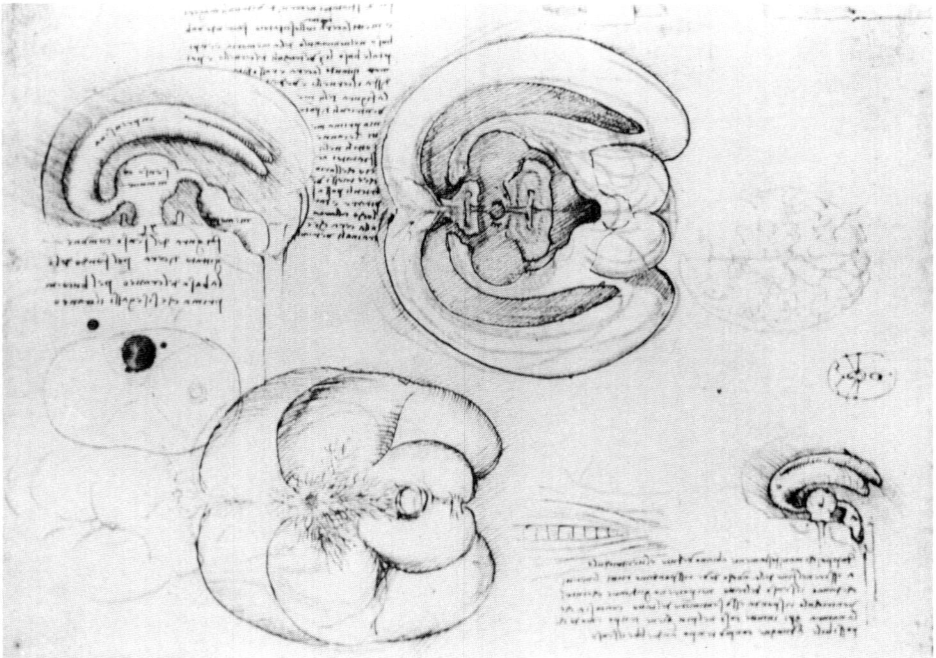

FIG. 7. Da Vinci's drawings of the brain.

The chalk drawings of da Vinci may make him the founder of iconographic and physiological anatomy.

Da Vinci drew one of the first diagrams of the cranial nerves, the optic chiasm, and the brachial and lumbar plexus. His most remarkable contribution to neurological anatomy was his successful wax casts of the four ventricles that were the first known attempts of anatomical injection. In Fig. 7, the intraventricular foramen as well as the cerebral aqueduct is represented. At the bottom of the drawing, the base of the brain shows the vascular rete mirabile, which was probably from the brain of an ox, since the human circle of Willis is not shown. Although da Vinci is said to have dissected 30 human bodies, this drawing of the rete indicates that he was also among those who included structures from animals in their drawings of human dissections.

The most fully illustrated of the pre-Vesalian brain dissections were those of Estienne (12), an anatomist and a prominent publisher of medical books during the Renaissance. Estienne's elaborate figures were composed in part of copies from contemporary artists. His eight dissections of the brain, made in 1539, give more anatomical detail than had previously appeared. The graphic representation (Fig. 8) of the difference between the convolutional patterns of the cerebrum and cerebellum is shown for the first time.

In Estienne's copper plates, it can clearly be seen that the plate of the brain dissection has been separately fitted into the overall plate. He shows the passage from the lateral third ventricle and that from the third to the fourth ventricle in addition to a representation of the cranial nerves. Without encroaching on anatomical clearness, Estienne shows a distracting predilection for poses and attitudes, which may be considered formally to unite art and neuroanatomy.

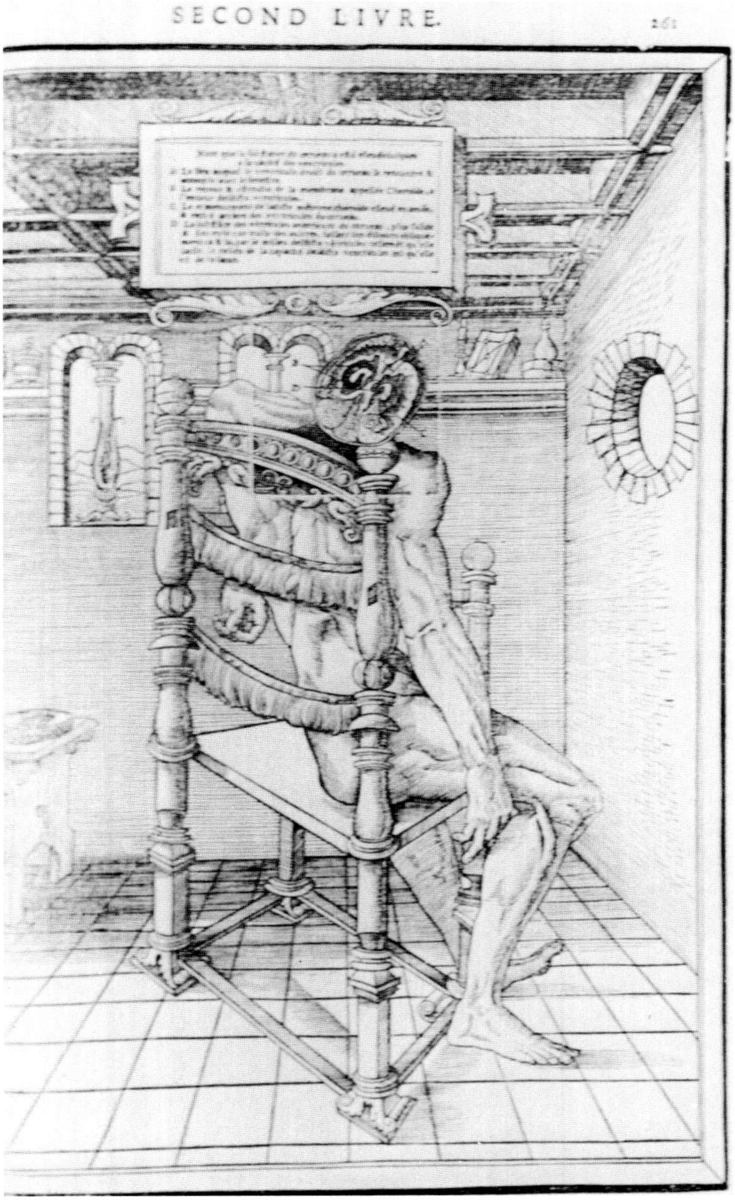

FIG. 8. Estienne's brain dissection.

Other early Renaissance artists and anatomists portrayed the brain and nervous system, but the height and beauty of anatomical illustration was reached by Vesalius in the publication in 1543 of his *De Humani Corporis Fabrica* (13,14). The artist who drew his work was Jan van Kalkar, who was a student of Titian. The fourth book of his *Fabrica* contains Vesalius' drawing of the overall anatomy of the nervous system. Opening with a view of the base of the brain, the cranial nerves are presented in a rather confused fashion, using

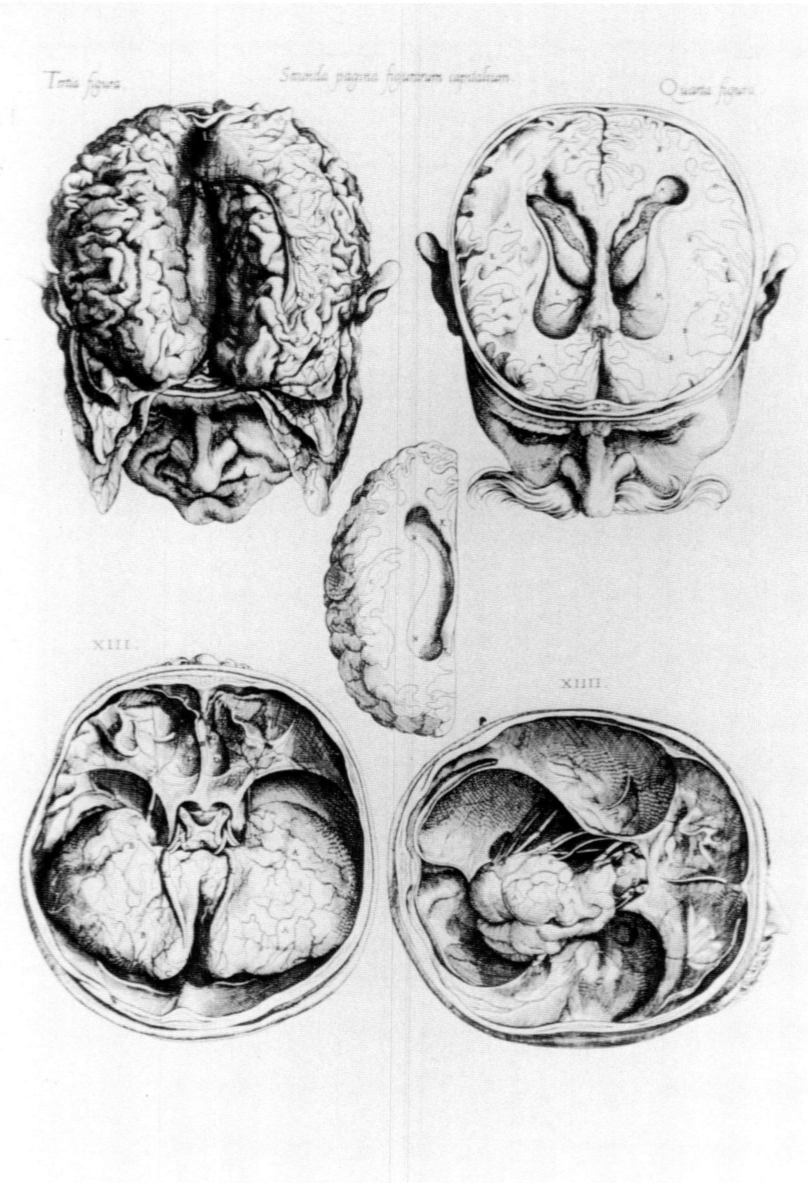

FIG. 9. Brain dissection of Vesalius.

the classıfication of Galen, into seven pairs. The structure of the lumbosacral plexus is one of the best to date. The brachial plexus, however, is imperfect. Two sets of roots of the spinal cord are not delineated and the description of the spinal cord itself is poor.

The seventh book of the *Fabrica* contains 15 diagrams of the brain, which are among the most outstanding drawings in neuroanatomy ever produced. The first dissection, representing a head from which the calvarium has been removed, accurately depicts the middle meningeal

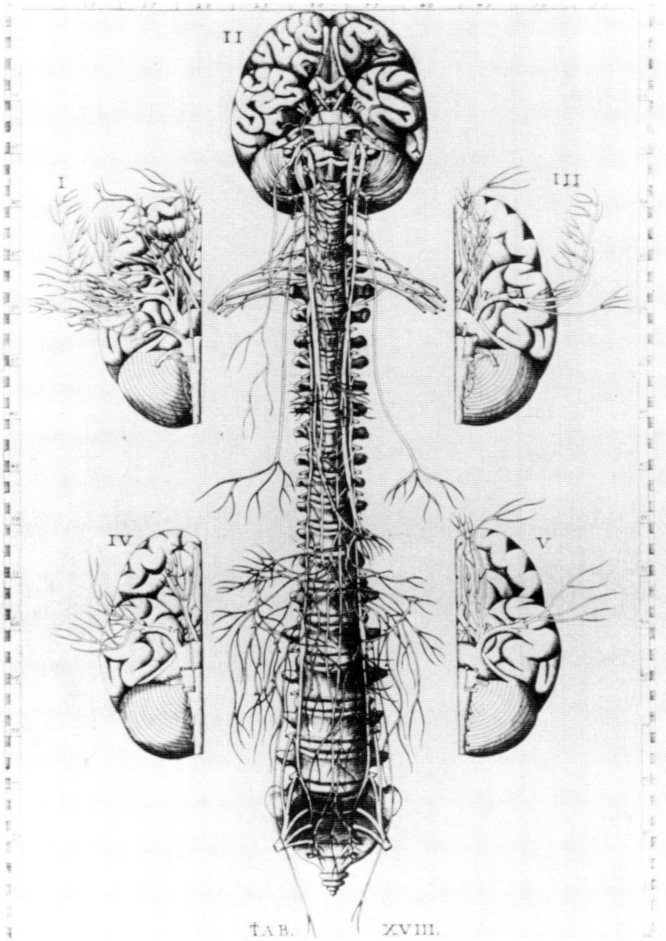

FIG. 10. Eustachius' portrayal of the nervous system.

artery meandering across the surface of the dura. In subsequent plates, horizontal sections through the brain at various levels reveal the entire internal structure of the human brain. Within the ventricular cavity, the engravings clearly portray the caudate nucleus, the thalamus, the stria terminalis, the fornix, and the choroid plexus. The distinction between gray and white matter structures is shown for the first time, including the cortical gray ribbon.

In the other engravings of the brain, the internal capsule and the lenticular nucleus are distinct, including the division of the latter into the putamen and globus pallidus. An admirable account of the midbrain with the pulvinar, the corpora quadrigemina, pineal gland, and the superior and middle cerebellar peduncles is also given. His description of the blood vessels in the brain is generally good, but for one reason or another he missed the hexagonal ring communicating vessels at the base of the brain.

Although Vesalius' concept of brain function was essentially Galenic, his anatomical detail was unique and held its accuracy through Willis in the 17th century and to Vicq d'Azyr in the 18th century. The English edition of the *Fabrica*, published in 1545 by Thomas Geminus, is one of the earliest (perhaps the second) works containing copper plates published

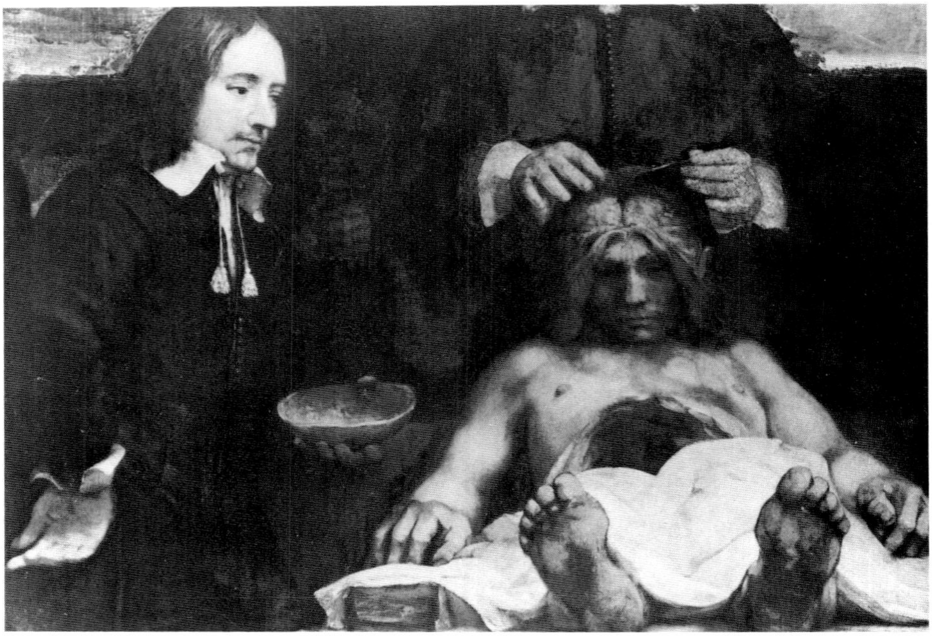

FIG. 11. Rembrandt's "Anatomy Lesson of Dr. Deymon."

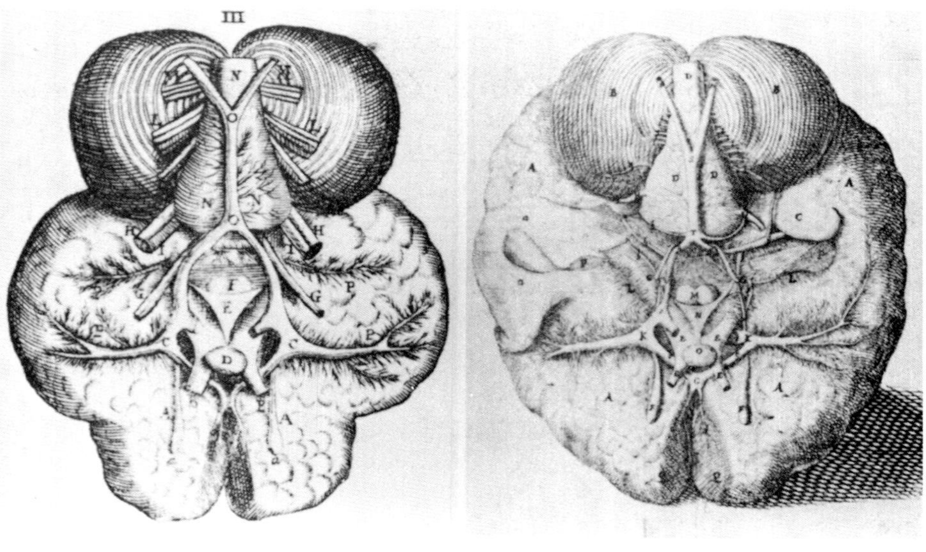

FIG. 12. The base of the brain shown by Vesling and Casserio.

in England. Figure 9, shown here, is of finer quality than its woodcut counterpart and shows in detail the structures described. Singer (14), has translated the seventh book into English. He pointed out that the most permanent achievement of Vesalius was his triumphant establishment of the graphic arts in the service of biological structure.

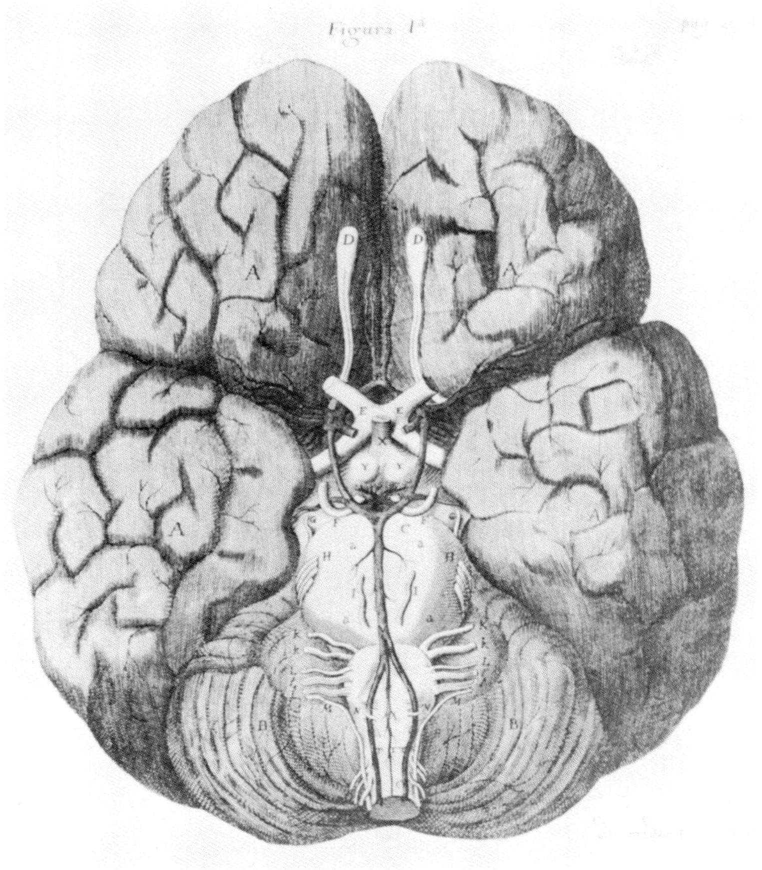

FIG. 13. Willis's engraving of the brain by Sir Christopher Wren.

A somewhat better Renaissance study of the base of the brain and sympathetic nervous system was made by Eustachius (15), second only to da Vinci and Vesalius. In anatomical illustration, Eustachius contributed significantly to neuroanatomy with his drawings of the sympathetic nervous system and the base of the brain. In the latter, the cranial nerves are more clearly and accurately rendered, and the pons is shown better than in earlier descriptions.

Eustachius' portrayal of the sympathetic chain shows it to be separate from the vagus nerve but rising from the abducens nerve, which he discovered. Although his fine copper plates were prepared in 1552, they were not published until the early 18th century. Figure 10, shown here, was so popular that it continued to be published in anatomical texts as late as Wister (16) in the 19th century.

The artistic epitome of neuroanatomy is Rembrandt's "Anatomy Lesson of Dr. Deymon," seen in Fig. 11. It was painted as a companion piece to his "School of Anatomy" for Dr. Nicholas Tulp, which is quite well known. Both paintings are in the Rijksmuseum in Amsterdam. This is only part of the original painting, as most of it was destroyed in a fire in 1723. All that is left is the portion showing the demonstration of the brain. Dr. Deymon is standing behind the corpse, but his head is not seen because it was destroyed in the fire.

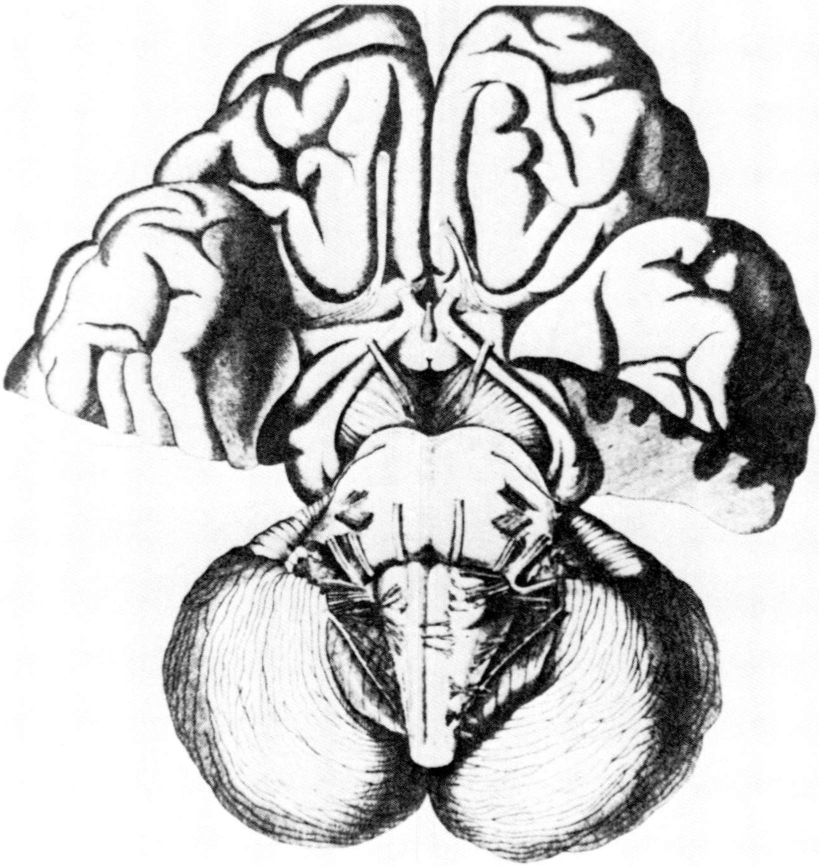

FIG. 14. Soemmerring's portrayal of the cranial nerves.

Traditionally, the most outstanding neuroanatomist of the 17th century was Thomas Willis, who was educated at Oxford with Richard Lower and Thomas Sydenham. Although Casserio (17) and Vesling (18) showed the arterial circle at the base of the brain (Fig. 12) in their works, it was named for Willis (Fig. 13). His portrayal of the neuroanatomical illustration in his *Cerebri Anatome* (19) was carried out by the noted artist and architect, Sir Christopher Wren. The word "neurology" was introduced by Willis and first appeared in Samuel Pordage's translation of Willis' *Cerebri Anatome* from Latin to English. Other 17th-century illustrated neuroanatomical works were those of Raymond Vieussens (20) and Humphrey Ridley (21). The spinal cord, showing differentiation between gray and white matter, was first illustrated by Geraud Blasius (22).

In the 18th century, one of the most remarkable works was that by Frederick Ruysch (23), who gave the earliest description of the arterial supply to the human brain using injection studies. He was the first to demonstrate the subarachnoid arterial anastomoses between the major cerebral arteries. Soemmerring (24) published a beautiful engraving of the base of the brain and was the first to portray the twelve cranial nerves (Fig. 14). In

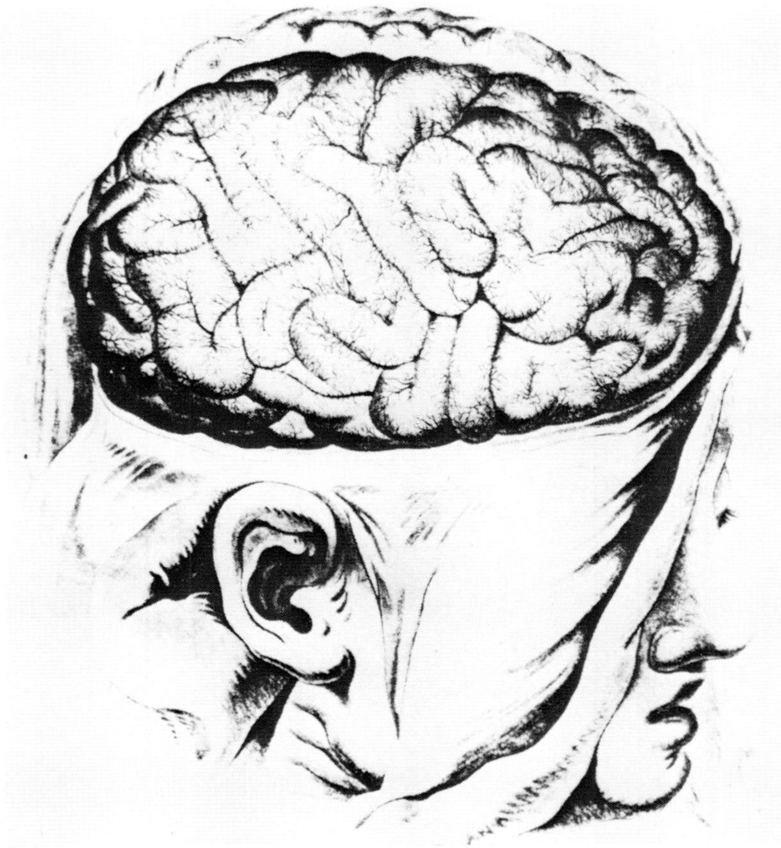

FIG. 15. Vicq d'Azyr's lithograph of the cerebral hemisphere.

Edinburgh, the three generations of the Monros contributed significantly to neuroanatomy. Specifically, Alexander Monro *secundus* published one of the best and up-to-date folio monographs (25). An Italian medical student, Francesco Gennari, was the first to portray artistically the laminar structure of the cerebral cortex. In his dissections, he was the first to observe a white line in the cortical substance of the occipital lobe, which was named for him (26).

The most significant achievement in the association between anatomical art and medical illustration using color came at the end of the 18th century with the invention of lithography or stone engraving. Up to this time, illustrations had been reproduced from woodcuts or from copper or steel engravings of one sort or another. This meant that the artist first had to make the drawing and an engraver then had to copy it and actually engrave or carve it into the wood, copper, or steel, a tedious and expensive process. Much of the quality and accuracy of the original drawing was sometimes lost in the engraving, and fine gradations of tone or shading were very difficult to reproduce. Lithography is a process of printing based on the mutual repulsion of oil and water. In the original lithographic process, the drawing was made on the stone with a grease crayon. The stone was then wet with water, but the water wets only the stone and not the greased areas. An oily ink was then applied,

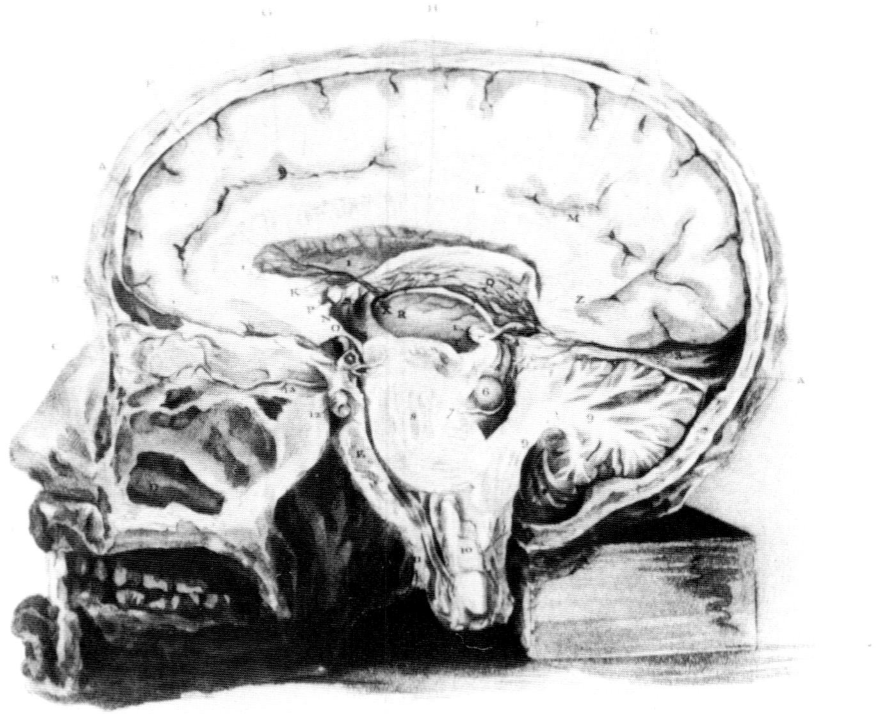

FIG. 16. Bell's drawing of a midline cut of the head.

and this in turn did not adhere to the wet stone but remained only on the crayon marks—the heavier the crayon the heavier the ink. The stone was then applied to the paper and a duplication of the drawing appeared. To reproduce colored illustrations, a separate drawing was made on a separate stone for each color, the drawing of course being very carefully and accurately registered. Each stone was then printed in a different colored ink, one superimposed on the other. Through lithography a number of beautiful and exquisitely illustrated anatomical, medical, and neurological texts appeared in the 19th century.

Lithography was first used in neuroanatomy by Vicq d'Azyr (27). Figure 15 shows a view of the head with the skull removed and the cerebral hemispheres exposed. The figure is interesting from the standpoint of anatomical eponyms. In this engraving, Vicq d'Azyr has shown for the first time the central fissure and the pre- and postcentral gyri. This plate was published in 1786. In 1829, Luigi Rolando described the pre- and postcentral gyri and the central fissure. Later, the anatomist Leuret named these structures for Rolando. When Leuret had prepared his treatise on the brain, he did not have a copy of Vicq d'Azyr's original edition that contained the plate showing the cerebral hemispheres. Leuret had only a later edition that, through faulty editorship, had lacked this plate. Thus, the cerebral convolutions that had been described over 50 years previously by Vicq d'Azyr were not named for him but for Rolando.

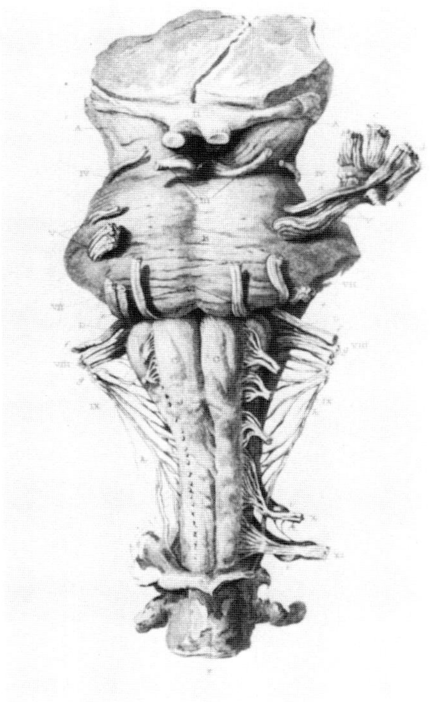

FIG. 17. Bell's drawing of the brain stem.

Anatomical illustration during the early part of the 19th century was characterized by the increased use made of color. Color printing after the style of Aselli or Gautier was not attempted. The finished impression, either copper plate or lithograph, was tinted by hand, either freehand or by means of stencils. Even with the cheapest of labor, it was an expensive process and quite unsatisfactory. Examples are shown of the use of hand-colored prints of various sorts. The plate of "Engravings of the arteries" by Charles Bell (28) is a stipple engraving, colored with a single color, red, along the course of the arteries. Some of the plates in Gall and Spurzheim's work (29) are in stipples strengthened by line engraving, a process very suitable to the reproduction of figures of the brain.

About 1830, steel plates gradually replaced copper. Line engraving was carried out after the main outlines and shadows had been worked onto the plate by means of etching. In this way, much time and much of the drypoint and engraver's work was saved. With the advent of the steel plate, finer lines could be etched or graved on the harder surface. Swan (30) published a series of plates of the sympathetic nervous system and the cerebral nerves. The plates were of steel and are of considerable artistic and anatomical merit.

From the standpoint of art and neurology, one of the outstanding combinations can be found in the work of Sir Charles Bell. Bell was born in Edinburgh in 1774 but later came to London and established himself as a surgeon. Not only are the illustrations in his neurological monographs of superb quality, but he also produced works for the artists, namely, "Anatomy of Expression" and "Anatomy and Philosophy of Expression as Connected with the Fine Arts." His works (31–33) on the nervous system were numerous and of extremely high quality, using the process of lithography (Figs. 16 and 17). His neurological works passed through several editions and many of them contained illustrations not used in earlier

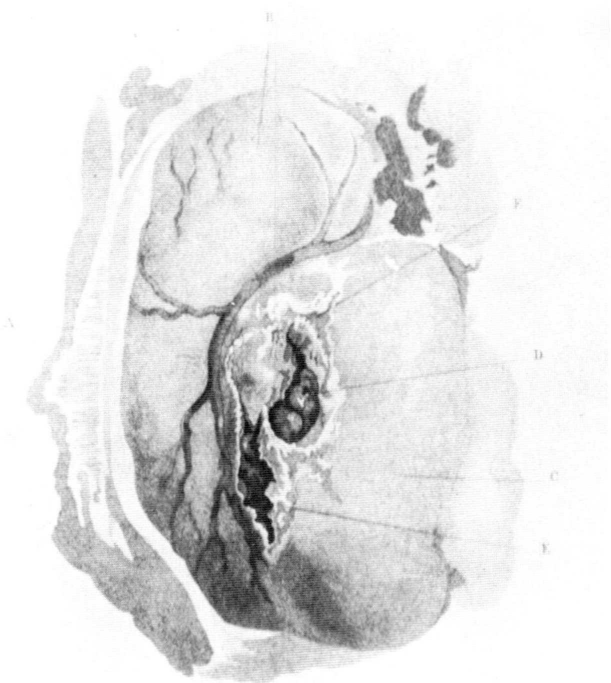

FIG. 18. Cheyne's drawing of a small hemorrhage in the basal ganglia.

editions. From a physiological standpoint, Bell is primarily remembered as the first to describe the functions of the anterior roots of the spinal cord. A controversy developed as to whether he or Magendie described the functions of the posterior roots. This dilemma is discussed at length in the recent publication of Cranefield (34).

During the remainder of the 19th century, many neurologists illustrated their own works. Copper and steel engraving were used as well as lithography and other methods of illustration. Beautiful neuroanatomical atlases were published in which lithography, photography, electroplating, and other devices of modern anatomical illustrations were utilized. In both neuroanatomy and neuropathology, the development of the microscope and different staining techniques inspired many anatomists and pathologists to illustrate their works themselves. Contributors to this field, along with the brothers John and Charles Bell, are Thomas Hodgkin, Jacob Henle, Wilhelm His, Lord Lister, Joseph Leidy, Alexander Auvert, James Hope, Hermann Lebert, and finally one of the most outstanding, Santiago Ramón y Cajal.

NEUROPATHOLOGY AND ART

Neuropathology as a separate science developed in the late 18th century with the work of Matthew Baillie. In the last chapter of his *Morbid Anatomy* (35) is a section on "Diseased appearances of the brain and it's membranes." Baillie's illustrations from an artistic standpoint leave something to be desired, but there are examples of tumors and cerebral hemorrhage as well as cursory descriptions of other brain lesions. Cheyne (36) was the first to

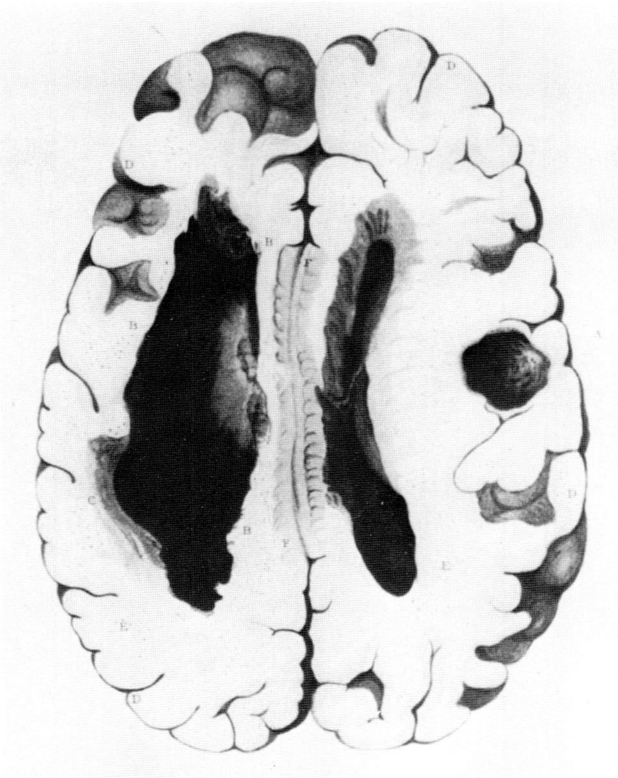

FIG. 19. Hooper's drawing of an intracerebral hemorrhage.

illustrate cerebral infarction (Fig. 18) with an engraving showing a lesion of the internal capsule and the thalamus. The corpus callosum, corpus striatum, and the thalamus, as well as the area of necrosis, are labeled.

Neuropathology as it is linked to art may be said to have begun with the work of Robert Hooper. He based his work (37) on over 4,000 autopsies performed at the St. Marylebone Infirmary over a period of 20 years. In his 1826 atlas, one of his main artistic contributions was a color lithograph of the base of the brain showing purulent meningitis. He also exhibited intracerebral hemorrhage (Fig. 19), brain abscess, tumors, and areas of softening. His *Morbid Anatomy of the Human Brain* is one of the first and, one might say, one of the most notable works in the early ancestry of neuropathology (38).

In France, Jean Cruveilhier, who became Professor of Pathology at the Faculty of Medicine in Paris, obtained his vast autopsy material from the dead house of the Salpêtrière. His atlas, *Anatomie Pathologique du Corps Humain* (39) contains the most beautiful colored lithograph that had yet been produced, truly a landmark in neuropathology. As well as describing the first epidermoid tumor, his plates give several views of a cerebellopontine angle tumor and a falx meningioma. There are splendid examples of intrinsic and extrinsic disease of the spinal cord, particularly multiple sclerosis (Fig. 20).

Cruveilhier's atlas contains clinical descriptions that have enough information in many of the case reports to allow us to arrive at our own diagnosis. More important is the fact that

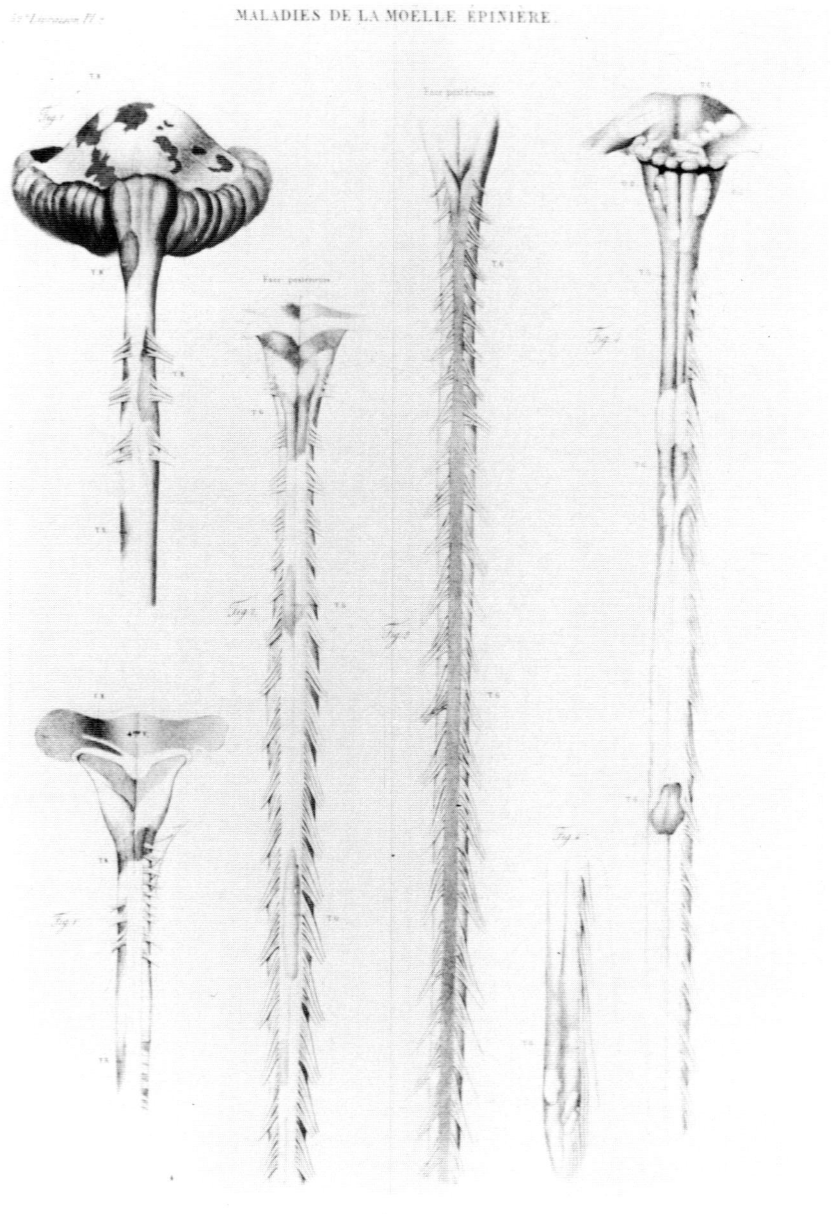

FIG. 20. Lithograph of the spinal cord showing multiple sclerosis by Cruveilhier.

Cruveilhier presented his material in a way that showed his understanding of certain basic differences in neurological conditions. For the most part, he was able to distinguish between patients with hemiplegia from a stroke and from a tumor. In cases of spinal cord disease, he distinguishes lesions of the cord itself from lesions compressing the spinal cord. Another of his contributions still valid today was his distinction between hemorrhagic cerebral infarction and ischemic cerebral infarction. From a clinical standpoint, he noted that hemor-

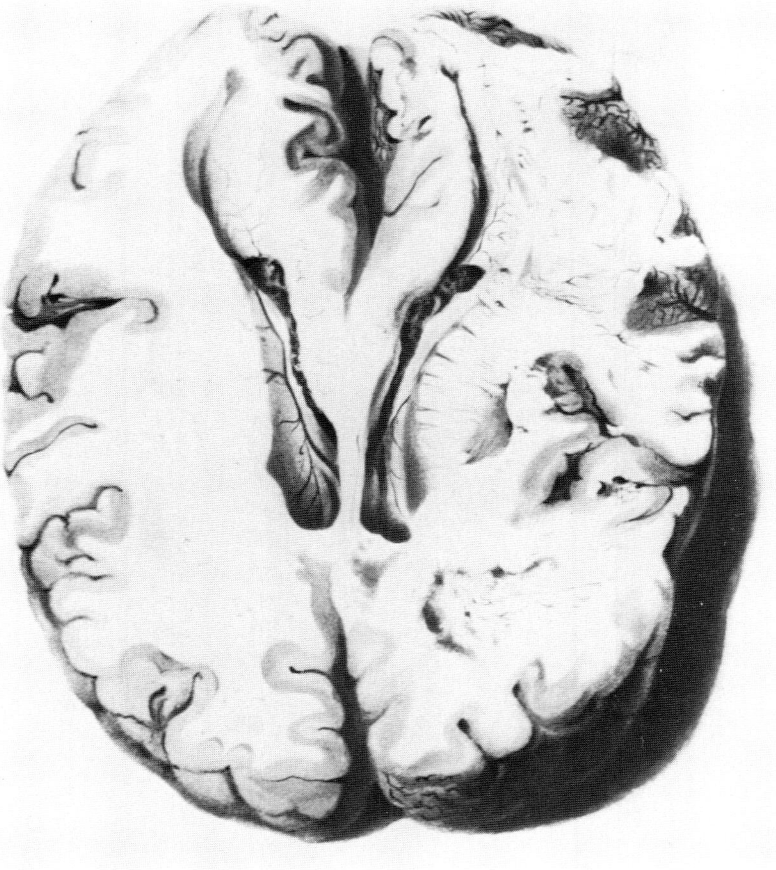

FIG. 21. A tumor of the right cerebral hemisphere from Bright's atlas.

rhagic infarction has a more abrupt onset in the clinical presentation than softening of the brain. His work was the first to unite clinical neurology and neuropathology (40).

One of the outstanding neuropathologists of the early 19th century was Sir Robert Carswell. After finishing his training in Glasgow, he went to Paris where he remained for three years, during which time he completed some 2,000 pathological drawings. These are preserved in the archives of University College in London and formed the basis of his *Pathological Anatomy* (41). Carswell himself prepared the lithographs of the colored drawings of disease structures that he had previously collected. Plate 4 of his atlas shows atrophy of the left cerebral peduncle and the left half of the pons and left pyramid from "Extensive destruction of the left copus striatum." His atlas also shows the first example of multiple sclerosis, described as "a peculiar disease state of the cord and pons Varolii accompanied with atrophy of the disc colored portion." This description appeared three years before Cruveilhier's classic portrayal of the same condition. Carswell's atlas falls somewhat short of the fine shades captured by Cruveilhier's, but both remain as lithographic milestones in neuropathology (42).

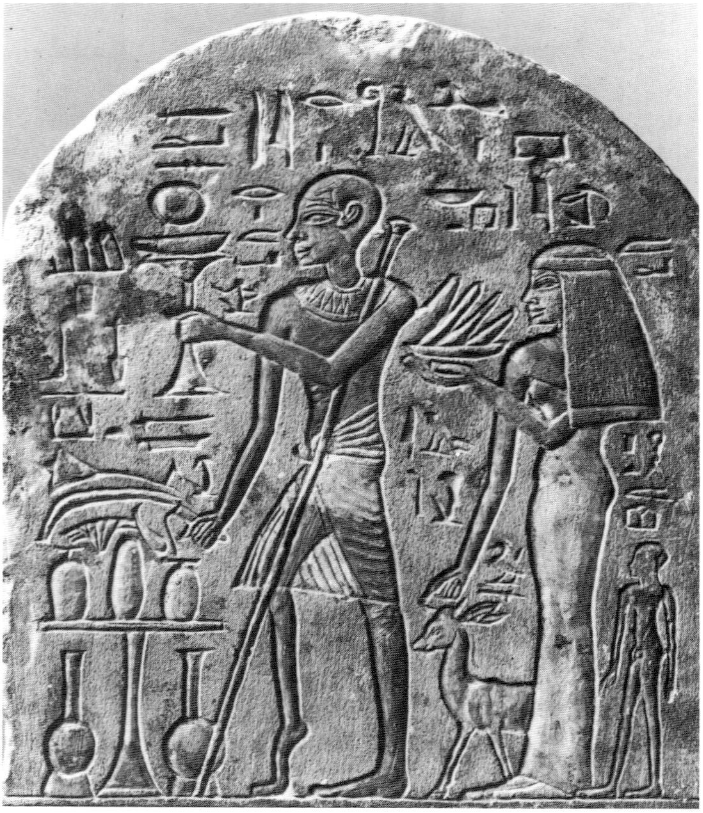

FIG. 22. The priest Ruma.

Although the works of Carswell and Cruveilhier appeared earlier, the remarkable neuropathology atlas of Richard Bright must be considered the most outstanding work of its type. Volume II contains his section on "Diseases of the brain and nervous system" (43), and although he is primarily remembered for his classic descriptions of glomerulonephritis and a differentiation between cardiac and renal dropsy, he nevertheless collected over 200 neuropathological cases, illustrated in 25 colored plates. These illustrations were accompanied by detailed descriptions which included the clinical history. Among these illustrative cases are examples of brain tumors (Fig. 21) along with a pontine glioma with hydrocephalus, staining of the meninges, but not of the brain, in jaundice, posttraumatic necrosis of the tips of the frontal and temporal lobes, a ruptured intercranial aneurysm, and cortical laminar necrosis from anoxic encephalopathy, as well as common examples of congenital, neoplastic, infectous, and vascular diseases of the brain.

CLINICAL NEUROLOGY AND ART

The earliest example of neurological disease portrayed in art is the funeral stele of the Priest, Ruma, from the 19th Egyptian dynasty. This 3,000- to 4,000-year-old work is the first example of what is probably the residue of poliomyelitis. The priest Ruma, accompanied by his wife, is shown in Fig. 22 approaching a small table carrying offerings to the god

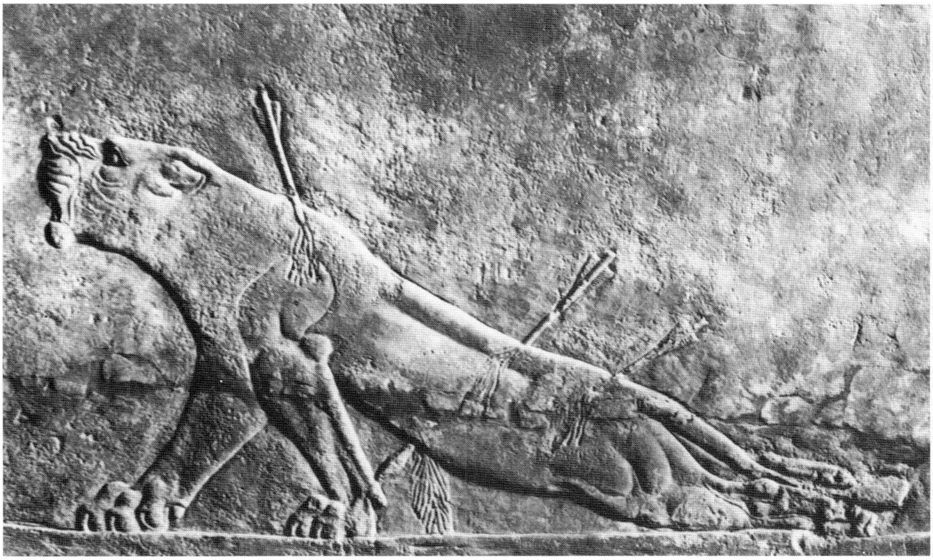

FIG. 23. The wounded lioness.

Astarta. His leg is shortened and his foot is atrophic; he is only able to walk on his toes using a cane. This work is in the Carlsburg Museum in Copenhagen. In the British Museum, there is a stone work dating from 650 B.C. showing a wounded lioness (Fig. 23). The animal's spinal cord has obviously been wounded by the arrows, yet in her dying anguish, the lioness still crawls forward snarling at her tormentors. The arrow on the right most likely has pierced the spinal cord causing paralysis of her lower legs.

There is little of specific neurological interest in Greek and Roman art; the votive tablets in the Asklepian Temples at Cos have recorded such items as paralysis of the extremities, but no votive tablets showing neurological disease have been uncovered. Figure 24 is a stone relief entitled "The Dying Bacchante." This most likely is an example of hysteria or perhaps someone starting to have a seizure. To the far right, the woman is swooning or has fallen. Seizures were called at this time "the Sacred Disease" and were well known in the Hippocratic era and later in the Roman period.

An unusual 15th-century carving in pink sandstone shows the head of a man with facial paralysis. This example (Fig. 25) of Bell's palsy is a piece of stonework from Saint John's Church in Strasbourg. The man has an obvious droop to the left side of his face, which gives him a rather grotesque appearance.

One of the most detailed examples of neurological disease portrayed artistically is in a fugitive sheet (Fig. 26) of 1620, at the bottom of which is a detailed history. The patient is a 40-year-old furniture maker from Innsbruck. He was healthy until six years previously, when he developed a toothache that was followed by stiffness of his neck. Three days later, he had severe pain in his left arm, in his back, and then in all of his limbs. Later, his arms and legs became stiff and paralyzed. For the next 15 years, with the exception of the ability to move his eyes and tongue, he was said to have resembled a wooden statue. The fugitive

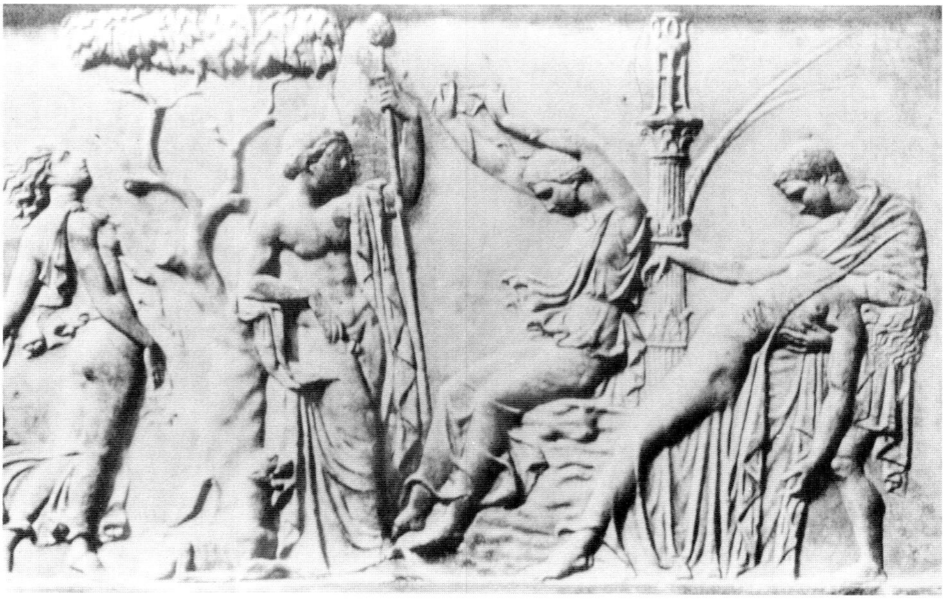

FIG. 24. The "Dying Bacchante."

sheet shows an asthenic man with atrophy of both arms and legs, with flexion contractures in his legs. There could be a number of neurological illnesses that could have caused his quadriparesis. With the exception of the ability to be able to move his mouth, he could be an example of akinetic mutism. Quite possibly, he may have had an attack of cervical myelitis or meningitis with inflammation of the meninges around the spinal cord producing subsequent damage of the cord. This could have originated from the septic focus in his tooth.

In the 16th century, Peter Brueghel the Elder did a number of subjects of medical interest; for example, Fig. 27 is an engraving of a painting in the Albertina in Vienna. This depicts a pilgrimage to Molenbeck. The engraving was made in 1642 by Hendrik Hondius. One can see men dragging women afflicted by St. Vitus' dance. This may be considered to be one example of mass hysteria, which occurred in repeated epidemics, particularly in the Rhineland in the 14th and 15th centuries. Although these patients show gait and movement disorders that could be hysterical, one might postulate this could well be a postencephalitic movement disorder that occasionally follows certain forms of epidemic encephalitis (44). Brueghel also painted contemporary scenes of persecutions, highway robbers, and punitive expeditions. These seem to be a form of protest against the arbitrariness and cruelty of his time. He added to his pictures as many cripples, beggars, and blind men as he could fit in. These pictures are primarily of interest because of their satirical content, their caricatural and symbolic execution, as well as their primitive and blunt style. They also have a medical pertinence that can be seen in the suffering and sick bodies that the artist observed in minute detail.

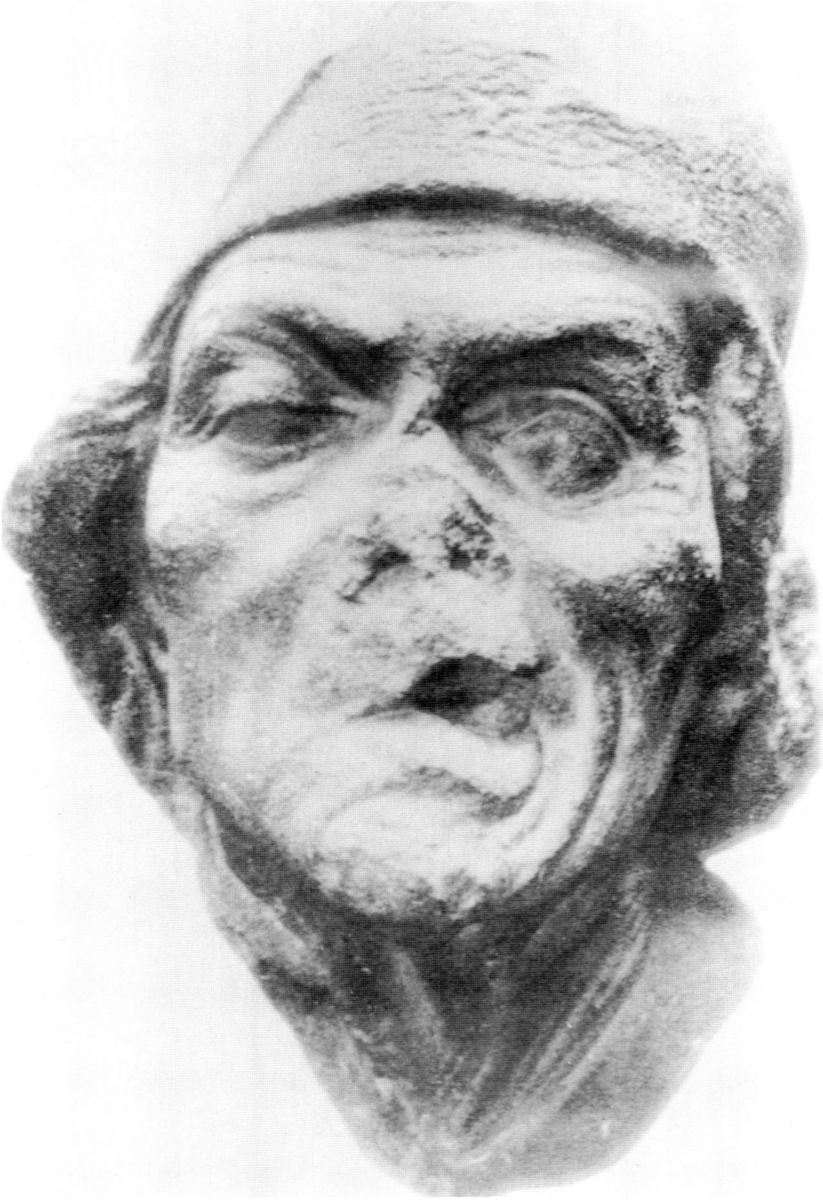

FIG. 25. Paralysis of the seventh cranial nerve.

The 17th-century painting shown in Fig. 28, by Jose Ribera is in the Louvre in Paris. It is entitled "The Clubfoot." The boy appears to have a right hemiparesis. The note in his left hand reads: "Give me alms, for the love of God"; it suggests that he cannot speak and thus may be aphasic. His intelligent expression, broad brows, and twinkled eyes seem to exclude the diagnosis of idiocy. The posture of his right hand and his clubfoot probably indicate a long-standing lesion of the left cerebral hemisphere. In fact, this is an example

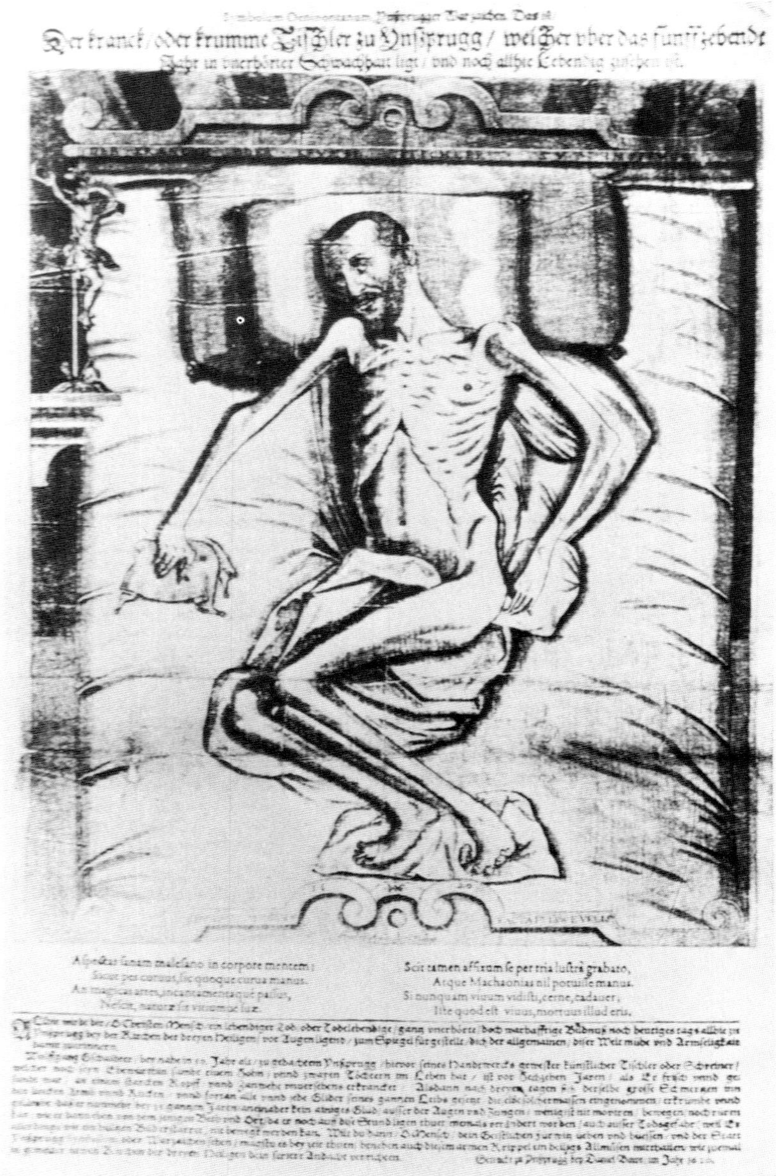

FIG. 26. Fugitive sheet of 1620.

of infantile hemiparesis. The painting also most likely represents the first and only graphic portrayal of aphasia.

Some diseases occur more often in artistic work than others. Hysteria and epilepsy are such examples, as in Fig. 29, an engraving entitled "Agitations du convulsionaires." As pointed out previously, epidemic hysteria was as common in the 17th century as it was during the Middle Ages and the Renaissance. One of the main problems that Charcot had

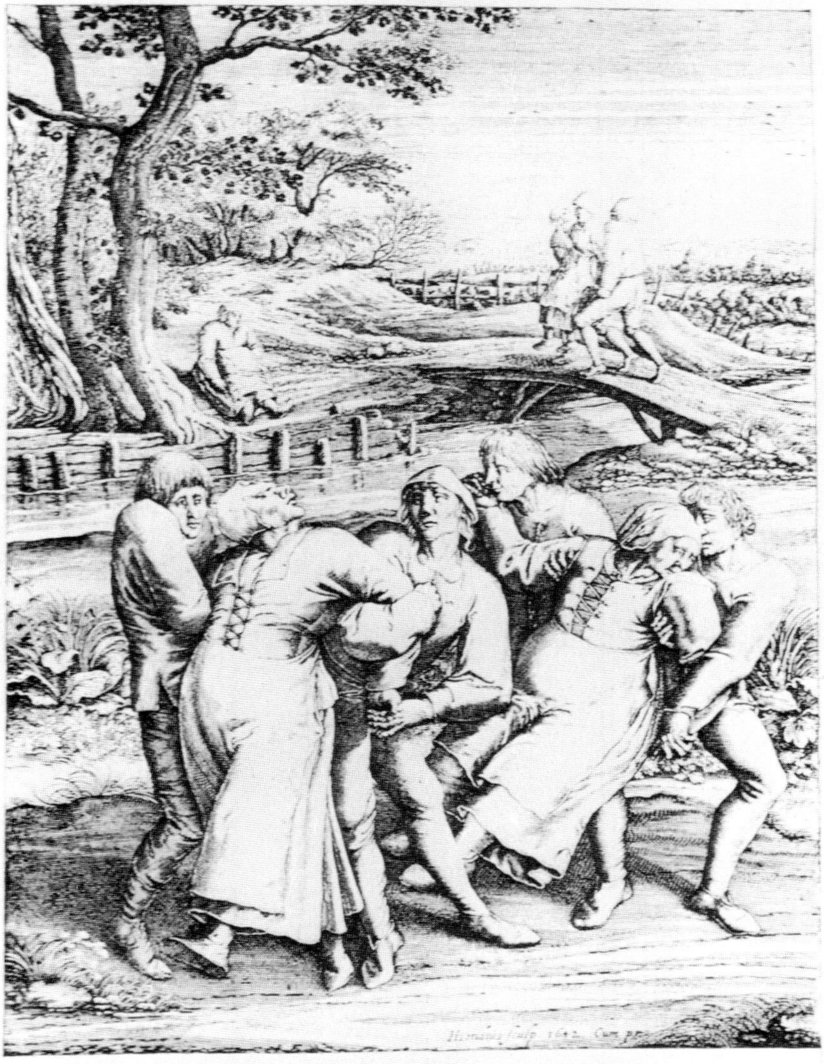

Fig. 148. Tanzwütige nach Pieter Brueghel d. Ä.
Radierung von Hondius (1642).

FIG. 27. St. Vitus' dance.

when he first took charge of the Salpêtrière was the separation of the malingerers and hysterics from the true epileptics.

One of the more amusing examples of neurological disease in art in the 18th century is in part of the engraving, "The Election," by William Hogarth. Figure 30 shows a man with an obvious severe neurological disease characterized by strabismus and postural movement

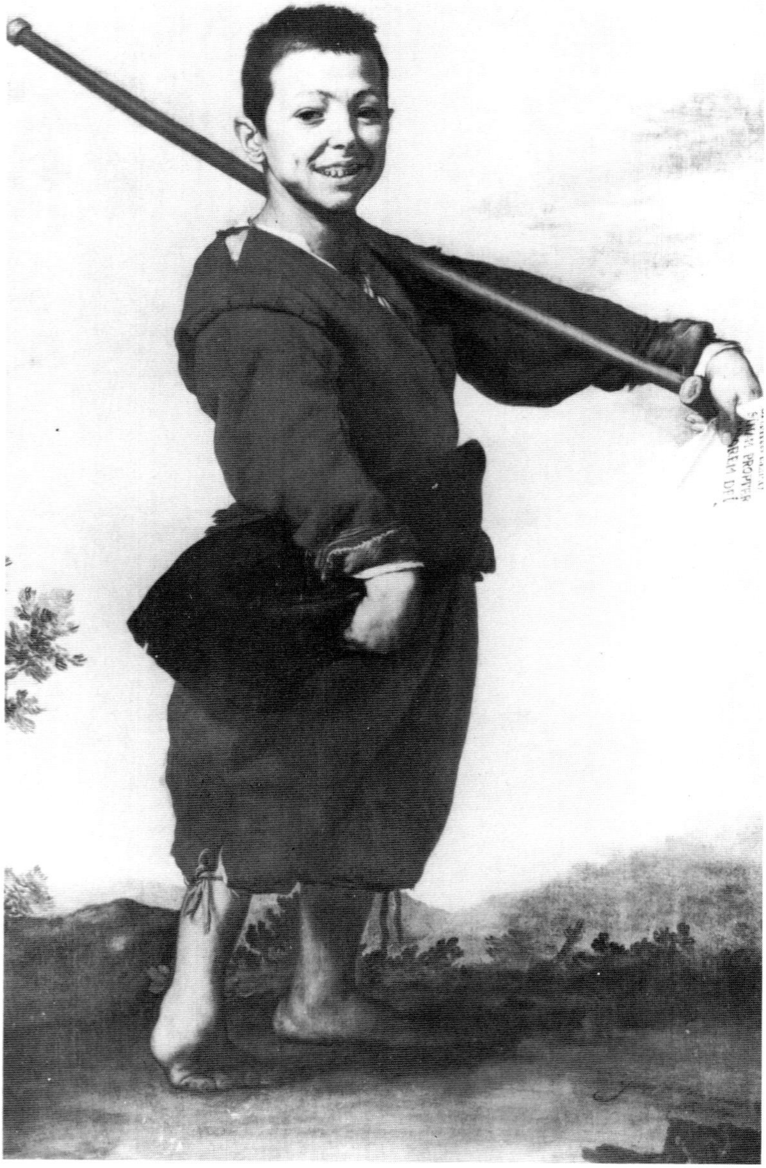

FIG. 28. "The Clubfoot" by Ribera.

abnormalities; he could well be a patient with Huntington's chorea. This engraving is a satire by Hogarth concerning the 18th-century election laws in England.

The formal union of art and neurology at its epitome can by seen in the work of Jean-Martin Charcot, the greatest neurologist of France. He became Professor of Pathology at the Faculty of Medicine in 1862. At the age of 36 years, he was appointed Chief Physician and Professor of Neurology at the Saltpêtrière. His descriptions of neurological disease

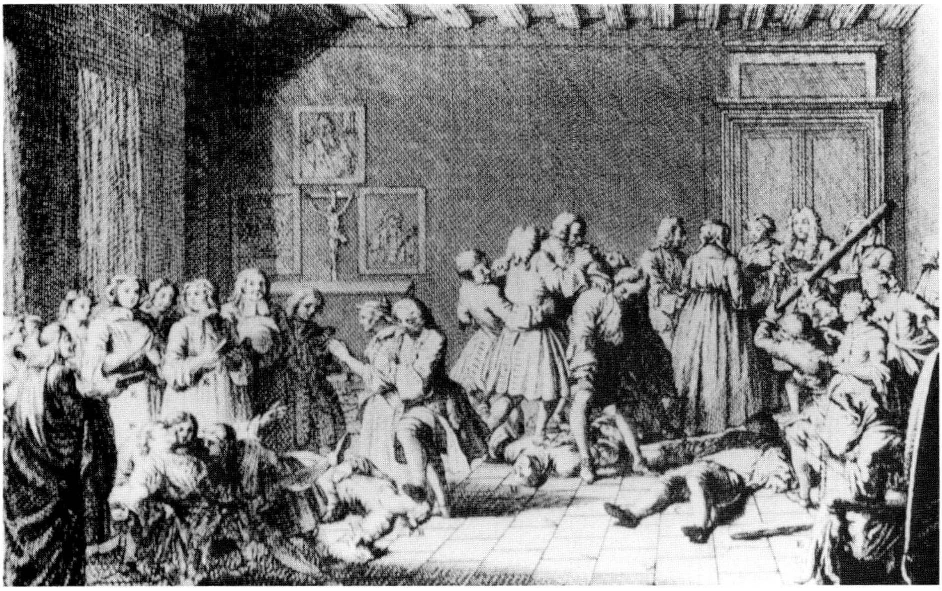

FIG. 29. Engraving of an epidemic of hysterical epilepsy.

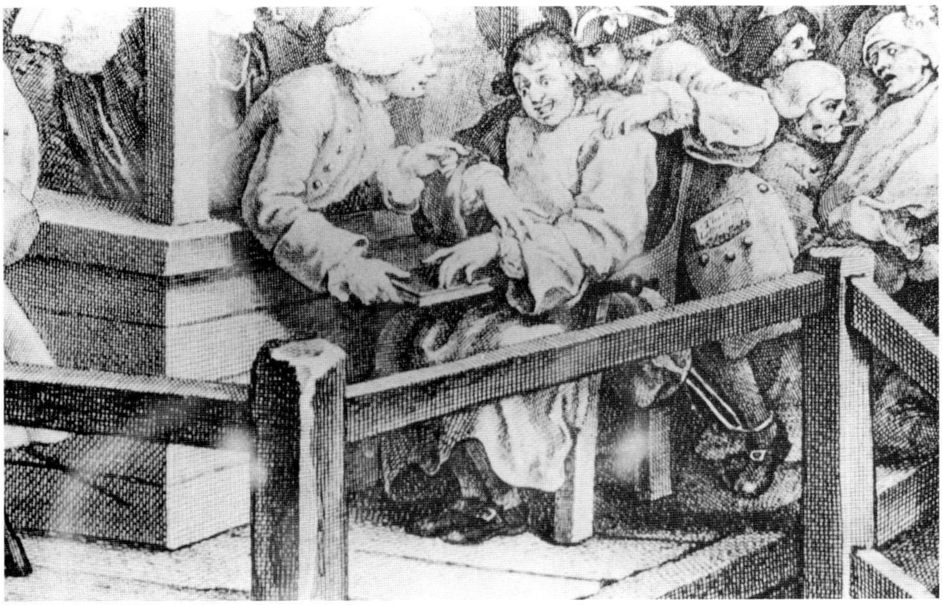

FIG. 30. Engraving by Hogarth.

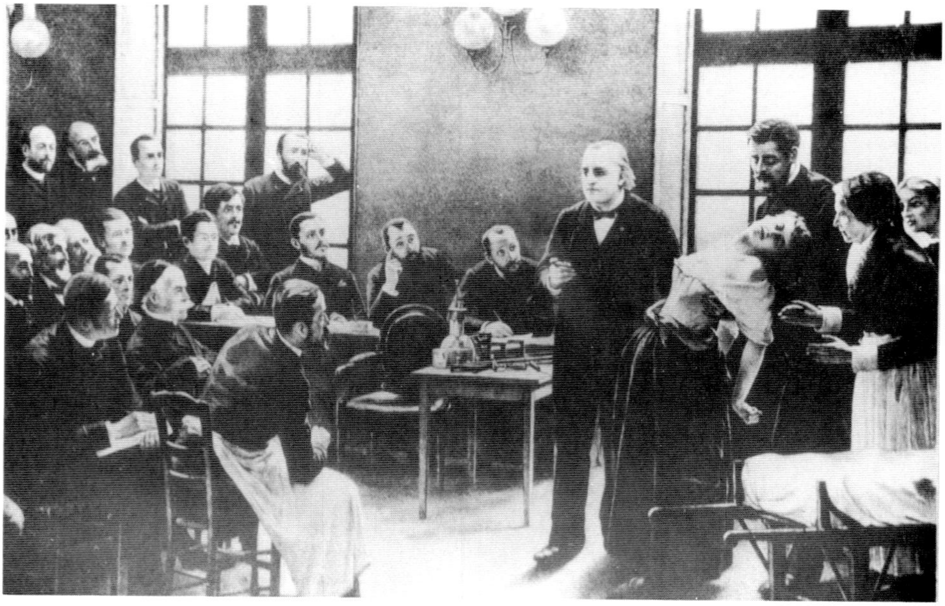

FIG. 31. Jean-Martin Charcot lecturing.

are legendary, as well as his neurological capability. In addition, he had an inherent unique artistic quality. From his youth, Charcot drew well. During his numerous voyages, he made sketches of churches, houses, unique buildings, sculpture, and of people native to the various regions in which he traveled. He always enclosed sketches in his letters to his family when he was traveling. His faculty to discern in a country scene or in a human body certain essential contours, to perceive instantly a pattern, and to be able to isolate from this pattern the elements necessary for its expression, and to do it exactly, in spite of all revelant details, was a faculty that Charcot possessed in a high degree. When he was in the hospital, he drew patients who exhibited unusual features.

At his famous Tuesday lectures (Fig. 31), Charcot appeared with his pupils and seated himself at a little table, sideways to the audience and looking across the stage. The patients were placed facing the audience behind footlights and sometimes further illuminated by spotlights from the calcium burner at the back. In a low, clear, distinct voice, Charcot proceeded to examine the patient, elucidating the case as he went by mimicking the various gaits, tremors, ticks, spasms, cramps, and postures, as well as sensory disturbances that were essential to the diagnosis. To locate individual abnormalities, anesthetic or hyperesthetic zones and the like, the patient was often examined nude. For chalk drawings of sensory abnormality and hysteria and other disorders, he was first to sketch the outline of the female figure that frequently appeared in textbooks of the period. He would also skillfully illustrate with colored chalk drawings on the blackboard the site and character of the lesion. He drew his own illustrations for his neurology texts, portraying both clinical and pathological lesions.

His ideals on painting and sculpture were very eclectic; he liked especially the sculpture of ancient Greece, the Italian paintings of the Renaissance, and Flemish and Dutch paintings. He admired the painter Delacroix and always kept in his office drawer an original album of this artist's watercolors and sketches. In his house at the Boulevard Saint Germain, he had

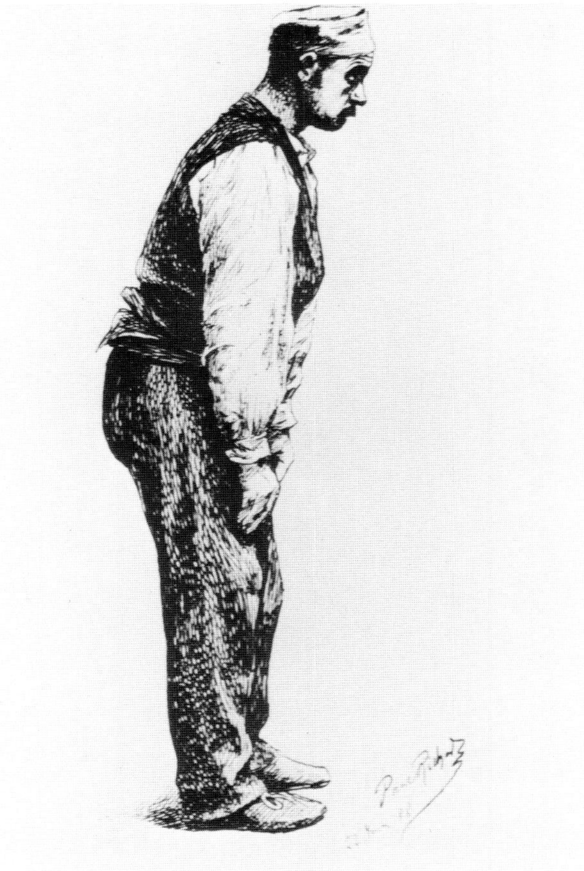

FIG. 32. Parkinson's disease.

a studio where he painted on porcelain or enamel. He copied several times the enamels of Leonard Limousin, showing the twelve apostles. In addition, he copied the "Dance of the Fools" of Albrecht Dürer on large porcelain slabs to decorate one of the facades of his house.

Charcot began to collect copies of paintings, engravings, and statuary representing nervous disease, the results of which were not published until some 34 years later. The albums of 1887 and 1889 with Richer are the work of a lifetime of steady research (45,46). In many ways, they are so exhaustive in scope that it would be impossible to improve upon them. They contain all the essential figurations that are unique in the combination of art and medicine. In 1888, Charcot began publishing the *Nouvelle Iconographie de la Salpêtière*. Most of the drawings were done by Charcot's distinguished artist, Dr. Paul Richer, formerly an intern of Charcot's and later Chief of the Laboratory at the Salpêtrière (47). Richer was also made Professor of Creative Anatomy at the National School of Fine Arts and was a member of the Institute and of the Academy of Medicine. One must agree with Strümpell and Erb that Charcot was an artist practicing medicine (48–50).

Figure 32 is a drawing of a patient with Parkinson's disease from Charcot's journal. The typical characteristics of this disorder are obvious. The patient has a stooped posture, his

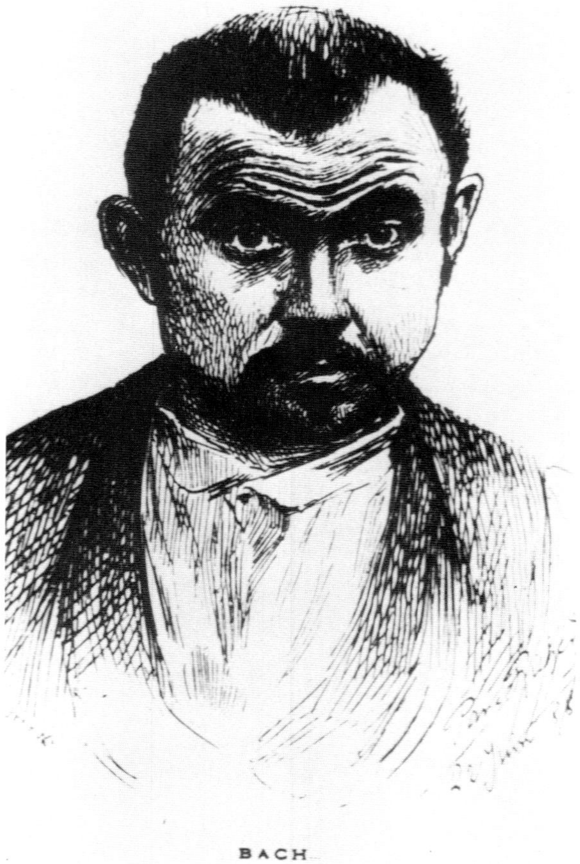

FIG. 33. Facial expression in Parkinson's disease.

arms are immobile, and his hands are held flat to his side. If he were to start to walk, one might imagine that his steps would be small and slow. Figure 33 shows the facial expression of the same patient. Here, graphically portrayed, is the masked immobile facies that are seen in any patient with Parkinson's disease. These drawings were done on July 22, 1888 by Richer.

Another artistic work is in the form of a sculpture. This bust (Fig. 34) was made by Richer and shows a woman with a glossolabial-pharyngeal form of bulbar palsy. In this condition, the muscles of the lips, tongue, and throat are paralyzed by a disease process that is similar to progressive muscular atrophy. The mouth hangs open and her tongue droops out, and she has the typical facies of a patient with progressive bulbar palsy.

In England, art and neurology were united in the works of Sir William Gowers, who was a clinician and, like Charcot, an artist. Gowers, onetime a professor of clinical medicine at University College Hospital, was appointed in 1870 as the first medical registrar of the National Hospital, Queen Square, and in 1872 he became physician to the hospital.

Gowers had great capabilities as an artist, which he developed during his youth. He was able to etch and draw general subjects as easily as medical. His drawings and etchings were often made during holidays in East Anglia and were exhibited once at the Royal Academy.

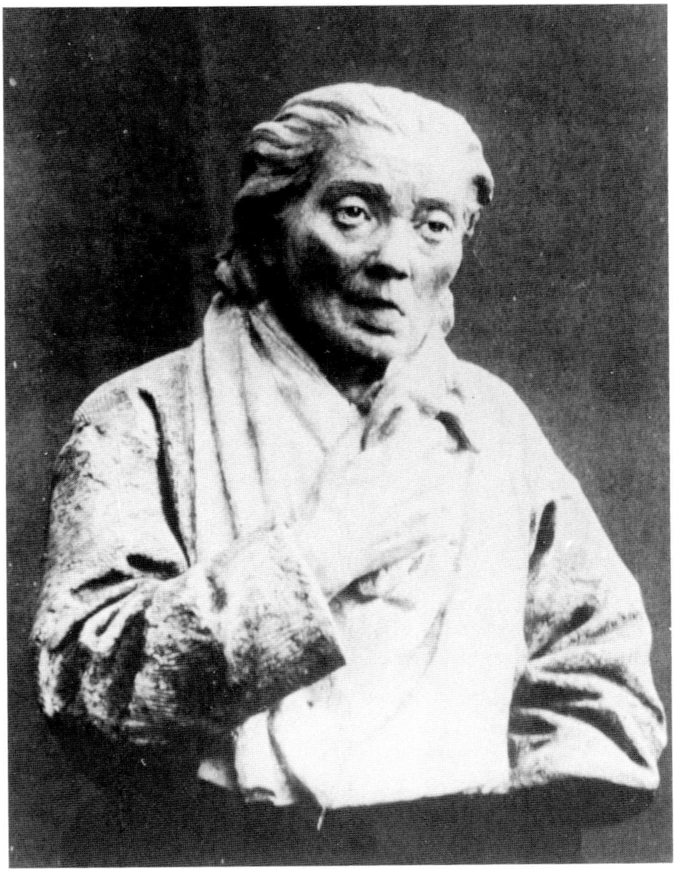

FIG. 34. Sculpture by Richer of a woman with progressive bulbar palsy.

Gowers made many original contributions to clinical neurology, which were brought together in his *Manual* (51). This was by far the most ambitious treatise on neurology that had so far been attempted in any language. The manual was essentially a personal accomplishment, for Gowers based his clinical descriptions on his own rich experience, shrewdly observing and carefully documenting the neurological disorders he encountered. Macdonald Critchley (52,53) called this work "the Bible of neurology." This has withstood the test of time in that those considering the report of a new clinical entity are advised to consult the *Manual* before claiming originality.

In this work and other writings, Gowers employed a prose style that was studiously clear and impressive. The illustrations were nearly all his own work, and by means of suppressing unnecessary graphic details, he was able to present cases in a manner that even modern photography cannot achieve. His illustration (Fig. 35) of a brain tumor in the posterior aspect of the cerebral hemisphere is as vivid as any of the clinical atlases previously described. One of his most interesting contributions is his drawing (Fig. 36) showing embolism of the basilar artery and occlusion of the left vertebral artery. The latter is shown cut open at l-v. The paler embolus, E, can be distinguished from the secondary thrombosis behind.

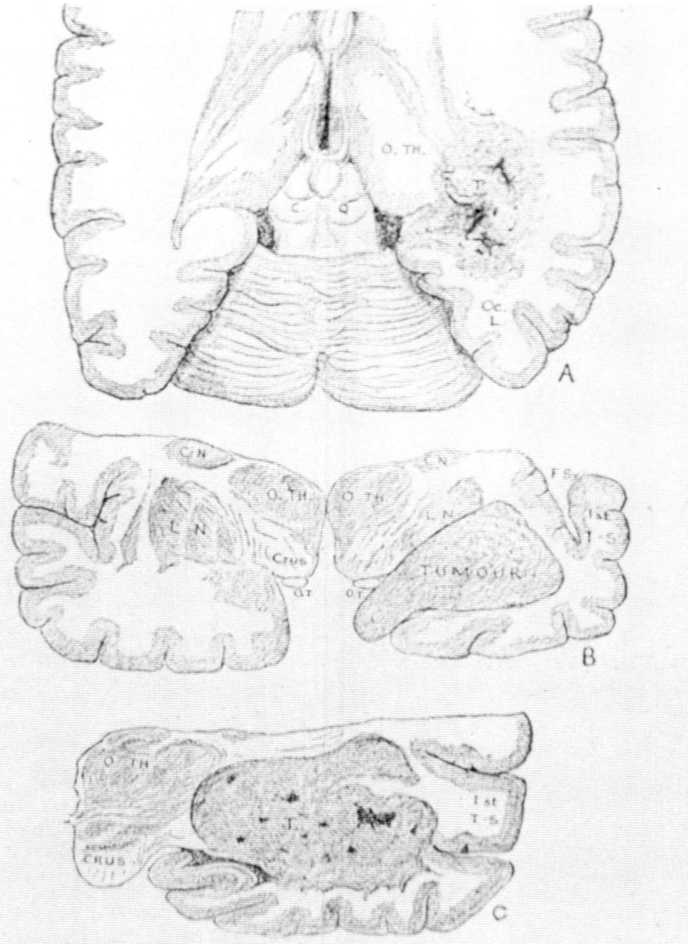

Fig. 136.—Tumour, beginning between the right optic thalamus and first temporal convolution and extending inwards from the temporal lobe, so as to compress the optic tract (Fig. 71, p. 145). A, horizontal section through the posterior parts of both hemispheres; T, tumour, with small irregular cavities, due to softening of its tissues; B, transverse section through the middle of the thalamus; C, through the posterior part of the thalamus. The patient suffered from hemianopia, fits beginning with an auditory aura (sound of bells referred to the opposite ear), optic neuritis, and hemiplegia.

VOL. II. 32

FIG. 35. Gowers' illustration of a brain tumor.

The history of the localization of cerebral function, described by Clarke and Dewhurst (4), had as its beginning a rather unique phenomenon called phrenology. The concept of the specific localization of function in the brain was approached in the early 19th century in a somewhat fantastic form by the anatomists, Gall and Spurzheim. Gall had noted that some individuals with certain intellectual qualities had interesting cranial prominences. From this notion, he and Spurzheim propounded phrenology, which was a belief that specific

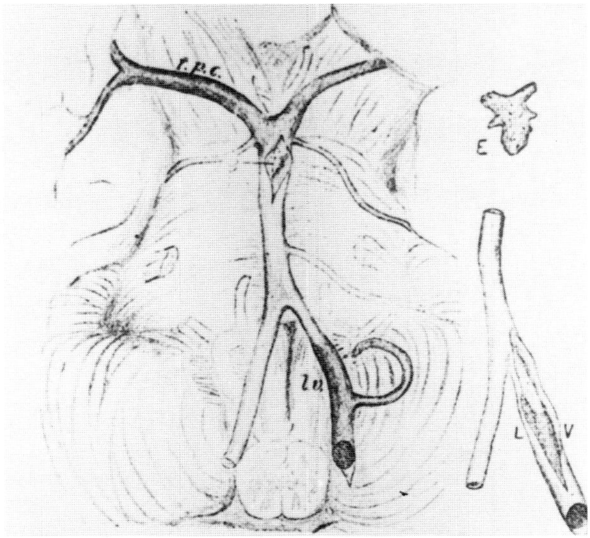

FIG. 36. Gowers' drawing of a basilar artery embolus.

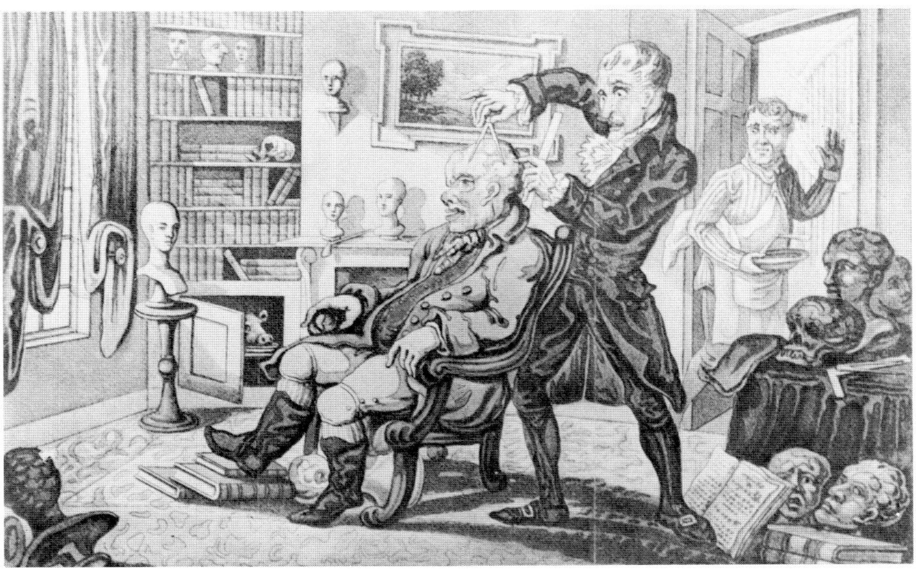

FIG. 37. Phrenology cartoon by Cocking.

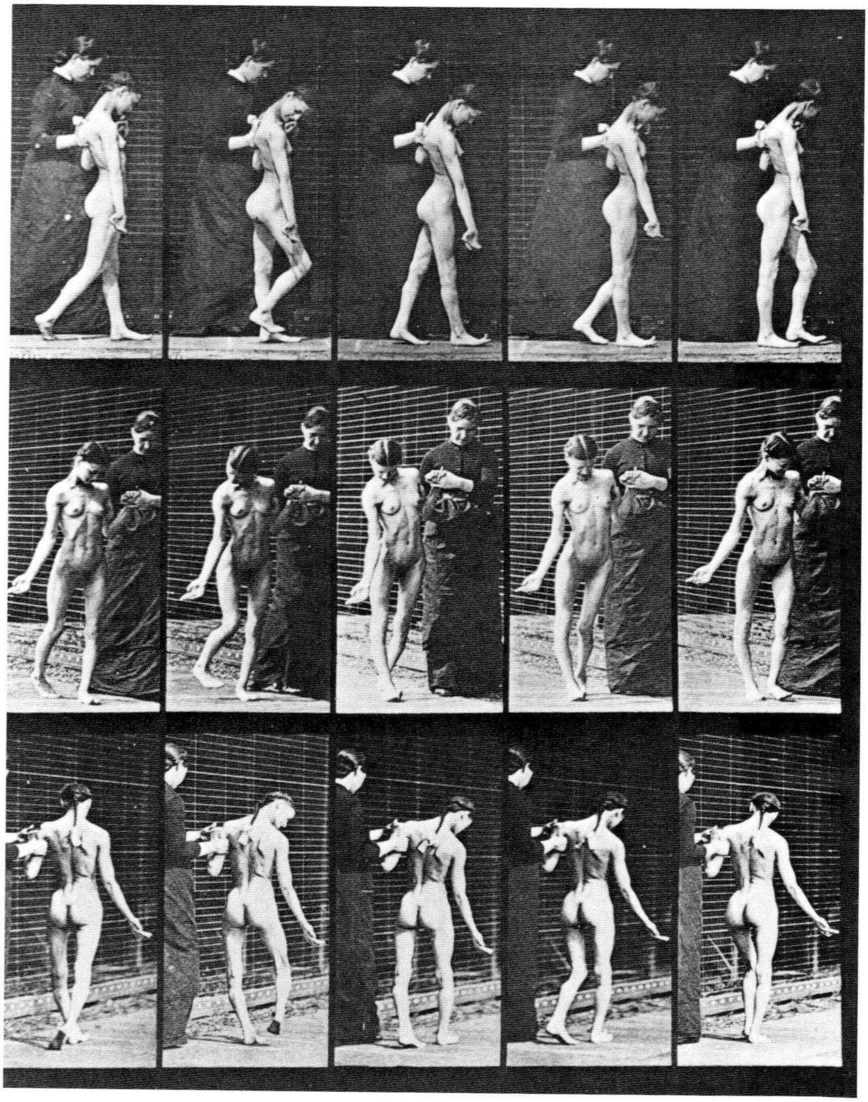

FIG. 38. Motion picture of spastic diplegia.

mental faculties were associated with certain bumps or prominences on the skull. This was quite the fashion, as shown in Fig. 37, during the latter part of the 19th century. Phrenology, however, soon became quite controversial, and Gall had to leave Vienna. Spurzheim's propagandism led to the formation of secret phrenological societies and journals in Great Britain and the United States. Exploited by quacks and charlatans, however, phrenology soon became an object of derision among scientific men and finally vanished as more scientific data were gathered on cerebral localization.

With the development of photography, neurology and art became a more exact science. The first photographic portrayal of neurological disease in art is said by Cuthdertcon (54)

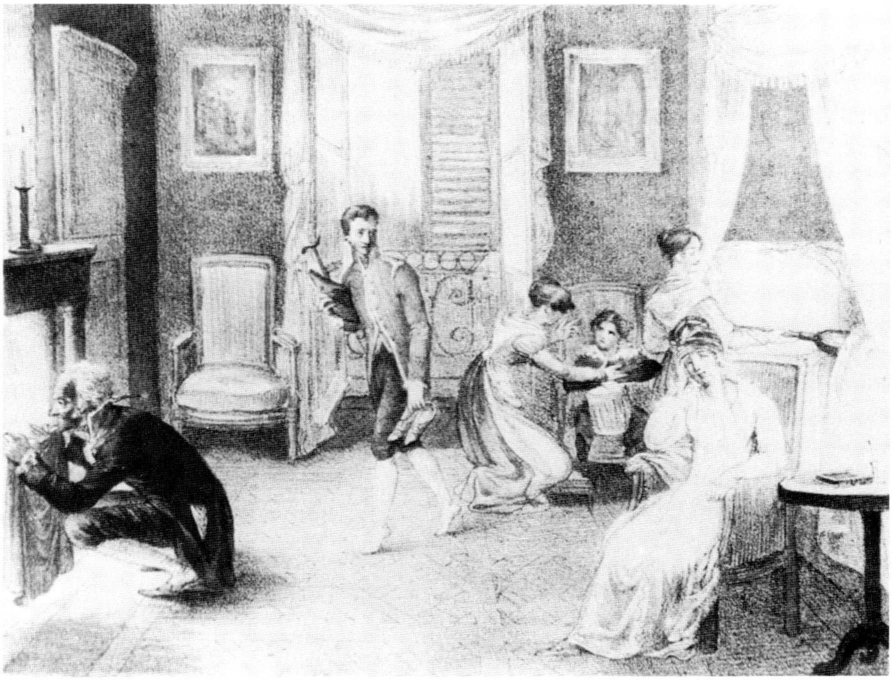

FIG. 39. Migraine.

to be in Duchenne's *Album* (55). This is primarily a photographic collection of patients with progressive muscular atrophy. A more graphic photographic or motion picture display of neurological diseases is in Muybridge's *Human and Animal Locomotion* (56). Muybridge, working in 1887 at the University of Pennsylvania, displayed various forms of walking, standing, and running in children and adults. He collaborated with Francis Dercum, Professor of Neurology at Jefferson Medical College, to show in motion pictures for the first time patients with neurological disease. The patient shown in Fig. 38 appears to have a scissor gait, which is characteristic of spastic diplegia. In addition, she has abnormal posturing and movements of her hands.

As a final example of neurology and the graphic arts, one cannot omit the cartoonists and caricaturists (Fig. 39). This early 19th-century cartoon depicts a woman with migraine. The lady who is seated on the chair is suffering from a severe headache. A servant is shielding the bright light of the fire while her husband quietly tiptoes away. Her child is being restrained from playing with his drum and another servant warms her bed.

In Fig. 40, we have a poor man struck down by apoplexy. The accompanying caption in this 1823 lithographic cartoon has an amusing but all-too-truthful expression. While his wife is away in the country, the man resolves to indulge his appetites. He invites a young cousin to join him in the festivities. Warm punch, a splendid meal, and the little cousin are too much, and our patient suddenly falls unconscious. The frightened cousin runs for the portress who summons the doctor. They prepare to bleed the patient while casting scolding glances

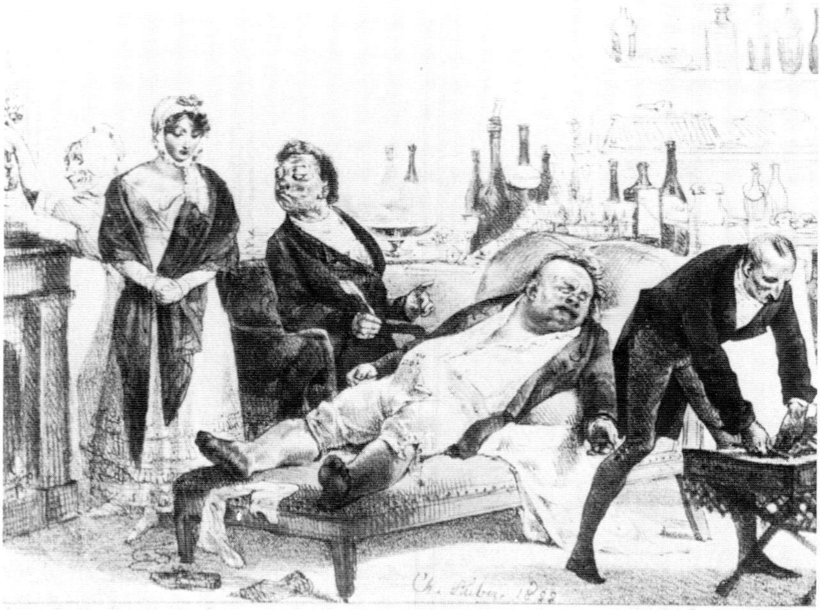

FIG. 40. Apoplexy.

at the little cousin. The author reflects that after death on the battlefield, which is living prompt and glorious, sudden death by apoplexy is the most beautiful.

ACKNOWLEDGMENT

I wish to thank Marion Laboratories, particularly Dr. Robert N. Henderson, for support in the preparation and presentation of this work.

REFERENCES

1. Herrlinger, R. (1970): *History of Medical Illustration*. Editions Medical Rara, New York.
2. Rousselot, J.: *Medicine in Art, a Cultural History*. McGraw-Hill, New York.
3. McHenry, L. C., Jr. (1969): *Garrison's History of Neurology*. Charles C. Thomas, Springfield, Illinois.
4. Clarke, E., and Dewhurst, K. (1972): *An Illustrated History of Brain Function*. University of California Press, Berkeley, California.
5. Singer, C. (1957): *A Short History of Anatomy and Physiology from the Greeks to Harvey*. Dover, New York.
6. Choulant, L. (1962): *History and Bibliography of Anatomical Illustration*, translated and edited by Mortimer Frank. Hafner, New York.
7. Dana, C. L. (1916): *Proc. Charaka Club*, 4:63.
8. Fries, L. (1519): *Spiegel der Artzny*. J. Grieninger, Strasbourg.
9. Berengario, J. (1523): *Isagogae Breves*, B. Hectoris, Bononie.
10. Keele, K. D. (1963): In: *Essays of the History of Italian Neurology*, edited by L. Belloni. Elli and Pagani, Milan.
11. Keele, K. D. (1964): *Med. Hist.*, 8:342.
12. Estienne, C. (1546): *La dissection des parties du corpus humain divisée en trois liures*. Simon de Colines, Paris.
13. Saunders, J. B. de C., and O'Malley, C. D. (No date): *The Illustrations from the Works of Andreas Vesaluis of Brussels*, World Publishing Co., Cleveland.
14. Singer, C. (1952): *Vesalius on the Human Brain*. Oxford University Press, London.

15. Eustachi, B. (1714): *Tabulae Anatomicae*. F. Gonzaga, Rome.
16. Wister, C. (1825): *A System of Anatomy*. Carey and Lea, Philadelphia.
17. Casserio, G. (1632): *Tabulae Anatomicae*. D. Buiretius, Frankfurt.
18. Vesling, J. (1647): *Syntagma anatomicum*. P. Frambotti, Patavii.
19. Willis, T. (1664): *Cerebri anatome*, V. Flesher, Londini.
20. Vieussens, R. (1685): *Neurographia Universalis*. J. Certe, Lugduni.
21. Ridley, H. (1695): *The Anatomy of the Brain*, S. Smith, London.
22. Blasius, G. (1666): *Anatomie Medullae Spinalis et Nervoruim inde Provenientium*, C. Commelinum, Amsterdam.
23. Ruysch, F. (1724): *Opera omnia anatomico-medico-chirurgica*, Janssionio Waesbergros, Amsterdam.
24. Sommerring, S. (1778): *De basi encephali et originibus nervorum cranio egredientium libri quinque*, A. Vanderhoeck, Gottingue.
25. Monro, A. (1783): *Observations on the Structure and Functions of the Nervous System*, W. Creech, Edinburgh.
26. Fulton, J. (1937): *Bull. Hist. Med.*, 5:895.
27. Vicq, d'Azyr, F. (1786): *Traité d'anatomie et de physiologie*. F. Didot, Paris.
28. Bell, C. (1801): *Engravings of the Arteries*. Longman, London.
29. Gall, J., and Spurzheim, J. (1810–1819): *Anatomie et physiologie du système nerveux en général et du cerveau en particulier*. F. Schoell, Paris.
30. Swan, J. (1834): *A Demonstration of the Nerves of the Human Body*. Rees, Orme Brown Green and Longman, London.
31. Bell, C. (1802): *The Anatomy of the Brain Explained in a Series of Engravings*. Longman, London.
32. Bell, C. (1803): *A Series of Engravings Explaining the Courses of the Nerves*. Longman, London.
33. Bell, C. (1830): *The Nervous System of the Human Body*. Longman, London.
34. Cranefield, P. (1974): *The Way in and the Way Out*. Futura, Mount Kisco, New York.
35. Baillie, M. (1793): *The Morbid Anatomy of Some of the Most Important Parts of the Human Body*. Johnson and Nicol, London.
36. Cheyne, J. (1812): *Cases of Apoplexy and Lethargy with Observations on Comatose Patients*. T. Underwood, London.
37. Hooper, R. (1828): *The Morbid Anatomy of the Human Brain*. Printed for the author, London.
38. Courville, C. (1945): *Bull. Los Angeles Neurol. Soc.*, 13:10.155.
39. Cruveilhier, R. (1835–1842): *Anatomie pathologique du corps humain*. J. B. Baillière, Paris.
40. Flamm, E. S. (1973): *Med. Hist.*, 17:343.
41. Carswell, R. (1838): *Pathological Anatomy: Illustration of the Elementary Forms of Disease*. Longman, London.
42. Courville, C. B. (1948): *Bull. Los Angeles Neurol. Soc.*, 130:143.
43. Bright, R. (1831): *Reports of Medical Cases Selected with a View of Illustrating the Symptoms and Cure of Diseases by Reference to Morbid Anatomy*. Longman, London.
44. Wilson, S. A. K. (1955): *Neurology*, 2nd ed. Williams & Wilkins, Baltimore.
45. Charcot, J.-M., and Richer, P. (1887): *Démoniaques dans l'art*. Lecronsier et Babe, Paris.
46. Charcot, J.-M., and Richer, P. (1889): *Les Difformes et les malades dans l'art*. Lecronsier et Babe, Paris.
47. Richer, P. (1902): *L'art et la médecine*. Gaultier and Magnier, Paris.
48. Guillian, G. (1959): *J.-M. Charcot, His Life and Work*, edited and translated by Pearce Bailey. P. Hoeber, New York.
49. Garrison, F. H. (1925): *Int. Clin.* (ser. 35), 4:244.
50. Meige, H. (1925): *Charcot Artiste*. Masson, Paris.
51. Gowers, W. R. (1886–1888): *Manual of Diseases of the Nervous System*, 2 vols. J. and A. Churchill, London.
52. Critchley, M. (1949): *Sir William Gowers, 1845–1915, a biographical appreciation*, W. Heinemann, London.
53. Critchley, M. (1958): *Central African J. Med.*, 4:212.
54. Cuthertcon, A. (1978): *Practitioner*, 221:276.
55. Duchenne, G. B. A. (1862): *Album de photographier complèmentaire du Livre intitule*. Baillière, Paris.
56. Muybridge, E. (1979): *Human and Animal Locomotion*, 3 vols. Dover, New York.

Macdonald Critchley

Honors, Titles, and Publications

Commander of the British Empire
M.D. (1st class Honours, Bristol University)
Fellow, Royal College of Physicians
Hon. Fellow, American College of Physicians
Hon. M.D., Zurich
Hon. D. en M., Aix-Marseilles

Consulting Physician, The National Hospital, Queen Square
Consulting Neurologist, King's College Hospital
Consultant in Neurology to the Royal Navy, 1937–1977
Consulting Neurologist to The Royal Masonic Hospital, 1935–1970
Served in World War II (1939–1946), travelling widely throughout the world as Surgeon Captain, Royal Naval Volunteer Reserve, Consultant in Neurology

President, The World Federation of Neurology, 1965–1973
Formerly Vice-President, The Royal College of Physicians
Formerly Dean, Institute of Neurology, Queen Square
Formerly Master, Worshipful Society of Apothecaries
Formerly President, International League Against Epilepsy
Formerly President, Association of British Neurologists
Formerly President, The Harveian Society
Member of the General Medical Council, 1957–1973
Founder Editor of *Journal of the Neurological Sciences*
Formerly Assistant Editor, *Brain*
Trustee, The Migraine Trust, since 1966

Hon. Fellow, Royal Society of Medicine
Hon. Member, Académie de Médecine de France
Hon. Member, Norwegian Academy of Science and Letters
Hon. Member, Royal Academy of Medicine, Barcelona
Hon. Member, Pan-African Association of Neurological Sciences
Hon. Member of 28 National Neurological Societies throughout the world

Goulstonian Lecturer, Royal College of Physicians, 1930
Long Fox Lecturer, University of Bristol, 1935
Hunterian Professor, Royal College of Surgeons, 1935
Bradshaw Lecturer, Royal College of Physicians, 1942
Croonian Lecturer, Royal College of Physicians, 1945
William Withering Lecturer, University of Birmingham, 1946
Tisdall Lecturer, University of Manitoba, 1951
Semon Lecturer, University of London, 1951
Sherrington Lecturer, University of Wisconsin, 1955
Orator, Medical Society of London, 1955
Hunterian Orator, 1957

Doyne Memorial Lecturer and Medallist, 1961
Victor Horsley Memorial Lecturer, 1963
Honyman Gillespie Lecturer, Edinburgh, 1963
E. H. Young Lecturer, University of Bristol, 1965
Hughlings Jackson Lecturer and Gold Medallist, Royal Society of Medicine, 1964
Schorstein Lecturer, 1964
Gowers Lecturer and Medallist, 1965
Harveian Orator, Royal College of Physicians, 1966
Veraguth Gold Medallist, Bern, 1968
Arthur Hall Memorial Lecturer, University of Sheffield, 1969
Rickman Godlee Lecturer, University of London, 1970
Patel Lecturer, Bombay, 1971
Samuel T. Orton Award, U.S.A., 1974
Cavendish Lecturer, London, 1976

Major Publications

Mirror Writing
Neurology of Old Age
Observations on Pain
Language of Gesture
Shipwreck Survivors
Sir William Gowers
The Parietal Lobes
The Black Hole (essays)
Developmental Dyslexia
Aphasiology
The Dyslexic Child
Silent Language
Music and the Brain
Dyslexia Defined
The Divine Banquet of the Brain (essays)

Papers on Aphasia and Language

On palilalia. *J. Neurol. Psychopath.* 1927. 8.
Aphasia. *Br. Encyc. Med. Pract.* Vol. I. London 1936.
"Aphasia" in a partial deaf-mute. *Brain.* 1938. 61.
The testamentary competency of a patient with aphasia. *Practitioner.* Feb. 1938. Vol. CXL.
Spastic dysphonia ("inspiratory speech"). *Brain.* 1939. 62.
Aphasic disorders of signalling (constitutional and acquired) occurring in naval signalmen. *J. Mt. Sinai Hosp.* 1942. 9.
Speech disorders arising from head injuries. *Proc. R. Soc. Med.* 1946. 39.
Speech iterations ('ting-a-ling' phenomenon). *Postgrad. Med. J.* 1948. 24.
Speech defects in children. *Proc. R. Soc. Med.* 1950. 43.
Articulatory defects in aphasia. *J. Laryngol. Otol.* 1952. 66.
Verbal symbols in thought. *Trans. Med. Soc. Lond.* 1955. 71.
Nature and content of aphasic utterance. Cent. papers. St. Eliz. Hosp. Washington. 1956. 207–220.
Premorbid literacy and the pattern of subsequent aphasia. *Proc. R. Soc. Med.* 1956. 49.
Animal communication. *Trans. Hunt. Soc. Lond.* 1958/9.
A critical survey of our conceptions as to the origins of language. *History and Philosophy of Knowledge of Brain and Its Functions.* 1958. 45–72.

The evolution of man's capacity for language. *Evolution After Darwin*. Univ. of Chicago Press. 1960.
Jacksonian ideas and the future, with special reference to aphasia. *Br. Med. J.* 1960. 1.
Testamentary capacity in aphasia. *Neurology*. 1961. Vol. II.
The everlasting "no"; the everlasting "yea." *Perspect. Biol. Med.* 1961. 5.
The nature of animal communication and its relation to language in man. *J. Mt. Sinai Hosp.* 1961. 28.
Head's contribution to aphasia. *Brain*. 1961. 84.
Speech and speech-loss in relation to the duality of the brain. *Interhemispheric Relations and Cerebral Dominance*. 1962.
Dyslexia in Braille-readers. *Bull. Johns Hop. Hosp.* 1962. Vol. III.
Regional "accent," demotic speech, and aphasia. *Livre jubilaire van Bogaert*. 1962. 182–191.
Kinesics: Gestural and mimic language. One aspect of non-verbal communication. *Problems of Dynamic Neurology*. Jerusalem. 1963.
The drift and dissolution of language. *Proc. R. Soc. Med.* 1964. 57.
Origins of aphasiology. *Scott. Med. J.* 1964. 9.
La controverse de Dax et Broca. *Rev. Neurol.* 1964. 110.
Creative writing by aphasiacs. *Neurol. Problems*. 1964. Sect. 5.
Aphasiological nomenclature and definitions. *Cortex*. 1967. 3.
The neurology of psychotic speech. *Br. J. Psychol.* 1967. 113.
Total speechlessness. *Mind and Brain Problems*. Rome. 1968.
Dysgraphia and other anomalies of written speech. *Pediatr. Clin. North Am.* 1968. 15.
Le langage est-il une fonction localisée du cerveau? *Rev. Med. Fonc.* 1970.
Lingua Adamica Restituta. *Perspect. Biol. Med.* Univ. of Chicago. Vol. 14. No. 4. 1971.
Communication: Recognition of its minimal impairment. *Scientific Found. of Neurology*. Chap. 7. Sect. VI. 1972.
Aphasia in polyglots and bilinguals. *Brain Lang.* 1974. Vol. I.
Some remarks upon the "localisation" of speech. Cent. vol. for Prof. O. Foerster. 1974.
Language. *Foundations of Language Development*. Chap. I. Academic Press. 1976.
Aphasiological research yesterday, today, and tomorrow. *Disorders of Central Language Processing*. Cairo. 1976.

Papers on Migraine

Migraine. *Lancet*. 1933. Vol. I.
Mechanism and treatment of migraine. *Practitioner*. 1934. 133.
Treatment of migraine. *Br. Med. J.* 1935. 2.
Mechanism and treatment of migraine. *Sind. Med. J.* 1935. 8.
Prognosis in migraine. *Lancet*. 1936. 2.
The malady of Anne, Countess of Conway. *K.C.H. Gaz.* April. 1937.
Migraine. *Br. Med. J.* 1950. 2.
Discussion on headache. *Trans. Med. Soc. Lond.* 1951.
History of migraine. 1966.
Migraine from Cappadocia to Queen Square. *Perspective in Migraine*. 1967.
The place of migraine within the systematic catalogues of medicine. *Migraine*. Migraine Trust. 1975.
Visual aurea and prodromes in migraine. 1979 lecture (to be published).

Papers on the Parietal Lobe, Agnosia, and Higher Nervous Activity

The phenomenon of tactile inattention, with special reference to parietal lesions. *Brain*. 1949. 72.
The parietal lobes. *Proc. Amst. Neurol. Vereen.* 1949.
The parietal lobes. *Proc. R. Soc. Med.* 1949. 44.
Parietal lobe syndromes. *Proc. R. Soc. Med.* 1951. 44.

Observations on parietal lobe function. *Tr. 5. I. Cong. Neurol.* 1953. 1.
Gerstmann's syndrome. *Acta Neuropsychol.* 1953. 2.
Parietal syndromes in ambidextrous and left-handed subjects. *Zbl. Neuroch.* 1954. 14.
Personification of paralysed limbs in hemiplegics. *Br. Med. J.* 1955. 2.
Observations on anosodiaphoria. *L'Encephale.* 1957.
Alterations de l'organisation visuo-spatiale dans les lesions occipito-parietales. *Les Grandes Activities du Lobe Occipital.* 1959.
Clinical investigation of diseases of the parietal lobes of the brain. *Med. Clin. North Am.* 1962. 46.
An appraisal of visual (object) agnosia. *Proc. 8. I. Cong. Neurol.* 1965. 5.
Disorders of corporeal awareness in parietal disease. *Acta Psychol.* 1964. 23.
The problem of visual agnosia. *J. Neurol. Sci.* 1964. 1.
The enigma of Gerstmann's syndrome. *Brain.* 1966. 89.
Impaired selectivity of mental processes in association with a lesion of the frontal lobe. (jointly) *Neuropsychol.* 1967. 5.
A personal account of a complicated case of parietal disease. *Proc. R. Virchow Med. Soc. N.Y.* 1968. 26 (Suppl.).
Disorders of higher nervous activity. *Handbook Clin. Neurol.* 1969. 3.
Misoplegia. *Mt. Sinai J. Med.* 1974.

Papers on Developmental Dyslexia

The significance of mirror-writing. *Proc. R. Soc. Med.* 1926. 397.
Some defects in reading and writing in children. *J. State Med.* 1927. 35.
L'écriture en miroir. *Ann. Med. Psychol.* 1929. 87. 323.
Inborn reading disorders of central origin. *Trans. Ophthalmol. Soc.* 1961. 81.
Developmental dyslexia: A constitutional dysymbolia. *Word-Blindness.* Pitman Med. Press. 1962.
The problem of developmental dyslexia. *Proc. R. Soc. Med.* 1962. 56.
Is developmental dyslexia the expression of minor cerebral damage? *Slow Learning Child.* 1966. 13.
Some observations on developmental dyslexia. *Mod. Trends Neurol.* 1967.
Developmental dyslexia. *Pediatr. Clin. North Am.* 1968. 15.
Specific developmental dyslexia. *Proc. Univ. Chic.* 1969. 14.
Developmental dyslexia. *Br. J. Hosp. Med.* 1969. 910.
Isolation of the specific dyslexic. *Dyslexia: Diagnosis and Treatment of Reading Disorders.* C. V. Mosby. St. Louis. 1968.
Language acquisition in developmental dyslexics. *The Child with Learning Disabilities.* A.C.L.D. Calif. 1971.
Developmental dyslexia: Its history, nature and prospects. *Reading Perception and Language.* York Press. Baltimore.
Specific developmental dyslexia. *Foundations of Language Development.* Vol. 2. Academic Press. 1975.

Papers on the Body Image

The body-image in neurology. *Lancet.* 1950. 1.
A phantom supernumerary limb after a cervical root lesion. *Arq. Neuropsiquiatr. (Sao Paulo).* 1952. 10.
Quelques observations relatives à la notion de la conscience du moi corporel ("Corporeal Awareness"). *L'Encephale.* 1955. 6.
Personification of paralysed limbs in hemiplegics. *Br. Med. J.* 1955. 2.
Disorders of corporeal awareness in parietal disease. *Acta Psychol.* 1964. 23.
Corporeal awareness. *Mod. Perspect. World Psychol.* 1968. 2.

Papers on Vision

The relation between eye movements and other cranial muscles. (jointly) *Br. J. Ophthalmol.* 1925.
Leber's optic atrophy and its relationship with the heredo-familial ataxias. (jointly) *J. Neurol. Psychol.* 1928. 9.
Ocular palsies. *Postgrad. Med. J.* 1934.
Neurological aspects of visual and auditory hallucinations. *Br. Med. J.* 1939. 2.
Metamorphopsia of central origin. *Trans. Ophthalmol. Soc.* 1949. 69.
Awareness or non-awareness of hemianopic field-defects. *Trans. Ophthalmol. Soc.* 1950. 69.
Visual perseveration. *Trans. Ophthalmol. Soc.* 1950. 71.
Types of visual perseveration: "Paliopsia" and "Illusory visual spread." *Brain.* 1951. 74.
Tactile thought, with special reference to the blind. *Brain.* 1953. 76.
Further remarks on the phenomenon of visual perseveration. *Ber. Phys-Med. Ges.* 1954. 67.
Acquired disorders of colour perception of central origin. *Brain.* 1965. 88.
Central disorders of colour perception and colour naming. *Riv. Patol. Nerv. Ment.* 1965. 86.
Modes of reaction to central blindness. *Cesk. Neurol.* 1965. 28.
Myopic derealization: An unusual visual neuropsis. *Wien Z. Nervenheilk.* 1967. 25.
Perseveration in the domain of vision. *Modern Neurology.* 1969.
Visual agnosia. *Medical Ophthalmology.* Chapman & Hall. London. 1976.

Papers on Old Age

Nature and significance of senile plaques. *J. Neurol. Psychol.* 1929. 10.
The pathology of the senile psychoses. *Proc. R. Soc. Med.* 1930.
Neurology of old age. *Lancet.* 1931. 1.
Neurologische Betrachtungen uber das Greisenalter. *Dtsch. Med. Wochenschr.* 1932. 58.
The mental and physical symptoms of the pre-senile dementias. *Proc. R. Soc. Med.* 1933. 83.
Jakob's syndrome (senile dementia with parkinsonism). *Proc. R. Soc. Med.* 1937.
Mental and physical symptoms of the presenile dementias. *Proc. R. Soc. Med.* 1938. 51.
Ageing of the nervous system. *Cowdray's "Old Age."* London. 1939.
Senile disorders of gait, including so-called "senile paraplegia." *Geriatrics.* 1949. 3.
Neurologic changes in the aged. *J. Chronic Dis.* 1956. 3.

Papers on Sleep

Disorders of nocturnal sleep in narcoleptics. *J. R. Nav. Med. Serv.* 1940. 26.
The syndrome of periodic somnolence and morbid hunger (Kleine-Levin syndrome). *Br. Med. J.* 1942. 1.
Sleeplessness. *Pharmacol. J.* 1948.
The predormitum. *Rev. Neurol.* 1955. 98.
Periodic hypersomnia and megaphagia in adolescent males. *Brain.* 1962. 84.
Le Syndrome d'hypersomnie et de mégaphagia periodique chez l'adulte male (Kleine-Levin): quelle est sa nature? *Rev. Neurol.* 1967. 116.

Papers on Epilepsy

Tuberose sclerosis and allied conditions. (jointly) *Brain.* 1932. 55.
On reflex epilepsy. *Ann. L.C.C. Rep.* 933. 4.
Uber reflex Epilepsie. *Schweiz. Arch. Neurol. Psychiatr.* 1935. 35.
Musicogenic epilepsy. *Brain.* 1937. 60.

Two cases of musicogenic epilepsy. *J. R. Nav. Med. Serv.* 1941. 28.
Troubles de la parole dans les cas d'epilepsie. *L'Encephale.* 1960. 2.
On reading epilepsy. *Epilepsia.* 1962. 3.

Papers on Epidemic Encephalitis

Respiratory disorders in epidemic encephalitis. *Brain.* 1925.
Hepatic aspects of epidemic encephalitis. *Lancet.* 1925. 1329.
Pathogenesis of respiratory anomalies after epidemic encephalitis. *Br. Med. J.* 1927.
Prognosis and results of post-encephalitic respiratory disorders. *J. Neurol. Psychopath.* 1928. 8. 191.

Papers on the Medical Complications of Boxing

Nervous disease in boxers. *Med. Ann.* 1935. 53.
Nervous disease in boxers. *Med. Ann.* 1937. 55.
Punch-drunk syndromes: The chronic traumatic encephalography of boxers. *Hommage à Clovis Vincent.* Paris. 1949.
Medical aspects of boxing, particularly from a neurological standpoint. *Br. Med. J.* 1957. 1.
Medical aspects of boxing: The punch-drunk state. *Trans. Med. Soc. Lond.* 1959–60. 76.

Papers on Sequelae of Lightning and Electric Shock

Effects of lightning with special reference to the nervous system. *Bristol Med. Chir. J.* 1932. 49.
Industrial electrical accidents in their neurological aspect. *J. State Med.* 1932. 40.
Neurological effects of lightning and electricity. *Lancet.* 1934. 1.
Injuries from electricity and lightning. *Br. Med. J.* 1935. 2.
Electrical injuries. *Trans. Med. Soc. Lond.* 1936. 59.

Miscellaneous Papers

Facial associated movements. *J. Neurol. Psychol.* August 1924. Vol. V.
Post-diphtheritic "Chorea." *Br. J. Child. Dis.* 1924. Vol. XXI.
The Parkinsonian syndrome: Some points in diagnosis and treatment. *Br. Med. Chir. J.* 1924.
A case of uveo-parotitic paralysis. *Lancet.* Nov. 1924.
The calcium content of the cerebrospinal fluid. *Brain.* 1924. Vol. XLVII.
The pathogenesis of tetany. *Arch. Int. Med.* 1925. 35.
Brain tumours in children. *Br. J. Child. Dis.* 1925. Vol. XXII.
Operative treatment of gastric crises in tabetics. *J. Neurol. Psychiatr.* 1925.
The diagnosis of cerebellar tumours in children. *Br. J. Child. Dis.* 1926. Vol. XXIII.
The hepatic aspect of epidemic encephalitis. *Lancet.* Dec. 1929.
Respiratory disorders after epidemic encephalitis. *Brain.* 1925. 48.
Sprengel's deformity with paraplegia. *Br. J. Surg.* 1926. Vol. XIV.
The mechanism of speech and deglutition in progressive bulbar palsy. *Brain.* 1926. Vol. XLVIII.
The pituitary adamantinomata. *Brain.* 1926. Vol. XLIX.
Forced grasping and groping. *Brain.* 1927. 50.
Cerebrospinal epidermoids (cholesteatomata). *Brain.* 1928. 51.
Discussion on disorders of the pituitary body. *Proc. R. Soc. Med.* Oct. 1929.
Clinical study of an heredo-familial disease resembling disseminated sclerosis. *Brain.* 1929. 52.
The Ayahuasca and Jagé cults. *Br. J. Ineb.* 1929. 26.
Spinal symptoms in chloroma and leukaemia. *Brain.* 1930. 53.
The anterior cerebral artery and its syndromes. *Brain.* 1930. 53.

A clinical study of congenital neurosyphilis. *Br. J. Child. Dis.* 1930. Vol. XXVII.
Some forms of drug addiction: Mescalism. *Br. J. Ineb.* 1931. 28.
Genius and mental defect. *K. Coll. Gaz.* 1931. 10.
Beitrage zur Anatomie und Pathologie der Arteria Cerebelli Superior. *Zeit. Neurol. Psychol.* 1933.
Huntington's chorea and East Anglia. *J. State Med.* 1934. Vol. XLII.
Some aspects of pain. *Br. Med. J.* 1934. Vol. II.
Observations on pain. *Bristol Med. Chir. J.* 1935. 52.
The symptomatology of tabes, as illustrated by the diary of Alphonse Daudet. *K. Coll. Gaz.* April 1936.
Alzheimer's disease. *Br. Encyc. Med. Pract.* Vol. I.
Neurological sequelae of spinal anaesthesia. *Proc. R. Soc. Med.* 1937.
Climate and the nervous system. *J. State Med.* 1937. Vol. XLV.
Climate and the nervous system. *Med. World.* March 1937.
Treatment of facial paralysis. *Trans. Med. Soc. Lond.* 60.
Neurological therapeutics. *Ir. J. Med. Sci.* Nov. 1937.
La physiopathologie de la douleur d'origine centrale. *Rev. Neurol.* 68.
Spasmodic torticollis: Spastic dysarthria: Tremor. *Proc. R. Soc. Med.* 31. 1938.
Observations on thirst. *J. R. Nav. Med. Serv.* 1943. 29.
Problems of naval warfare under climatic extremes. *Br. Med. J.* 1943. 2.
A medical study of the Black Hole of Calcutta. *J. R. Nav. Med. Serv.* 1945. 31.
Remarks on acclimatization. *J. R. Nav. Med. Serv.* 1945. 31.
Semon's law. *Proc. R. Soc. Med.* 1946. 39.
Problems of naval warfare under climatic extremes. *Mil. Surg.* 1946. 98.
Los problemes de la guerra naval bajo condiciones climaticas extremas. *Rev. San. Mi. Buenos Aires.* 1946. 45.
Discussion on idiopathic recurrent laryngeal nerve palsies. *J. Laryngol. Otol.* 1947. 61.
Effects of climatic extremes. *Br. J. Ind. Med.* 1947. 4.
Olivo-ponto-cerebellar atrophy. *Brain.* 1948. 71.
Observations on essential (heredo-familial) tremor. *Brain.* 1949. 72.
The muscular dystrophies. (Myopathies). *Practitioner.* 1950. 164.
Heredopathia atactica polyneuritiformis (Refsum's syndrome). *Proc. R. Soc. Med.* 1951. 44.
The "idea of a presence." *Acta Psychol. Neurol.* 1955. 30.
Volitional movement. *Proc. R. Soc. Med.* 1954. 47.
Congenital indifference to pain. *Ann. Int. Med.* 1956. 45.
Dyssynergia cerebellaris progressiva. *Trans. J. Am. N. Assoc.* 1962.
Observations on the so-called idiots savants. *Lehoczky Fest.* 1968.
Die sich Ausdehnenden Grenzen der Neurologie. *Psychiatr. Neurol. Med. Psychol.* 1971.
Interhemispheric partnership and interhemispheric rivalry. *Scientific Foundations of Neurology.* 1972.
Great Britain and the early history of Huntington's chorea. *Advances in Neurology.* Vol. I. 1973.
Fear of music. Birthday vol. *Academician Sarkisov.* 1975.
The training of a neurologist. *Horizons in Neurological Education and Research.* 1975.
Ecstatic and synaesthetic experiences in association with musical appreciation. *Music and the Brain.* 1976.
Musicogenic epilepsy. *Music and the Brain.* 1976.
Occupational palsies in musical executants. *Music and the Brain.* 1976.
Cacoethes scribendi. Birthday vol. Walter Riese. 1976.
Frontal lobe syndromes. Egas Moniz Centenary. 1977.
Butterworths medical dictionary. Editor-in-Chief. 1978.

Subject Index